OCCUPATIONAL MEDICAL MANAGEMENT

A Guide to the Organization and Operation of In-Plant Occupational Health Services

OCCUPATIONAL MEDICAL MANAGEMENT

A Guide to the Organization and Operation of In-Plant Occupational Health Services

Jean Spencer Felton, M.D.
Clinical Professor, Community and Environmental Medicine, University of California, Irvine, California College of Medicine; Clinical Professor, Emeritus, Preventive Medicine, University of Southern California School of Medicine, Los Angeles

Little, Brown and Company
Boston/Toronto/London

First Edition

Library of Congress Catalog Card No. 89-84861

ISBN 0-316-27775-4

Printed in the United States of America

MV

To the memory of Jan,
and to Gary, Keith, and Robin

CONTENTS

PREFACE

The latter half of the twentieth century has witnessed the greatest growth and maturation of occupational medicine in the United States. While previous decades saw the establishment of health services in industry and their periodic enlargement necessitated by production for war, the tenor of descriptive writings has changed from the early reviews of departmental organization and anecdotal case reports of work-initiated illness and injury to variations of research findings in toxicology and epidemiology. A sophisticated delineation of physiologic and functional impairment occasioned by untoward inhalation, ingestion, or absorption of toxic work materials is necessary for a program of occupational disease prevention, the essence of health programs in commerce and industry.

The task of disease prevention is delegated to a single division of the employer's institution—the occupational health service (OHS), which is the locus of the professional personnel, their health care delivery systems and equipment, the programs offered in the promotion of wellness, and the evaluation, maintenance, betterment, or restoration of an employee's health status. That such an operational unit requires skilled management is an organizational truism, for no societal entity can be effective without a systematized scheme of operation.

Occupational Medical Management has as its objective the definition and clarification of an OHS—the contemporary designation of choice of the time-honored medical department—and of its many activities, programs, functional relationships, and working philosophies. As the OHS comprises people who interact with other people, attitudes and behavioral insights are extremely important in the successful provision of preventive and therapeutic care. Emphasis is given to these aspects of program building and execution, for irrespective of the decorous beauty of the physical plant or the educational or experiential qualifications of the staff, abrasive, unfeeling, denigrating, or discriminatory behavior will nullify any positive attributes otherwise possessed by the personnel. Rapport, understanding, and compassion are mandatory ingredients of a true service and are to be nurtured and exercised in every procedure undertaken by staff members.

While effort has been made for contemporaneity in the references cited, many vintage writings are quoted or listed, for the principles given in these pieces have not been frayed by time. Further, recent publishing in the occupational health disciplines seemingly has shied from material relative to the administration of an in-plant OHS. It is fitting that the principles imbuing the management process are reflective not only of today's needs and options but also of the author's personal body of experience in several practice situations. In these different settings, the cast of employed characters may change, but the theme of sound worker-oriented service remains the same. The concepts offered will prove helpful to both the newcomer to industry's health arm and the veteran who may wish to freshen up a slightly tired activity.

The text may seem to bear the message that the company's medical director carries the responsibility for the health of the labor force. Such is not the reality, for, as in any institution, there is a hierarchy in the leadership scheme, and it is the chief executive officer (CEO) who is ultimately accountable not only for the well-being of the employed body but also for its morbidity and mortality, as given testimony by the managers' messages to the media and the public in such situations as the Bhopal disaster or the *Challenger* explosion. It is, however, the task of the medical director to formulate the philosophy, the policies, and the spirit of the health program for serious and concerned articulation by the CEO. Anything less than congruence between the expressed thoughts from the executive level and actual practice in the OHS can only be counterproductive, if not destructive. The medical director provides sage counsel in an area where he or she is particularly skilled and wise and to persons unknowing of the core of occupational health knowledge. In these days of readily generated litigious action and sharply codified legal constraints and mandates, managers must have the best, the most current of discerning advice. The text offers helpful milestones in the structuring of policy that is honest, unbiased, and supportive of the health of both the employees and the organization. No longer can today's managers in corporate industry be neglectful of human rights, irrespective of the area of involvement—employment, safety, or health. More than ever before is well-honed guidance needed through the mine fields of the considerable amount of federal and state legislation.

Even minor entries in a monograph can benefit from a modicum of explanation. Why quotations to lead the chapters?—merely to recall some earlier voices that gave thoughtful consideration to topics that were as pertinent in the past as they are currently. Much of what concerns today's health care professionals loomed as problems in decades past when technologies were simpler and the products less hazardous. An occasional spotlight reminds one that not everything was created yesterday.

Occasionally commercial devices are mentioned, as are sources of information, training packages, or educational materials. Their inclusion does not imply endorsement in any sense, and their being named does not necessarily mean that the catalog is all-inclusive. Unquestionably, there are other agencies, producers, and manufacturers, and nothing of a negative view is implied through an unintentional omission.

The same principle is applicable to the periodic literature that is indicated and the monographs that are cited. The body of publications germane to occupational health is vast and growing constantly, not only through new issues of long-established journals, but also through the appearance of new periodicals and hardcover books. Reference to all is impossible.

Although mentioned previously that much of this book's content derives from a personal practice background, it must be emphasized that all of the case examples are the stories of real people who underwent real experience and, in their way, served as mentors in the author's personal professional growth. There is no instruction to equal the product of a living laboratory.

Finally, if there is a baring of one's soul in this writing, it is intended to be just that illuminating and disclosing. If such exposition lends substance to the belief that the expressed principles do work, that is precisely what the author wishes to transfer to the reader. May one person's rewards and pleasures be shared.

J. S. F.

ACKNOWLEDGMENTS

No contemporary health care publication is ever the product of an author working in isolation. There is need of many individuals to assist in the preparation of a manuscript from the filing of references to the completion of the final draft. Particular appreciation is expressed to Janet M. Torpy, who recently added *M.D.* to her name; Moonhee Song; Kimberly Yen; and Jeff Farrow, all of whom diligently pursued references in several libraries and verified the many minutiae required in bibliographic citation. Word processing of the early chapters was accomplished by Pamela Swick, and many of the latter chapters were put into manuscript form by Betty Ulery and Donna Bohegian. The final draft was prepared by Christine Jasiewicz; I am particularly grateful to her for extremely careful attention to detail and for establishing a consistent style. In addition, she has been of immeasurable help in locating sources of information, in verifying many of the nonmedical details, and, with a peculiar kind of prescience, in staying ahead of the author in recognizing lacunae that required filling. Any amount of gratitude would fall far short of that which is deserved.

Continuing support and encouragement were provided by my first editor at Little, Brown, Curtis Vouwie, and more recently by his successor, Christopher Davis.

The gracious cooperation of the many authors, agencies, professional societies, companies, and publishers who granted permission to reproduce or cite from their material is acknowledged, and particular thanks is given to the many medical directors who shared material from their programs early in the preparation of this work.

Last, thanks are due to the faculty and staff of the Southern Occupational Health Center, University of California, Irvine, whose association and efforts made many difficulties disappear.

It is to these many individuals that I owe much in the readying of this volume. Without them there would be no publication.

J. S. F.

OCCUPATIONAL MEDICAL MANAGEMENT

A Guide to the Organization and Operation of In-Plant Occupational Health Services

1. INTRODUCTION

"Where shall I begin, please your Majesty?" he asked. "Begin at the beginning," the King said, very gravely, "and go on till you come to the end: then stop."

Lewis Carroll
Alice's Adventures in Wonderland

Life without industry is guilt, and industry without art is brutality.

John Ruskin

EARLY EFFORTS

Characteristic of American industry since its birth with glass production in Virginia in 1607 has been a generally continuous linear growth. Apart from temporary cyclic recessions or extraordinary growth demands made by wars, this steady expansion has persisted. The lunar landings, the space shuttles, the energy shift, and altered work methods and facilities of the future augur further development. The conversion to a postindustrial or service society bespeaks changes in the work settings and the risks to which the labor force might be subjected.

Work has been traditional to human beings for survival and continuation of the species, and what was once the effort of a single primitive being is now the activity of vast numbers of persons grouped by type of industrial enterprise. In the time frame of our maturation, the move from an agrarian economy to collective production spans but a small segment of history. Yet, with the establishment of factories, the growth of cities around them, and the spread of unused or once-used waste materials over the land, people may become an endangered species, undergoing slow pathologic obliteration through the incredible process of self-destruction and uncontrolled use of irreplaceable natural resources.

The early years of the twentieth century saw the introduction into the manufacturing operation of great aggregates of materials hazardous to the health of the worker. In a few instances, the toxicity of certain substances was known, but as the numbers of raw materials and intermediates multiplied, little effort was expended in defining the noxious attributes of newly synthesized or added ingredients.

With a rising awareness of the hazards to the health and safety of the worker, mature legislation brought certain sanctions into the industrial scene. Workers' compensation insurance coverage, safety codes, and protective time and place constraints for women and young employees, among others, were introduced as deterrents to further deleterious inroads into the health of work personnel. Medical controls in the form of preventive programming took shape early in the 1900s. As the century approached its three-quarters mark, a significant legislative rebirth in the maintenance of the worker's well-being was seen in the passage of the Occupational Safety and Health Act of 1970 (OSHA 1970). Although attacked vigorously and with considerable emotion and rhetoric by Ralph Nader [1], who saw the law as beneficial to employers, the Steiger-Williams Act is the strongest codification to appear that has been concerned with occupational health. President Nixon [2] alluded to this enactment in his 1971 health message when he stated, "We must begin immediately to cut down on the 14,000 deaths and more than two million disabling injuries which result each year from occupational illnesses and accidents."

The conception, institution, and continuation of medical controls have taken the form of various preventive health programs, both within industry and in the communities surrounding the physical plants themselves. Normally supported by the employer, such an occupational health program is considered part of the cost of doing business—of manufacturing a marketable product, of providing a publicly utilizable service, of executing a governmental charter, of selling or distributing a wide assortment of commodities, or of furnishing us with a new law or a truth freshly derived from a research facility. The type, size, philosophy, and method of offering such a service to a group of employees are dimensions of an activity determined by a spectrum of factors, some measurable, some intangible.

THE CONTEMPORARY SCENE

GROSS NATIONAL PRODUCT

Higher than in previous years, the gross national product for 1986 was $4,180 billion in current dollars, or about $2,393 billion in the dollars of 1972 [3]. Total personal income exceeded $831 billion in 1970 and rose to over $3,314 billion 15 years later. The per capita income averaged $13,850 in 1985 [4].

LABOR FORCE

By July 1987, the civilian labor force totaled over 121 million persons, and 7.2 million were unemployed, a rate of 5.9 percent. Adult men over age 16 years who were working represented 55.6 percent (67.656 million) of the employed segment of the labor force, and adult women in the same age group made up nearly 44.4 percent (54.016 million). Of 11 large states, unemployment varied from a low of 3.8 percent in Massachusetts to 9.3 percent in Texas. Manufacturing averaged 41.0 weekly hours of work, with an average overtime superimposed of 3.8 hours, both figures slightly lower than for the comparable period of 1 year before. The average weekly earnings level for private nonagricultural payrolls was $311.85 [5].

Goods-producing industries (mining, construction, and manufacturing) utilized over 24.8 million workers (nearly 29.3 percent), while service-producing industries, including government, had more than 77.2 million employees (75.7 percent), indicating the shift to the service society mentioned earlier [5]. Consistently, over the years, the number of businesses with few workers has exceeded the number of firms with large labor forces. It has been the small business that has utilized the services of outside health care consultants in preference to any form of in-plant health facility because of the lesser costs of ad hoc medical care.

POPULATION

The population of the United States increased by 2.32 million, or 11.4 percent, from 1970 to 1980, so that the decennial analysis showed a total of 226,545,805. The greatest increase was in the West at 23.9 percent. The estimated population for 1990 is 249.203 million, or nearly a 10-percent increase over the 1980 census [3]. During 1985 there were 3.749 million births, 2.084 million deaths [3], and 570,000 in net immigration [4].

It is anticipated that by the year 2000 the population of the United States, including the Armed Forces overseas, will increase to 268 million and may reach 309 million by 2050, representing an increase of 17.7 percent between 1980 and 2000 and 15.2 percent in the following 50 years. The greatest growth will be in the ages 65 and over, from a 1980 level of 25.708 million to 67.06 million by the year 2050, a rise in percentage from 11.3 to 21.7. The under-25-years segment will diminish from 93.988 million to 90.457 million in the 70-year span.

While 1980 data show females per 100 males in the top age bracket at 148.1, the figure will rise until the year 2000, when it will reach 155, and then return to 148.0 in 2050, still representing about 8 percent more women [6].

Indicative of altered technology is the drop in agricultural workers from 7.057 million in 1960 to 3.115 million in 1985 [4].

The current mean longevity expectation at birth is now 71.0 years for men and 78.3 years for women [7].

A CHANGING SOCIETY

Planning an occupational health program for a commercial, industrial, or governmental institution involves a sensitivity to the many constraints within which business is operating today. The milieu of secrecy that prevailed in previous decades regarding risks and hazards has given way to the employee's "right to know." Active efforts, particularly by the Occupational Safety and Health Administration (OSHA), have been targeted toward orientation and education of the worker, in compliance with OSHA 1970, which states that "the Secretary [of Labor] . . . shall provide for the establishment and supervision of programs for the education and training of employers and employees in the recognition, avoidance, and prevention of unsafe or unhealthful working conditions. . ." [8]. Tepper [9], in a Sappington Memorial Lecture before the American Occupational Medical Association, stated that when information is lacking, the void is filled by the potential for harm or dangerous misinformation. Without accurate, substantive instruction, myths regarding alleged occupational disease or innumerable symptoms accredited to work exposure will arise and spread rapidly through a laboring group and soon become fixed as real and causally true.

New chemicals appear for use both as raw materials and as intermediates and less frequently as finished products. With a growing body of knowledge of the presence and effects of industrially used carcinogens, mutagens, and teratogens, genetic changes have been observed that require immediate industrial hygiene control, if not substitution of nonhazardous substances. New metals, comparably, have put certain work groups at risk.

The Rehabilitation Act of 1973 [10] and the supportive regulations of Sections 503 and 504 of the Act [11] have made possible the acceptance for employment of physically limited job applicants, with the mandate that there shall be no discrimination against such persons in their hiring, promotion, upgrading, award of tenure, demotion, transfer, layoff, termination, right of return from layoff, or rehiring. Even though American business and industry had advanced in the employment of handicapped job aspirants, there were still many who had not had an equal chance to work or advance, once employed. This type of affirmative action has required, on the parts of many employers, the development of a new philosophy that slowly would penetrate to all levels of supervision.

Labor has a new role in the conduct of an enterprise. Health insurance and occupational medical demands have entered into negotiations, with federal mandates supporting such demands. Trade union leaders themselves have become sophisticated in occupational safety and, through their own staff specialists and training programs, have apprised their members of the nature of the work substances that they face daily and the surveillance procedures and precautionary actions needed to prevent the incurrence of work-generated illness. In fact, unions are now being sued by their members or the families of members for failure to inform them of workplace hazards [12].

The industrial scene is not the peaceful and affluent setting of the post–World War II days. Bombings of manufacturing and financial establishments, kidnapping of American industrialists abroad [13], a skewed balance of trade, the closing of plants, the raiding of long-established companies, excessive and ever-increasing profits of a single industry, inflation, governmental precedent-setting support of companies about to fold, weakening of antitrust legislation, and diminished federal spending have changed both the growth and continuation of American business and industry and also have made careers in this arena less attractive.

Superimposed on these alterations have been certain additional negative factors with medical relevance—increased workers' compensation benefits*, the rise of cumulative injury claims, the augmented medical care costs as reflected in industry's share of the worker's health insurance package, and the many more applications for disability retirement by employees who, for reasons often unrelated to an impaired health status, wish to cease working and derive a tax benefit from this form of separation.

These circumstances make the planning of a health service somewhat more complex than in former years and more demanding of greater medical participation in the structure of company policy related to health issues. The times are not peaceful.

As indicated previously, the population will continue to increase, immigration will persist, and these factors, in addition to many others, will influence the kinds of enterprises that will flourish and the jobholders who will be the recipients of occupational health services.

Determinants of the size and variety of working groups go beyond the demand for certain goods and services. As examples given by the Bureau of Labor Statistics, employment of carpenters increased greatly in the mid-1970s because millions of new homes were built. During the same years, the number of shoe repairers decreased because people discarded shoes rather than having them repaired. Mechanization can increase a product output while decreasing the need for workers, for instance, the change in the technology of binding books. Although until 1980 credit buying was rising, the employment of credit managers declined because of the centralization of credit operations [14].

It is anticipated though that employment will increase in almost all occupations, and total employment by 1990 may rise to 114.0 million workers, an increase of almost 18 million new jobs. More openings are expected through departures from the labor force because of family duties, early and regular retirement, illness, or death. The need for new personnel in environmental protection, energy development, and health care will increase openings for professional workers. The expansion of retail trade will lead to greater numbers of salespeople. The largest growth is expected among service workers, and because businesses want and need better security systems, more protective service persons will be sought. But new work methods will increase, such as computer-aided design and numerical-control machine-tool operation. New positions will open by the year 2000—in space manufacturing and ocean development, as examples. Computer manufacturing, in contrast to a decline in general manufacturing, will rise, and there will be a greater need of robotics technicians, laser technicians, housing rehabilitation technicians, and solar technicians, the last in the expanded effort to utilize new sources of energy [14].

With the delay of the retirement age until 70 and the increase in the number of older persons, the data indicated may change. New industries will appear and present challenges to the directors of occupational health programs. It is hoped that the examples set by older industries that are accustomed to in-plant health units will percolate through to new organizations undergoing formation or merger.

*In 1984, workers' compensation benefits reached $19.529 billion, in contrast to the 1970 level of $3.031 billion [3].

WORKER MORBIDITY

The Black Lung Benefits Reform Act of 1977 directed the Secretary of Labor, in cooperation with the National Institute for Occupational Safety and Health (NIOSH), to conduct a study of all occupationally related pulmonary diseases. While the resulting report [15] related almost solely to respiratory disease, certain findings are illuminating. It was learned that almost 2 million workers are either severely or partially disabled from an occupationally related disease, and one-third of this group is suffering a long-term total disability. In 1978 alone, the income lost because of disabling work-generated disease amounted to $11.4 billion.

An analysis of the effects of exposure to 10 substances* known to cause pulmonary disease and cancer of the respiratory tract, in large groups of workers, indicates that the number of deaths and disabling disorders resulting from these exposures presents a major challenge for all the health care systems and programs of income maintenance. Responsible in great part for this financial burden is the long period of latency between exposure and the onset of the disability or death. In such a situation, it is difficult to plan adequate reserves, for the severity and duration of disability are not so predictable as they are in cases of traumatic injury. Public and private income support programs replace only about 40 percent of the wages lost by persons disabled by occupational disease, while individuals who have sustained work injuries experience a 60-percent replacement rate. One in four of the severely disabled receives no income support payments, while one out of every three receives benefits from multiple sources.

Through workers' compensation benefit payments, about two-thirds of the lost income should be recaptured. The fact that only 5 percent of occupationally diseased workers collect such benefits results partly from the difficulties involved in establishing the work-relatedness of the illnesses and partly from the defensive litigation strategy used by some insurers [15]. A further comparison of inequity is in order. Persons injured at work receive benefits and the claim is settled in an average of 2 months, while the worker disabled by disease waits a year before the first benefits arrive. Further, first claims for occupational disease were denied in 60 percent of cases, while such denials only went to 10 percent of individuals filing because of injury. Occupational disease claims are settled in 50 percent of the cases through the mechanisms of compromise and release, wherein the attorneys representing the claimant and the defendant meet and agree on a small sum settlement rather than going through lengthy and costly hearings. Only 16 percent of injury awards undergo such a procedure.

In a successful occupational disease claim in the case of a permanently disabled worker, total compensation benefits average about $9,700, in contrast to expected future earnings of $77,000. Implicit in this finding is the fact that the disease-disabled worker has but one-eighth of his wages replaced through workers' compensation.

Lastly, as pointed out in the Department of Labor report [15], about 40 cents of every dollar collected in workers' compensation premium is used for legal and administrative costs. Since disease claims lead more often to litigation, it is likely that the costs associated with these claims are even higher. With a view at another system, occupational diseases cost the social security and welfare systems about $2.2 billion annually.

Emphasis is given the fate of the illness-afflicted worker because the primary objective of any occupational health program is the prevention of occupational disease, rather than injury. The prevention of accidents and accident-caused injuries among workers is the province of the safety specialist. However, the provision of emergency medical care to the traumatized worker is a function of an occupational health program. The National Safety Council estimates that there were approximately 10,800 deaths arising from accidents at work in 1986 [16]. Fatalities in the major industrial groups varied from 5 per 100,000 workers in trade to 52 per 100,000 workers in agriculture.

In addition to the deaths, there were 1.9 million work-related disabling injuries and 70,000 permanent impairments following injury. Total work accident costs for 1984 were estimated to reach $32.4 billion. The direct, or insured, costs—wage losses, medical expenses, and insurance administration costs—totaled $15.1 billion. The indirect, or uninsured, costs were estimated conservatively to equal the direct costs and include the money value of time lost by workers, other than those employees sustaining the disabling injuries, who are directly or indirectly involved in the accidents. Fire losses in industrial and business establishments came to about $2.2 billion. Accidents incurred away from work further compounded the loss in human resources and productive capacity. Those injuries sustained in accidents both on and off the job resulted in 45,200

*Asbestos, cotton dust, silica, beryllium, cadmium, chromium, arsenic, nickel, coal tar products, and diisocyanates.

deaths and 4.4 million disablements. In 1984, 40 million workdays were lost from on-the-job death and disabling injuries, and an additional 50 million workdays were lost from production time due to off-the-job accidents. In the 10-year period from 1974 to 1984, the accidental death rate of workers declined 31 percent, from 16 to 11 per 100,000 workers.

These data are given to lend a sense of dimension to the problem of human loss at the worksite. The prevention of this astounding number of mishaps is a sizeable task, but not beyond the capability of skilled health professionals, working with supportive employers, with alert safety personnel, in controlled environments, with understanding cooperative trade unions, and in a milieu where it is believed that there is worth in the individual worker. Further, it is expected that part of the cost of production will come from a program of protection mounted not solely for compliance with regulation but for the preservation of a force of experienced employees, unhampered by preventable illness and capable of ever-increasing productivity. In substance, it is good business.

THE FUTURE

Demographic moves and morbidity and mortality data do not tell the entire story of industrial change. The post–World War II years were characterized by recessions, mergers, diversification, and growth in the nuclear energy industry and later in aerospace activity. In the 1960s and early 1970s, other elements entered as stressors to industrialists. An awakening concern over the environment has led to operational changes for many employers and the institution of new systems of waste management. The growing strength of consumerism brought about automobile callbacks, pharmaceutical recalls, and broadening of the functions of the Food and Drug Administration in addition to structural changes in political parties, university board and committee systems, student and patient government, and joint provider-consumer health service planning.

The several new federal bills relating to worker health, in addition to the Steiger-Williams Act, have led to positive employer action—adding health and safety personnel—or to strong negative energy, in the form of defeatist lobbying. Initially, the Target Health Hazards Program brought to immediate focus for study five of the most health-hazardous substances in common use or productive of serious pathologic change. The materials designated were asbestos, cotton dust, silica, lead, and carbon monoxide, and the use of four of these substances is now governed by standards promulgated by the Department of Labor (DOL). It is obvious that with this setting of priorities and writing of regulations, employers have begun to feel the impact of the legislation.

There will unquestionably be some change in the structure of corporate activity, as already given evidence by the giant hostile takeovers. Few people believe that business is striking a good balance between profit and service. Public confidence is being eroded, and this loss of faith is given solidity by the assumption of the ombudsman role by so many radio and television stations. The appeal of the show "Consumer Buyline" bespeaks the public's resentment against overpriced, short-lived, inferior products and misleading advertising. The consumer movement and the pollution-ecology movement, which Yankelovich [18] believes have become one, are solidifying the public's mood of dissatisfaction and are channeling it against business, particularly the extraordinarily high-profit industries. What are the feelings of the workers who turn out inferior products and who realize that they themselves are purchasers of these very goods?

Values previously found in religion, sex, the family, and the work ethic continue to be challenged, and youth somehow has related its anger and disenchantment against business as the power source responsible for all of today's ills. The denims worn by young attorneys and physicians as the garb of office convey some of the attitude of resentment against what has been. The overadvertising of industry's efforts at pollution control, the subsidization of public television programming, and the counter-commercials sponsored by the manufacturer of an ill-fated airplane do not ameliorate the feelings of distrust among the consumers. The closure of plants and the moves abroad further the sense of animosity generated each day at the supermarket checkstand and by the source labels on clothing.

The feelings of the public regarding industry have been given, for a credo of community obligation is still to be developed by many employers. The nurturing of such a belief unquestionably will involve industry's health services, for therein are professionals long accustomed to facing people with deep personal needs, with multiplicities of problems, and with long-persisting social hurt. In light of a potential restructuring of occupational health services to meet more contemporary demands, it is vital to know about the public's opinion of business, of the quality of health care, or of the impersonalization of the governing process. One's employees are part of the larger community that verbalizes its attitudes, and frequently they extend these feelings to their own employers. In developing an occupational health service, it must be remembered that the responses to ineptness, rudeness, impoliteness, prejudice, or inequitable treatment will surface as readily within the plant as outside to the pollsters. It is as important to structure a service of warmth and welcome as it is to devise an efficient physical facility.

While much can be done in abating job-related injury and death by the organization and its managerial and health service personnel, the primary task remains with the individual workers to conserve their health and maximize their working lives. It was expressed well in an unsigned editorial [19]:

> In theory occupational diseases are wholly preventable, but in practice so long as society requires an industry's products some men will fall ill and even die as a result. A cost in terms of illnesses and accidents is exacted for the benefits provided by most productive industry. Society and its elected representatives need to be informed of the risks in order that work can be made as safe as possible, consistent with the need to continue or increase production; but the ultimate responsibility in a democratic society for occupational morbidity and mortality rests with every individual.

In the interim, in spite of much adverse comment, the NIOSH list of the 10 leading work-related diseases, based on the criteria of frequency of occurrence, severity, and amenability to prevention, remains as follows [20]:

1. Occupational lung diseases: asbestosis, byssinosis, silicosis, coal workers' pneumoconiosis, lung cancer, occupational asthma.
2. Musculoskeletal injuries: disorders of the back, trunk, upper extremity, neck, lower extremity; traumatically induced Raynaud's phenomenon.
3. Occupational cancers (other than lung): leukemia, mesothelioma, cancers of the bladder, nose, and liver.
4. Amputations, fractures, eye loss, lacerations, and traumatic deaths.
5. Cardiovascular diseases: hypertension, coronary artery disease, acute myocardial infarction.
6. Disorders of reproduction: infertility, spontaneous abortion, teratogenesis.
7. Neurotoxic disorders: peripheral neuropathy, toxic encephalitis, psychoses, extreme personality changes (exposure-related).
8. Noise-induced loss of hearing.
9. Dermatologic conditions: dermatoses, burns (scaldings), chemical burns, contusions (abrasions).
10. Psychological disorders: neuroses, personality disorders, alcoholism, drug dependency.

A full task in creative occupational health remains, with the goal, as expressed by Roemer [21], of "the restoration of the patient to social usefulness."

REFERENCES

1. Nader task force blasts the safety establishment. *Occup Haz* 34:54, 1972.
2. Nixon, R. *Special Message on Health.* Release from the Office of the White House Press Secretary, Feb 18, 1971. P. 12.
3. *Reader's Digest 1987 Almanac.* Pleasantville, NY: Reader's Digest Association, 1986. P. 200.
4. *Statistical Abstract of the United States 1987* (107th ed). Washington, DC: U.S. Department of Commerce, Bureau of the Census, 1986.
5. The employment situation: July, 1987. *NEWS.* U.S. Department of Labor, Bureau of Labor Statistics, Aug 7, 1987.
6. United States population outlook. *Stat Bull Metrop Life Insur Co* 65:16, Jan–March 1984.
7. Gains in U.S. life expectancy. *Stat Bull Metrop Found* 65:18, July–Sept 1984, as amended.
8. Public Law 91-596. Occupational Safety and Health Act of 1970. Approved December 29, 1970, Sec. 21(c)(i).
9. Tepper, L. B. The right to know; the duty to inform. *J Occup Med* 22:433, 1980.
10. Public Law 93-112. The Rehabilitation Act of 1973. Approved September 26, 1973.
11. Nondiscrimination on basis of handicapped programs and activities reviewing or benefiting from federal financial assistance. *Fed Reg* 42:22675, May 4, 1977.
12. Unions increasingly being sued by own members for unsafe conditions. *Occup Health Saf Lett* 10:1, July 22, 1980.
13. Williams, R. M. The rise of a grim new business. *Saturday Rev* 7:13, Jan 5, 1980.
14. Nardone, T. The job outlook in brief. *Occup Outlook Q*, Spring 1980. Pp. 2–21; Looking at the future. *Occup Outlook Q* 28:14, Fall 1984.
15. *An Interim Report to the Congress on Occupational Diseases.* Submitted by the United States Department of Labor, December 1979.
16. Hoskin, A. F. Preliminary accident report: 1986 work deaths decreased. *Saf Health* 135:58, May 1987.
17. Who's counting right? *Natl Saf News* 130:8, Dec 1984.
18. Yankelovich, D. Business in the '70's: Decade of crisis. *Michigan Bus Rev* 24:27, Nov 1972.
19. Smoking, coal, asbestos, and the lungs. *Br Med J* 283:457, Aug 15, 1981.
20. Lung diseases are top concern of NIOSH list. *Occup Health Saf* 52:9, May 1983.
21. Roemer, M. S. Medical ethics and education for social responsibility. *Yale J Biol Med* 53:251, 1980.

2. HISTORICAL DEVELOPMENT OF OCCUPATIONAL MEDICINE IN THE UNITED STATES

The history of medicine investigates and teaches how medicine, including its individual branches, developed from its beginnings and gradually became what it is today; and it does this in relation to the general history of mankind of which the history of medicine is only a part.

J. F. Hofacker

Life can only be understood backwards, but it must be lived forwards.

Søren Aabye Kierkegaard

Tracing the growth of occupational medicine in the United States can only be accomplished by following the maturation of industry and the human problems that such evolution created. There have been significant milestones in this country's past that indicate early concern with the effect on the employee's health of contact with work substances and manufacturing processes. Any recounting of the events composing a traceable past must undergo certain abbreviation and condensation, for a view of the developmental years, even in this perspective, can stand as a work unto itself.

THE BEGINNINGS

In any new land being settled, a system of support for its colonizers must be established. Such sustentation comes from the soil, so that agriculture represents the first effort at survival. This country's seminal years saw the clearing of the land and the planting and harvesting of crops that would nurture the agrarian economy of the seventeenth and early eighteenth centuries. It would be later that the colonies would oppose the production constraints laid on them by the mother country and begin their own manufacturing in parallel with the beginnings of the Industrial Revolution in England.

The first industrial activity in the colonies was initiated at Jamestown, Virginia, in 1607 when, at the "glass house," glass trinkets were made for trade with the Indians [1]. Archeologic diggings conducted centuries later revealed a conversion to the fabrication of bottles and other utilitarian objects. As the need for iron tools, ship fittings, and household appliances grew, investment was sought from Britain, and eventually an iron works was built on the Saugus River in Massachusetts.

In the seventeenth century, the new society was based on farming, fishing, maritime activities, and the few small manufacturing industries that had sprung up. The first legislation concerned with child labor was that of a Massachusetts Bay court order that called for the town magistrates to look into the possibility of teaching all boys and girls the spinning of yarn. Labor unrest appeared early when Polish workers in Jamestown protested their being denied the right to vote, but by action of the Council of London, they were enfranchised in 1619. A few years later, in 1636, fishermen on an island off Maine struck to protest the withholding of a year's wages. Boston shoemakers and coopers formed the first labor organization in 1648 under 3-year charters, which were not renewed because of complaints by local rural artisans of alleged hindrance of free trade by the guilds.

Although it would be more than 250 years later that workers' compensation legislation would be passed, the piratical Captain William Kidd made an agreement with his crew that "if any man should lose a leg or arm in ye said service, he should [receive] six hundred pieces of Eight, or six able slaves."

The workforce continued to be built by indentured servants who bound themselves for employment in the new land in return for their passage across the Atlantic. America was still a nation of farmers, for the first census in 1790 showed that only 5 percent of the 3.929 million population lived in towns of 2,500 or more persons. To meet the needs of farmers and plantations growing the tobacco, rice, indigo, and wheat and the requirements of both the Navy and the whaling and fishing fleets, production was soon seen of brick, tile, and pottery; of masts, spars, and yards; of staves for the cooperages and of hard woods for cabinetry; and of tar, pitch, and turpentine.

Parliament passed a law in 1765 forbidding the emigration of skilled workers and subsequently enacted measures prohibiting the deportation of textile machinery, plans, and models from England. In turn, the poor, the unskilled, vagrants, and criminals were encouraged to move out. Meanwhile, skilled workmen flowed into the colonies from western Europe, even up to the outbreak of war with England.

The proscriptions against the use of the essentials of industry were counteracted in part by Samuel Slater, a one-time worker in Arkwright's British mills who, after an empty-handed arrival in the colonies, was able to design equipment comparable to that developed in England and by 1789 reproduced complete cotton-making machinery in a mill in Pawtucket, Rhode Island. Within 20 years, hundreds of spinning mills made their appearance in New England.

As this concentrated industry grew, an interesting experiment began in Lowell, Massachusetts, where starting in 1814 many young women came to work in the mills, in a manner comparable to the short stints at sea put in by their brothers. These workers were given such benefits as educational and religious programs, and after a few years they began publishing *The Lowell Offering,* which carried their own writings on such subjects as "Solitude," "Beauty," and "Twilight Musing." The alleged idyllic existence attracted visitors from abroad, including Charles Dickens, all of whom compared the working conditions most favorably with the wretched circumstances of the British mill worker. The Lowell Hospital, established in a "spacious and elegant mansion house," was set apart for sick operatives of the mills by the corporations of the community. A practitioner from Lowell was appointed the physician, and he resided there. Seventy-five percent of the costs were underwritten by the corporations. A dispensary was also created for "relief of the poor, by affording medicines and medical attendance gratuitously."

In time, there were voiced demands for increased pay and shorter hours—14 hours composed the workday—and by the 1840s and later, immigrants from the early waves out of Europe took the places of the young women. No valid morbidity data were available, for when the operators became ill, they usually would return home and cease employment.

Little is known of work-caused disease in the seventeenth and eighteenth centuries, unless one considers scurvy as labor-related. In 1671, Governor Berkeley testified that "there is not oft seasoned hands (as we term them) that die now, whereas heretofore not one of five escaped the first year" [2]. Nearly 75 years later, Cadwallader Colden wrote that "the scurvy is exceedin[gly] common in North America & hardly anybody [is] free of it & often mistaken for other diseases" [2].

LEGISLATION

As a result of Benjamin Franklin's claim that the "West India gripes" was actually lead colic resulting from the drinking of Jamaican rum distilled in equipment where the still heads and worms were made of lead, the Massachusetts Legislature enacted a measure in 1776 prohibiting the use of lead in those parts of the stills.

Legal recognition of the need for compensating an injured worker was first encountered in 1797, when through "An Act for the Relief of Sick and Disabled Seamen," Congress provided partial pay to personnel of the Navy who were wounded or disabled in the line of duty. One year later, the Marine Hospital Service, the antecedent of today's U.S. Public Health Service (USPHS), was created to provide medical care for seamen. The costs were borne through payroll deduction of 20 cents from the wages of persons so employed. This early system of prepayment explains the placement for so many years of the USPHS in the Department of the Treasury.

The next significant legislation was encountered in 1836, when Massachusetts passed the first child labor law, which required that each child under 15 years of age be given at least 3 months of schooling during the year preceding any year of employment. Six years later, an amendment to the act mandated that children under 12 years of age could not work more than 10 hours daily in manufacturing establishments. Concomitant with this action was the passage in Connecticut of a law limiting the work of children under 14 years of age in cotton and woolen mills to 10 hours.

The hours of work drew first regulatory attention in 1840 when an executive order issued by President Van Buren called for a 10-hour day in government navy yards. Seven years later, the first state law was passed in New Hampshire establishing 10 hours of work a day as the standard for all workers unless there would be in force "an express contract requiring greater time." The operatives "would be allowed that time for intellectual and moral culture."

Massachusetts maintained its position of primacy in protective legislation through several actions. In 1850 it became the first state to study occupational safety. Factory safeguards were required through legislative edict in 1877, and after another 2 years, factory inspections were mandated. By 1886, industrial accidents had to be reported.

The 8-hour workday was first called for by a union in 1859 at the time of the annual convention in Philadelphia of the machinists' and blacksmiths' unions. Recognition of the shorter day was given in 1867 by Connecticut, Illinois, Wisconsin, New York, Missouri, and California. Federal legislation followed the next year when laborers, workers, and mechanics employed by the federal government were given the 8-hour day. State and municipal workers were accorded the same ruling in New York in 1870.

Among other laws relating to the length of the work span was the federal legislation of 1907, which now extended into the private sector when trainmen were prohibited from working longer than 16 consecutive hours. It was the Walsh-Healey Act of 1936, though, that called for time-and-a-half pay for overtime and a 40-hour week for workers employed under government contracts exceeding $10,000. By 1938, workers engaged in interstate commerce came under the 40-hour week standard as required by the Fair Labor Standards Act.

MEDICAL DOCUMENTATION

As in most Western countries, writings pertinent to the diseases produced by work were appearing slowly. While there were sixteenth-century essays that recorded the observations of Agricola and Paracelsus, and Ramazzini's book on *Diseases of Workers* was in its first edition in 1700, American pieces were late in reaching the medical community. Although defended and published by a native South Carolinian, William Bull's 1735 dissertation, "De Colica Pictonum," was written as part of the requirement for the medical degree at the University of Leyden [3]. The first paper on occupational medicine appeared in response to a prize offered by the Medical Society of the State of New York. The $50 award was garnered in 1837 by 23-year-old Benjamin McCready, who produced his 50-page essay under the title of "On the Influence of Trades, Professions, and Occupations in the United States, in the Production of Disease" [4]. Using British data and citing that country's Thackrah extensively, he warned about the dangers of child labor, long working hours, and impaired ventilation. He was later to participate in the establishment of Bellevue Hospital Medical College and become its first professor of materia medica and therapeutics.

J. Addison Freeman of Orange, New Jersey, is identified as the first contributor in America to industrial toxicology by way of his 1860 paper on mercurialism [5]. Although probably incomplete, McCord's 1955 listing gave 200 titles of writings published before 1900 [6]. There were discussions and case reports of anthrax, decompression illness (caisson disease), the pneumoconioses, industrial injuries, noise-induced hearing loss, arsenic poisoning, lead poisoning, dermatosis, illness-absenteeism, occupational morbidity, nitroglycerin intoxication, phosphorus necrosis, fatigue, the "cramp" of various occupations, and the general effects of certain kinds of employment.

INDUSTRY

The country was growing. Iron and steel were being produced in eastern centers, the transcontinental railroad was being joined at Promontary Point west of Ogden, Utah, sail was giving way to steam, and newly discovered Pennsylvania oil was soon to move from use as a nostrum to a fuel for the early automobiles. To staff these growing industries, immigrants settled in cities, which rapidly were becoming overcrowded and unsanitary, with enclaves of different expatriates who retained much of their native culture, ethos, and language.

Workers' compensation was yet to come, so that the trilogy of defenses against injured workers, the assumption of risk, contributory negligence, and the fellow-servant rule—particularly the assumption of risk—still proved effective in the courts, and they were left disabled and jobless. The movement of people into the United States continued until World War I.

Sick-benefit programs sponsored by unions began to appear in the 1870s, and the first major prepayment medical care scheme in industry was initiated in Sacramento by the Southern Pacific Railroad Company in 1869. The hospital originally built in that city burned, and it was rebuilt in San Francisco, where it functioned deep into the twentieth century until the jet age made its incursion into railroading.

About the same time, Massachusetts established the first state Bureau of Labor Statistics, and about 12 comparable units appeared in other states between 1872 and 1884. In most cases, these bureaus became the State Labor Departments; in recent decades, many have changed to the euphemistic designation of Departments of Industrial Relations.

At the federal level, nearly 100 bills were introduced into the Congress between 1864 and 1900 to establish a labor department. All were unsuccessful until 1884 when a bill was passed and signed by President Arthur creating a department of labor statistics, called the Bureau of Labor, headed by a commissioner and placed in the Department of the Interior. There was considerable support for a move to change the bureau to a cabinet-level department. In 1888 a redesignation to Department of Labor was approved but without the desired cabinet status. After weathering and assisting in the resolution of many strikes and in response to commercial interests, a new Department of Commerce and Labor was established. Its heads were prominent in business and finance, subordinating the interests of labor. On President Taft's last day in office, in 1913, he reluctantly signed a bill creating the Department of Labor [7].

HEALTH CARE IN INDUSTRY

Late in the nineteenth century, the beginnings of an industrial outreach to medicine were seen. In 1882 the Northern Pacific Railway Beneficial Association was founded, an employee-sponsored mutual benefit association that developed a program of complete medical care and other benefits financed by employer-employee payments. Medical care was provided through group practice in the Northern Pacific Hospital in St. Paul and through arrangements with physicians in communities along the line of the railroad.

In 1885 the Macy Mutual Aid Association was created, and a part-time physician was appointed to offer counsel on sick-benefit claims and to give care for "minor ailments." The Domestake Mining Company of Lead, South Dakota, established an employer-financed medical department in 1887, with a full-time staff that provided complete medical service to workers and their families. The first record of a "plant surgeon," by name, is that of Dr. William J. Middleton, appointed by the Pennsylvania Steel Company in 1884 in Shelton, Pennsylvania.

The first professional society that related work to health was the American Association of Railroad Surgeons, founded in 1888. The progenitors of today's occupational health organizations were not to appear until the second decade of the century ahead.

The Barber Match Company and the Armstrong Cork Company developed in-plant dental programs in 1890, and that of the Metropolitan Life Insurance Company was established in New York in 1915.

By 1893 there was some concern being manifested regarding the health of working women. California passed the first law that required a weekly rest day for women workers. In 1895, in a milestone move, the Vermont Marble Company of Proctor, Vermont, employed a young nurse, Ada Mayo Stewart, to provide health care to its employees at home and in the small company hospital. The John Wanamaker Company of New York followed with similar action in 1897, the Brooklyn Department Store of Frederick Loeser in 1899, the Emporium in San Francisco in 1900, the Plymouth Cordage Company in Massachusetts and the Anaconda Mining Company in Montana in 1901, and in 1902 the Chase Metal Works of Connecticut and the Broadway Store in Los Angeles. Dr. Robert T. Legge, long associated at a later date with the University of California at Berkeley, brought professional nurses into the lumber camps of McCloud, California, in 1900. Such action was not uncommon around the turn of the century, for lumbering, mining, railroading, and other labor-intensive industries with great potential for injury were functioning in remote areas where medical facilities were not available. As dependents frequently accompanied their working husbands or fathers to these sites, the first prepaid medical care plans provided care for both the workers and their families. Joint participation by employer and employee was frequent.

Andrew M. Harvey, chief surgeon of the Crane Company of Chicago, provided safety glasses for workers in 1897. Although only tangentially related to medical care but significant in the prevention of dermatosis, it can be pointed out that baths were installed in 1893 in the Brooklyn plants of the J. H. Wilson Company.

The first federal report on industrial hygiene was prepared in 1903 by Dr. C. F. L. Doehring, a former student of Dr. George M. Kober*, for the Bureau of Labor Statistics and was titled, "Factory Sanitation and Labor Protection." Children under 16 years of age were limited by a 1903 act in Illinois to an 8-hour day of work, and by 1914 such a standard was found in 23 jurisdictions. In the year following, because of continuing concern over the welfare of children, the National Child Labor Committee was formed, later to be incorporated through congressional action, which served to investigate working conditions, build public opinion, and promote protective legislation.

Other official writings began to appear, and in 1905 the Massachusetts State Board of Health issued a brief report on the health and safety of workers in factories and other establishments. Two years later, this initial account was supplemented by a lengthy study of dusty trades by Dr. William C. Hanson, who was shortly to join Dr. Kober in preparing a significant monograph on the health of workers. Some 90 photographs from the study, along with charts and

*Later to be identified closely with occupational health through investigations of working conditions and preparation of a significant early text.

samples of dust and other work materials, were put on display in Boston, and thus was created the first occupational health exhibit in the United States.

Teaching of industrial health was initiated in 1905 at the Massachusetts Institute of Technology in the Department of Biology and Public Health by Dr. Charles-Edward A. Winslow. One year later, the Medical Department of the University of Pennsylvania, in conjunction with its doctoral program in public health, placed considerable emphasis on industrial hygiene, with attention being given plant inspections, in-plant emergency medical service, and the Occupational Disease Clinic of the University Hospital.

WORKERS' COMPENSATION

Rage was building in the United States in the early years of the new century over the injuries and deaths encountered among workers, particularly in heavy industry. Crystal Eastman, in her 1910 book *Work-Accidents and the Law* [8], pointed out that in 1 month, in a single county of industrialized Pennsylvania, there were 50 on-the-job fatalities. In 1906, the first federal law relating to compensation for injuries sustained in the course of employment in interstate commerce was passed for railroad workers, but it was declared unconstitutional in 1908; a revision of the original law was enacted and interpreted as constitutional in 1912.

Certain federal employees were granted a right to compensation for injury in 1908, and in 1916, the act was replaced by one that covered all civilian employees of the government.

As a sense of need grew in the United States regarding compensation, a few states passed employers' liability acts, which were short-lived. Several state commissions were formed to study the issues involved, and finally a group went abroad to view directly the method of underwriting work injuries, as Germany had had such social legislation since 1884.

Simultaneous with the ferment in workers' compensation was a tragedy that took place in a building that still stands near New York University at Washington Square. Early on a Saturday afternoon at closing time on March 25, 1911, a fire broke out on the ninth floor, occupied by the Triangle Shirtwaist Company, trapping workers in this loft factory, which just shortly before had been inspected for means of worker egress during a fire and had been put on notice. At the end of the melee of ineffective escape, arm-in-arm jumpings from the building, and entrapment of employees in adjacent floors, 146 workers, mostly young immigrant women, died. The same day, the 1910 compulsory Workers' Compensation Act passed by the New York state legislature was declared invalid, the opinion of the jurists reading, in part, "The statute, judged by our common-law standards, is plainly revolutionary," and ". . . violates private right by taking the property of one and giving it to another without due process of law . . ." [9]. The fire has since been memorialized in a television show and in a monograph [10].

The public and the labor unions were incensed by this juxtaposition of events, and eventually, by amendment to the Constitution in 1914, a compulsory Workers' Compensation Act was passed. The first state act was approved in Wisconsin in 1911; in the same year, seven other states took similar action, and California made it mandatory to report occupationally incurred diseases. Mississippi, in 1948, was the last state to pass a Workers' Compensation Act, some 37 years after the inception of such state legislation.

OCCUPATIONAL HEALTH PROGRESS

The year 1908 saw the first official involvement of Dr. Alice Hamilton, then a disciple of Ludwig Hektoen in Chicago, in matters relating to work and health hazards. As an associate of Jane Addams and a resident of Hull House, she knew the immigrant families in that area of the city and their lack of redress in the event of work-caused illness or injury. She was appointed by the governor of Illinois, Charles S. Deneen, to lead a commission on industrial diseases, and while she investigated lead poisoning, Dr. Emery R. Hayhurst studied copper, and Dr. Peter Bassoe, caisson disease. The final report appeared in 1911, and Dr. Hamilton went on to conduct many investigations for the U.S. Department of Labor until 1921.

She was the first woman to be appointed to the faculty of Harvard School of Medicine, where she taught from 1919 to 1935. It was through her efforts that a research project on the action of lead in the human body was endowed there, funded by industry and conducted by Dr. Joseph C. Aub [11].

Examinations had begun to appear as an early component of occupational health efforts, and in 1906 Massachusetts required, by law, the physical examination of all children applying for employment certificates. Dr. Frank T. Fulton gave examinations to workers of a large saw works in Providence, Rhode Island, for the detection of tuberculosis, and by 1909, Dr. Harry L. Mock had instituted such a procedure with the employees of Sears, Roebuck & Company of Chicago, Illinois, 2 years later, enacted legislation requiring monthly physical examinations of workers in hazardous industries. With the continued engineering required in bridge and tunnel construction, New York passed the first law, in 1909, specifying that all applicants for work in compressed air must be found physically qualified by a physician paid by the employer. In that same year, as a demonstration, the Milwaukee Visiting Nurse Association placed a nurse in a local industrial plant to show the employer the economic value of a public health nursing service.

At the suggestion of Lillian Wald, the Metropolitan Life Insurance Company, later to develop a strong occupational health team for service to its assureds, began using visiting nurses from the Henry Street Settlement House as a service to holders of industrial policies in a section of Manhattan.

Characterizing the early years of the twentieth century was the appearance of clinics specifically for the diagnosis of, and presumably treatment of, occupational diseases. The first of such clinics was begun at the outpatient department of the Cornell Medical School in New York City in 1910 by Dr. W. Gilman Thompson, who wrote a lengthy text 4 years later. The clinic was discontinued in 1916. A second comparable facility was started in 1911 at the Sprague Memorial Institute of the University of Chicago and the Rush Medical College under the direction of Dr. Emery R. Hayhurst. It was he who was to conduct the first statewide survey of industrial health problems in Ohio for the State Board of Health. Begun in 1913, the results were published in 1915 as a report entitled *Industrial Health Hazards and Occupational Diseases in Ohio*.

An organization that became extremely active in the area of occupational diseases was the American Association of Labor Legislation (AALL), whose motivating force was its secretary, John B. Andrews. Considerable attention focused on the effects of work with phosphorus, and it was the Andrews report for the Department of Labor, *Phosphorus Poisoning in the Match Industry in the United States,* that eventually led to the unusual control measure that put an end to the so-called phossy jaw. As an economist, Andrews conceived the idea of a tax, and after much educational campaigning and many hearings, President Taft signed the Esch Act, which authorized the use of the government's taxing power for the protection of the worker. The bill placed a tax on each box of matches made from white phosphorus, thus making their manufacture infeasible. Without any difficulty, the makers substituted the harmless sesquisulfide for the phosphorus, and the mandibular necrosis left the work scene as a disfiguring, painful, industrially caused lesion. The AALL continued its inaugural work, published 52 issues of its *Review,* and promoted the first National Conference on Industrial Diseases, which was held in Chicago in June 1910. The emphasis was on occupational hygiene, as the subject was called, and reports ensued on the health effects of lead, mercury, anthrax, compressed-air illness, methyl alcohol, and arsenic [12]. In 1911, the AALL presented a memorial on occupational diseases to President Taft, and 1 year later published Dr. Thompson's *Classification of Occupational Diseases*.

ORGANIZATIONAL BEGINNINGS

As Doyle has pointed out [13], government programs have strange origins, some arising in response to compelling demands, some resulting from public or political pressure, and others being inspired by the dreams or foresight of one person. It was through the last mechanism that the first federal office concerned with worker health came to be. The U.S. Bureau of Mines had already been established in 1910 with Joseph E. Holmes as director. Studies of silicosis among miners in the Joplin, Missouri, area and later Pueblo, Colorado, led most likely to later involvement of the USPHS because of the tuberculosis that so often accompanied silicotic changes. Because of pressure to extend the studies conducted in the mines and in plants of the United States Steel Corporation, in 1914, the USPHS formally established in its Hygiene Laboratory the Office of Industrial Hygiene and Sanitation with Joseph W. Schereschewsky, M.D., as its first chief.

Studies of this office in the New York garment district in search of tuberculosis led to the eventual elimination of the "sweatshops." As a consequence of this entire effort, the International Ladies Garment Workers Union Health Center was established under Dr. Leo Price and later was continued by his son, Dr. Leo Price, Jr. Apart from the prepaid health programs mentioned previously, this development marked the first large-scale involvement of a labor union in the delivery of health care.

The silicosis studies were later to be continued by Dr. Anthony J. Lanza (who was to become head of the Army's effort in industrial medicine during World War II*), Dr. Royd R. Sayers, and Dr. Frank Merriwether. Further investigations were conducted of the

*Initially in 1942, Dr. Lanza directed an Occupational and Military Hygiene Subdivision (of the Division of Preventive Medicine, Office of the Surgeon General), and later he became head of the Occupational Hygiene Branch, subsequently to be redesignated the Occupational Health Division [14].

granite industry, the anthracite mines, the use of radium, tetraethyl lead, and industrial dermatoses. The office was to become the Division of Industrial Hygiene and, after many name changes, to be designated by the Occupational Safety and Health Act of 1970 (OSHA 1970) as the National Institute for Occupational Safety and Health (NIOSH).

In Milwaukee, in late 1912, the first National Safety Congress was organized, and 2 years later it became the National Safety Council. About this time, the physicians employed in industry were seeking a forum for exchange of experiences, and in 1914 the Conference Board of Physicians in Industrial Practice was formed in the eastern states, and its transactions were published during the next several years. In 1916 the American Association of Industrial Physicians and Surgeons was formed with nearly 200 members. This group underwent changes in designation and until 1988 was the American Occupational Medical Association (AOMA). Later in that year, it underwent a merger with the American Academy of Occupational Medicine to become the American College of Occupational Medicine.

The XV International Congress on Hygiene and Demography, presided over by Dr. Kober, was held in Washington, D.C., in 1912, and a large section of the program was devoted to industrial hygiene. Concern over workers' health was increasing. Proceedings of the conference attest to a broad range of topics in the 64 presentations and marked the beginning of an American body of literature in occupational health. Additional early programming was seen in the 1915 annual meeting of the American Medical Association (AMA), when the first scientific symposium on industrial hygiene and medicine was held.* Just the year before, the section on industrial hygiene, now the section on occupational health and safety, was organized in the American Public Health Association as its fifth section.

LEGAL ACTIVITY

With World War I on the horizon, many legislative attempts were made in the way of human conservation at the worksite. A federal child labor law was enacted in 1916 but was declared unconstitutional on June 3, 1918, and a second act passed February 24, 1919, was reversed similarly on May 15, 1922. An amendment to the Constitution on child labor was proposed June 2, 1924, but only 28 of the needed 36 states ratified the change.

Both the compulsory and elective types of state workers' compensation statutes were declared valid by the United States Supreme Court in 1917, and Hawaii was the first jurisdiction within the United States to enact occupational disease compensation legislation, and legal support of rehabilitation was encountered in the passage of the Vocational Education Act of 1917, followed 1 year later by the Vocational Rehabilitation Act.

The only significant effort targeted toward protection of the World War I production worker was the establishment in 1918 of the Working Conditions Service within the Department of Labor, which attempted to improve the working environment of those persons engaged in defense production. This agency functioned cooperatively with the office of Industrial Hygiene and Sanitation of the USPHS.

BETWEEN THE WARS

World War I left no great heritage in occupational medicine. The early hospital clinics did not survive, but the labor movement was undergoing strengthening. In 1919, the University of Cincinnati established a 1-year course leading to a certificate of public health in industrial medicine. Courses were offered also at Yale and Johns Hopkins universities.

Several writings began to appear. The *Journal of Industrial Hygiene* was born in 1919, the first serial publication in occupational health to appear in the United States. Dr. Clarence D. Selby, then a consultant to the USPHS, and later to become Corporate Medical Director of the General Motors Corporation, conducted a significant nationwide survey of the health services in contemporary industry. P.H. Bulletin No. 99 is a valued collector's item. The first work for industrial nurses, written by Florence Swift Wright, was published in 1919, *Industrial Nursing. Industrial Medicine and Surgery,* written by Dr. Harry E. Mock, was based on both his military and civilian experiences. The same year saw the creation in New Jersey of six clinics for the rehabilitation of injured industrial workers, two of which were under the direction of Dr. Henry H. Kessler, who was to provide such outstanding leadership in rehabilitating the Navy amputees of World War II.* An early effort

*Organizational recognition of occupational medicine was not given by the AMA until 1937, some 22 years later, when the Council of Industrial Health was created.

*Dr. Kessler's 50 years in rehabilitation medicine are related with great humor in his 1968 autobiographic publication, *The Knife is Not Enough* (W. W. Norton & Co.).

at studying the health and welfare of women in industry was seen in the establishment in 1920, in the U.S. Department of Labor, of the Women's Bureau.

The delayed effects of work with radium carried on during World War I came to professional notice with the deaths encountered in 1924 of the watch-dial painters who had tipped their brushes with their lips, thus absorbing the radium salts. Dr. Harrison Martland of New Jersey and the USPHS conducted the pertinent studies of the hazard. Dr. Alice Hamilton's work, *Industrial Poisoning in the United States,* published in 1925, was the first American text on industrial toxicology.

Headed by Dr. V. V. Anderson, a team studied the emotional health problems of the employees of R. H. Macy & Company of New York, and the work was described in his 1929 book, *Psychiatry in Industry.* During the great depression, *Industrial Medicine,* a monthly journal, appeared and was edited for many years by Clarence O. Sappington, M.D., and is still published under the name of *Occupational Health and Safety.* The *Journal of Occupational Medicine* appeared in 1959 as the official publication of the AOMA and currently is in its thirty-first volume in 1989. *The American Journal of Industrial Medicine* made its appearance in 1980.

The American College of Surgeons (ACS) in 1926 appointed its Committee on Industrial Medicine and Traumatic Surgery, and the product of that committee, *Minimum Standard for Medical Service in Industry,* was the criterion for many years by which the ACS judged and approved the medical departments of industry. As an early venture in recuperation from the depression, the 1933 National Industrial Recovery Act, in its industrial codes of fair competition, included regulations governing work hours and safe and healthful working conditions, but these segments were declared unconstitutional in May 1935. The eminent reports on 5 years of study submitted by the Committee on the Costs of Medical Care and issued in 1933 contained 4 of 28 reports dealing with industrial prepayment medical care plans.

The passage of the Social Security Act in 1935 made funds available to the USPHS for the extension of research efforts and grants-in-aid to the states for public health work, including industrial hygiene, which led to the development of industrial hygiene units within the state agencies, most of which remain active today. In the same year, a study by the USPHS, conducted in Pennsylvania at the request of the governor and with the joint support of the anthracite coal operators and the United Mine Workers of America, resulted in the publication of *Anthraco-Silicosis Among Hard Coal Miners.*

Silicosis was beginning to attract further attention elsewhere during the 1930s when a large hydroelectric tunneling project was undertaken in West Virginia, near the small community of Gauley Bridge. As jobs were unavailable in those depressed years, workers with their families came from all over the United States to be involved in the totally uncontrolled dusty dry drilling through 3 miles of sandstone and shale, representing almost pure silica. The medical data from this tragedy have been scant, but the acquisition of "acute silicosis" by presumably hundreds of men and the unconscionable hurried burying in total anonymity of those workers who died led to congressional hearings. Although no evidence exists of the scope of the "epidemic" apart from the reconstruction of Dr. Martin Cherniack in his epic review, *The Hawk's Nest Incident: America's Worst Industrial Disaster* [15], the claims resulting were numerous and costly, and from this activity sprang the so-called silicosis racket. Frances Perkins, then Secretary of Labor in 1936, called the first National Silicosis Conference because of the publicity given both the Gauley Bridge and the Oklahoma-Missouri-Kansas episodes of this work-generated disease. With the final reports emerging in 1938, at long last considerable attention was now being given to job-related lung disease. Following these extraordinary events in the tri-state and West Virginia areas, the Air Hygiene Foundation, later to become the Industrial Hygiene Foundation (IHF), was organized, supported by some of the country's largest industrial concerns. Highly contributive annual meetings and efforts in continuing education have marked some of the foundation's subsequent activities.

In 1939, the Indiana State Health Department became the first such agency to employ an industrial nurse consultant, and Michigan followed the next year. The Walsh-Healey Act of 1936 (Public Contracts Act), although never given strong enforcement, was a significant piece of federal legislation, which set safety and health standards for workers employed in government contract work exceeding $10,000.

Just prior to the entry of the United States into World War II, a landmark agreement was reached in late 1941 in Connecticut among the owners who were processing hatters' fur, the labor union, and the state health agencies, and at the instigation of the Surgeon General of the USPHS, to eliminate mercurial compounds from the carroting process then in use. This action put an end to the cases of mercurialism arising in that industry until, with the emergence of hatless John F. Kennedy as President, the industry itself nearly disappeared. Mercury became a hazard again when imported hat bodies were found to have been felted by the age-old mercuric nitrate method.

WORLD WAR II

Although production of war goods had increased greatly through the Lend-Lease Agreement with Great Britain, who was already at war with the Axis countries, and many plants had converted to such manufacture, intense buildup of both the military and the civilian labor force did not take place until early 1942. With the great need of manpower in the defense plants and with the absorption into the armed forces of so many employed men and women, new categories of workers were now appearing, as they did in World War I—women, oldsters, and the physically impaired. The required examinations of such applicants, the necessity to lower the absenteeism—which became an outstanding problem in light of the need for some personal-business time—the downtime resulting from long queues at private physicians' offices, and the onslaught of work injuries demanded either the institution of in-plant medical facilities or the buildup of the meager installations that existed during the 1930s.

Physicians, nurses, and support personnel were recruited, and as the Army and Navy* became employers of large numbers of civilians, many medical officers in uniform were assigned to arsenals, depots, ports of embarkation, air stations, shipyards, staging areas, and other ground and shore facilities where civilians were replacing uniformed personnel. A great number of the physicians who received their first experience in occupational medicine during the war years remained in this type of practice or entered specialty training, later to become medical directors in industry. In the meantime, in 1942 all authority over employment and employment training was consolidated within the War Manpower Commission. In the same year, the American Association of Industrial Nurses, later to become the American Association of Occupational Health Nurses (AAOHN), was founded to improve the standards of nursing practice in industry.

MATURING IN THE MID-CENTURY

By the post-war 1940s and 1950s, occupational health had assumed a position of permanence in nearly all of the large corporations listed annually by *Fortune,* although a few companies held out, electing not to have in-house medical consultation or direction. The number of health services staffed by a single nurse grew, and the occupational health effort began to attain stature as evidenced by the content of the annual conferences of the AOMA, the AAOHN, and the more recently created American Industrial Hygiene Association (AIHA) and the American Conference of Governmental Industrial Hygienists (ACGIH).

As noted, in 1948 Mississippi passed a workers' compensation act, thus making such legislation nationwide. One year later, the USPHS conducted a significant study of the health effects of air pollution in Donora, Pennsylvania; and in the same year, the Presidential Board of Inquiry studying the labor dispute in the basic steel industry concluded that social insurance and pension programs should be considered as a part of normal business costs to care for the temporary and permanent "depreciation" in the members of the labor force.

Establishing a precedent in 1950, the University of Pittsburgh conferred the degree of Doctor of Industrial Medicine upon three graduates who had completed a special course of study. In keeping with the increasing recognition of the need for training in occupational medicine, the Council on Medical Education of the AMA approved the establishment of residencies at the Saginaw General Hospital in Saginaw, Michigan.

By 1951, the AOMA took over from the ACS the evaluation and certification of medical services in industry, effecting such functions through the American Foundation of Occupational Health, later to be known as the Occupational Health Institute, the educational arm of the AOMA. Teams of recognized specialists conducted visits to applicant companies and would recommend or disapprove accreditation.

The early post-war years gave substance to the belief that the disabled World War II veteran could work, having been rehabilitated under the concepts promulgated by Dr. Howard Rusk. The restoration of the injured civilian was undertaken by the more concerned casualty insurance companies, and the state vocational rehabilitation agencies began active placement of their clients in industry. Amendments to the Vocational Rehabilitation Act in 1954 provided a more effective use of federal funds.

An important step in support of specialized education was seen in 1951 when the General Motors Corporation gave $1.5 million to the University of Michigan to establish the Institute of Industrial Health, emphasizing the broad concerns of research,

*The Air Force did not become independent of the Army until 1947.

education, and service. An even greater milestone was erected in 1955 when the Council on Medical Education and Hospitals of the AMA authorized the American Board of Preventive Medicine to create a subspecialty, with examination and certification, in occupational medicine. This ultimate recognition came primarily from the ceaseless efforts of Dr. Adolph G. Kammer, who finally was able to demonstrate that residencies in occupational medicine could be established in certain industrial or governmental facilities that were approved for that purpose and that hospital training, characteristic of nearly every other medical specialty, was both unattainable and inappropriate.

Labor began to realize the need for interest in the health of the worker—beyond the usual concern over hours, pay, and other work amenities—and at its founding convention in 1955, the American Federation of Labor and Congress of Industrial Organizations (AFL-CIO) established a Standing Committee on Safety and Occupational Health. In the 1970s, several of the component international unions would add occupational safety and health specialists to their staffs.

Certification of specialists in industrial hygiene was made possible in 1960 through the chartering of the American Board of Industrial Hygiene (ABIH) under the laws of Pennsylvania.

Recognition must be given the dual contributions to the growth of occupational medicine by the then Atomic Energy Commission (AEC). Outstanding preventive medical programs were in existence in the plants and research laboratories under its jurisdiction and operated by leading prime contractors from industry. Secondly, the AEC created fellowships for physicians, enabling them to pursue residencies in occupational medicine, with some hope that, on completion, the graduates would seek placement in AEC installations.

Although the Federal Employees Health Service Act had been enacted in 1946 to provide government workers with preventive medical programs, agency heads were slow in effecting such additions to their activities. In 1964, though, the U.S. Civil Service Commission expanded the health programming for federal employees, and growth was seen in installations of 300 or more workers.

CHANGES IN INDUSTRY

During the years following World War II, the methods of industrial production were changing. Mechanization was giving way to automation, soon to be followed by a gross expansion of the use of the computer. New occupations in operation and maintenance were created, and fewer unskilled jobs remained. Agriculture had been mechanized, and what "stoop" labor was residual was assumed by immigrants or aliens who came into the United States either legally or without authorizing documents. The Space Age, given impetus by Russia's Sputnik, came to its peak with the 1969 moon landing. Deemphasis on the program released innumerable highly skilled technical persons, who went jobless or took menial work for the purpose strictly of family maintenance. The Vietnam effort increased production but threw the 1960s into rebellious shambles, which had its toll on industry and academe through bombings and other antiestablishment actions.

Big business became bigger, with mergers and expansion of conglomerates, in some instances increasing the occupational health component, in others diminishing what had been outstanding efforts. Programs in public employment were given birth, training was offered to the undereducated, and the move to lessen the spending by government, in addition to certain agency malfeasance, have slowed such supportive undertakings. Unemployment has risen, and artificial stimuli through proposed defense projects meet with extremely mild responses. Added to this confusing social state have been the questions of alternative energy sources, the status of the automobile and other smokestack industries, the insolvency of municipalities, and continuing interracial tensions emerging frequently in the inner city. But even with this gross instability, occupational health has taken new form.

NEW LEGISLATION

Most important in the health of the worker has been the passage of OSHA 1970, in which full cognizance was taken of the many needs in the worker's safety and health. Standards have been promulgated at federal and state levels; employers, professionals, and workers have been educated and trained; and research has been greatly expanded. Health records have been given new meaning in their creation, retention, and availability. Surveillance programs of workers at increased risk have been mandated.

In spite of these positive moves, there are constant efforts among lawmakers, subject to external pressures, to attenuate the strength of OSHA 1970 in the name of freeing industry of governmental regulation and allowing the free enterprise system to flourish.

Although the United States has progressed remarkably far from the days of child labor, the 12-hour day, and abbreviated longevity of workers, there is still an insensitivity to the need for controls that will allow one to earn a living without sacrifice of health. Further corrective legislation is seen in the Federal Coal Mine Health and Safety Act, the Black Lung Benefits Act, and the Toxic Substances Control Act.

THE CURRENT YEARS

In recent decades, epidemiology has flourished, and detailed studies of groups at risk have demonstrated many heretofore unrecognized associations between work exposure and certain untoward health effects. Workers in some industrial operations have shown greater than expected rates of cancer, some at highly unusual sites.

Studies have brought a greater knowledge of the asbestos-related diseases and of the effects of fibrogenic inhalants, and the continued use of the chlorinated hydrocarbons, metals, pesticides, and such substances as 1,3 dibromochlorpropane (DBCP) has indicated that our body of toxicologic information is lacking. We have learned from untoward clinical effects rather than from laboratory investigation.

The consumer movement has allowed both a demand for and a spread of existing data, and the Freedom of Information Act has brought disclosures not previously possible. The public has been sensitized to the potential harm present in many industrial operations, and supportive, at times overzealous, media have highlighted the dangers of the workplace.

THE 1980s

The body of literature has increased greatly, both in monographic and periodic publications, and the data banks of NIOSH and others allow almost instant response to questions concerning toxicity. The number of industrial hygienists has increased greatly, and graduates of university programs in occupational safety or health are finding no dearth of employment opportunities.

The Educational Resource Centers established by NIOSH have made continuing education for professionals both possible and substantive, as the Labor Occupational Health Programs supported by OSHA have made training for workers understandable and attractive.

Research in all areas—epidemiology, toxicology, clinical occupational medicine, the overt and subclinical behavioral effects of harmful work exposures, and work physiology—continues. Through the promulgation of the Hazard Communication Standard at the federal level, and the subsequent state "right-to-know" laws, workers are being apprised of the toxicity of the materials with which they are working and the precautions to be taken in their use. For the communicative process, good translations from the technical literature in appropriate lexicons have been developed so that information previously guarded has become common currency in various work groups.

A greater role in occupational medicine is envisioned for primary care physicians by their own professional organizations, and inroads are being made in their learning through inserted segments at continuing education courses on worker health.

REFERENCES

1. Cooke, D. C. *Marvels of American Industry.* Maplewood, NJ: Hammond, 1962. P. 231; Cotter, J. L. *Archeological Excavating at Jamestown.* Washington, DC: U.S. Department of the Interior, National Park Service, 1958. Pp. 98–102.
2. Duffy, J. *Epidemics in Colonial America.* Baton Rouge: Louisiana State University Press, 1953. Pp. 12–13.
3. Beck, J. B. *Medicine in the American Colonies.* Albany: Horn and Wallace, 1966. Pp. 47–48.
4. McCready, B. On the influence of trades, professions, and occupations in the United States in the production of disease. *Trans Med Soc NY* 3:91, 1837. Reprinted by the Johns Hopkins Press, Baltimore, MD, 1943.
5. Freeman, J. A. Mercurial disease among hatters. *Trans NJ State Med Soc,* 1860. Pp. 61–64.
6. McCord, C. P. Occupational health publications in the United States prior to 1900. *Ind Med Surg* 24:363, 1955.
7. Grossman, J. *The Department of Labor.* New York: Praeger, 1973. Pp. 3–11.
8. Eastman, C. *Work-Accidents and the Law.* New York: Charities Publication Committee, 1910.
9. *Ives* v. *South Buffalo Railway Co.,* 201 NY, 271.
10. Stein, L. *The Triangle Fire.* Philadelphia: Lippincott, 1962.
11. Aub, J. C., Fairhall, L. T., Minot, A. S., and Reznikoff, P. *Lead Poisoning.* Medical Monographs. Baltimore: Williams & Wilkins, 1926.
12. Arluck, M. S. (Ed.). *Guide to the Microfilm Edition of the Papers of the American Association for Labor Legislation 1905–1943.* Glen Rock, NJ: Microfilming Corporation of America, 1974.

13. Doyle, H. *The Federal Industrial Hygiene Agency: A History of the Division of Occupational Health, United States Public Health Service*. History of Industrial Hygiene Committee, American Conference of Governmental Industrial Hygienists. P. 1. 1974.
14. Cook, W. L., Jr. Occupational Health and Industrial Medicine. In *Medical Department, United States Army: Preventive Medicine in World War II*. Washington, DC: Office of the Surgeon General, Department of the Army, 1971. Vol. IX, Special Fields, p. 107.
15. Cherniack, M. *The Hawk's Nest Incident: America's Worst Industrial Disaster*. New Haven, CT: Yale University Press, 1986.

3. DEFINITIONS

A definition is the enclosing a wilderness of ideas within a wall of words.

Samuel Butler

To understand the raison d'être of a medical program of any type or size in an industrial or commercial establishment, it is desirable that the terms in common parlance be defined. In early 1961, an editorialist in the *Journal of the American Medical Association* [1] attempted to realign the nomenclature used in occupational medicine several months after the AMA's council had changed its designation from industrial health to occupational health. Subsequently its congress and pertinent reference committee followed.

This move from a family of long-familiar terms to a set of new language tags had bred confusion not only among lay readers and listeners, but among professional colleagues as well. Efforts toward modernization and shortening are always welcome. As various conglomerates alter their logotypes in keeping with the redirections of their research, manufacturing, or diversifying activities, so should a profession, which speedily adopts new diagnostic tests and therapies, update its distinguishing marks.

Without belaboring further the historic aspects of a specialty's development, it is sufficient to say that physicians who found their way into occupational medicine in the early years of this century were designated as industrial physicians. The particular worksites where the original workers' compensation insurance acts were applied and where medical practitioners first implemented the new programs were, in fact, industrial installations. The term *industrial,* however, omits the inclusion of workers in construction, agriculture, civil service, education, retail trade, transportation, the armed services, or even housewifery (homemaking to today's lexicographer). The term *occupational* is all-inclusive and encompasses not only all of the vocations mentioned but also such persons as students, astronauts, and retirees whose hobbying frequently involves hazardous chemical exposures.

These comments compose a preamble offered to support the editorial writer referred to above, who invited use of some "strange-sounding terms."

DEFINITIONS OF ACTIVITIES

OCCUPATIONAL MEDICINE

Occupational medicine is defined as a specialty field of medicine concerned with (1) the assessment, maintenance, restoration, and improvement of the health of the worker through the application of the principles of preventive medicine, emergency medical care, rehabilitation, and environmental medicine; (2) the promotion of a productive and fulfilling interaction of workers with their work, through the application of the principles of human behavior; and (3) the active appreciation of the social, economic, and administrative needs and responsibilities of both the worker and the work community.

The use of the term *occupational medicine* is given substance by the American Board of Preventive Medicine, which designates the subspecialty as one of four in which certificates of special knowledge are issued by the board* [2].

Other definitions have been devised, for example that of the AMA's former Council on Occupational Health: ". . . that branch of medicine practiced by physicians in meeting medical problems and needs within occupational health programs" [3]. This statement, while accurate, is a global assertion without the specifics that point up the multiple arenas of concern of the practitioner.

Many years ago, a more inclusive identification was provided: "Occupational Medicine is that branch of medicine which deals with the relationship of man to his occupation, for the purposes of the prevention of disease and injury and the promotion of optimal health, productivity and social adjustment" [4]. Injected into this interpretation is the sense of involvement with more than medical needs, which

*Aerospace medicine, general preventive medicine, occupational medicine, and public health.

really characterizes the operational world of most of today's medical directors.

Example: A civil service firefighter is found to have myocardial ischemia, necessitating his removal from active duty and placement on sick leave status. Services to be provided: medical consultation; supportive psychological counseling; rehabilitation (testing, training, and placement); education of patient and spouse regarding coronary artery disease; reconditioning program (diet, exercise, smoking cessation); continuing liaison with treating physician; guidance regarding disability retirement.

Example: A 28-year-old with diabetes type I, mother of three children, develops retinitis and near-total blindness within 2 months. Services to be provided: referral to welfare agency for assistance and child care; transportation for medical care; referral for training at Braille Institute (reading and writing of Braille, mobility or other training, use of special "reading" devices); psychological counseling; diet guidance.

Other terms now in rather restricted use include *industrial medicine,* which is limited in most instances to clinics where the treatment of patients presenting with industrially caused injuries is offered, and *industrial health,* which is equivalent to occupational health but has remained with its older companion designation.

OCCUPATIONAL HEALTH

Occupational health is the extension of the principles and practice of occupational medicine, to include the conjoint preventive or constructive activities of all members of the occupational health team.

On occasion, occupational medicine may be defined in its narrowest sense as a professional undertaking or activity of a specially prepared and experienced physician. Occupational health implies the cooperative functioning of all professional, paraprofessional, and semiprofessional members of the group charged with the operation of a program in occupational health.

The term *occupational health* is frequently used also in a public health context, in keeping with the titles given other public health activities. Persons engaged in such programs in official health agencies most frequently provide services to organizations not having fully staffed medical departments of their own. The objectives are identical to those of in-plant programs, but more environmental studies and analyses are conducted, and little individual direct medical service is offered employed persons apart from mass or case-finding surveys or specific epidemiologic studies relative to unidentified etiologic agents possibly responsible for new occupational diseases.

Occupational health, for much the same reason, in addition to wanting a health objective, was the legislative designation of choice for the Occupational Safety and Health Act (OSHA 1970) and its agencies, Occupational Safety and Health Administration (OSHA) and National Institute for Occupational Safety and Health (NIOSH).

OCCUPATIONAL MEDICAL PROGRAM

An occupational medical program is a program of preventive medical care provided by management to deal constructively with the health of employees as it relates to their work.

The definition is adapted from the AMA statement, *Scope, Objectives and Functions of Occupational Health Programs** [3]. This concept of programming is applicable to the in-plant medical activity, and although in rare instances such a program may be created by a physician at some distance from the plant premises in an office or clinic, the usual connotation is that of a service carried out in a special facility located physically within the complex of buildings constituting the industrial or commercial enterprise.

OCCUPATIONAL HEALTH SERVICE

Occupational health service is the composite of the personnel, the services offered, and the physical plant wherein the occupational health program is carried out for the employees of the organization.

Other terms in use may include *medical department, medical service, health service,* or in strangely archaic facilities, *hospital.* An equivalent title of considerable currency is *employees' health service,* used particularly in health care institutions. To be expunged from contemporary lexicons are such inappropriately used appellations as *clinic, dispensary,* or *infirmary,* which may be fitting in other settings, but in the sense of occupational health ring only of decades past.

Never to be employed, particularly when professional personnel are on duty, is *first aid* or *first aid room.* The term connotes the temporary therapeutic use of wrested fence rails and torn shirting and not the delivery of sophisticated personal health services. Travers [5] has written her feelings regarding the incorrect application of this term in modern industry. She emphasizes that the nurse is a member of a distinguished and dedicated profession and is not a "first aider."

*This statement, prepared by the Council on Occupational Health of the AMA, was approved by the Board of Trustees and was adopted by the House of Delegates.

OCCUPATIONAL PHYSICIAN

The occupational physician is a physician engaged in the practice of occupational medicine. One term now in limited use is *occupational health physician.*

In keeping with the need for preciseness in definition, an editorialist [6], most likely the late Dr. Carey P. McCord, speaks directly to the point: "The terms 'company doctor' and 'contract doctor' carry opprobrious connotations in occupational medicine. They call up the vision of a physician who has sold his soul and his integrity to a Mephistophelean third party, to the detriment of the individual patient he serves. Happily these terms are falling into disuse."

The physician, in many settings, works jointly with an occupational nurse and an occupational hygienist (synonymous terms used currently include *occupational health nurse* and *industrial hygienist*). To strengthen the nomenclature, it is pointed out that the pertinent societies in England are the Society of Occupational Medicine and the British Occupational Hygiene Society.

OCCUPATIONAL NURSING

Occupational nursing is a specialty in nursing that applies the principles of professional and public health nursing to the development and conduct of a nursing service tailored to the changing environment of the work organization and the specific needs of its employees* [7].

The most commonly used title for such an activity is *occupational health nursing.* The former designation was *industrial nursing,* but the newer term is seen in the name of the professional organization The American Association of Occupational Health Nurses. When such a service is offered on a part-time basis through a public health agency, it has been termed community health nursing for working people [8], and formerly this activity was part-time nursing in industry [9].

In this designation, as in the identifying tag of occupational physician, the word *health* has been omitted merely for brevity. The extension of nursing roles leads to unduly long terminology, such as occupational health nurse practitioner or clinician. The excision of "health" neither changes the concept of the specialty nor alters the functions of its practitioners. Tightening and convenience are the sole objectives.

OCCUPATIONAL NURSE

The occupational nurse is a professional nurse who practices occupational nursing in a work organization.

As already indicated, the title *industrial nurse* is still encountered. The modifying adjective of *occupational* is preferred for the same reasons given previously.

With the current scrutiny being given the allocation of all health resources, the health sciences are undergoing restructuring, with the transfer of certain functions to persons at lower levels of skill and with less formal education or training.

New rubrics have been devised for members of the health services, and as skills have been passed down, those persons at the top of the professional nursing ladder have acquired functions formerly executed solely by the licensed physician. The role of the nurse has been extended in several of the specialty areas in health care, such as pediatrics and emergency service, and in the categories of primary care, acute care, and long-term care [9].

OCCUPATIONAL NURSE PRACTITIONER

More discussion of this occupational health professional will be offered later, but the term *occupational nurse practitioner* is cited as a relatively recent arrival in the health care categorizations. Such a professional person is an occupational nurse who, by additional education, is able to assume a greater share of responsibility for the provision of occupational health service or care through increased interaction with occupational physicians and who will augment the ability of physicians and other occupational health professionals in meeting the demands for care at the worksite [9].

OCCUPATIONAL ENVIRONMENTALIST

The occupational environmentalist is a professional member of the occupational health team, frequently from an engineering or chemistry background, who is involved in the recognition, evaluation, and control of those work environmental factors or stressors—chemical, physical, biologic, and ergo-

*A variation of this description is seen in ". . . the application of nursing and public health procedures for the purpose of conserving, promoting and restoring the health of individuals and groups through their places of employment" (Brown, M. L. *Occupational Health Nursing.* New York: Springer, 1956. P. 15). In the second edition of *Occupational Health Nursing* (Springer, 1981), Brown adds the primary goal of occupational health nursing practice as "assist[ing] the worker to attain and maintain optimal physical and psychological functioning."

nomic*—that may cause illness, impaired health, or significant discomfort to employees or residents of the community [10].

More commonly heard, and more traditional, is *industrial hygienist,* but with the concern over community pollutants and the interest in the interrelationship of pollution and mental health,† the field of the knowing hygienist has broadened. Infrequently, as the late Professor Philip Drinker pointed out many years ago, the environmentalist may also be a physician [11]. Eckardt [12] has underscored the great need for the physician to supply management with counsel regarding the effects of the chemical environment on health.

The federal compliance officer fills a significant role in the administration of OSHA 1970, and many such persons, at higher levels, may be occupational environmentalists (industrial hygienists). In some governmental jurisdictions, environmentalists are termed engineers for certain fiscal or administrative reasons, rather than for strict adherence to functional roles or educational preparation.

HEALTH PHYSICIST

The health physicist is a professional person engaged in radiation protection activities that are directed toward minimizing the exposure of persons to sources of ionizing radiation, such activities to include, primarily, evaluation of exposure or contamination levels, decontamination, shielding design, radiation protection training, personnel monitoring, and the supervision of activities or persons involved in these areas [13,14].

Equivalent terms that may be encountered are *radiologic health specialist, radiation protection specialist,* or depending on specificity of task assignment, *medical physicist, radiation safety officer, reactor health physicist,* or *radiologic physicist.* As indicated previously, a physician (frequently a radiologist or occupational physician) or an industrial hygienist may serve in this capacity [14].

OCCUPATIONAL EPIDEMIOLOGIST

The occupational epidemiologist is an epidemiologist concerned with the identification of the host, agent, and environmental factors, and their correlations, present in the work setting, in the study of cause and effect relationships in such diverse areas as absenteeism, disability retirement, environmental toxins, health service utilization, labor turnover, morbidity (present and projected), mortality (present and projected), nonoccupational injury, occupational disease, and work-generated injury. The primary contribution of the epidemiologist in the workplace is the identification of the cause of a particular occupational disease. Such a person has been termed by Dr. Lloyd Tepper as an "etiologist." Professional activities of this nature may be performed also by biostatisticians or, on occasion, by environmental epidemiologists.

OCCUPATIONAL OPTOMETRIST

An occupational optometrist is engaged in the investigation of all physiologic optical defects of the vision, including the deficits of refraction, and ocular muscle function; corrects or aids these defects by means of lenses, prisms, muscle training or other measures; and conducts this practice in the work setting.

OCCUPATIONAL HEALTH EDUCATOR

The occupational health educator is a professionally trained person whose mission is to effect an alteration of health behavior so as to elevate the health status of workers, including both those employees exposed to specific occupational health hazards and those employees whose work does not put them at special occupational disease risk. The educator is engaged, in addition, in conducting programs in compliance with the right-to-know legislation.

OCCUPATIONAL MENTAL HEALTH SPECIALIST

The occupational mental health specialist is engaged in the diagnosis and treatment of behavioral and emotional disorders of employed persons at the place

*Ergonomics, as defined by the International Labour Office and cited by Zenz (in Ergonomics: Work Effort, Determination of Energy Expenditure, and Fatigue, in C. Zenz [Ed.], *Occupational Medicine—Principles and Practical Applications*. Chicago, IL: Year Book, 1975. P. 423), is the "application of the human biological sciences in conjunction with the engineering sciences to achieve the optimum mutual adjustment of man and his work, the benefits being measured in terms of human efficiency and well-being."

Innumerable related fields interdigitate with occupational health, particularly in the study of the many aspects of the work environment. Further, a particular manufacturing process or a specific kind of end product may dictate greater utilization of the knowledge of one science or another. The disciplines from which certain knowledge is needed periodically are aerospace medicine, anthropology, anthropometry, biomechanics, biometeorology, biotechnology, environmental physiology, industrial engineering, information theory, human factors engineering, product design, submarine medicine, systems safety, and work physiology. These fields among others are cited by Zenz.

†As an example, see *Pollution: Its Impact on Mental Health*. Rockville, MD: National Clearinghouse for Mental Health Information, National Institute for Mental Health, 1972.

of work and may be a psychiatrist, a psychologist, or a psychiatric social worker. Such a person may be part of the employee assistance program team.

OCCUPATIONAL (INDUSTRIAL) TOXICOLOGIST

The occupational (industrial) toxicologist is an investigative scientist who is engaged in the study of the harmful actions on living systems of chemicals and other agents encountered in work processes and contacts, using experimental data to develop, test, and refine theoretic models that can be used to predict the effects of untested materials, focusing on a quantitative relationship between the measurable properties of a toxic material and the resultant measurable harmful effects [15].

OCCUPATIONAL LICENSED VOCATIONAL NURSE

The occupational licensed vocational nurse is a licensed vocational nurse (LVN) who provides basic and personal nursing care to employee-patients that requires a knowledge of standardized procedures in an occupational health service or in an occupational setting [16].

Many of the duties performed by the occupational LVN are those customarily executed in a variety of health service formats, such as the preparation of patients for examination, determination of patients' needs, recording of blood pressure, or under medical direction, such duties as venipuncture for the collection of blood specimens, administration of immunizing injections, application of dressings and bandages to traumatic injury sites, or assisting a nurse or a physician with a diagnostic or therapeutic procedure.

In one study [17], it was learned that 1,007 LVNs were functioning in industry, many presumably serving in places either formerly filled by graduate nurses or in newly created positions that call for LVNs at a lower salary level. An alternative designation is *occupational licensed practical nurse.*

OCCUPATIONAL PHYSICIAN'S ASSISTANT

The occupational physician's assistant is a skilled person qualified by academic and practical training to provide patient services in an occupational health setting under the supervision and direction of a licensed physician who is responsible for the performance of that assistant.

This definition is recommended by the AMA [18]. Other terms are utilized to which the modifier occupational might be added, such as *surgeon's assistant, physician's associate, allied health person,* or *physician's aide.*

OCCUPATIONAL ENVIRONMENTAL TECHNICIAN

The occupational environmental technician is a technician, appropriately trained, who serves under the direction of an occupational environmentalist and who conducts the simpler, more repetitive tests in environmental hazard assessment or control, utilizing instruments or equipment that provide direct reading of values measured or that, with certain calculations, can give meaningful measurements of the level of potential health hazards in the ambient air of workrooms.

With the great demand for skilled occupational environmentalists, there will be an increasing need for team associates at a technician level to perform standardized, less complicated mensuration procedures. They may be termed industrial hygiene technicians in certain institutions.

OCCUPATIONAL HEALTH TECHNICIAN

The occupational health technician is a technician trained to perform certain instrumented tests or laboratory procedures used in the medical examination of work applicants or employees, such as urinalysis, recording of blood pressure, electrocardiography, measurement of visual and auditory acuities, determination of height, weight, and skinfold thickness, and completion of the microhematocrit procedure.

OCCUPATIONAL HEALTH ADMINISTRATOR

Nearly all of the positions defined so far reflect personnel with professional or technical education or training in health care or whose operations involve primarily an interface with applicants or patients in a diagnostic or therapeutic sense. Relatively new to the occupational health scene is the administrator, whose concerns are with the overall operation of the service and with its personnel and rarely, if ever, with the patients seen by the professional staff.

The administrator is a member of the directorate of an occupational health service whose background, education, or experience might be in personnel, hospital administration, or business management, who carries out, under the supervision of the medical director, such nonmedical functions as personnel and salary administration, budget preparation and review, procurement of supplies and equipment, orientation of nonprofessional personnel, supervision of medical record systems, communications, and quality control [19].

OCCUPATIONAL DISEASE
Occupational disease is a disease arising out of, or in the course of, employment—resulting from the exposure to, the absorption of, or intoxication from harmful chemical, microbiologic, or physical agents to which the general public normally would not be exposed. Other terms in use include *industrial disease* and *industrial illness*.

OCCUPATIONAL INJURY
Occupational injury is an injury arising out of, or in the course of, employment, resulting from the action of physically or chemically traumatizing agents. The other term in use is *industrial injury*.

A rubric frequently employed for this clinical condition is "industrial accident." This designation is not correct, for there can be accidents without injuries and accidents with attendant injuries. Confusion is heightened by the loose use of the term, for in the compilation of data in occupational safety management, an industrial accident may imply a collision of company vehicles.

ENVIRONMENTAL HEALTH
Environmental health is that aspect of public health that is concerned with those forms of life, substances, forces, and conditions in surroundings that may exert an influence on human health and well-being [20].

This definition is included because, with the compliance by industry with the provisions of OSHA 1970, some companies have designated directors of environmental health to serve in the oversight of programs in occupational health, safety, occupational hygiene, and infrequently, fire protection. The incumbent might have been either the medical director, the safety director, or the industrial hygiene manager. The terms *occupational health* and *environmental health* are not clearly distinguished in most usage. The confusion is increased because of the conversion in many institutions of the label *sanitation* or *industrial sanitation* to *environmental health*; the former term seemed to be considered opprobrious with the new emphasis given ecology, the environment, and the safety and health of the worker. Most sanitarians are now classified in official health agencies as environmentalists or environmental health specialists.

PATIENT
It may appear to be facetious to offer the definition of a patient, but because each occupational health activity is patient- or employee-oriented, it is logical to provide a common understanding.

A patient is any person, well or sick, who is receiving the services of a professional provider of health care for the purpose of promoting, maintaining, or restoring health or minimizing the consequences of illness [9].

REFERENCES

1. What's in a name? (Editorial). *J.A.M.A.* 175:321, 1961.
2. See *Directory of Medical Specialists, 1985–1986* (22nd ed.) Chicago: Marquis Who's Who, 1985. Vol. 2, pp. 2791–2792.
3. *Scope, Objectives, and Functions of Occupational Health Programs* (rev. Dec 1971). Chicago: American Medical Association, 1971.
4. Kammer, A. G. Reporting on panel on the training of physicians for industry at the graduate level. In The Education of Physicians for Industry. *J Med Educ* 31(2):58, 1956. See also Occupational Medical Practice Committee. Careers in occupational medicine. *J Occup Med* 23:122, 1981.
5. Travers, D. The significance of a name. *Am Assoc Ind Nurs J* 14:20, Feb 1966.
6. Semantics and taboos. *J Occup Med* 7:475, 1965.
7. *Functions and Qualifications for an Occupational Health Nurse in a One-Nurse Service.* New York: American Nurses' Association, 1968.
8. *Community Health Nursing for Working People.* Cincinnati, OH: U.S. Department of Health, Education, and Welfare, Public Health Service, Environmental Health Service, Bureau of Occupational Safety and Health, 1970.
9. *Extending the Scope of Nursing Practice.* A Report of the Secretary's Committee to Study Extended Roles for Nurses. Washington, DC: The Committee (U.S. Department of Health, Education, and Welfare), Nov 1971. P. 7.
10. Olishifski, J. B., and McElroy, F. E. (Eds.). *Fundamentals of Industrial Hygiene.* Chicago: National Safety Council, 1971. P. 1. See also Industrial hygiene: Definition, scope, function and organization. *Am Ind Hyg Assoc J* 20:428, 1959.
11. Drinker, P. The practice of industrial hygiene. *Am Ind Hyg Assoc Q* 11:101, 1950.
12. Eckardt, R. E. The role of the industrial health physician in environmental health problems. *J Occup Med* 13:161, 1971.
13. Little, M. S. Professional status of radiation protection personnel. *Am J Public Health* 61:1947, 1971.
14. Moeller, D. W. Meeting radiological health manpower needs. *Am J Public Health* 61:1938, 1971.
15. Courtesy of Robert F. Phalen, Ph.D. (Personal communication, 1986.)
16. *Position Classification Standard for Nursing Assistant Series GS-621.* Washington, DC: U.S. Civil Service Commission, Bureau of Policies and Standards, June 1970. P. 13.
17. Marshall, E. D., and Moses, E. B. *LPN's, 1967 An Inventory of Licensed Practical Nurses.* Bethesda,

MD: U.S. Department of Health, Education and Welfare, Public Health Service, National Institutes of Health, Bureau of Health Manpower Education, Division of Nursing, Jan 1971. P. 33.

18. Todd, M. D., and Foy, D. F. Current status of the physician's assistant and related issues. *J.A.M.A.* 220:1714, 1972; *Physician's Assistant Q & A*. Chicago: American Medical Association, March 1980.
19. Petry, P. M. and Hilker, R. R. J. The medical administrator: A new person in the industrial medical department. *J Occup Med* 13:339, 1971.
20. Purdom, P. W. *Environmental Health* (2nd ed.). New York: Academic, 1980. P. 6.

4. PROGRAM OBJECTIVES AND CONFIGURATION

Having . . . strolled into a narrow path that led to no goal . . . I see the idleness of my journey.

Hugh Walpole

How people behave is dramatically influenced by how we organize . . . institutions.

Elliott Jaques

With the introduction in the early 1960s of management by objectives, with periodic review and redefinition, business and governmental administrators have become accustomed to the delineation of specific program goals. Accompanying each described objective is a date when such an objective might be reached or its task elements completed. When the objectives are spelled out, all activities within a unit are then related to them, with each particular program item being subsumed under one of a series of objectives. The system allows for improved planning, frequent updating, more refined budgeting, the introduction of alternatives when necessary, and a sharper identification of costs and benefits accrued. The process of management by objectives and results has been described by Odiorne [1] as the process in which ". . . the superior and subordinate managers of an organization jointly identify its common goals, define each individual's major areas of responsibility in terms of the results expected of him [sic], and use these measures as guides for operating the unit and assessing the contribution of each of its members." The principle concerned is the direction of all effort and behavior within an organization toward the achievement of the identified objectives.

Objectives can be recognized in occupational health, as in any other group undertaking, subobjectives or subgoals can be assigned, and specific actions or elements or tasks can be attached to each objective.

Before detailing program structure, it would be helpful to provide the objectives of an occupational health program (OHP) as viewed by the American Medical Association [2]:

To protect employees against health and safety hazards in their work situation.

Insofar as practical and feasible, to protect the general environment of the community.

To facilitate the placement of workers according to their physical, mental, and emotional capacities in work that they can perform with an acceptable degree of efficiency and without endangering their own health and safety or that of others.

To ensure adequate medical care and rehabilitation of the occupationally ill and injured.

To encourage and assist in measures for personal health maintenance, including the acquisition of a personal physician whenever possible.

Added to these objectives are certain basic program requirements that have been stated by the American Occupational Medical Association (AOMA) [3], in that an OHP must, as a minimum:

Obey all relevant laws and regulations.

Take all feasible steps to keep industrial operations and/or products from having an adverse effect on the health of employees, customers, and the public.

Accept responsibility and assist in the provision of necessary care in cases where health is harmed due to industrial operations and/or products.

In an Occupational Safety and Health Administration (OSHA)–sponsored conference on OHPs, there was consensus as to certain elements and characteristics of any effective health program. The following met agreement by all participants [4]:

Top management and labor commitment to the program: Management should endorse and actively support the program, providing the necessary resources for its operation. Labor commitment should be manifested by active participation in and support of the program, whether the employees are organized or not.

The program should contain a hazard anticipation, recognition, evaluation, and abatement plan, including such items as materials inventory, regular internal inspections, complaint investigation procedures, and the like.

The program should contain a written statement of goals and objectives, written policies and procedures, and specific directions for implementation. It should contain also a plan for regular monitoring and auditing of its operation, with provisions for periodic evaluation and deficiency correction. Implementation must be in accordance with these written policies and procedures.

The program should contain an active employee training and education plan.

Consensus began to lessen with the following elements:

The program should be carried out by qualified and competent professional personnel, in adequate number and coordinated properly.

The program should contain an active data collection and retrieval system with both workplace and employee statistics necessary for the proper monitoring and assessment of occupational health hazards. The records must be retained for a reasonable period. Employees should have access to the data, but individual employee health records should be protected from undue disclosure.

The program should provide for access and use of industrial hygiene monitoring, preferably with board-certified overview.

The program should provide for access to and use of medical surveillance, including baseline and periodic evaluation.

The program should provide emergency procedures.

The program should require communication of hazard information to employees.

With the following elements, consensus dropped substantially:

The program should prescribe specific work practice procedures.

The program should require the application of feasible [term undefined] engineering controls.

The program should require the existence of appropriate workplace facilities and equipment in adequate number and of adequate quality. Facilities should be properly maintained and instruments properly calibrated.

The program should require the availability of medical care, internally or externally.

The program should require compliance with existing health standards, assuming that such standards are adequate.

The program desiderata provided by the conference, while sound and ideal, are stated with the word *should,* which used in an auxiliary function loses the strength of its present tense of *shall.* A series of elements can be prescribed but, when weakened, serve solely as gentle reminders. The inclusion of other qualifiers—“adequate” and “properly”—without definition, further attenuate the good intentions of the listing. The differences in priority of the elements among the three sets point up varying points of view of the arbiters.

The objectives and the elements given form the framework of a program, but to understand the full potential of occupational health, it is necessary to match activities against goals. One schema follows.

PROGRAM SCHEMA

MISSION, OBJECTIVES, AND FUNCTIONS IN OCCUPATIONAL HEALTH

MISSION OR PURPOSE

The conservation of human resources at the place of employment.

OBJECTIVE

The improvement of worker productivity, morale, and socially adaptive behavior.

FUNCTION

The assessment, preservation, restoration, and improvement of the health of workers at the place of employment,* with appropriate adjunctive activities to support this function.

FUNCTION 1
Assessment of the health of workers.

Objective
Placement and retention of workers in, or upward movement to, positions commensurate with their physical, mental, and emotional capacities.
Actions to Achieve Objective

1. Conduct medical† examinations of job applicants, and forward recommendations regarding their placement to the employment authority.
2. Conduct periodic medical examinations of employees, and assist personnel managers in the placement of employees with medical, physical, or functional limitations.

FUNCTION 2
Preservation of the health of workers.

Objective
Increase of individual work effectiveness with maximization of environmental and personal health potentials.
Actions to Achieve Objective

1. Conduct programs of communicable disease control.
2. Conduct programs for the prevention or early detection of cardiac, respiratory, and other chronic or degenerative diseases.
3. Conduct health education or promotional activities concerning physical and emotional health.
4. Provide information concerning potential occupational health hazards.
5. Conduct a hearing conservation program.
6. Conduct a vision conservation program.
7. Conduct nutrition counseling.
8. Conduct drug-abuse and alcoholism screening programs.
9. Identify, control, or eliminate the health hazards or hazardous work processes present in the employment environment, in keeping with both policy and mandates.
10. Promote healthful and safe work behavior.
11. Provide administrative counsel to managers and supervisory personnel on specific physical and emotional health problems of individuals and groups, without compromise of privileged information.

FUNCTION 3
Restoration of the health of workers.

Objective
Maintenance of an effective, contributing, productive workforce with minimal loss of the economic and human resources of the organization.
Actions to Achieve Objective

1. Provide emergency medical care to ill or injured employees.

*May be interpreted in more customary terms as the detection, treatment, and prevention of illness and injury and the rehabilitation of the employee with post-injury or postillness disability.

†The term *medical* is used in preference to *physical*, for it is more inclusive. If objections to psychological evaluations are raised because such procedures are not encompassed by a *physical* examination, it is clear that a *medical* examination may include many different assessments.

2. Provide referrals of ill or injured employees to community physicians, specialists, or other health care agencies.
3. Conduct quality control of extramural medical care given ill or injured employees through review of the treatment provided and liaison with sources of care.
4. Provide counseling for employees with emotional problems.

FUNCTION 4
Improvement of the health of the worker.

Objective
The release of the human energy or potential entrapped by residual physical disability, faulty personality structuring, or congenital impairment with discovery of new sources of individual growth and contribution to the mission of the organization.
Actions to Achieve Objective
1. Conduct program in physical restoration and vocational rehabilitation.
2. Conduct alcoholism rehabilitation program.
3. Conduct drug-abuse rehabilitation program.
4. Conduct physical reconditioning or wellness program.
5. Conduct individual and group counseling for employees whose performance is restricted or altered by deep emotional problems.
6. Assist in the adjustment to the work scene of the previously unemployed or currently underemployed minority members, including women, the handicapped, and the aged.
7. Effect liaison with community agencies to increase employment of physically limited job applicants.
8. Inform managers of mechanisms of "reasonable accommodation"* that will enhance the employment of physically limited or impaired job applicants.

FUNCTION 5
Provision of administrative support.

Objective
Facilitation of all occupational health programming through use of appropriate administrative procedures.
Actions to Achieve Objective
1. Initiate and maintain a computerized medical records system with capability for retrieval of information.
2. Provide secretarial, clerical, and technical support to professional health team.
3. Provide personnel management support, in conjunction with the functions of the personnel department.
4. Provide systems of compliance with health and safety codes of all governmental jurisdictions relating to the organization.
5. Provide a system for the cost analysis of all program actions and for subsequent budget preparation, review, and adjustment.
6. Provide a system for the obtaining, receipt, storage, inventory, and issue of medical and office supplies, with the assistance of the procurement authority.
7. Identify and quantify the morbidity and mortality experience of employees, and quantify the provision of services by the program.
8. Initiate and maintain systems of evaluation (epidemiology).
9. Devise and carry out in-service training programs for program employees, and build experience for students from extramural sources.
10. Initiate and participate in research efforts.

*Reasonable accommodation, in general, is the effort made by the employer, who is a recipient of federal funds in any form, to accommodate the handicapped person through the provision of accessible facilities, job restructuring, modified work schedules, special devices, provision of readers, and so on. See *Federal Register* 42:22680, §84.12, 1977, Reasonable Accommodation (Regulations to Sec. 504, Rehabilitation Act 1973).

This material may serve several purposes. It can be a base for management by objectives, for cost analysis and budget preparation by program element, and for assignment of staff responsibilities. Details of certain of the actions will be given in later chapters.

AN ALTERNATIVE PROGRAM SCHEMA

A second format, which delineates the services offered by program and which provides the details of program elements, follows. In either framework, all possible service actions are listed. No individual program will include all suggested procedures, but from such a listing the ideal program for one's particular point of reference can be built, using the elements pertinent to the undertaking and deferring or discarding those program units not germane to the industry, the company, or the local or community situation.

MODEL OCCUPATIONAL HEALTH PROGRAM

I. *Total occupational health program*
   A. *Objective.*
      The objective of a comprehensive occupational health program is the conservation of human resources through the evaluation, protection, promotion, and restoration of the health of employees.

II. *Program of preplacement medical examinations*
   A. *Objective.*
      The objective of the program of conducting medical examinations on job applicants is to minimize the incidence and severity of employee injuries and illness by means of placement of employees in positions in accordance with their physical and emotional capacities and the physical and environmental demands of the job.
   B. *Elements of the program.*
      The examination comprises several components—examinations and tests conducted by both medical and health-service personnel. The elements follow:
      1. *Preplacement medical examination.* Systems inventory, health status appraisal, and functional capacity determination by review of medical history, occupational history, and physical examination findings or yield.
      2. *Preplacement diagnostic procedures**
         a. Audiometry (and speech discrimination testing, if indicated by job).
         b. Visual skills determination through use of precision stereoscopic instrument.
         c. Electrocardiography, as indicated by age, physical demands of position, or related clinical cardiovascular findings.
         d. Chest radiography.†
         e. Hematologic studies—complete blood count.
         f. Blood chemistry studies, as indicated.
         g. Urinalysis.
         h. Serodiagnostic test for syphilis.
         i. Tonometry.
         j. Other radiographic studies as indicated by previous history, residua of job-related injury or illness, findings on examination (such as blood or urine levels of absorbed environmental contactants or toxicants), or specific job to be held.
         k. Psychodiagnostic tests or special interview, as selected or indicated, by mental-health specialists.
         l. Dynamic electrocardiography, as indicated.
         m. Pulmonary function determina-

*One or more of these test procedures may be conducted in keeping with the need for early worklife reference points or the need for baseline levels before exposure to toxic work materials.

†Although so-called routine radiography of the chest has been decried because of the factor of exposure to ionizing radiation, such a study is considered necessary in certain situations in light of the innumerable pneumoconioses or pulmonary sensitivity responses to which a worker may be subject.

tion, as indicated by past work experience or currently applied-for position.

3. *Summation of physical and emotional capacities for the job.*
4. *Matching of functional capacities against physical and environmental demands of job and classification of applicant, without use of excessively rigid standards that may preclude acceptance.*
5. *Additional preplacement procedures*
   a. Administration of immunizing injections, as indicated.
   b. Initiation of confidential health records.
   c. Formulation and forwarding of recommendations regarding placement.

III. *Program of periodic medical examinations*

A. *Objective.*

1. *Medical examinations for reevaluation, or for determination of fitness for duty, of employees.*
   Determination and evaluation of possible abnormal or defective physical or emotional factors in relation to poor work performance, disturbed interpersonal relationships, or excessive absenteeism.
   a. Interval medical and work histories.
   b. Physical measurements—height, weight, pulse, respiration rate, blood pressure, and so on.
   c. Vision measurements, including visual acuity, visual fields, color discrimination.
   d. Audiometry.
   e. Complete medical examination.
   f. Radiographic examination—chest and other areas as indicated by interval histories, physical examination findings, or work assignment.
   g. Pulmonary function determination.
   h. Laboratory examinations—urinalysis, hematologic and blood chemistry studies, as indicated by history, physical findings, or work exposure.
   i. Cardiac evaluation, including electrocardiography, when indicated.
   j. Specialty consultation.
   k. Preparation and forwarding of release forms to obtain information regarding interval illness or injury experience from private physician, clinic, hospital, or other source of care.

   Full consideration of all abnormal findings in relation to reason for requested medical reevaluation, and formulation and forwarding of work limitations or statement regarding examinee's medical capability of meeting job requirements.
2. *Postillness or postinjury return-to-work reviews or examinations.*
   Determination of employee's physical or emotional capability to return to normal work activity following a nonoccupational illness or injury.
   a. Medical history of illness or injury.
   b. Inspection or medical examination related specifically to illness or injury.
   c. Preparation and forwarding of release forms to obtain more complete information on illness or injury from treating physician, clinic, or hospital, when appropriate.
   d. Full evaluation of findings and forwarded information to determine employee's capability of returning to normal work activity.
3. *Periodic examinations of personnel exposed to work hazards* and of key executives. Repeated examinations at intervals most appropriate to the work of employees in special category, to determine the employees' continuing physical and emotional capacity to perform their work assignments.*
   a. Interval medical and occupational histories.

*The designation "work hazards" implies exposure to jobs where potential health hazards exist, such as excessive noise, toxic chemicals, fibrogenic dust, or ionizing radiation, or where peak sensory capacity is required, such as in the operation of cranes or motorized equipment, law enforcement, firefighting, or diving.

b. Physical measurements—weight, height, pulse, respiration rate, blood pressure.
c. Vision measurements, total and near vision acuity, color discrimination, visual fields, and other procedures, as indicated.
d. Tonometry.
e. Complete medical examination with special attention to bodily organ systems that might be involved through exposure to potentially hazardous agents.
f. Audiometry.
g. Chest and other radiographic studies, as indicated by the occupational history, physical examination findings, and the potential hazard involved, such as chest radiographs in case of fibrogenic dust exposure, long-bone studies in case of diving personnel, and the like.
h. Resting, 12-lead electrocardiography.
i. Complete hematologic study.
j. Blood chemistry battery.
k. Special bioassay procedures as determined by work exposure, such as blood and urinary levels of absorbed work substance, blood cholinesterase, and the like.
l. Urinalysis.
m. Test of stool for occult blood.
n. Consultation in special areas, for example, cardiology, orthopedic surgery, urology, when indicated.
o. Abnormal findings due to pathologic or aging processes are weighted, and if necessary, limitations are formulated to maintain the employee at work, whenever possible.
p. All findings considered in light of potential hazards involved and in consultation with occupational hygiene specialists concerning possible corrective actions that might be necessary in light of environmental deficits.

IV. *Program of cardiopulmonary evaluation (physical fitness)*

A. *Objective.*

The objective of the cardiopulmonary evaluation program is the preservation of the effective health status of key personnel, in the hope of obviating the development of cardiac disease.

B. *Elements of the program.*

1. *Physical fitness evaluation.*

a. Height determination, weight determination, and skinfold measurements—triceps, subscapular, biceps, and suprailiac.
b. Spine mobility—trunk flexion, rotation, lateral flexion, and extension.
c. Muscular strength—hand grip, back, and leg.
d. Pulmonary function determination.
e. Twelve-lead electrocardiography.
f. Continuous heart rate measurement.
g. Continuous ECG monitoring by oscilloscope, tape, and printout.
h. Periodic blood pressure measurement.
i. Ergometric (exercise) measurement at heart rates of 100, 120, 140, and 160.
j. Oxygen uptake.
k. Overall evaluation of test scores.
l. Instructions and counseling regarding specific conditioning program to improve physical fitness, when necessary.
m. Counsel regarding diet and negative elements in life-style.
n. Counsel regarding definitive medical care, when indicated.

V. *Program of emergency medical care*

A. *Objective.*

The objective of the emergency medical care program is to limit employee ineffectiveness caused by illness or injury while at work.

B. *Elements of the program.*

1. *Primary elements.*

a. Furnish emergency medical care to all employees, visitors, and vendors, as required.
b. Emergency medical care, upon request, to the acutely ill or injured in work facilities at some distance from the occupational health service (OHS).

c. Provision of emergency medical care in satellite health care facilities in areas of high employee density.

2. *Program details.*
   a. Medical history of incident.
   b. Physical characteristics (vital signs)—temperature, pulse, respiration rate, blood pressure.
   c. Physical examination of body part involved.
   d. Radiographic examination of area involved.
   e. Provision of appropriate emergency treatment, as indicated.
   f. Arrangement for follow-up care in OHS or referral to patient's private physician or outside consultant when appropriate.
   g. Arrangement through personal physician for follow-up visitation to the hospital by a representative of OHS.
   h. In cases of nonoccupational minor injury or illness of employees, care in OHS, when appropriate, or referral to personal physician.
   i. Consultations in specialty areas—orthopedic surgery, cardiology, social and emotional health counseling, or occupational hygiene service regarding work environment.
   j. In cases of occupational injury or illness, preparation and forwarding of indicated reports, including supplementary reports and release-to-work forms for departmental use as needed.
   k. Development of health care segment of disaster plan.

VI. *Program of counseling*

A. *Objective.*

The objective of the counseling program is to identify and counsel employees presenting emotional or behavioral disorders that impair their job performance.

B. *Elements of the program.*

1. *Assessment of psychological status of applicants for work, when indicated by the discovery of unique historic episodes or by the findings on medical examination.*
   a. Review of records prior to interview.
   b. Conducting 45- to 50-minute detailed interview, for determination of life background.
   c. Administration of psychological test battery, when indicated, followed by interpretation.
   d. Reduction of findings to recommendations regarding placement.
   e. Entry of findings in the medical record or confidential file, or both, as indicated.
   f. On short-term qualification, conducting of postemployment follow-up, consisting of individual counseling sessions, review of reports from supervisor, and possible initiation of counseling sessions for applicant or group sessions for applicants.
2. *Psychological reevaluation of employee or transferring employee.*
   a. Detailed review of recent health problems of employee, including medical records, supervisor's reports, and psychological or psychiatric data.
   b. Conducting of interview to determine current psychological status of employee.
   c. Administration, when indicated, of psychological tests, followed by interpretation.
   d. Forwarding of recommendations to examining or treating physician in OHS.
   e. Semi-monthly follow-up through individual counseling sessions.
   f. Recommendation of removal from worksite and referral to extramural sources of care when recurrence of work-precluding symptoms is noted.
   g. Recommendation of transfer, when indicated, with follow-up.
   h. Entry of findings in medical record or confidential file, or both.
3. *Emergency care—crisis intervention.*
   a. Evaluation of acutely disturbed person.
   b. Informing physician of degree of disturbance.
   c. Holding of ventilative or supportive sessions with employees or applicants as indicated.

d. Referral to extramural sources of mental health care.
e. Factoring out of psychological deficits in cases of injury, and institution of counseling, if indicated.
f. Entry of findings in medical record or confidential file, or both.

4. *Counseling.*
Counseling activities are conducted on those employees whose emotional deficits, irrespective of etiology or precipitating event, cause impaired job performance.
a. Individual and group counseling for employees with emotional problems.
b. Group counseling for employees who are grossly obese or who request diet assistance.
c. Group counseling for employees with marital problems.
d. Individual or group counseling for employees who have recently sustained a loss of an immediate family member.
e. Individual or group counseling for problem drinkers, former drug abusers, compulsive gamblers, and compulsive smokers.

5. *Consultation.*
Consultative and educative conferences with managerial personnel regarding crisis intervention. Understanding of job adjustment of the handicapped, injury repetition, and resolution of problems in behavior.

VII. *Program of health education/information communication*

A. *Objective.*
The objective of the health education program is the alteration of health behavior. Implicit in this is the promotion of the continuing health of the well, the education and counseling of employees with specific risk factors, the explanation and clarification of disease patterns and their accompanying treatment plans, when required, and the presentation of information concerning toxicants and hazardous exposures in the workplace.

B. *Elements of the program.*
1. Development of audiovisual materials (such as videotapes or slide/sound tapes) specific to the organization in areas of occupational health risk, such as asbestos-related disease, noise-induced hearing loss, mercurialism, lead poisoning, dermatitis.
2. Development of graphic materials (brochures, leaflets, and wallet cards) for use by, and distribution to, involved employees in specific risk areas, such as work in contact with fibrogenic dust, in areas of high noise level, or with cutting oils, solvents, abrasive materials, epoxy paints.
3. The conducting of individual educational conferences with employees in need of specific health guidance.
4. The conducting of group educational programs for employees at risk for certain nonoccupational diseases, such as coronary artery disease, chronic obstructive pulmonary disease, obesity, hypertensive heart disease.
5. Conducting of individual and group conferences covering exposure to potential occupational health hazards, such as heavy metals, solvents, increased atmospheric pressure.
6. Individual or group conferences relating to the prevention of specific injuries, such as back injuries, eye injuries.
7. Conducting of group conferences for the interpretation of periodic medical surveillance procedures, such as chest radiographs, pulmonary function studies, liver function studies.
8. Preparation of health column for weekly newspaper or monthly magazine (house organs).
9. Obtaining and distribution of extramural publications on health covering nonoccupational disease entities or preventive health care, for example, alcoholism, heart disease, immunization programs, communicable disease, skin disorders, compulsive behavior.

VIII. *Program of health record documentation*

A. *Objective.*
The objective of the health record documentation program is to provide for clinical, legal, and administrative use a set of health records that will be useful as a segment of support to the administrative arm

of the organization in the completion of its mission.

B. *Elements of the program.*

1. The initiation, maintenance, updating, distribution, retrieval, and refiling of health records, and preparation of statistical summarizations of entries from both active and inactive health records, constantly updated with notes arising from examination, treatment, workplace environmental evaluation, administrative action, reported care from extramural sources, news clippings, or official organizational documents when there is pertinent application to employee-patient.
2. Through the use of specialized forms for medical examination, radiograph requests and reports of interpretation, laboratory test reports, and correspondence, a sequential history is maintained of significant medical events in the life of the employees that can, and frequently do, affect their work performance.
3. The temporary storage, inventory, and selection for extramural filing of certain inactive health records, and in accordance with federal or state mandates, the orderly retention of records of employees exposed to specific occupational health hazards.
4. Maintenance of correspondence developed with sources of health care in the community (within the state or out of state) regarding past medical data on applicants or employees.
5. Development of codes to allow conversion of record data to computerization for research, epidemiologic study, and program planning.

IX. *Program of administration*

A. *Objective.*

The objective of the administrative program is to provide direction for the total OHP, which consists of activities in the primary OHS branches, medicine, nursing, occupational hygiene, counseling, environmental health, optometry, health education, and administration, and the subsets of medical record administration, emergency medical care, radiology, clinical laboratory, pharmacy, supply, and such other units as may be germane (epidemiology, ambulance service).

B. *Elements of the program.*

1. Maintenance of files and records relating to personnel and personnel actions, supply, controlled medications, budget, space allocation, planning, and official correspondence.
2. Administrative support to the program of emergency medical care in the form of correlation of efforts of occupational medicine and nursing, workers' compensation administration, and departmental personnel administration.
3. Direction to primary branches and secondary units regarding justification for and documentation of personnel actions.
4. Obtaining of justification and specifications regarding equipment or supplies to be ordered, and preparation of requisitions or purchase orders.
5. Maintenance of inventories and related documents pertaining to controlled medicinals.
6. Arrangement of staff meetings and in-service training programs, in cooperation with the health educator.
7. Documentation of current space usage, and initiation of plans for expansion of available work areas.
8. The correlation of feeder reports for the preparation of periodically recurring reports (monthly, quarterly, semiannual, or annual) in occupational health activities, radiation and other untoward exposures, and individual special reports of illness or injury.
9. Facilitation of receipt, preparation, logging, and forwarding of administrative and professional correspondence and documents.

X. *Program of epidemiology*

A. *Objective.*

The objective of the epidemiology program is to provide the administrators of the OHP with reliable, valid information on the prevalence and incidence among employees of all major classes of disease and disability and causes of death, occupational and nonoccupational, and the health factors causing special placement of applicants for positions with the organization, in addition to other such studies concerning response of employees to health-hazardous exposures.

B. *Elements of the program.*

1. Establishment of channels through which reliable and valid data, which are required from departments and divisions, may be secured on a continuing basis.
2. Institution of optimal means of gathering health data within the OHS on a reliable, valid, and continuing basis.
3. Institution of indexes of diseases, disabilities, and causes of death, on a basis that will permit meaningful comparison with state and national statistics, particularly as these indexes relate to work-generated illness.
4. Provision of appropriate records to the administrators of the OHS to obtain the indicated benefits.
5. Assessment of the value and role of computerization of epidemiologic data and of the extent to which this may supplement the data systems of other departments of the organization.
6. Participation in in-service education on the value of epidemiologic data, and the organization of adequate data collection systems.

XI. *Program of immunization*

A. *Objective.*

The immunization program objective is to prevent the acquisition by employees, in the domestic organization or abroad, of those communicable diseases that are preventable by the injection or ingestion of protective vaccines, sera, or other specific biologics.

B. *Elements of the program.*

1. Review of existing medical records to determine need.
2. Orientation of work groups regarding need.
3. Selection of work groups at greatest risk, such as field engineers, laboratory workers, exploration personnel.
4. Arrangement for space and time at work unit, when indicated, for administration of immunizing injections.
5. Transportation of personnel and supplies when injections are to be administered in the work area.
6. Administration of injections.
7. Entry of procedures in individual health records.
8. Establishment and maintenance of recall appointment file by means of computer printout.
9. Maintenance of clinical and statistical records of injections.
10. Provision of personal immunization records to all employees.

XII. *Program of occupational hygiene*

A. *Objective.*

The objective of the occupational (industrial) hygiene program is to prevent the acquisition by employees of occupational illnesses derived exclusively from work contacts with toxic materials or health-hazardous environments.

B. *Elements of the program.*

1. Conducting of surveys of worksites with potential occupational health hazards in the form of noxious chemical, physical, biologic, social, or emotional agents.
2. Measuring with precision instruments in the workroom area the level of toxic materials or the level of physical energies, such as noise or radiant energy.
3. Collecting samples of fume, dust, gas, vapor, or mist for laboratory analysis.
4. Detecting sociologic or psychological stresses impinging themselves on the workers, which they may interpret erroneously as secondary to contact with physical or chemical agents.
5. Comparing findings of air mensuration with threshold limit values for chemical substances, airborne contaminants, and physical agents to determine if a potentially hazardous situation exists.
6. Conducting of studies in ergonomics to alter the working environment and effect greater comfort or eliminate hazards for the employee.
7. Submitting of recommendations for the correction of hazardous exposures through the use of exhaust ventilation, dilution ventilation, improved housekeeping, substitution of toxic

materials with nonhazardous agents, isolation of the process generating the hazardous substances, or provision of personal protective devices.

8. Conducting subsequent inspections to determine compliance with the recommendations.
9. Submitting of work materials such as reagents, solvents, or additives for analysis to determine toxicity, with particular attention to their potential carcinogenesis, mutagenesis, or teratogenesis.
10. Conducting surveys regarding the safety of certain equipment procured through purchasing sources.
11. Determining the level of community air pollutants, which in certain areas may be inhaled by employees who are on duty where high levels of atmospheric contamination exist or where there is juxtaposition of a work area to an abandoned, leaking toxic waste dump site.
12. Obtaining of occupational histories in conjunction with the clinical survey of exposed personnel.
13. Operation of occupational (industrial) hygiene laboratory to meet needs of program elements listed above.

XIII. *Program of environmental health*

A. *Objective.*

The objective of the program in environmental health is to control those factors in the environment that may adversely affect the public health of the employed personnel, through the introduction and enforcement of sanitation in the areas of food and drink consumption, water supply, solid- and liquid-waste disposal, toxic-waste disposal, community air pollution, recreation facilities, and insect and rodent control.

B. *Elements of the program.*

1. Sanitary surveillance of foodstuffs, food preparation, food dispensing, food storage, including surveillance of ice manufacturing and distribution.
2. Sanitary evaluation of eating places, including cafeterias, special dining rooms, vending machine areas, bag-lunch rooms, and coffee preparation facilities.
3. Sanitary evaluation of company living quarters, if present, and surveillance of portable sanitary facilities if used at temporary remote work locations.
4. Surveillance of potable water, including all sources and points of use.
5. Evaluation of recreation and physical fitness facilities, including swimming pools.
6. Surveillance of change-room facilities with special attention to segregation of contaminated work clothing and clean street clothing.
7. Surveillance of systems of solid-waste management.
8. Surveillance of liquid-waste management, including liquid industrial wastes.
9. Participation in community air pollution control programs when effluents, if any, contaminate surrounding community.
10. Rabies control.
11. Control of rodents and insects.
12. Liaison with federal, state, and local health agencies.

XIV. *Program of occupational optometry*

A. *Objective.*

The objective of the program in occupational optometry is to conserve the vision of personnel, to prevent occupationally incurred injuries and illnesses of the eyes, and to detect, through screening measures, early evidence of constitutional disease.

B. *Elements of the program.*

1. *Conservation of vision.*
   a. Periodic updating of visual job analyses.
   b. Field screening of employees to determine present state of visual acuities.
   c. Conducting of refractions basic to the provision of protective corrective eyewear.
2. *Prevention of occupational injuries of the eyes.*
   a. Procurement, inventory, and issue of protective corrective eyewear.

b. Repair and maintenance of previously issued safety glasses.
c. Publicity of Wise Owl program.
d. Educational program in the prevention of eye injuries.

3. *Conducting of screening programs for the detection of constitutional disease as exemplified by hypertensive retinitis, diabetic retinitis, and glaucoma.*
4. *Conducting of counseling in association with screening programs for the teaching of vision conservation.*

XV. *Program of staff development*

A. *Objective.*

The objective of the staff development program is to maintain the highest level of professional skill in the disciplines that form the occupational health team and to refresh periodically the skills needed in the practice of these disciplines.

B. *Elements of the program.*

1. Provision and maintenance of a current library of the recognized monographic literature.
2. Provision and maintenance of a current library of the periodic literature in occupational health and related fields.
3. Conducting of periodic in-service training programs in all areas of occupational health practice, including emergency medical procedures such as cardiopulmonary resuscitation, field emergency care, and the like.
4. Provision of staff time to allow conducting of a journal club.
5. Provision of staff time to allow attendance at rounds conducted at community teaching hospitals.
6. Provision of staff time to allow library research and preparation and publication of articles for the professional literature.
7. Provision of field learning experience for students in affiliation from community colleges and universities in the fields of occupational and environmental health, occupational health nursing, social work, and rehabilitation.
8. Availability of funds to permit attendance at refresher seminars and conferences.

XVI. *Program of research*

A. *Objective.*

The objective of the research program is to establish a body of knowledge referable to the risks and diseases unique to the mission of the organization.

B. *Elements of the program.*

1. To establish cooperative teaching and research efforts with universities in the community, particularly those institutions where occupational safety and health educational resource centers may be based, or where teaching is conducted in the disciplines of occupational health.
2. Preparation and submission of applications for supportive research grants.
3. The provision of research opportunities and material for theses, dissertations, and publications for students in affiliation from colleges and universities in the community.
4. Establishment of an annotated data bank referable to environmental characteristics and health variables of the labor force.

ENTRY INTO MANAGED OPERATIONS

To the physician new to the world of large organizations, the complexities of the industrial society initially may seem incomprehensible and baffling. Although all practitioners of medicine have had associations with universities, hospitals, and in some instances, the armed services, they rarely have shared in the administration of a business institution. In most instances their functions have related to professional medical activities. They may have had some contact with the scheme of management of an organization as members of an advisory committee or board of directors of a community agency. Although proximity to administrators, in the main, has been narrow, with entry into occupational health, physicians find themselves for the first time in the dual position of staff and line officers—"staff" to their immediate superiors, and "line" to their own work group members.

SITING OF OCCUPATIONAL HEALTH PROGRAMS

Although some in-plant medical services were offered employees in the nineteenth century at locations where care was not readily available, the greatest impetus to the establishment of occupational health programs came with the passage of workers' compensation legislation beginning in 1911. Apart from legal obligation as a motivation for the creation of health services, there has been a movement of welfare work in industry that dates as far back as manorial days. Initially seen as philanthropy, these activities began to coalesce, so that various employment arrangements guaranteeing security to masters of handicraft, as well as to their journeymen and apprentices, appeared in medieval industry [5].

About two centuries ago, Robert Owen initiated experiments in employee welfare during the early days of modern industry. In-plant care has emerged from these multiple sources, so that today one finds programs in a broad variety of institutions, many of which are related only by the common thread of the daily reporting of groups of employees to the worksite, to assist in the completion of the organization's established mission.

The parent body that is the "company," a term to be used generically, may take many forms. Occupational health services will be found, in one format or another, in such private sector employment sites as communications, educational institutions, construction, finance, hospitals, power production and distribution, publishing, transportation, and wholesale and retail sales, among many others.

Similarly, in the public sector, OHPs will be encountered at all levels of government, from the federal to the municipal. A variety of functions will be executed by government agencies, many comparable to activities within the private sector, with others unique to the public arena. The recipients of occupational health services in governmental settings will be engaged in such activities or installations as administration, airport operation, animal control, forestry services, jails, museums, protective services, road maintenance, wildlife preserves, and zoos, many of these functions not seeing replication in private business.

The extent of the service provided, the number of health care personnel employed, and the type of program offered—in-plant, out-of-plant, consultations by a physician in absentia—will vary among the kinds of enterprises listed. For example, an aircraft assembly plant may have a full OHS with a large health staff, while a professional football team may have only an orthopedic consultant who will attend all games, conduct the examinations, and perform the surgery indicated in the injuries sustained by the players.

Howe [6] conducted a census of companies retaining physicians who were members of the then Industrial Medical Association, now the AOMA. While not all physicians providing occupational health services were members, the results gave a partial indication of the loci of health programs. Irrespective of the numbers involved, occupational physicians were encountered in nearly every kind of enterprise in both the public and private segments of social organizations. The point being emphasized is that the sites for OHPs are highly diverse, and reasons for the presence of such supportive health services may be equally varied, if at all definable.

INDUSTRIAL MANAGEMENT AND MEDICINE

The former Council on Occupational Health of the American Medical Association has published several reports in which it has attempted to introduce business managers and physicians to the ways of each other. Many industrial executives are familiar with the practice of medicine only in their personal role as patients, and even if their undergraduate or graduate majors were business management, extremely little would have been inserted into the curriculum relating to the place of medicine in corporate administration. Much of what is to follow will be drawn from the former council's valuable publications.

The physician, individualistic and only a team member intermittently, will appreciate the usual pyramidal managerial structure but initially may find his or her staff role frustrating, as well as the usual custom of having to follow the vertical courses of communication. The council has delineated well some of the basic concepts of organization [7]:

Organization is the grouping of activities necessary to obtain enterprise objectives, with the assignment of each grouping to an executive having the authority necessary to manage those activities.

Organization involves establishment of authority relationships with provision for coordination among them, both vertically and horizontally, in the enterprise structure. Each part of an organization should be judged in light of how well it contributes to the objective of the enterprise.

Organization planning is the process of logically grouping activities, delineating authority and responsibility, and establishing working relationships that will enable both the company and the employee to realize their mutual objectives. Responsibility should always be coupled with corresponding authority.

Organization is efficient if it meets its objectives with minimum unfavorable consequences or unnecessary costs—all costs, not merely such measurable items as dollars or man-hours.

All organizations have *line* and *staff* functions, personnel, and units, and the entire medical activity operates in a *staff* role. The line-staff concept is traditional in the armed forces, and the designation "line officer" further substantiates the concept. The council has differentiated the two in the following manner [7]:

Line (*operating*)	*Staff* (*service*)
Information passes downward in the "chain of command"	Information tends to pass upward in the "chain of command"
Authority to command	Authority of "ideas"
Makes decisions and issues instructions	Advises, does not command
Tells	Sells
Acts	Thinks
Instructs	Recommends

The two functions have been defined also as follows: *Line* connotes the work, functions, or organizational components that are accountable for fulfilling the economic objectives of the organization, while *staff* implies the work, functions, or organizational elements required to supply information and services to the line segments [8].

The physician, in a *staff* function, has authority to command,* make decisions, or issue instructions only within his or her own service, as do section heads or supervisors in relationship to their subordinate personnel.

Companies differ in the designations of the groupings within the structure. A *department,* or its equivalent tag such as *division,* is that distinct unit over which a manager has authority for the performance of specified activities [7]. In many organizations, the primary subdivision is a department or, in some, a directorate, such as comptroller, manufacturing, engineering, international, or public relations. The next level, within a department, frequently is the division; for example, within an industrial relations department, there may be the labor relations, insurance, employee relations, safety, or personnel divisions. Further bifurcation, upward or downward, may utilize such designations as system, bureau, service(s), section, branch, or unit.

The pattern of reporting to top management is of considerable significance to the physician who serves an enterprise, and the larger the company, the more important is the physician's position in the managerial stratification. Many surveys have been conducted [9–13], and a slim majority of the findings points to the placement of the medical activity in the industrial relations department, which is frequently headed by a vice-president.

The OHS might be a part of the personnel division, a functioning segment of the industrial relations department, and if so, might be placed on the same level as the safety section. In other configurations, it might be placed equally with the personnel division. In rare instances, the medical director is in the same echelon as the industrial relations director, particularly if the physician is a vice-president. Although this does exist in a few extremely large corporations, it cannot be considered usual.

In more recent years, with greater attention being given the "environment," the vice-presidential title has been used more frequently. In one large manufacturing organization, the physician is designated Vice-President—Health and Environment and reports upward to the one executive vice-president, as do those officers holding other portfolios, such as personnel, engineering, and purchasing, among others. He has a five-point control base, with the managers for medical programs, environmental health services, workers' compensation, psychiatric services, and resource recovery in reporting positions. At the next level of management within the health and environmental pyramid is the manager of safety.

A second multi-interest, multinational corporation has a physician vice-president as Director of Medical Relations and another physician as vice-president who is Director of Health Affairs, the latter reporting to the former. Although a recent change altered its structure, a mammoth corporation had its chief physician serving under the title Vice-President, Health Services, who reported to an Administrative Vice-President, whose superior was an Executive Vice-President for Personnel Services, directly under the President. A more recent change, which effected certain organizational shifts, shows the medical chief as Vice-President, Personnel and Health Services, re-

*The term is a harsh one; in practice one frequently "requests" or "asks." There even has been occasional discomfiture experienced with the use of the age-old "physician's orders."

porting to an Administrative Vice-President, Labor Relations, Personnel, and Health Services. It is conjectural if this particular format will endure.

Some organizations have given the medical director responsibility for both health and safety, and occasionally, when there are indications for a unit in radiation health or safety, the physician will head all three activities. Periodically, one encounters the placement of the physician in a unit reporting to the safety director. This may be found in older companies where the development of an accident prevention activity antedated the addition of a medical program or where the physician visits the plant for part of a day or for a few mornings each week.

The desirable line of reporting for medical directors (or consultants as they may be called, especially if they execute an out-of-plant medical program) is directly to top management. If the reporting is to the president, it is ideal. The second choice is the chief executive officer, if that person is the executive vice-president or plant manager. Such a scheme is not designed as a matter of prestige, power, or vanity. It is strictly one of practical efficiency in accomplishing the missions of the medical department. The greater number of persons through whom one must report or seek action, the greater the delay in accomplishment. The lower the position of the physician, the less is the capacity of the next administrative echelon to act. As policies are made at the top, time is lost in transmitting a medical communication or request. Furthermore, for one reason or another, one of the managers in the "layering" might have a negative, prejudicial, or even religious feeling against the health service and delay decision-making in a medical matter or stop the communication at that level. With each additional waypoint, there are needs for interpretation, explanation, reasoning, and justification; while this process goes on, valuable time that could be devoted to medical action is unnecessarily sacrificed. The closer to the top executive the physician is on the organizational ladder, the more expeditiously will medical programs move forward with the manager's support.

In one of the studies cited [9], the issue of reporting levels was displayed in telling fashion: of companies reviewed, 14.3 percent (11) had no higher level; 48.0 percent (37) reported one level above; 24.7 percent (19) indicated two levels; 7.8 percent (6) showed three levels; and 5.2 percent (4) told of four reporting levels.

With no levels intervening, the medical director enjoys immediate interchange with the president of the company, can construct a philosophy for the executive to adopt and expound or espouse, and is able to obtain direct support for a proposal when comprehension is the significant variable and there are funding and personnel available for the issue. When the upward gap widens, the health service head may encounter disinterest or actual lack of knowledge. In some instances, a proposal sent through the layers may be halted because it is antithetic to the individual work goals or ambitions of the person heading the next higher echelon, may be contrary to personal beliefs, or may demand greater temerity in forwarding and explanation than possessed by the intervening superordinate person. Often, a medical matter can be given a more adequate representation to top management by a physician, particularly if the issue requires technical information or if the subject encroaches on areas of high human sensitivity.

One point polar to these arguments must be presented. It has been stated to the author by a medical director who reports directly to the company president that although he enjoys the directness and proximity of the relationship, the president is away from headquarters so much of the time that often decisions must be delayed for undue lengths of time.

In substance, the more direct the reporting interchange in the span of management, the more accurate and more feeling will be the presentation of need, and the more comprehending, authoritative, and prompt will be the responsive action.

ETHICS

The placement of the medical director and the OHS within managerial ranks provides signals to the labor organizations of a plant that the health activity operates exclusively as a protective device of the company. Such an argument frequently is verbalized with the accompanying question of "Well, who pays the doctor's salary?" Strangely, the inquirer loses sight of the irrefutable fact that the employee's salary comes from identically the same source.

Practice in the past, prior to the writing of occupational safety and health legislation, often saw a single stance adopted by the health director—right or wrong, the company was always right, and specious arguments would be devised, in concert with corporate counsel, to support such a position. A physician of this ilk could rightly be accused of unilateral loyalty. Forgotten, however, was the real role of the medical director, that of advisor to managers on all matters pertaining to the health of employees. The physician, or the professional staff representative, has been engaged to serve the occupational health needs of the enterprise, and it is the physician's responsibility to identify areas of deficit within that disciplinary and organizational jurisdiction. Further, it is the physician's task to direct attention to these deficiencies and make recommendations for resolution or correction.

If the lack in the cited issue is that of management or supervision, the medical director must seek correction through channels appropriate for such action. If there is a break in the use of personal protective devices or in the application of exhaust ventilatory equipment because a union official has indicated noncompliance, it is the duty of the medical director to bring remedial processes into play, this time involving union leadership through the accepted communication chain. The director's loyalty is primarily to the health of the worker and the principles of occupational medicine and not to one embattled side or another, or to one adversary or another. Frequently, this ethical position is not understood by either managerial or trade union personnel. The climate that results is one in which managers feel that physicians (or their programs) are totally union-oriented, while the labor organizations believe them to be completely dedicated to the company. It is difficult for either side to understand the impartial position of the physician, irrespective of the clarification given to both contesting parties.

Enmeshed in this situation is the expectation by managers that, because the medical director is "one of them," some or all clinical information involving certain employees will be shared, irrespective of its obviously confidential content. It is difficult for certain department heads to accept refusals to share medical information because they believe that any information obtained on a worker should be placed in the public domain. One has to personalize the issue before the pressure is released. The author has many times asked, in a rather banal manner, "If you had high blood pressure, quadruple syphilis, and galloping gonorrhea, how many people here at the plant would you want me to tell?" Usually, little discussion follows.

The solution for this frequently arising dilemmatic situation is to familiarize all personnel with whom one has contact that one will offer an opinion completely reflective of a thorough study of all facets of a problem and of the conclusion derived from such a thoughtful review. Some opinions and recommendations will favor the employer, some the worker. This variation will persist if there is honesty at all times. If the physician is persuaded once to shade his conclusion, or to reverse a decision without scientific or experiential support to warrant such a change, then he or she may expect innumerable requests in the future to yield to such requests. When one's position is established initially and clearly of calling things exactly as one sees them, then one will not be approached again to offer a favoring, but unfounded, opinion.

RELATIONSHIP WITH ORGANIZED LABOR

In keeping with their nonpartisan positions, physicians must establish equal relationships with both labor and management. Although it may seem difficult at first to be the impartial professional counselor to both groups, one can attain this role and maintain it, provided one is honest, is consistent, and retains confidentiality.

The author had a fascinating experience in this area when he became director of an unimpressive OHS in heavy industry with the objective of building it into a strong, effective department. The first week on the scene, a meeting was requested, through the industrial relations office, with the presidents of the three unions—two were unions, and the third was a trades council representing a dozen craft locals.

For 1½ hours, one listened to all of the complaints regarding the past and all of the solicited ideas for the configuration of the program to be developed. Pages of notes were taken. This session was followed by a period of 3 months, during which time the new medical director was tested. The council referred many of its members with unresolved medical and placement problems, and at the end of that period, the referrals stopped abruptly except for a continuing few. The opinions offered, the recommendations made, and the actions taken were consistent and in parallel with the philosophy expressed at the meeting—the cases would be judged on sound conclusions derived from valid clinical and work data. Although one was unaware at the time of being tested, the cessation in the flow of referrals soon illuminated the game that was being played.

From this initial contact stemmed the designation of one council agent as the medical liaison with the OHS. Through many daily telephone calls and weekly or more frequent conferences, problems were solved and impasses eliminated. As a measure of the success of the system, one can recast the situation numerically. Prior to the new program, there were regularly two grievances filed per month based on medical actions or lack of action. Subsequent to the appointment of the union representative, there were no medically caused grievances in a 4-year period.

Consonant with this ongoing working relationship with the unions was the monthly meeting of an occupational health advisory committee, with representatives of all levels of management and labor and various employee groups. A forum of this kind permitted an interpretation of expressed needs and the early apprisal, particularly of the union leaders, of the medical programs being planned. There were several "meet and confer" sessions with union officials prior to institution of the programs, so that they would be fully knowledgeable in advance of any change and would be supportive when queried by the rank and file.

Although this program has been described in some detail elsewhere [14], suffice it to say that good relationships with both managers and labor unions can be kept in equilibrium provided one does not take union opinions for granted, one keeps the officials informed of changes being contemplated, and one remembers that union officials are as important to their constituents as physicians are to their clientele.

The position of the medical director is often described as "neutral," meaning that he or she does not side with one group or the other. But there cannot be neutrality, for that implies the absence of an opinion. Conclusions must be formulated and recommendations forwarded, fall where they may. One cannot be neutral when numerous issues await definitive action.

DEPARTMENTAL ORGANIZATION

Within each OHS, there is an organizational pattern in which the functions, span of control, and reporting lines are indicated. The design of a medical department staff deployment will differ from one company to another and will change over time. Figures 4-1, 4-2, 4-3, and 4-4 show the organizational configurations for four large corporations, as examples. These charts, like similar depictions from other companies, should be considered as being in dynamic, rather than fixed, modes.

PROGRAM FORMAT

The dimensions of an OHP are determined in several ways. Without a background of experience, managers may designate a specific budget that the physician is to use in the manner that the physician believes most productive of employee health. The physician will determine the services in greatest need, and the personnel equipment, supplies, and outside consultative assistance required for program support, and apportion the funds appropriately.

If a company has been informed bluntly by its workers' compensation insurance carrier that its losses are too high owing to numerous serious accidental injuries, the single objective established for the OHP could be the reduction of these costly occurrences. Such a move will imply emphasis on accident prevention, a greater degree of early and continuing in-plant care for trauma, and a minimum of concern with general health promotion.

Frequently an employer expects the medical costs to be expressed as a certain number of dollars spent per employee per year, and a sum will be made available based on the number of workers in a company.

There might be certain contractual arrangements (such as those involved in defense or wartime production) that permit considerable sums to be expended for industrial relations on a cost-plus basis, and managers will utilize this means to polish up its corporate image, and an enriched medical program will result.

Or it might be that extraordinarily dangerous materials or processes are being used or developed, and there will be legal requirements to be met in the form of highly sophisticated in-plant medical surveillance, as in the case of asbestos fabrication or installation [15], work with a hepatotoxic agent, or an operation hazardous to the reproductive system. On the same planking, a trade union may demand increased protective measures in the form of good medical facilities. Other reasons play significant roles in determining the scope of a program, not the least of which might be the president's or manager's personal emotional involvement with medicine, a specific disease, or a memory of alleged medical negligence.* In one program with which the author has had close identification, it was the surfacing social concern of a thoughtful personnel director that led to the creation of a fully facetted program in occupational health.

On occasion, one might endeavor to learn of the rationale for the initiation of an in-plant activity. In a great number of instances, contemporary medical staff members are unfamiliar with the beginnings of their own departments, and no company archives can be located that might contain significant board minutes of managerial decisions that brought about medical programming. Apart from the time of American industry's adolescent years, such as those of the Lowell mills of Massachusetts [16] when operators allegedly were concerned with worker welfare, few programs were begun because of altruistic motivations.

As indicated previously, most programs resulted from enactment of workers' compensation laws in

*This point is exemplified by the late President Kennedy's interest in mental retardation and the reflection of this interest in both increased research appropriations and intensified research activity.

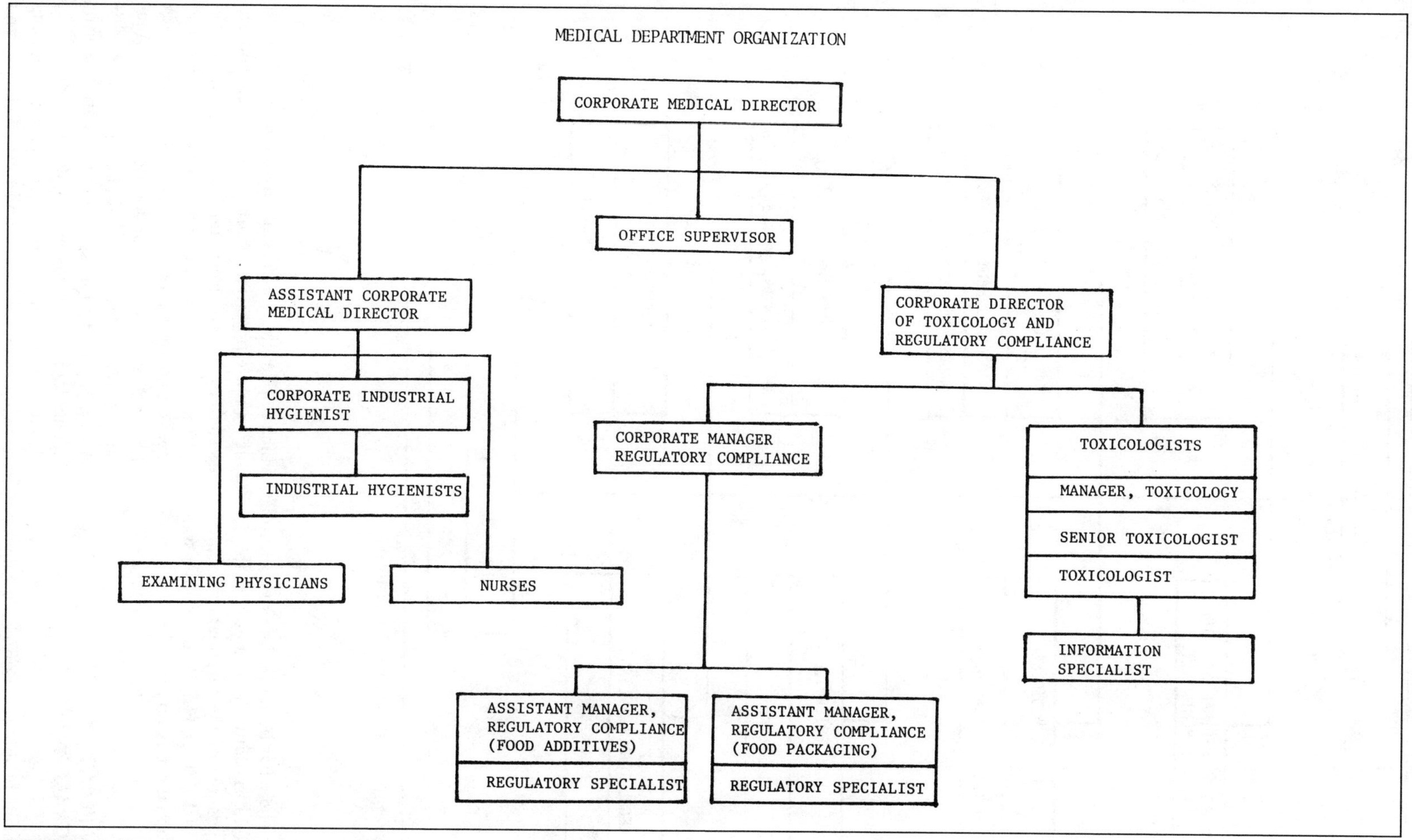

FIGURE 4-1. *Organizational structure of Medical Department I.*

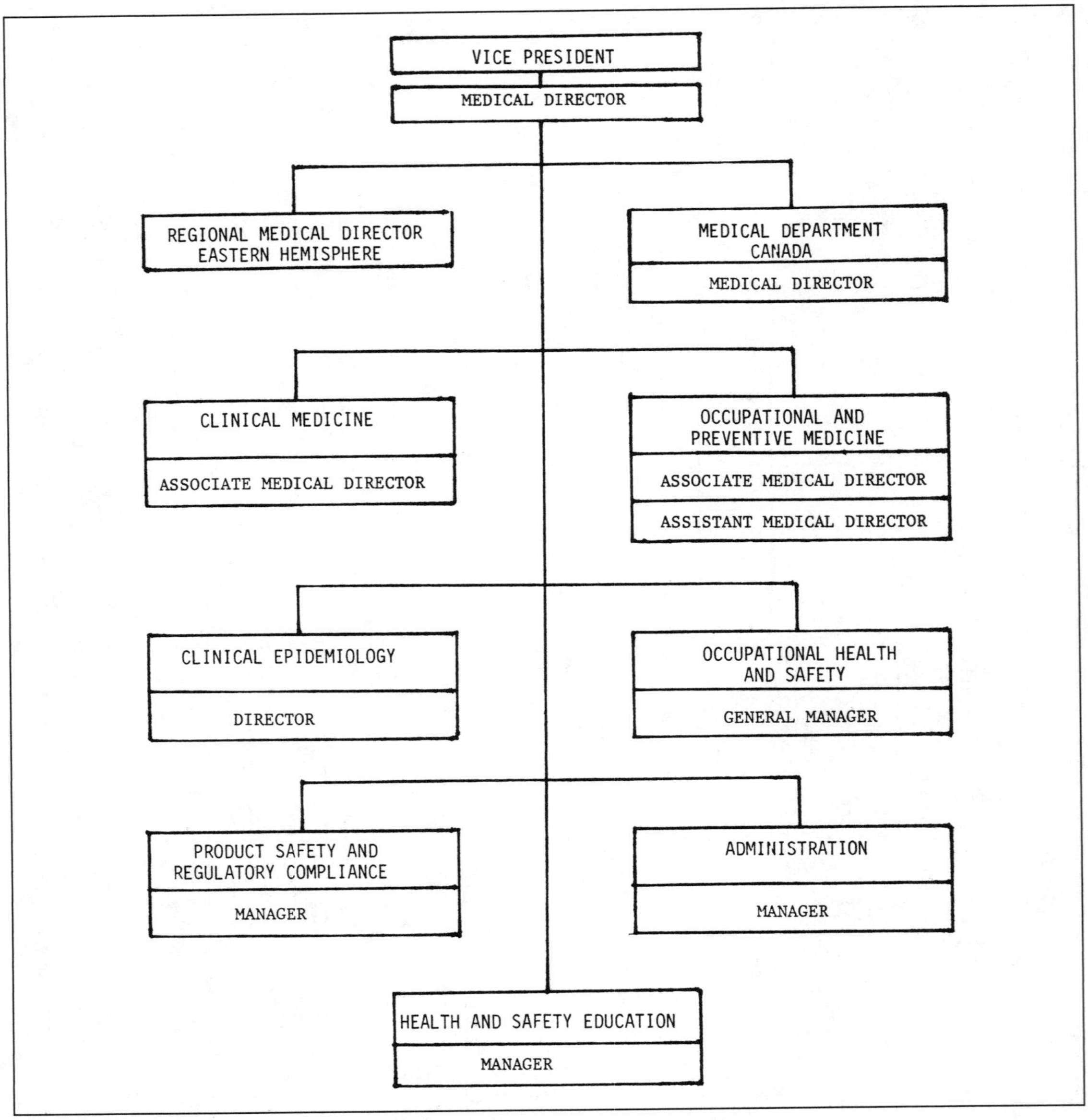

FIGURE 4-2. *Organizational structure of Medical and Health Resources Division.*

the early 1900s. There has been evidence of a second surge in response to legislative mandates with the development and passage of the Occupational Safety and Health Act of 1970 (OSHA 1970) and the state plans in occupational safety and health.

COMPLETE IN-PLANT HEALTH PROGRAM

A complete in-plant health program is the fully developed multiservice program in occupational health, which implies the presence of physicians at all times. One or more physicians staff a department and are assisted by occupational nurses, occupational hygienists, medical or radiology technicians, medical records administrators, clerks, and if required, such additional persons as psychologists, health information specialists, health physicists, ophthalmic dispensers, physiotherapists, sanitarians, statisticians or epidemiologists, and custodians, among others.

Such a service may provide occupational nursing coverage during odd shifts and over weekends, and may have smaller satellite facilities (fixed or trans-

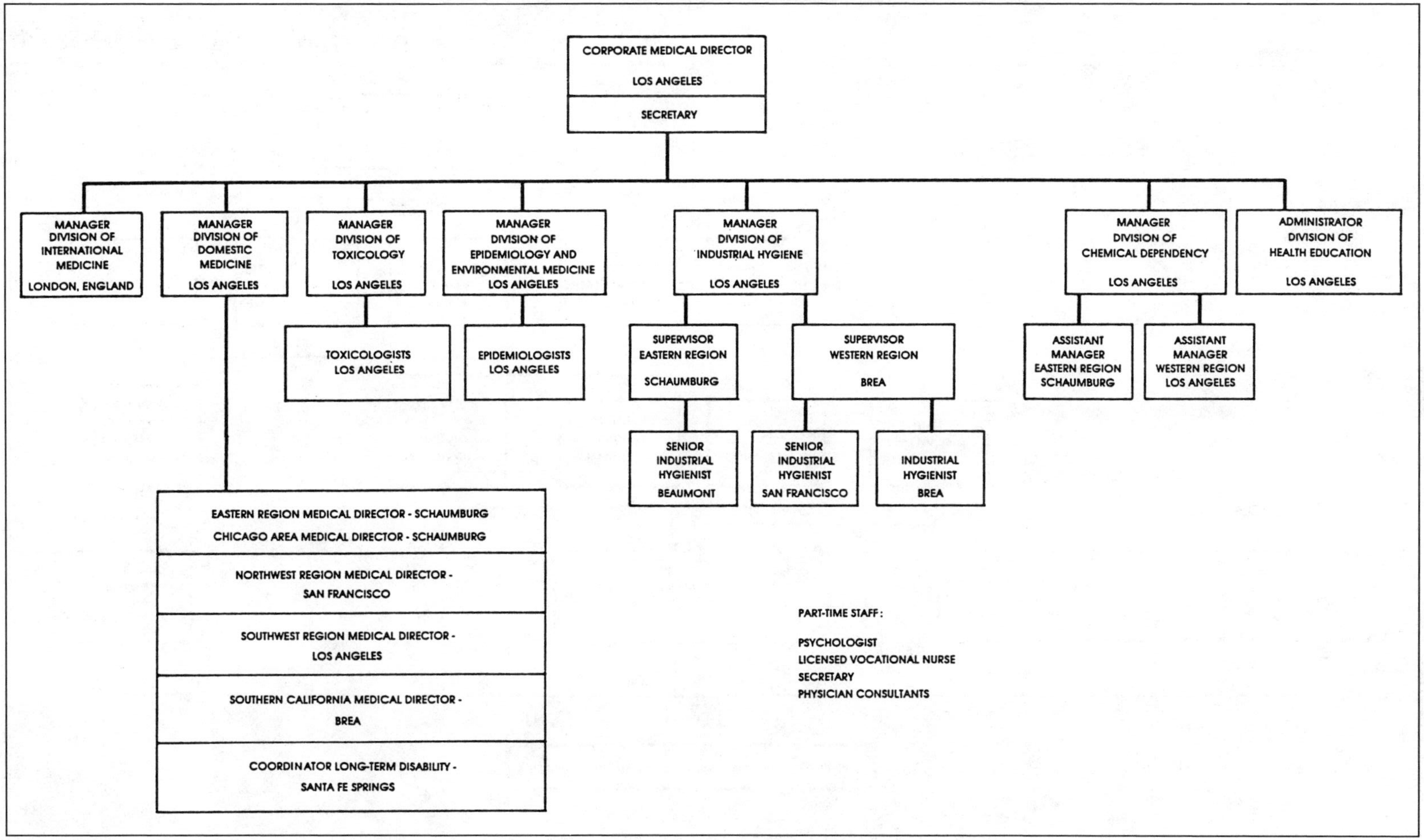

FIGURE 4-3. *Organizational structure of Medical Department II.*

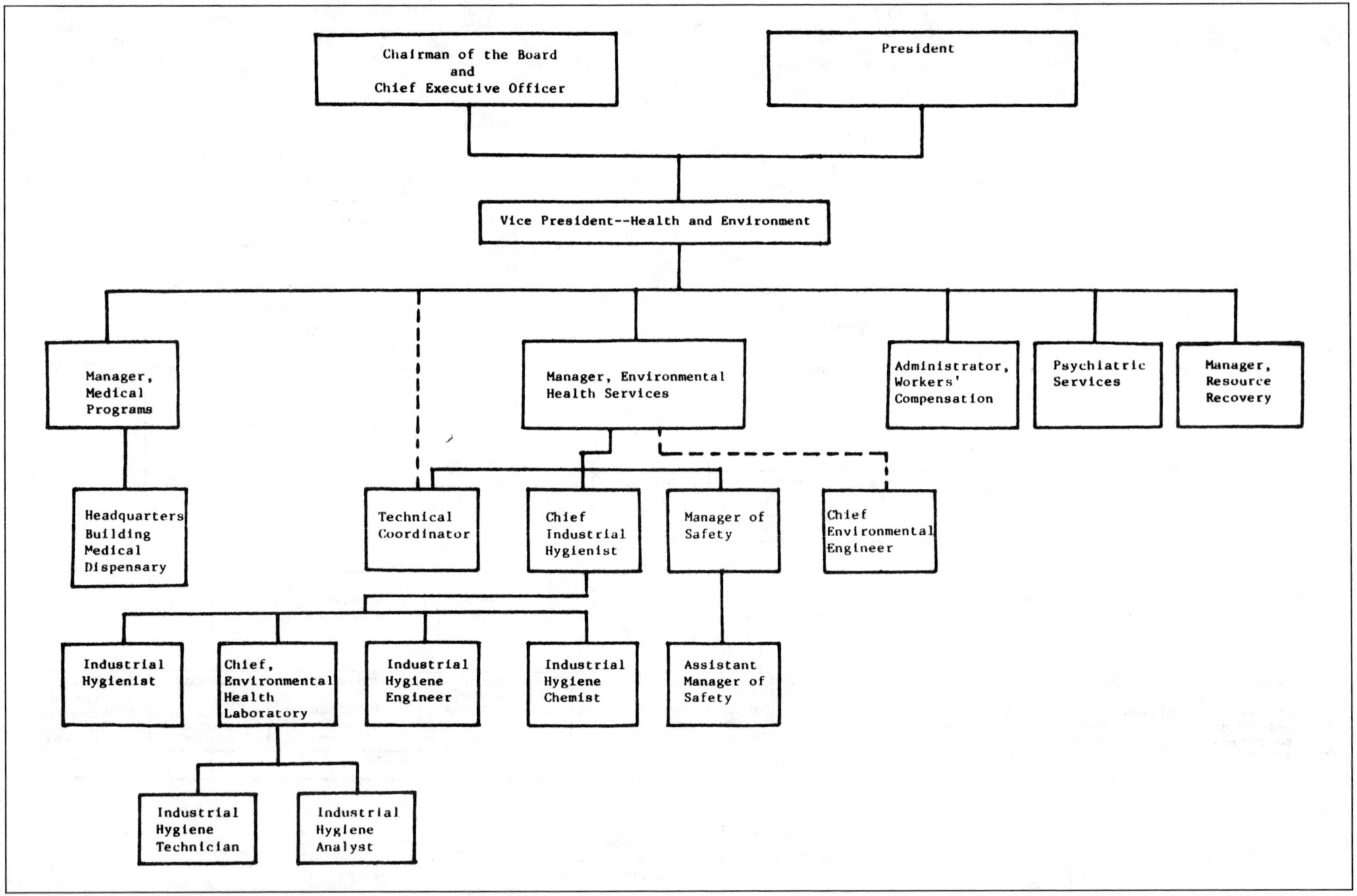

FIGURE 4-4. *Organizational structure of Health and Environment (department).*

portable) peripheral to the main medical department, and may operate a mobile unit for distant work groups* [17]. If the company manufactures chemicals, it may have a toxicology laboratory as part of its medical facility† [18].

A complete in-plant program usually has its policies and procedures collected in an operating manual, which will include guiding principles for occupational nurses (see Chapters 13 and 15) [19].

CENTRAL FACILITY

A company that occupies a large area with numerous buildings or other work facilities covering many acres, or several square miles, may have its primary health installation close to the central administrative offices or in that area of the plant nearest the greatest number of employees. It is most convenient for the examination of job applicants if the OHS is adjacent to the personnel activity. The medical examination can be conducted at a location close to the site of the employment interview and the completion of the application and written examination, if one is given. Organizations involved with sensitive research and development or with contracts requiring security clearance of workers will find this adjacency of functions extremely convenient. If industrial espionage is of concern, the juxtaposition of all employment processes to the entrance, and outside the restricted areas of the plant, will be desired.

In companies that have less security restriction, the medical department may be in its own building or in part of a large manufacturing structure that houses many of the employees. Although visitors may be admitted to a central location, escort personnel frequently may be required, particularly if hazardous production processes or equipment might be encountered en route. Further, in certain plants, the time-consuming issue of protective eyewear or hard hats may be required for applicants. The various elements regarding location will be discussed later.

In the main facility, there will be centralized capabilities in administration, medicine, nursing, medical records, radiology, clinical pathology, environmental health, health education, epidemiology and statistics, and possibly a cardiopulmonary exercise test facility. Special features such as multiphasic testing stations, ophthalmic dispensing, and an executive health examination suite may also be based here.

*This format is seen in the large mobile units operated by the major petroleum companies.

†The Eastman Kodak Company, Dow Chemical Company, and the E.I. duPont deNemours Company have such facilities.

SATELLITE FACILITIES

When employees or worksites are dispersed over a large area, with many members of the labor force at a considerable distance from the main occupational health installation, it is advisable to establish satellites or branches of the main OHS. Ordinarily, these units are staffed by occupational nurses or occupational nurse practitioners who function under medical directives prepared jointly with the medical director and signed by him or her. In some instances, physician's assistants or emergency medical technicians may be found in such work locations.

The indications for a satellite should be explored in light of the size of the population to be served, the distance from the central facility, transport availability, the type and extent of physical and health hazards, and even certain demographic variables, such as the percentage of women or the age of the employees. A workforce of 400 employees can utilize a one-nurse satellite provided a good rapport exists between the professional person and the clientele, the nurse is willing to tour the work area periodically, service is rendered promptly, and the nurse is skilled in counseling. An aloof nurse concerned solely with the care for trauma would be idle with a work group triple the size suggested.

A system of record interchange and the retention of an auxiliary set in the satellite obviate difficulties in the maintenance of sequentially recorded observations.

An occupational nurse in the satellite setting can provide emergency care, offer individual health counseling, group health education, and certain screening procedures, and conduct physical examinations, if prepared as an occupational nurse practitioner. The nurse may, in addition, refer employees to their own sources of health care in the community or to specialized agencies.

DEPARTMENTAL LIAISON NURSES

A concept developed by the OHS of the Personnel Department, County of Los Angeles, has been that of the liaison nurse. The particular population served and the structure of the county workforce lent themselves to a new need-response in occupational health. At the time, there were nearly 70 departments, districts, and separate administrative units composing the government of the county, with over 70,000 employees scattered throughout a 4,000-square-mile area. It was not possible to reach all employees, so the idea of a liaison nurse for a single department was conceived to provide a service to a group particularly in need of health care guidance.

The first department selected was that of Building Services, with a staff of nearly 1,700 custodians, working in innumerable county buildings, all at a low wage level, and with large families, most coming from a background of extremely limited health care.

A senior occupational nurse was assigned to serve as health ombudsman for the department and was given office space in both the department and in the OHS. In the period of trial, she visited nearly all of the primary worksites, met with both supervisors and employees, initiated immunization programs, reviewed the cases of undue absenteeism, referred many workers either to the OHS or to community sources of care, and conducted courses in first aid. Although no formal evaluation accompanied the effort, many employees were brought to sources of health service, and better health behavior was detected in many of the department's staff. An assignment of this type allowed an OHS representative to have a specific knowledge of a group's health needs, and in a large organization this format is worthy of trial.

MOBILE UNITS

There are specific indications for the use of mobile units in the provision of occupational health services. Employee groups may be too small for the assignment of personnel to a fixed facility. Workers may have job assignments over a large area, and their needs could be met best by a professional who could "circuit ride" the company's installations. If there are budgetary constraints, it might be best to establish a facility in a transportable building rather than construct a permanent unit.

When so-called demountables are used, they can be moved readily from one site to another as the numbers of workers change, or as work missions are completed and employees are moved to other locations.

An early experience of the author consisted of providing service to the many army-operated piers on the San Francisco waterfront during World War II. No single pier had sufficient employees to warrant a full-time occupational nurse, so a mobile unit was developed that made rounds, putting in at selected piers twice daily and at regularly scheduled times. The unit was replenished early each morning at the main medical facility at the San Francisco Port of Embarkation.

Mobile units or trailers may be used for long periods of time, for they are readily adapted and equipped for OHS use. Removal of adjacent side walls permits the joining of two or more such units. Their utilization by space-hungry universities and overcrowded hospitals testifies to the worth of such structures.

In essence, their employment should be considered when work projects are of short duration, budgets preclude costlier permanent installations, immediate facilities or services are required, workers are of insufficient number to justify full-time, on-site health care, or worksites are located over large expanses of land. To be remembered is the fact that mobile units can be truly mobile and can constantly be involved in a visitation service, or they can be impermanently fixed for the duration of need, subject to removal as indicated. Mobile facilities in the form of a tractor and semitrailer are utilized in multiphasic test programs and will be discussed later.

PARTIAL IN-PLANT HEALTH PROGRAM

Although a partial in-plant health program may be in operation for a full workshift, a physician will be in attendance for only a portion of the day. The time will be divided between private practice and the occupational medical practice, which is carried on at the plant medical department. In the physician's absence, the occupational nurse will be in charge of the OHS or the satellites, and other persons in the department will function in accordance with written, guiding principles. When there is only a partial program, there will rarely be additional personnel beyond other nurses or a clerk. Although first-aid attendants are to be found in many companies in the United States and elsewhere and such positions are described in some of the governmental personnel classification systems, their employment is not recommended, for there is no organized system of training, examination, registration, or licensing as there is, for example, with physician's assistants. The addition of these workers as full-time members of an occupational medical program bespeaks either ignorance on the part of management or the persistence of a practice long rendered obsolete by the contemporary availability of skilled professional personnel for program assignments.

The most recent development in the training of ancillary personnel has been that of the physician's assistant. Allied health workers of this classification, like licensed vocational (practical) nurses, are coming into occupational health and, one day, may provide serious numerical competition to the occupational nurse unless additional curricula continue to be established in occupational nursing in the Occupational Safety and Health Educational Resource Centers (ERCs) and opportunities for continuing education are made available at those centers.

No accurate data exist as to the exact number of physicians who serve industry on a part-time basis. When practitioners are employed for a span of time each morning, they may be engaged fully in performing preplacement medical examinations, in providing emergency medical care, or in both types of services. On occasion they may offer health counseling to workers and are consultatively helpful to the occupational nurse. A partial service of this nature has many limitations. Most often, the physician is young, has had no training in occupational medicine, and is just beginning to practice, so that the relationship with the company will be of short duration—until the practice is self-sustaining.* Or, at the spectrum's other end, the physician may be retired and may not be especially innovative in the ideas he or she brings to the organization.

Irrespective of age, there remains the truism that part-time physicians are only part-time interested and see their task solely as one of income supplementation. Rarely do they visit the work areas to learn the processes of manufacturing or to observe the employees at work. Their knowledge of the work environment is restricted. On one occasion, the author was on a tour of a plant with a group of students, the tour ending in the plant OHS. A leading question was presented regarding the level of noise exposure of a certain high-decibel operation. The part-time physician knew nothing of the process, and the full explanation had to be provided by the personnel manager who, fortunately, was keenly knowing of the problem.

In one plant in a small community, distinctly the opposite was seen with a partial program. A physician, whose office was but three blocks distant, visited the company three half-mornings each week. On the third day, he spent the full 2 hours walking about the work areas, studying the assembly lines, talking with employees, and following up on patients. A company with insightful managerial personnel will see the wisdom of such a schedule.

The other disadvantage lies in the discrepant schedules of the physician and the nurse. The physician is the visitor, the outsider, not "one of us," as is the nurse who is full-time and known to all personnel. The nurse becomes the true counselor, which is entirely to the worker's benefit; however, such a situation lessens the value of the physician's visits, for the employees will not come in so readily for consultation. The physician's hours are fewer and usually are more crowded, so that the worker is more hesitant in seeking opportunity for counsel or listening.

The partial program conducted by an occupational health nurse makes an invaluable contribution to employee health, and this issue will be discussed further in Chapter 15.

OUT-OF-PLANT MEDICAL PROGRAM

Implicit in the classification of an out-of-plant medical program is the program executed almost exclusively in the offices of private physicians who serve in a consultative capacity to an organization. Rarely do they visit the company for which there is this responsibility, for prospective employees are referred out for physical appraisal, as are workers who have been injured. This type of program is strictly expediential.

It is conducted as "occupational medicine" when, in actuality, it is one of traumatic surgery and rather perfunctorily performed medical examinations—with little knowledge of the work environment or of the job demands built into the examination or treatment situation. For intelligent medical guidance to management, the physicians must visit the plant's operating area so that the examination and treatment procedures can be carried out with logical goals and objectives.

Another disadvantage lies in a relationship of this type; reports that are generated by the physician are usually sent to the industrial relations or personnel managers, who are lay persons and may misinterpret recommendations made in good faith. Further, confidentiality is broken in this scheme of communication, a factor that may tend to provide certain constraints in the physician's reporting system. Whereas the outside consultant always plans to visit the plant to review certain case records for which they have consultative responsibility, rarely do these physicians go on site.

CONTRACT HEALTH PROGRAM

With the birth of the space age, new methods of providing "housekeeping" services to the research, assembly, or launching bases were devised. Companies in diverse fields would bid on packages of services for the space program, one of the services included for bid being an employee health program. If a company were successful in obtaining the bid, an OHP would be established much as if the parent organization were to open a plant and provide on-site ser-

*This situation is undergoing some modification as instruction in occupational medicine is introduced into the residency programs in family medicine and as a position paper of the American College of Physicians (Recommended Core Curriculum Guidelines in Occupational Medicine for Family Practice Residences) attains greater distribution.

vices for a new labor force. The program personnel would relate to counterparts at the company's corporate level and also to counterparts in the headquarters of the National Aeronautics and Space Administration.

The programs were sound, staffed by experienced or trained professionals, but were in constant jeopardy of change. Periodically, toward the close of a certain contract-covered time span, bids would be resought, and it was entirely likely that a second company would be successful in obtaining the bid, so that staff changes would be made. Further, with the deceleration of the space effort, medical support groups were lessening greatly in size. In a sense, the situation was not dissimilar to that of the war production plants of 1941 to 1945; the programs were intense, but of short duration, although many persisted with the return to peacetime production. Greatly affected were the medical services of the supporting companies that developed and produced various systems for the space program. As aerospace engineers were reduced in force at the end of the 1960s, so were medical staffs. The success or failure of these contract methods of delivering occupational health care is yet to be evaluated by the practitioners involved or by the participant companies [20]. It is believed that possibly as a result of the continuing impact of OSHA 1970, this form of practice might once again be on the rise.

A second form of in-plant programming to appear in the same period and remain in the early 1970s is one utilized by medium-sized companies. Rather than employing its own health staff, purchasing equipment, and the like, an organization will contract for full services with a medical corporation, which will provide the staff, obtain equipment, maintain records, bring in supplies, handle payroll, and conduct all the supportive services normally cared for by the client company. Little has been published regarding the quality of such a contract program, and as before, neither of the participants (provider or consumer) has as yet evaluated the services provided, nor have good cost-benefit analyses, or even cost analyses, been developed [21].

It is believed that a different esprit must exist in such a setting, for the health team could readily be viewed as an outsider group, bearing no enduring relationship to the employees.

PROGRAMS FOR SMALL PLANTS

Traditional in the writings on occupational health has been the term *small plant*. To the purist, a "plant" most likely connotes a factory.* The Council on Occupational Health of the American Medical Association, in its *Guide to Developing Small Plant Occupational Health Programs* [22], used the designation *plant* to mean any industrial, business, or commercial establishment, which may be independent or a branch of a larger establishment. The same sense of definition will be followed here. To delimit the dimension implicit in the modifier *small,* the *Guide* specified plants with fewer than 500 employees, and a similar round figure will be implied in this discussion. Writers in the area of small plant programming have used a multiplicity of synonyms, some implying labor forces of 500, others staffs of as few as 20 [23–29].† The size of the workforce does not necessarily relate to the type of OHP provided, for some small plants offer well-developed and broad programs, while some companies with larger populations have minimal occupational health activity.

Recent data [30,31] show that small plants (under 500 employees) represent 99.7 percent of all work establishments and have 78.7 percent of all the workers in the labor force, exclusive of government employees, railroad employees, and the self-employed.‡

The development of in-plant medical services with full-time physicians and nurses and the focus of this kind of practice for the graduates of residency programs have adumbrated somewhat the potential role of the private practitioner in small plant medicine, in spite of the huge population in need. It is these estab-

*One of the most respected dictionaries gives this definition: "The fixtures, implements, machinery, and apparatus used in carrying on any industrial process" (*The Compact Edition of the Oxford English Dictionary.* Oxford, England: Clarendon, 1971. Vol. II, p. 2197). Another lexicon defines *plant* as "the equipment, including machinery, tools, instruments, and fixtures, and the buildings containing them, necessary for any industrial or manufacturing operation" (*The American Heritage Dictionary of the English Language.* Boston: American Heritage and Houghton Mifflin, 1969. P. 1003).

†A speaker once defined a small plant as one independent of the number of employees but one that could not afford the services of a full-time medical director.

‡Data for 1982 reveal that 328,932 manufacturing establishments had 19,572,113 employees. Some 314,500 establishments employed from fewer than 20 to 249 persons, or 78 percent of that segment of the labor force. The plants with 250 to 999 employees represented 9 percent of the manufacturing workers, while establishments of 1000 workers or more accounted for 13.9 percent of the employees. Assuming that plants with staffs under 250 workers have no occupational health services and that only some of the companies in the 250 to 999 grouping had occupational health personnel, it may be concluded that the majority of today's workers have no in-plant occupational health activity.

lishments that have had little medical coverage and about which so much has been written to stimulate managers toward the initiation of some health services and to motivate practicing physicians to consider small plants as sites of professional activity. No easy or umbrella type of plan will cover all situations, and no well-documented studies of costs and savings have been published for employers to review.

The kinds of services that can be rendered on a part-time basis differ little from most of those offered by the larger full-time operation. Preplacement, periodic, hazardous-employment, and return-to-work examinations are conducted. Injured employees are given care, emergency medical care is given workers with minor medical conditions, and health counseling is carried out in these plants, where a great variability exists as to the number of hours of coverage provided.

Metcalf [32], in writing for the Small Business Administration, has outlined the following basic points for recognition by the small business owner:

Efficiency of employees is dependent on proper selection, utilization, and maintenance. Employees who are properly selected, properly placed, and helped to keep healthy are *productive* employees.

Recognition of the importance of health by management and the provision of health services build incentive among the workers the employer desires to retain.

Reduction of labor turnover, sickness absenteeism, and errors accountable to ailing workers gives the employer greater control over production and sales.

Elimination of potential hazards from the workplace and proper precautions taken with accident-prone workers help to cut workers' compensation costs.

FORMATS FOR RENDERING MEDICAL SERVICE

There are several configurations for the provision of partial in-plant programs for small organizations.

Central Health Facility

A single facility can be established and maintained by a group of small companies, and such a service can be staffed by a number of physicians, nurses, and paramedical personnel. The initial investment can be borne by the companies receiving services, and the costs of operation are divided among the firms in proportion to the numbers of their employees. The center can be augmented by small satellites in the individual companies, where a visiting nurse (or physician) can see certain patients.

The physicians are expected to tour the plant facilities periodically to survey the physical conditions and to remain aware of the work environment of the people they treat. If the service is a large medical undertaking, there should be a business manager who can be in charge of accounting, promotional or marketing activities, and other administrative functions and who can add new subscribing companies.

Control is vested in a group selected by and from the managements of the supporting organizations, and an advisory board consisting of local physicians can be created to advise on all medical policies and procedures.

Associated Health Units

A group of firms may wish to have a physician regularly on their premises on specified days, for a certain number of hours. Each company will build its own service unit, equip it, and pay the salaries of the occupational nurse or nurses and of the physician, who may visit, as an example, one half-day per week. There is a fixed schedule among the industries, so that if the physician is needed urgently at another plant in the group, he or she can be called [32]. Several writers have reviewed the experience of the prototypical "Hartford Plan" and other cooperative programs [33–39].

Individual Contracts

A third variation is the contract entered into by a single company and a physician. The services might be provided in the company's health unit or in the physician's office [32].

Other Formats

In some industrial areas, a large clinic will have several of its physicians visit a group of firms on a regular schedule. Usually the same physician will visit the same company week after week, so that the employees and nurses can have a more solid physician-patient or physician-staff relationship. This kind of program usually has deficits in counseling and health education on the part of the physician, and little attention is given potential health hazards. The arrangement commonly meets minimal needs in examinations and care for injuries only.

A rare industrial clinic will have most of the workers referred to its own facility for attention, but the director, who usually has a broader knowledge of occupational medicine, will visit the plants' premises and provide counsel on hazardous materials, control measures, or problems of absenteeism or alcoholism.

Rieke [29], the late pioneer in the concept of the broad-scope industrial clinic, which in addition provides community leadership in health understanding, wrote extensively of the service to small companies. He summarized his experience:

> We have provided services at the Clinic and at various plants. We have supervised nurses in nearby industrial plants, supplied immunization teams to the workplace and to ships in the harbor. Continuous emergency service has been maintained at the Clinic or the nearby hospital for twenty-four years. For various reasons, demand for surgical care of injury has fallen off. Work at the Clinic is still surgical but is shifting noticeably to the preventive and consultative. For many years large employers have sent special problems for assessment and decision: the post-surgical back [patient] for placement; the convalescing heart patient for adjustment to graduated work; the spiritually or emotionally troubled for counseling; the aged for retirement planning; the driver for certification; or the lead worker for surveillance. In recent years individuals and those from small plants have come increasingly for the same kinds of examinations, for planning and adaptation to demands of the job and community.

He commented further on the problem of the location of the industrial clinic and viewed globally the clinic's role in the changing central city:

> We are caught in an era of change; large and small plants are becoming have-nots, short on clean air and surrounded with unsightly blight. This Clinic and its nearby major hospitals are at the center of the city. Workers and businesses are rapidly scattering to distant suburbs, leaving a disproportion of the poor, the elderly and the black. These changes are apparent in the clients we serve.
>
> Health manpower is presently clustering at central city hospitals but will gradually move to suburban clinics and hospitals. Rapid production of physician generalists may ameliorate some imbalances but will not quickly change service potentials in the central city or in remote villages. Utilities and many large employers remaining within the central city report increasing difficulty in securing quick, simple medical and health services.
>
> Business and industry are inextricably woven into the life of the surrounding community. As goes the community, so goes industry. Discontent of young Americans, deterioration of the environment, failure of the city as a social organism, or inappropriate health and social services are instantly reflected in performance at the workplace. The health of this symbiotic relationship is constantly under review in this industrial clinic. For twenty-five years we have tried to sustain a comfortable interaction by constantly adapting our work to the needs of individuals, employers, associations, government and other providers of service. I anticipate further continuous shifts in the role of the clinic, but am encouraged by the track record to think we shall remain useful and relevant, whatever the changes.
>
> I think we have also demonstrated that the private medical clinic of medium size is a most flexible, responsive and acceptable provider of preventive and community level health care, both for occupational and for general health problems.

Finally, as a source of service to small firms is the official health agency. Bartlett [40] discussed the role of the county health department in stimulating OHPs for smaller companies and businesses, which actually had created new opportunities for physicians and occupational environmentalist personnel in private occupational health practice. He cited the role of the Santa Clara County (California) Health Department's Bureau of Occupational Health in assisting both in-plant health service personnel and small plant management. The bureau's functions were outlined as follows:

Locating professional medical and nursing personnel.
Setting up first-aid stations.
Obtaining first-aid training for designated employees.
Establishing records designed to meet compensation insurance requirements and ethical medical considerations.
Providing health education and counseling.
Giving orientation and guidance in fundamental principles of occupational health nursing and medical services.
Helping to plan for a part-time nurse and physician as needs justify.
Providing consultation to part-time physicians and plant nurses.
Helping to plan for physical layout, equipment, and supplies.
Evaluating present programs in terms of present needs, accomplishments, and future requirements.
Consulting on in-plant nutrition and food services.
Helping to arrange in-plant multiphasic screening visits or single procedures such as mobile-unit chest x-rays, mobile-unit audiometric testing, glaucoma clinics, diabetic clinics, and immunizations.

The bureau's staff also promotes the "best practical environmental controls at work" in this way:

Providing general plant hygiene surveys.
Making recommendations for general improvements in mechanical safety procedures, equipment, ventilation, and safer production techniques.
Making special industrial hygiene surveys to evaluate environmental noise hazards, toxic hazards, lighting and heating problems, ionizing radiation exposures, and air pollutants.
Analyzing chemicals and other materials used in manufacturing to determine possible health hazards.
Making recommendations for selection of personal

protective equipment, such as respirators, goggles, and clothing.

Reviewing construction plans to evaluate industrial hygiene equipment in view of current experiences in other companies and with the purpose of reducing health hazards in new plants.

Referring plant management to private laboratories for industrial hygiene or radiation evaluation services that appear to be indicated on a regular repetitive basis.

Ordinarily, it is the larger county that will give emphasis to an occupational health consultative service in its health department. An excellent guide, now out of print, was made available in this segment by the American Public Health Association [41].

One last site for the provision of service to small plants is the community general hospital. This format has been utilized more successfully in England than in the United States, and Hill [42] has reviewed some seven group OHSs of that country, anticipating in all instances continuing growth of the established units and of five new services being planned or started. Hill believes that group OHSs "form a part of New Town thinking which could be a pattern for their gradual natural growth." The United States has only partially built this idea into the planning of its new industrial parks or estates. However, more and more hospitals are now adding an OHS to their outpatient departments, for considerable income potential is seen in the utilization of such a department.

FUNCTIONS

In *Guide to Developing Small Plant Occupational Health Programs* [22], certain activities are cited that can be selected for inclusion in an OHP.

It is pointed out first that an OHS derives from five distinct disciplines: the clinical practice of occupational medicine, occupational toxicology, industrial hygiene and safety, epidemiology, and occupational medicine administration. From these disciplines the following various program elements can be developed, as indicated by local need and through professional consultation [22].

The Occupational Health of the Worker
- Diagnosis, treatment, and rehabilitation of (workers sustaining) occupational injuries and diseases
- Preplacement examinations
- Biologic monitoring
- Environmental control
- Secondary prevention (emergency first-aid training, cardiopulmonary resuscitation training, disaster planning)
- Epidemiology
- Diagnosis and [limited] treatment of (workers presenting with) nonoccupational injuries or illnesses

The Personal Health of the Worker
- Periodic health appraisals
- Fitness programs
- Smoking withdrawal programs
- Substance abuse programs
- Nutritional counseling
- Stress management programs
- Return-to-work evaluations
- Immunizations
- Health education and counseling

Attention is also directed in the *Guide* [22] to the health of the corporation (which involves):

Product liability
Environmental emissions
Health costs
Absenteeism control
Other issues: Increase of productivity through proper job placement and ergonomics
Reproductive hazards

PERSONNEL

Formulas have been proposed for the amount of time to be given a single company by the physician. One provides for 2 hours of time per week for the first 100 employees and one additional hour for each additional 100 workers. There cannot be a rigid adherence to this schedule, for needs differ among plants as determined by the many variables cited previously. Rarely should this formula be foreshortened. Additional time will be required for completion of medical records and workers' compensation reports, telephone consultations, correspondence, conferences with managers, and plant visits [22].

One full-time nurse, if fully knowledgeable and concerned, can be completely occupied with a plant population of 300 to 400. Below the 300-employee level, a part-time visiting service would suffice.

A physician's assistant can serve in a small plant OHS and will extend the physician's work capacity by 75 percent [22].

FACILITIES

In *Guide to Developing Small Plant Occupational Health Programs* [22], these requirements are cited, with some modification:

In general, there should be about 1 square foot of floor space per employee.
Assured privacy, quiet, cleanliness, and immaculate housekeeping.
A minimum of one room to serve as an examining room; it may also function as a records room.
A larger room divided by screens into several areas for partial examinations and treatment.
A waiting and reception area.
Room with a bed—compulsory in some states.
Adequate toilet facilities.
Interior painting in light colors.
Sink with hot and cold water supply and elbow-, foot-, or knee-operated faucets.
Shower for whole-body cleansing following contamination by harmful chemicals.
Dust-free and locked instruments and storage cabinets.
Locked records cabinet and nurse's and physician's desks.

PROBLEMS

The consistent programming at professional society meetings of presentations on occupational health for the small plant bespeaks continuing difficulties without total solution. Braun [43] has pointed up some of the unresolved problems in this arena of care. As indicated previously, there have been inconsistencies in the definition of a small plant. The Small Defense Plants Administration was authorized by statute to determine which concerns were to be designated as "small business." An automotive parts concern was regarded as small if it employed fewer than 1,500 persons, and a producer of women's apparel with 200 workers was deemed as large for that industry.

Further, extremely small firms may have no special health hazards and, in some states, may not even come under the Workers' Compensation Act, negating one incentive for program inauguration. In small companies, also, the relationship of worker to owner is often close and the morale high. It is not feasible, therefore, to use increased morale as an objective of an OHS. An OHP would be superfluous, truly. Braun [43] asks, "Have we, then, been assigning a magnitude to the problem of occupational health in 'small plants' which in truth does not exist? If so, our figures have been exaggerated and like all exaggerations, have tended to lose force and to be less than convincing to the people we are trying to impress." Suggested, then, is the idea that a comprehensive program replete with sophisticated segments may be much too elaborate for the small firm. This problem has been emerging in the backlash to the enforcement of the provisions of OSHA 1970.

There are additional problems encountered by the contemporary part-time physician in industry, as voiced by Patterson [44]. There is variance in the preemployment process. One company employs highly skilled and educated individuals, while a second has need only for laborers. Further, can the examining physician accommodate him- or herself to different medical standards as he or she examines for a variety of companies?

The addition of strong "long-term disability coverage" to the fringe benefit program makes the acceptance of an applicant headed for serious physical or pathologic change precarious, even though one cannot reject a job candidate on the basis of future risk. The employment of the handicapped may be viewed incorrectly in the same light by some employers. The desiderata of the Rehabilitation Act of 1973 will be discussed later. Patterson [44] comments on another organizational disadvantage to part-time physicians: their lack of line control over full-time paramedical personnel, for they operate outside the company's table of organization and thus have no supervisory capacity.

Finally, touching once again the policy variations among companies, Patterson [44] points up differences in duration of maternity leave* and the great disparities among private physicians in regard to their postillness or postinjury return-to-work recommendations. It is these antithetic problems that part-time practitioners must face if they provide service to several small companies.

ETHICS

If physicians serving small industries use this professional activity as a means of building private practice, they will be subject to censure and will find themselves in the position of conflicting interests. They cannot see, as private patients, those employees they examine or treat at the plant. In the first edition (1973) of the *Guide to Developing Small Plant Occupational Health Programs* [see also 22], this point was stated conclusively: "The plant physician should never use his industrial affiliation improperly as a means of gaining or enlarging his private practice. If he observes these ethical relationships, the plant physician should experience no difficulty in establishing cordial relationships with other physicians in the community and gaining their cooperation on mutual problems." The Code of Ethical Conduct for Physicians Providing Occupational Medicine Services [45], developed by the AOMA, emphasizes this point in another way: "Physicians should . . . avoid allow-

*The redesignation of maternity leave as sick leave will be discussed later.

ing their medical judgment to be influenced by any conflict of interest."

Einert [25] has epitomized the attributes and convictions of the part-time provider of health services as including "a willingness to practice only the same quality of medicine inside the plant [as] . . . outside; a willingness to become a member of the production team, but not its leader, except in medical matters."

Not too long ago, the New York County Medical Society condemned direct solicitation of contracts from industrial management personnel. Much of the content is still germane. The full statement in support of its position is discussed in the sections *Independent Industrial Clinics,* through *General Responsibilities of the Occupational Physician* [46].

[Independent industrial clinics] generally serve a number of smaller companies which would not otherwise maintain such facilities and, in most cases, provide capable and thorough care. The policy of the group and the actions of the individual physicians are expected to conform to the principles set forth in this statement. The solicitation of contracts for such medical care from management personnel by any person in or acting for the group is not ethical.*

[Union health groups, usually joint management-union trusteeship] originally provided diagnostic study only of non-occupational disease. An increasing number have now been authorized to provide complete diagnosis and treatment for union members and their families. It is urged that such comprehensive groups arrange to provide adequate medical service at *all* times and not merely during clinic hours, since they have assumed the role of a family physician. It is, of course, desirable that medical policy decisions remain in the control of physician administrators.

[Health evaluation groups—independent or hospital affiliated:] Many firms have arranged for a program of periodic health evaluation of key personnel by medical groups specializing in this service. In many cases the employee must sign a prior authorization for release of the findings to the company. It is desirable and the Committee urges, that with the employee's consent a complete copy of the examination be provided to the employee's private physician and, equally important, to the company's medical officer, if there is one. Such information should not be released to non-professional management personnel.

More serious, however, is the increasing frequency with which such groups refer patients to specialists for treatment of diseases found on such health examinations. This is not the proper function of such a group and [patients] should be referred to the employee's family physician.

Lastly, the active advertising or direct solicitation of new contracts for such services (whether by newspaper articles, direct mailing, etc.) is unethical. It cannot be condoned, regardless of the status of the individual who does so. Professional members of such groups, whether full or part-time, must accept responsibility for such unethical conduct.*

[Primary aims of an OHP:] Whether medical services are offered to plants on a full-time or part-time basis, the same primary aims of an occupational medical program, as outlined by the Council on Occupational Health of the AMA should be pursued. It is with a view to pointing up these basic principles in their application to the special types of services indicated above that the present policy statement is presented:

To facilitate by careful pre-placement examination the proper placement of new employees in assignments compatible with their health.

To cooperate in the development of effective measures to prevent occupational disease and injury.

To provide for the competent treatment of diseases and injuries arising from the occupational environment, when so requested by the employee.

To provide for emergency care of serious non-occupational illness occurring on the job until the employee can be seen by his private physician.

In addition, but secondary to those functions listed above, management may wish to provide for minor treatment of non-recurring non-occupational illness to enable employees to complete their work shifts. Provision may also be made for periodic health evaluation of employees for the early detection of disease.

[General responsibilities of the occupational physician follow:]

The physician in industry (whether full- or part-time) must, of course, maintain the highest standards of professional ethics and competence in the handling of the employee patient.

He must be alert to current medical developments as well as those legal, social and economic factors relating to medical care in industry.

He must insist on control and complete confidentiality of all employees' medical records, releasing to the employer or to others only such information as the law requires. In other cases it might be released only upon written consent of the employee.

He must supplement, not interfere with or attempt to replace the relationship of the employee with his private physician.

He should not use his position in industry to solicit employees or their families to become his patients in his private practice.

To summarize, occupational health programs which conform to the principles outlined above are essential to the health and safety of the employee at work. In their fullest degree, they supplement the patient-family physician relationship and together best achieve a common goal—the continued good health of the workers.

*A Clinic administrator or business manager is expected, however, to seek now accounts.

*In many jurisdictions, advertising by professional persons has been accepted or restrictive legislation has been nullified. In fact, in many metropolitan newspapers such advertisements have become common.

CONCLUSION

To conclude a discussion of small plant medicine, the thoughts of a late eminent Midwest part-time practitioner [47] bear reproduction:

Medicine in industry is not very different from the private practice of good medicine. In both types the welfare of the patient is the prime consideration. The added requirement for the industrial physician is familiarity with the industry itself, its machines, its chemicals, its processes, and its exposures that might result in traumatic injury or in occupational diseases. This requirement can be met only by the regular devotion of time to the plant itself, to the work environment. The plant becomes one of his patients. If this particular requirement be fulfilled then any good private practitioner of medicine may become equally successful as the small plant industrial physician.

In substance, the arrangements under which small firms have obtained *in-plant* health services have been epitomized by Meigs [48]:

1. Individual, management-sponsored, full- or part-time in-plant services.
2. Cooperative, full- or part-time, in-plant services for several companies, sponsored jointly by the different managements.
3. Part-time, in-plant nursing services sponsored by visiting nurse associations in cooperation with local physicians or medical associations; or offered by individual nurses.
4. Part-time, in-plant medical and nursing services sponsored by physicians or groups of physicians, usually with a central clinic or dispensary.
5. Central clinic services provided by insurance companies or hospitals.
6. Services available through union health centers.
7. Services available through health departments.
8. Mobile dispensaries, operated out of a central clinic by appropriate agencies.

CONTRACTUAL AGREEMENTS

At best it is difficult for a physician to seek a company that might be in need of medical services. Tradition and medical ethics, as indicated previously, preclude an actual solicitation of patients or groups, but through consultants, the ERCs, or county medical societies, one might learn of positions available in industrial plants where the services of a physician on a part-time basis are desired.

Referring once more to *Guide to Developing Small Plant Occupational Health Programs* [22], one learns that the physician can serve under one or a combination of several contractual arrangements.

One can be paid a salary on an annual, monthly, weekly, or hourly basis, for which it is agreed that a certain amount of time will be spent in the plant medical department and that the physician has responsibility for the administration of the OHP in which other personnel will be engaged and for the provision of clinical services. This method is preferred.

A second method consists of one's being paid a retainer, plus a fee for specific services, which might include preplacement physical examinations, treatment of injured or ill employees, or disability evaluations. These procedures may be carried out at the plant or in the physician's private office. The visits that are made to the plant are not conducted on a regularly recurring basis but are made as needed to provide direction and maturity to the OHP.

In the third type of agreement, the physician is remunerated only for the services that are rendered, such as emergency medical care, physical examinations, or treatment of work-injured employees. There may be several physicians rendering this kind of service, functioning exclusively on an ad hoc basis, and assuming no responsibility for directing the general OHP. The physicians do not visit the plant and have little awareness of the overall health needs or the working conditions.

The best of these systems is, of course, the first method because a good occupational health activity can result. As described previously, if one plant cannot afford this level of service, it can join with other plants and provide the physician with several companies for the development of preventive medical services. In the second scheme (retainer plus fee for services), there is the advantage that there will be an occasional visit to the plant made by the physician, for exposure to some of the health problems. The third type of contract is actually an ineffective one from the company's point of view, and about the only advantage accruing is to the physician, in that there is additional income for each individual service rendered.

An additional arrangement that is increasing in the United States is seen in the participation of group clinics in occupational medicine. One or more physicians in such a clinic will serve a department designated "Occupational Medicine" and will provide services to many industrial organizations, but again usually these services will be obtainable only at the clinic. Many of these groups are used for executive health examinations, but other program elements may be carried out by them.

It would be desirable for a contract to be drawn up and signed by both the employing company and the physician, for in such a document, there can be stipulations as to the services expected, the working conditions of the physician, and the attendant responsibilities. Renewal of the contract on an annual basis can provide for program growth and readjustment of any one of the contractual elements.

It must be borne in mind that, in certain states, contractual arrangements are illegal. Therefore, one should verify the legality of these arrangements with the state department of labor, industrial relations, social welfare, or health or the industrial accident board or commission, whichever might have jurisdiction.

IN-PLANT OCCUPATIONAL NURSE VISITATION

One other program design may be seen in the part-time utilization of occupational health nurses for visitation at a number of establishments. The origins of this type of service date to 1908 when a contract was drawn between the Lowney Chocolate Factory and the Boston Visiting Nurse Association of Milwaukee and the Pfister & Vogel Leather Company [49]. The role of such a nurse in the Chicago Visiting Nurse Association scene was described warmly by Foley in 1927 [50].

Most visiting nurse associations are in large industrial cities, and services on an hourly cost basis can be arranged by contract or by an individual visit charge. A sample format for a contract between an agency and a company can be found in Lee [49].

Although many of the nurses undertaking visitation from visiting nurse associations may be public health nurses, it does not necessarily hold that they are knowing in the specialty of occupational nursing. In Canada, the Victorian Order of Nurses (VON) provides part-time services to companies too small to require a full-time nurse [51–54], and currently 24 VON branches of its 85 are servicing 30 organizations, the time given varying in duration from 1 hour per week to half-time. The companies covered had 7,629 employees, and 3,710 separate sessions of service were provided. In some instances, the written agreements have called for home visitation of sick employees. All of the VON nurses are public health nurses. It is the belief of the VON that the minimum single unit of nursing time for a plant employing over 35 workers should not be less than 2 hours. Further, a ratio of 1 hour of physician's time to 3 hours of nurse's time per 100 workers is suggested.

IN-PLANT PUBLIC HEALTH NURSE VISITATION

Emerging from demonstration-program origins has been the use of public health nurses (PHNs) for visits to industrial establishments. The PHN has added the workplace to her visitation sites, frequently meeting with expectant mothers; gradually, other functions were included in the more customary PHN battery of services.

An early experiment was carried out in Hillsborough County, Florida [55], where 92 percent of the plants employed 50 persons or fewer and where many of the workers were black or Spanish-speaking. The nurses became involved in health counseling, immunizations, safety programs, dermatitis prevention, and referrals for family planning.

A second trial was launched in southern Clay County, Missouri [56], where the following program objectives for PHNs were formulated and met: (1) to understand an occupational health program in a county health department and help the Community Health Nurse (CHN) consider her new role in the occupational setting; (2) to increase the CHN's knowledge of the industrial environment and the health needs of adult workers; and (3) to increase the CHN's ability to extend nursing skills to workers at the workplace.

The CHN selected a target company in her area, made her own contact with the plant manager, and personally presented the nursing services available. Programs of prevention were introduced, including diabetes and vision screening; tuberculin testing, followed by chest radiography; tetanus immunization; education in cervical cancer detection; and correction of environmental health deficits. In Wisconsin [57], efforts were directed toward multiphasic testing and counseling. The Health Department of Pasadena, California [58] introduced a broadened program for PHNs through joint efforts with occupational health nursing consultants, and activities have been extended to industry in tuberculosis control, chronic disease control, health education, and in-service education.

The role of the PHN in occupational health was well delineated in a committee report that was an outgrowth of the 1959 California Conference of Local Health Officers. The conference recommended that OHPs be included as a basic element in all local health departments. The Nursing Directors Group of the California State Department of Public Health appointed a special committee that developed a set of guidelines for PHSs [59].

In substance, service provided by a visiting PHN to a small plant should be in accordance with the premise suggested by Lee [49] and earlier by Brown [60]—6 hours per week of nursing time per 100 employees, as a minimum service. Variables that might alter this ratio would be the type of industry represented by the company, the composition of the workforce, and the geographic location [59].

REFERENCES

1. Odiorne, G. S. *Management by Objectives.* New York: Pitman, 1965. Pp. 55–56.
2. *Scope, Objectives, and Functions of Occupational Health Programs.* Chicago: American Medical Association, Department of Environmental, Public, and Occupational Health, 1971. P. 6.
3. Occupational Medical Practice Committee, American Occupational Medical Association. Scope of occupational health programs and occupational medical practice. *J Occup Med* 21:497, 1979.
4. *Report on the Proceedings of the Conference on Occupational Health Programs.* Sponsored by the Occupational Safety and Health Administration—October 6–8, 1982, Washington, D.C. Washington, DC: The Administration, 1983. Pp. 8–10.
5. Boettiger, L. A. *Employee Welfare Work: A Critical and Historical Study.* New York: Ronald, 1923.
6. Howe, H. F. Distribution of occupational physicians among industries. *J Occup Med* 11:191, 1969.
7. Council on Occupational Health: The role of medicine within a business organization. *JAMA* 210:1446, 1969.
8. *Concepts of Organization Planning.* NICB Studies in Personnel Policy, No. 183. New York: National Industrial Conference Board, 1962. P. 7.
9. Sappington, C. O. Industrial Health Department Functions and Relationships: A Quarter of a Century of Progress in Industrial Health Administration. In *Medical Bulletin No. VIII.* Pittsburgh: Industrial Hygiene Foundation, 1948. Pp. 43–44.
10. Goldstein, B., and Chernick, J. *In-plant Medical Programs in New Jersey.* New Brunswick, NJ: Rutgers—The State University, Research Program, Institute of Management and Labor Relations, 1961.
11. Goldstein, B., Northwood, L. G., and Goldstein, R. L. Medicine in industry: Problems of administrators and practitioners. *J Health Hum Behav* 1:259, 1960.
12. *Company Medical and Health Programs.* NICB Studies in Personnel Policy, No. 171. New York: National Industrial Conference Board, 1959. Pp. 45–46.
13. Freedman, A. Staffing and Managing. In *Industry Response to Health Risk.* Report No. 811. New York: National Industrial Conference Board, 1981. Pp. 31–44.
14. Felton, J. S. Occupational health relates to management and labor. *Navy Lifeline* 6:18, 1977.
15. Levine, R. J. (Ed.). Control of the Asbestos Hazard: Medical Management. In *Asbestos: An Information Resource.* Bethesda, MD: National Cancer Institute, May 1978. Pp. 89–97.
16. Miles, A. *Lowell, As It Was, and As It Is.* Lowell, MA: Nathaniel L. Dayton—Merrill & Heywood, 1846.
17. Mobile industrial medical clinics. *Ind Med Surg* 23:545, 1954.
18. *Haskell Laboratory for Toxicology and Industrial Medicine.* Wilmington, DE: E.I. duPont deNemours, 1954.
19. Council on Occupational Health. Medical directives for occupational health nurses: Guide for development. *Arch Environ Health* 5:631, 1962.
20. LaRoche, P. Occupational medicine at Cape Canaveral: An eight year review. *South Med J* 57:509, 1964.
21. Howe, H. F. Personal communication, 1973.
22. *Guide to Developing Small Plant Occupational Health Programs* (2nd ed.). Chicago: The American Medical Association, 1983.
23. Bond, M. B. Occupational health services for small employee units. *Rocky Mountain Med J* 68:31, 1971.
24. *Cooperative Medical Programs: A New Solution for Small Companies.* NICB Studies in Personnel Policy, No. 134. New York: National Industrial Conference Board, 1953.
25. Einert C. Part-time, in-plant medicine in modern general practice. *Ind Med Surg* 31:121, 1962.
26. Howe, H. F. Preventing occupational health and safety hazards in small employee groups. *Am J Public Health* 61:1581, 1979.
27. Metra, S. D., and Banerjee, A. K. Health and safety of workers in small factory establishments: Need for statutory regulations. *Indian J Public Health* 6:179, 1962.
28. Pyle, H. Promotion of occupational safety and health in small undertakings. *Ind Med Surg* 39:42, 1970.
29. Rieke, F. E. Industrial clinic services to small industries. *Am J Public Health* 62:69, 1972.
30. *County Business Patterns 1982.* Washington, DC: U.S. Department of Commerce, Bureau of the Census, Oct 1984. Pp. 1, 3, 10.
31. *Statistical Abstract of the United States 1985* (105th ed.). Washington, DC: U.S. Department of Commerce, Bureau of the Census, 1984. P. 758.
32. Metcalf, W. O. *Health Maintenance Programs for Small Business* (2nd ed.). Small Business Management Series, No. 16. Washington, DC: Small Business Administration, 1964.
33. Buchan, R. F. Small plant medical services: Will-o'-the-wisp? *Arch Environ Health* 9:111, 1964.
34. Klem, M. C., and McKiever, M. F. *Small Plant Health and Medical Programs.* Washington, DC: U.S. Department of Health, Education, and Welfare, Public Health Service, Occupational Health Program, 1952 (reproduced Jan 1958). Pp. 77–103.
35. Larke, A. G. Smaller Plants Share the Health. *Dun's Rev Mod Ind* 65:44, 1955.
36. Thompson, D. M. New Haven small plant medical program. *Calif Health* 15:57, Oct 15, 1957.
37. Smaller plant: Here's a medical service for you. *Occup Hazards* 14:28, Oct 1952.
38. Small plant health program. *Mo Ind Health Bull* 10:1, Dec 1952.
39. Stalker, W. W., Stalker, V. G., and Rosenblatt, A. L. A multi-plant program in employee and environmental health. *Am Ind Hyg Assoc J* 24:462, 1963.
40. Bartlett, J. P. Community health resources for small plants. *Arch Environ Health* 9:117, 1964.
41. *Local Health Official's Guide to Occupational Health.* New York: American Public Health Association, 1968.
42. Hill, R. N. With one eye on the accounts: Group oc-

cupational health services today. *Trans Soc Occup Med* 22:24, 1972.
43. Braun, D. C. Occupational health programs for small plants. *Arch Environ Health* 12:457, 1966.
44. Patterson, R. B. Problems faced by the less than full time occupational physician. *J Occup Med* 13:277, 1971.
45. Code of Ethical Conduct for Physicians Providing Occupational Medicine Services, Committee on Ethical Practice in Occupational Medicine. *J Occup Med* 18:703, 1976.
46. Ethical practices for independent industrial medical clinics. *J Occup Med* 7:294, 1965.
47. Jones, E. J. What constitutes a part-time industrial physician?—Down to earth industrial medicine. *Ind Med Surg* 32:248, June 1963.
48. Meigs, J. W. cited in 34 above. Pp. 32–33.
49. Lee, J. A. *Community Health Nursing for Working People* (revised). Cincinnati, OH: U.S. Department of Health, Education, and Welfare, Public Health Service, 1970.
50. Foley, E. L. The place of the visiting nurse in industry. *Nation's Health* 9:29, 1927.
51. Small plant health services provided by V.O.N. *Occup Health Bull* (Ottawa). 11:1, Oct 1955.
52. McEwen, A. E. Personal communication, March 16, 1973.
53. MacArthur, M. C. Visiting nurse north of the border. *Nurs Clin North Am* 4:333, 1969.
54. MacArthur, M. C. New challenges for visiting nursing. *Nurs Clin North Am* 6:467, 1971.
55. Dowling, E. B. "We cover every aspect of our patients' lives." *RN* 30:57, Jan 1967.
56. Lindquist, P. A. Community health nursing for people who work. *Am J Public Health* 61:2015, 1971.
57. Chambers, C. Potential contribution of public health nursing [to Occupational Health]. *Am J Public Health* 53:1894, 1963.
58. Ochiai, M. Role of the public health nurse in an occupational health program. *Calif Health* 21:201, 1964.
59. Occupational health guidelines for public health nurses. *Calif Health* 21:205, 1964.
60. Brown, M. L. Occupational health problems in small employee groups. *Arch Environ Health* 3:79, 1961.

549401

5. PROGRAM ACTIVITIES RELATING TO PROSPECTIVE EMPLOYEES

Which of us . . . is to do the hard and dirty work for the rest—and for what pay? Who is to do the pleasant and clean work, and for what pay?

John Ruskin

One of the earliest functions assigned to the first physicians in industry was the examination of applicants for work. Because of the passage of workers' compensation legislation in 1911 and the years following, employers grew concerned over the physical quality of the persons brought in to staff their plants. Fitness was the operating word, for there was great fear that any physical defect manifested by a worker at the time of hire would, one day, return as a claim of job-related injury. So the protocols executed by the physicians were, in truth, preemployment examinations. The examiner made a single dichotomous choice of "accept" or "reject," no consideration being given special placement in light of physical, mental, or behavioral illness residua or concomitants. A candidate for work had to be physically perfect, preferably strong of muscle, male, white, and young. More than 60 years had yet to elapse before the baseless bans on certain employee groups were to be lifted through civil rights legislation.

PREPLACEMENT HEALTH EXAMINATION

Much discussion has been generated over the titles for these determinations of health status. In many companies they are designated "preemployment" physical examinations. The concept of "preplacement" procedures grew with the emphasis given utilization of the physically handicapped worker, and to bring about a suitable and safe employment, the physical examination was done before placement. The medical appraisal was undertaken to permit the personnel department to "place" candidates for work in jobs for which the applicants were physically and emotionally fit. If they were not suited for the positions applied for, additional efforts would be made for placement in jobs that would match individual capabilities.

The objectives of the placement examination have been given by the American Medical Association [1] as follows:

To evaluate the medical fitness of individuals to perform their duties without hazard to themselves or fellow workers, *or to the employer's property* [phrase added].

To assist employees in the maintenance or improvement of their health.

To detect the effects of [past or present] harmful working conditions and advise corrective measures.

To establish a record of the medical condition of the employee at the time of each examination.

In a sense, the changeover from the long-standing "employment examination" was necessary to free the process of the commonly associated stigma of misuse. In unscrupulous hands, the examination frequently was utilized as an instrument of administrative policy to reject an "undesirable" person. This individual was "undesirable" not because of any physical deviation, but because of certain trade union affiliation, a history of conflict with other companies, a history of repeated injuries, or suspected, alleged, or proved inimical political attachment.

In keeping with the Rehabilitation Act of 1973 as applied to federal contractors, the applicant for employment cannot be required to have a physical examination before a job is offered. The preplacement medical examination can be conducted after a job offer is made provided such an examination is required of *all* persons seeking work. This action is aimed at precluding rejection of a potential employee on the basis of a "failed" examination.

Today, the health status evaluation is conducted to aid the appropriate utilization of capabilities brought to the job and not to determine feasibility for employment. This decision is an administrative one, reached after the weighing of *all* evidence, only part of which is the physician's classification—a recommendation offered by a professional staff person and not a definitive act, order, or command as though issued by a line executive.

The examination is one of several kinds of health evaluations. The term *health examination* is actually preferred to either of the other taggings, *physical examination* or *medical examination,* particularly if certain psychological tests are to be included, even though preference was given *medical examination* in an earlier discussion. In some instances, the addition of such procedures has been contested, for they are not measurements of a "physical" or "medical" condition. They do measure emotional health in a broad sense, and thus the designation *health examination* provides a wider umbrella to cover all tests and procedures.

The examination must be authorized by the employing arm of the company, and a written authorization or request to the physician is needed to proceed with the evaluation. This step is accomplished usually through use of a completed form that will include the date, the applicant's name, the department in which it is anticipated the applicant will be working, and the prospective job title and number. The reason for this requirement is to avoid the examining of either the wrong individual—a substitute may have appeared surreptitiously—or a person seeking an examination at no cost.

The examination should include not only a personal and family medical history but also a carefully documented occupational history indicating all jobs held, their dates and places, and the kinds of work exposures sustained by the applicant. If any occupational disease has been experienced, the circumstances should be described in detail.

The assessment of physical status should be carried farther than the usual organ inventory with notations of major or minor physical changes, for it should include an evaluation of functional capacity. There should be clear descriptive statements of the applicant's ability to perform in light of missing extremities, impaired skill in ambulation, elevated blood pressure, partial sightedness, or any other deviation from the physical, physiologic, emotional, or mental mean customarily associated with the candidate's age or other influencing variables.

The scope of the examination will vary with certain factors, such as the nature of the company's mission (hazardous exposures, unusual physical demands), the type of position sought (clerk-typist versus police officer), the history of the applicant (previous institutionalization, stabilized tuberculosis), the industrial injury experience of the company (residua of back injuries), the location of the job site (applicant who has paraplegia), or the duration of employment (summer job of a college student), among others.

MEDICAL HISTORY

In recent years, the traditional, locally devised paper-and-pencil history questionnaire has undergone change. Commercially available now are printed history forms that present questions to the subject for response with a "No"/"Yes" choice, the correct response to be circled or checked. In some of the forms, through designed overlap systems and the use of noncarbonized, chemically treated copy paper, the last sheet will carry all the responses in code. A visual sweep of the page will identify instantly questions, areas, or bodily organ systems with clinical problems, past or current.

The Cornell Medical Index Health Questionnaire has been used by the author for many years with extreme satisfaction. The edition used is one copyrighted in 1949,* before it was changed by the omission of certain questions relating to behavior. This questionnaire has some defects that are difficult to compensate for, unless there is the usual follow-up interview. Many persons, particularly scientists accustomed to finite quantification, have difficulty answering questions carrying such qualifiers as *seldom, sometimes, ever, often, usually, frequently,* or *occasionally.*† Often the person completing the form will write in clarifying notes, in addition to the "Yes" or "No" choice. The emotionally sick individual either will answer all significant questions positively or reply "No" to every one of the 195 questions. Physician-applicants almost never will circle a "Yes" response, irrespective of positive medical histories or the presence of visible physical variance.

Certain more specialized history questionnaires are available, the Diagnostic Inventory for example, which can be used for such discrete entities as back pain, joint pain, eye complaints, fatigue, dizziness, and the like.

A variation of this theme is seen in the automated history wherein the examinee may face a display screen and respond to questions by depressing keys on a console. A hard-copy printout is produced that records all of the positive history in complete sentence format.

*Cornell Medical Index Health Questionnaire copyrighted 1949 by the Cornell University Medical College, 1300 York Avenue, New York, New York 10021.

†A study has been published illustrating the variability in interpretation of words used to indicate frequency. See R. M. Kenney, Between never and always. *N Engl J Med* 305:1098, 1981.

A further variation of the paper-and-pencil health questionnaire is one that utilizes mark-sense technique and is computer-generated and computer-processed. Multiple levels of the test permit more detailed inquiry into positive responses, thus individualizing the questionnaire. An optical scanner reads the forms and produces a printout for the physician, in slightly telegrammatic English.

Printed questionnaires can be lengthy and capable of combination with the concept of Health Hazard Appraisal (HHA). While the utilization of HHA is frequently associated with fitness or wellness programs, a comparable protocol can be used as part of the preplacement examination. The seminal work in "prospective medicine" has been identified with Dr. Lewis C. Robbins and ultimately with the Methodist Hospital in Indianapolis, Indiana [2–5]. While the beginnings date to the early 1960s, the concept has matured so that with the computerization of data, an individual—or a group of employees—after supplying basic information concerning family, medical history, patterns of health behavior, and methods of coping, can be given in essence a health forecast. Information is developed that provides one's risk of contracting or dying from such major diseases as cancer, heart disease, or stroke; a comparison of one's risks with similar persons; knowledge of the impact of habits, good and bad, on health and life expectancy; the direction for changes that can control the risks and increase life expectancy; and the number of years that can be added to a life with altered health behavior patterns.

The reason for indicating the use of the HHA in industry and business is that the preplacement examination as it is presently carried out in many institutions represents little return to the examinee. There may be a form letter that assures the new employee or incumbent that there were no findings meriting attention or that certain examination or laboratory test results warrant further study by the individual's personal physician. While the use of the HHA adds to the cost of the preplacement (or periodic) examination, it does give the person a product that is meaningful, has significant numbers, and has the capability of motivating changes in life-style or health behavior. It can alter the concept that many employees have that the examination is "strictly for management" and that they really derive nothing of value from it.

While there has been criticism of the reliability of the HHA [6], of the problematic scientific basis for the risk predicting [7], and of the appropriateness of the health education messages for all persons [8], it is felt that the device offers the respondents a tangible return for their participation in the examination process and a set of goals toward which they can work. The last becomes somewhat more feasible in that there is now a printed document that can be shared with spouses for potentially greater proaction.

The form of medical history record selected or the method of obtaining personal history data can be determined by weighing a number of influencing factors. The time-tested printed form is in successful use and will continue to be when the number of job applicants seen daily is low or, in other words, where the labor turnover of the company is minimal. If there are many applicants seen each day, without an appointment system, much more waiting room space will be required as prospective examinees complete the questionnaires. If candidates are seen by appointment, a smaller waiting area will suffice.

Some employers (and clinics) send the medical history questionnaire in advance so that the completed form can be brought to the examination facility. The concern regarding a response provided jointly by helpful spouses or other family members may have been reversed so that the answers given to questions might be more accurate when two or more interested and related adults pool their recall capabilities.

Many companies have issued guides to their medical examiners that outline particular points to be observed in the history, particularly as they relate to reactions to stressors, difficulties in adjustment or adaptation, or participation in antisocietal movements. Life norms are changing, and what might have been considered maladaptive behavior a decade or two ago may now be viewed as merely the forthright expression of feelings that heretofore were contained and not allowed to surface. Police records on applicants are scanned and currently are being given less weight as contraindications to employment than they were formerly. School dropouts or former student dissenters may be suspect of philosophies contrary to one or more "establishments," but personal beliefs of this nature may bear no relationship to future job performance and may actually have lost their fervor. We cannot remain totally fixed or rigid in our views, and we must not assume that because the occupational health facility is management-supported that medical history data must parallel in behavioral philosophy that of the policy-making body. Were this inflexibility to characterize the medical operation, the rehabilitation potential in work would soon be lost.

A final word of caution by Levinson [9] is offered, in light of the mechanization and automation that seem to be overtaking the history portion of the preplacement examination procedure. He questions whether any device, no matter how sophisticated, can substitute for the physician-obtained history. The interview, he states, is more than an information-gathering activity; it is the means by which the physician and patient establish the quality of their personal relationship. A physician who does no more, Levinson observes, than look over a computer printout or a checklist may compromise or destroy his or her identity as an understanding human being capable of responding to the needs of the patient. He goes on to comment, "No substitute for the human mind has yet been devised which can elicit, interpret, and respond to the complexities of past and present events which culminate in an illness and do so in a way which, in itself, can often be therapeutic." Technology, as he views it, best serves mankind when it supplements, rather than substitutes for, human effort and liberates man from routine so that he may do those things that are uniquely human.

The physician-historian can use the computerized printout, but there must be feeling inquiries made of the patient that provide the detail, color, and emotions attendant upon the clinical disorder noted initially by the pencil-checking or key-pressing of the item presented for questioning.

PRELIMINARY TEST PROCEDURES

Several tests can be performed by ancillary or paraprofessional personnel prior to an applicant's being examined by the physician. Many of these procedures compose the multiphasic test protocol, to be reviewed in Chapter 6, but mentioned briefly here. One may select specific assessment modalities from the group, or utilize all of them, depending on how complete a health baseline is desired at the time of hire. These reference point data are secured before exposure to certain toxic materials and prior to the onset of the effects of stressors, aging, illness, injury, or the late appearance of damaging genetic factors. The following procedures can be carried out preliminarily:

Height and weight determination
Skinfold thickness measurement*
Audiometry
Visual skills determination through use of a precision stereoscopic instrument
Electrocardiography, resting, 12-lead
Chest radiography*
Pulmonary function testing (spirometry)
Hematologic studies (complete blood count, hematocrit or microhematocrit, or such portions as are considered relevant)
Urinalysis (including chemical and microscopic examinations)
Blood chemistry battery, and subsequent phenotyping in hyperlipidemia or lipid fractionation, if desired
Serodiagnostic test for syphilis
Blood typing and Rh-factor determination
Tonometry by standard contact technique or applanation
Other radiographic studies as indicated by previous history, former job-related injury or illness, or findings on examination (particularly, blood or urine levels of absorbed environmental contactants or toxicants) as indicated by history or by specific job to be held†
Psychodiagnostic tests as indicated and selected by consulting psychometrician
Sickle cell trait and disease screening, with follow-up electrophoretic studies for the presence of disease in certain applicants at risk, that is, with job-related hazardous exposures
Urinalytic drug screening on selected groups
Malaria smears on certain veterans or immigrants from Southeast Asia.

All of the above procedures remain as options of the medical program, and the worth of the results must be weighed against the costs. One particular program director may wish to give emphasis to physical fitness, another to reduction of risk factors in disease, another to eradication of nutritional anemia, while another may wish to underscore a hearing or vision conservation program. To all of the above may be added clinical photographs to serve as referents in future comparisons of (1) skin lesions, areas of pigmentation, or depigmentation, healed post-traumatic scars, tattoo-bearing areas of skin sensitive to chemicals; (2) congenital anomalies; (3) amputation stumps; or (4) body configuration (as in anorexia

*In a query to *JAMA* (Glazier, E. H. Are girth measurements necessary in a routine physical examination? *JAMA* 213:2278, 1970), it was asked if chest and abdominal measurements were essential. A specialist in sports medicine (F. L. Allman, Jr.) responded that such measurements, including those of extremities, should be included, for they can indicate such disease states as ankylosing spondylitis, a herniated disk or other spinal or peripheral nerve injury, or a knee disorder. Also such mensuration can provide evidence of physical deterioration. A gerontologist (F. C. Swartz) thought them to be without worth. In light of the injury and illness potential of contemporary industry, such measurements can provide meaningful baselines.

*The views to be selected may be determined by the subject's previous contact with fibrogenic dusts.
†For example, a scout film of the abdomen may be taken to detect the presence of aortic calcification when a total cardiovascular study is required.

nervosa, rheumatoid spondylitis, or in achondroplasia, among innumerable other clinical states).

EXAMINATION BY THE PHYSICIAN

The actual examination to be completed by the physician does not differ from the traditional review of bodily organ systems and estimation of functional capacities. A preface to the protocol, though, is a discussion with the applicant of the significant elements of the history, as recorded. There may be revealed the need for copies of records from previous sources of care or hospitalization, particularly when placement is being considered of candidates with static impairments, recent surgical intervention because of malignant disease, or sensitive, labile, chronic disease states such as diabetes or the convulsive disorders. Many times applicants will discuss problems with a physician that they had been reluctant to indicate in a history form, handled initially by other personnel.

An opportunity to gain insight into the applicant's personality is frequently lost to the examiner in industry who fails to observe the candidate's behavior while the latter is undressing for the procedures. Meares [10] has pointed out the many advantages to the practitioner of being present during this period of preparation. The applicant discloses himself in a way that was done only in part while dressed. As Meares expressed it,

> The psychological effects of physical examination are largely brought about by the mechanisms of symbolism. There is symbolic significance in uncovering the body. It is a laying bare . . . a voluntary disclosure of the self. The secrets of the body are exposed; there is no hiding anything. The symbolic effect of this laying bare of the body is to facilitate the laying bare of the mind. . . . Every day we see patients who hold back something in the formal part of the interview. In physical examination the secrets of the body are disclosed. Then, with no additional prompting, and for no apparent reason, the secrets of the mind are spontaneously disclosed.
>
> Physical examination is more than laying bare the body; it is a matter of being examined by some other person. It is really more than a matter of being examined, it is a matter of being scrutinized.

Liebman [11] offers an opposing view, but both opinions make sense, as determined by the situation:

> In too many clinics and doctors' offices, practically all patients are placed in a small room or cubicle and told to undress and wait for the doctor. Later, the doctor takes the history while the patient, wrapped in a sheet, sits on the edge of the examination table. To many women this is so embarrassing that they don't always give the complete story to the doctor. In many private office practices or working in the health department prenatal and family-planning clinic, I always talk to the patients in a private room—while they are dressed—before sending them to the examining room. They appreciate the respect for their privacy and the courtesy of not being made to feel they are on an assembly line.

To perform appropriately in the preplacement evaluation, the examining physician must be furnished with the title of the job the applicant is seeking, a brief description of the duties, the environmental demands made on the incumbent, and the physical and emotional capacities required. It is the latter capacities against which the physician matches the findings derived from the organ inventory, functional evaluation, and results of all the adjunctive tests. Without knowledge of the job to be obtained, the examination process is purposeless.

COMPONENTS

The components of the examination are the same as those used in any other physical examination, but some points differ. The *skin* must be examined carefully because of the plethora of dermatogenic agents in industry. *Ophthalmoscopy* should not be omitted. Some physicians are hesitant to dilate the pupil to facilitate examination of the ocular fundus because of a fear of precipitating acute glaucoma, even though it is understood that significant systemic and ocular disease may go unrecognized. Friedman [12] has pointed out, with full explanation, that it is likely that many more patients have been harmed by the failure to dilate the pupil than have been injured by iatrogenic angle-closure glaucoma.

If the *external ear* shows ceruminosis, the canal should be lavaged so that the structures become visible and, more importantly, an accurate measure of auditory acuity can be obtained. *Breast examination* should be included in both men and women. A *rectal examination* should be performed on both male and female applicants, but a pelvic examination should not be done. If the abdominal examination leads to suspicion of a pelvic lesion, the applicant should be referred to her own physician.

Frequently the vital signs are recorded as the first step of an examination, and elevations or depressions in the level of *temperature* cause concern. Benzinger [13] of the National Bureau of Standards has stated unequivocally that there is no general norm or range for body temperature. Each person has his or her own norm, and a range in setpoint variation between individuals varied from 97.5 to 98.8°F (36.4–37.1°C), with the feeling that, pending investigation of larger groups, the range may be wider. In spite of well over a century of clinical rectal thermometry, more reference data on ranges and rhythms are still wanting.

Sphygmomanometry has had its accuracy questioned. In a study [14] in which both aneroid and mercury instruments were calibrated against a new mercury manometer, it was learned that 68.4 percent of 310 aneroid devices and all of the mercury manometers were accurate within ± 3 mm Hg tolerance. It was stressed that aneroid instruments must be calibrated periodically against a mercury manometer standard with a simple Y-tube connection. Aneroid instruments should be used in blood pressure mensuration only when there is regular careful maintenance and calibration. For accuracy, special arm cuffs should be used on obese subjects, and such large cuffs should not be used on subjects whose arm circumference is greater than 32 cm. Use of the inappropriate large cuff resulted in a lowering of the systolic reading by an average of 4.4 ± 1.66 mm Hg and 3.52 ± 1.25 mm Hg for the diastolic measure [15].

Iatrogenic factors in blood pressure measurement have been known to many practitioners and their patients for decades. A group from Milan [16] monitored patients by use of a continuous intraarterial recorder. When a physician repeatedly arrived at the bedside and measured the pressure by the cuff method, the levels peaked within 1 to 4 minutes—both systolic (mean 26.7 ± 2.3 mm Hg) and diastolic (mean 14.9 ± 1.6 mm Hg). The heart rate rose an average of 15.9 ± 1.5 beats per minute. Another report by one of the same investigators [17] concluded that the best assessment of resting blood pressure was that made by the patient using a self-monitoring device. The next best method was for a nurse, not a physician, to measure the pressure over at least a 10-minute period.

Position is important. The official recommendation of the American Heart Association is that the arm be "slightly flexed and with the whole forearm supported at heart level on a smooth surface." The heart level was indicated as the fourth intercostal space at the sternum. This position will avoid the rendering of spurious results [18].

Practitioners differ in their personal systems of blood pressure determinations, some obtaining the level in one upper extremity, others checking bilaterally. It is the recommendation of Hagelsten, Jessen, and Knudsen [19] that in "health examinations" there is no need to perform the procedure on both sides. In a study of 472 Philips employees in Copenhagen, only three persons, all asymptomatic and disease free, showed a difference of 15 mm Hg or more between the two arms.

Seth [20] has warned against the blind acceptance of the 140/90 normalcy standard for blood pressure in women. He recorded the pressure in 3000 women applicants for work in Bexley, England and concluded that the accepted figure of normal blood pressure as given in the literature is not only an assumption but also a figment of imagination of a clinician. In comparing United Kingdom data with those of the Actuarial Society of America, he found the British levels for both systolic and diastolic pressures to be of a difference of between 5 and nearly 8 mm. He asks for a standard to be established on an environmental, geographic basis, rather than a cultural one. It would be wise to have norms for every area where preplacement examinations are being conducted.

Neumann [21] has suggested that the examinee can be relaxed prior to recording the blood pressure by having him take a few preliminary deep breaths. This procedure, in his experience, has led to a reduction of both apprehension and blood pressure. The explanation lies, he believes, merely in muscle relaxation combined with the diversion created by the deep breaths.

STANDARDS AND CRITERIA

As indicated previously, employers, through the actions of their medical examiners, may display greater concern over self-protection than over the appropriate utilization or employment of persons seeking work. Whether it is wanted or liked, unwanted or disliked by industry, legal constraints to rigidity in hiring have come about through the passage of various bills aimed at the elimination of discrimination in employment. In the public sector, particularly, where the appeal process is built into all merit systems, there has been considerable criticism of certain standards involving weight, height, sex of the applicant, and the integrity of the cardiovascular system.

The issue was given substance through the passage by the Congress of the Rehabilitation Act of 1973 (Public Law 93-112), and as amended by Public Law 93-516 of 1974 and the promulgation of regulations implementing Sections 503 and 504 of the Act. The essence of the mandates can be stated simply. The Rehabilitation Act guarantees the civil rights of persons with disabilities, and the pertinent sections are specific. Section 503 states that federal contractors and subcontractors may not discriminate against any employee or candidate for employment on the grounds of physical or mental disability for any position for which the applicant is otherwise qualified. Such contractors with procurement contracts of $2,500 or more are required further to take affirmative action to employ and promote qualified disabled persons at all job levels.

In Section 504, the language of Titles VI and IX of the 1964 Civil Rights Act is used in extending to all handicapped persons the guarantees of equal treatment of racial minorities and women. The final wording in Section 504 succinctly spells out the mandate: "No otherwise qualified handicapped individual in the United States . . . shall, solely by reason of his handicap, be excluded from the participation in, be denied the benefits of, or be subjected to discrimination under, any program or activity receiving Federal financial assistance," which includes money, services, and property.

In view of the federal fiscal support in research, defense, education, environmental preservation, small businesses, and the like, it is seen readily that extraordinarily few institutions are totally free of contractual relationships with the federal government, so the requirements of the Rehabilitation Act may be considered as reaching nearly every employer in this country.

While not immediately related to current employment, but germane in the light of future employment is the case of an applicant to a school of nursing who was accepted initially, but rejected after a physical examination revealed that she had Crohn's disease. She sought relief under Section 504, as the school received federal financial assistance. A federal appeals court granted an injunction ordering the nursing school to accept the candidate and later ruled in favor of the appellant and against the school [22].

In a second case, a woman was refused employment in 1974 because of overweight; the examining physician noted "gross obesity." She was 5 feet 6 inches tall and in that year weighed 249 pounds. After 10 years in the courts, the New York State Court of Appeals ruled in May 1985 that the employer had no right to refuse her employment. Estimated compensation due her was approximately $100,000. She got full insurance benefits and was not required to take a second examination. Further, the company paid moving expenses from Staten Island to Rochester when she began work September 9, 1985 [23].

Further clarification is helpful in understanding the process of compliance. First, the personnel actions implicit in the proscription of discrimination include not only initial hiring, but also promotion or demotion, transfer, layoff, rehiring, and application of all benefits such as leaves of absence, sick leave, training programs, and any other fringe benefit offered by the employer.

Secondly, once the handicapped individual is hired, the employer is required to take reasonable steps to accommodate to the disability, unless such action would cause undue hardship. "Reasonable accommodation" includes the provision of accessible facilities, job restructuring, modification of work schedules, the provision of special devices, the addition of readers for the blind if paperwork is required, and so on [24]. It can be expected that employees with compensated defects, postillness or postinjury residua, congenital anomalies, sensory deficits, or certain static impairments will require such accommodation. A deaf worker requiring telephone contacts may be supplied an interpreter, a user of a wheelchair must have adequate workspace and access, and an employee who must visit a methadone clinic daily may need a minor adjustment in working hours.

Current thinking divides consideration of the individual's disability into elements that are job-related or employment-related. For example, if a certain machine requires bimanual operation and no redesign is feasible, then an uncompensated upper-extremity amputee would not be able to function in that position effectively because the use of two arms is definitely job-related. An applicant who presents with controlled hypertension or has diabetes cannot be rejected because it is believed that the disorder may adversely affect the retirement program or the life insurance program. Such a condition is thought of as "employment-related" and cannot serve as a basis for rejection in the employment process. Actuarial data, company experience, costly benefit packages, and the like have no role in the hiring of handicapped persons. In essence, one cannot use so-called future-risk criteria in considering applicants for employment, as such practice would be contrary to the legislation cited previously.

Particular efforts have been made by the former U.S. Civil Service Commission (currently the Office of Personnel Management) and the President's Committee on Employment of the Handicapped to bring into service persons who have static limitations and, in some cases, persons with progressive disease. The push-pull movement still continues between proponents for acceptance and the hiring authorities. A second difficulty is to be found with examining physicians of an older vintage to whom physical variance means disability, ergo inability to work. Another block to more liberal hiring is the employment interviewer who is inclined to discourage the visibly different applicant—the paraplegic, the amputee, the blind—and, infrequently, the candidate whose limitation cannot be seen but who has answered truthfully certain medically oriented questions insinuated into the employment application.

Strongly favoring employer acceptance of the so-called handicapped have been personnel of the disease-identified voluntary health agencies—heart, cancer, multiple sclerosis, epilepsy, and the like—who campaign wisely and usually with foundations of good research supporting their platforms. The basis of opposition to these movements is to be found primarily in workers' compensation decisions that, in many situations, punish the employer for having hired the individual with heart disease, epilepsy, or pneumoconiosis by granting excessive awards. Further, the existence of the so-called presumptive clause in California provides all firefighters, sworn police personnel, and district attorney investigators, among others, the presumption under workers' compensation law, although rebuttable, that their heart disease, pneumonia, tuberculosis, hernia, or cancer arose out of or in the course of their employment. Frequently, lobbying to make the presumptive clause conclusive, thus nonrebuttable, is carried on. Awards for heart disease, with corrective surgery and lifelong pensions, are extremely costly.

Suggestions are offered for certain yardsticks to be applied when appraising an applicant's ability to work. Common to all situations, though, is the plea that all candidates be given a thorough, individual review and that their capacities be matched against the demands of the job. Not every man or woman seeking work need meet the requirements laid on the astronauts. For example, there are many jobs that the brace-wearing, 50-year-old individual who has had polio can fill without having to undergo excessive ambulation while at work.

In essence, preplacement examinations are conducted to determine that job applicants will be able to carry out their assigned tasks without harm to themselves or others and, if a chronic or static disorder is present, to assure the employer and the employee that such tasks repeatedly performed will not aggravate the condition. Further, the findings on such a medical review make up a statement of health that will serve as a baseline or standard against which to match future estimates of well-being. Health, being relative, must be viewed in the context of the human capacity to cope, to survive, and to grow. A person with one kidney can be in excellent health, as can be a functioning individual with paraplegia. It is the role of the physician and the other members of the occupational health team to ascertain that this health will not be destroyed in the course of the employee's pursuit of a wage.

The legislative mandates cited earlier do not eliminate the need for criteria or standards to be used by the examiner, for job demands vary, and certain positions can be filled by persons with a variety of physical limitations, while others because of certain stressors or needs for strength or endurance may be carried out only by workers free of most illness residua.

The issues of employment and standards should not be left without some reference to the oft-quoted "healthy worker effect (HWE)." Much actuarial calculation has been based on the concept that, because of the method of selection used in adding personnel, the worker is in better health than the general population. The belief has been reviewed critically by Wen and co-workers [25], who point out that the HWE is the composite result from factors such as selection of workforce, changes in lifestyle accompanying employment, and methodologic characteristics of the standardized mortality ratio (SMR). The writers indicate that other factors, beyond selection, are important. They include such employment-associated benefits as economic gain, medical insurance, lifestyle changes, the proportion of active workers, the calculation method, data completeness, length of follow-up, and certain characteristics of SMR methodology. Some of the "effect" is traceable to SMR methodology, and the strength of the HWE depends on the proportion of active workers in the cohort being followed. The disappearance of the HWE may result from such factors as aging of the cohort, totally unrelated to the true increase in mortality risk. They conclude that its disappearance may be an artifact of SMR methodology, thus explanatory of the observed mortality deficit.

MEDICAL STANDARDS—SAN BERNARDINO PROJECT

While there have been efforts dating to World War II to identify the physical and environmental demands of jobs so that applicants' physical and emotional capacities could be matched against them in the process of selective placement [26], it has only been in recent years that a new system has been devised that has met considerable enthusiastic response in the public sector. The Medical Standards Project developed by the County of San Bernardino, California produced standards that were job-related as determined by an assessment of the physical demands of a wide variety of jobs, the procedure termed physical abilities analysis. Job-related standards are based on job requirements, "those factors that relate directly to the applicant's immediate ability to perform the essential functions of the job" [27]. When these demands and requirements become known, they can be used as the basis for the development of a comprehensive set of preplacement standards or guidelines [28]. The system should be applicable to nearly all jobs; it should be practicable and understood by users such as physicians, nurses, managers, and personnel specialists; and the results should be quantifiable, reliable, and objective.

Initially, 15 benchmark jobs were chosen for rating, jobs that represented the range of physically demanding positions in the county. Of three groups of raters—supervisor, incumbents, and personnel specialists—it was found that the actual jobholders were the best groups to rate the jobs, as manifested by the

TABLE 5-1. *Scale and Activities of Dynamic Flexibility*

Dynamic flexibility	*Scale*	*Activity*
Requires many fast and repeated body-bending, twisting, or stretching movements.	7	
		Do the butterfly stroke in a championship swim competition at the Olympics
	6	
	5	Saw dead wood
	4	
		Milk cows
	3	
		Fill a bag with shells at the seashore
Requires few repeated bending, twisting or stretching movements where speed is not important	2	
	1	

SOURCE: Modified from S. W. Nylander and G. Carmean, *Medical Standards Project Final Report* (3rd rev. ed.). San Bernardino, CA: County of San Bernardino, Personnel Division, Oct 1984. Vol. I.

highest interrater agreement level among the three groups.

Of the physical abilities judged, the ones eventually used in the project were the following:

Strength—static strength, explosive strength, dynamic strength, trunk strength;
Stamina—stamina, effort;
Flexibility—extent flexibility, dynamic flexibility, durability, speed of limit movement, gross body coordination, gross body equilibrium;
Use of hands and arms—arm-hand steadiness, manual dexterity, finger dexterity;
Vision—near vision, far vision, visual color discrimination;
Hearing—ability to hear and understand conversation in a quiet environment, the same in a noisy environment, the ability to tell where a sound is coming from, the ability to discriminate among environmental nonspeech sounds

Each of the physical abilities is defined, and the differences between a single ability and others possibly akin to it are clarified. For example, *dynamic flexibility* (No. 8) is defined as follows: "[T]he ability to bend, stretch, twist, or reach out with the body, arms and/or legs both quickly and repeatedly" [29]. The difference between dynamic flexibility and other abilities is illustrated in this manner [29]:

Dynamic Flexibility: Involves both *speed and repeated* bending or stretching;	vs	*Extent Flexibility* No. 7: Requires no speed, just degree of bending or stretching in *single* movements.
And involves the degree to which the *muscles "bounce back"* during repeated bending or stretching.	vs	*Stamina* No. 5: Involves the degree to which *one does not get winded* when doing physical work over time.

TABLE 5-2. *Working Conditions*

1. Inside	19. Silica dust
2. Outside	20. Allergenic [substances]
3. Low temperature	21. Toxic conditions
4. High temperature	22. Chemical irritant
5. Sudden temperature changes	23. Oily [conditions]
6. Low humidity	24. Odors
7. High humidity	25. Explosives
8. Wetness	26. Electrical hazards
9. Slippery surfaces	27. Ionizing radiation
10. Body injuries	28. Infections
11. High elevations	29. Air pressure
12. Confined spaces and/or cramped body positions	30. Working with others
13. Moving objects	31. Responsibility for persons
14. Vibration	32. Job complexity
15. Noise	33. Role ambiguity
16. Burns	34. Irregular or extended work hours
17. Non-ionizing radiation	

SOURCE: S. W. Nylander and G. Carmean, *Medical Standards Project Final Report* (3rd rev. ed.). San Bernardino, CA: County of San Bernardino, Personnel Division, Oct 1984. Vol. I.

Each ability is given a seven-point scale with examples of various physical activities positioned on the scale to illustrate the range of energy expenditure. For example, still using *dynamic flexibility*, the scale and four activities are shown in Table 5-1 [29]:

The *working conditions* are also defined and are divided over a four-point range: no effect, little, moderate, or great. The working conditions are shown in Table 5-2. The four-point range used to evaluate or rate the extent of each working condition is exemplified by the levels given for *high elevations* (No. 11) [29]:

0. No effect—is not a condition of the job.
1. Little—work from platforms or fairly stable surfaces up to 4 feet above floor or ground level.
2. Moderate—work from ladders or other surfaces from 4 to 12 feet above floor or ground level.
3. Work from ladders, scaffolding, rigging, bosun's chairs, or other equipment more than 12 feet above floor or ground level.

In the development of standards, the bodily organ systems were listed individually as follows:

Skin
Nose and mouth
Ears and hearing
Eyes and vision
Respiratory system
Heart
Peripheral vascular system
Gastrointestinal system
Genitourinary tract
Musculoskeletal system
Nervous system
Endocrine, metabolic, and nutritional systems
Hematopoietic and lymphatic systems

An example of the rating of physical abilities with a particular physical finding is taken from the standards for the musculoskeletal system [28]:

No. 41: Spondylolisthesis, without operation, Category B, acceptable if the demands of the job do not exceed:
3 on Static Strength
4 on Explosive Strength
3.5 on Dynamic Strength
4 on Trunk Strength
3 on Stamina
3.5 on Extent Flexibility
3 on Dynamic Flexibility
3.5 on Speed of Limb Movement
3 on Body Coordination
2.5 on Body Equilibrium
4 on Mobility

Illustrative of the use of the working conditions scales is the following standard from the division on the heart:

No. 11: *Coronary Heart Disease, Functional Class I* (asymptomatic, positive exercise ECG or coronary angiogram with obstruction of 50 percent or less proximately) is acceptable if the demands of the job do not exceed:*
4.5 on Stamina
4.5 on Dynamic Strength
4.5 on Trunk Strength
5 on Explosive Strength
5 on Static Strength;
and working conditions do not exceed:
2 on Extreme Heat
2 on Extreme Cold

In organ systems where the use of a numerical scale is infeasible, the standard is given in the form of a statement accompanied by a rationale. For example, under the gastrointestinal system, one finds the following [27]:

No. 10: Chronic Regional Enteritis (Crohn's Disease) is acceptable other than safety positions if the symptoms permit the applicant to perform the essential functions of the job.
Rationale: This condition is subject to remissions and relapses; symptoms include abdominal pain, diarrhea, and extra-intestinal symptoms such as arthritis, which pose significant placement problems.

In the published standards more than 400 medical disorders were included, based on these criteria: (1) the occurrence of the disease or condition in the applicant population, (2) the significance or nonsignificance for employment of a disease or medical condition, and (3) evidence that the disorder was incorporated into the medical standards of various California employers [28].

As the methods of analyzing the working conditions and physical abilities necessary to perform a job are included in the project report, the system can be applied to and developed in any employment situation. The technique is recommended, for the basis of acceptance or rejection of an applicant for work is strictly job-relatedness, and it allows the employment of persons previously denied work because of perceived "future risk" and legitimately permits the denial of candidates whose clinical condition might readily produce incapacity in them or others [28].

The system used in the central San Bernardino project has been extended to and validated successfully in several other jurisdictions by OCCU-MED,†

*Rationale for scalar values lies with relationship between a person's maximum oxygen consumption and maximum cardiac output, which in turn relates to a person's ability to perform the job.

†OCCU-MED Corporate Health Services, 95 N. Marengo Avenue, Pasadena, California 91101, telephone (818) 795-8666. It is headed by James Johnson, the original project director for the San Bernardino study.

a firm specializing in the development of medical standards for municipalities, governmental agencies, and companies in the private sector.

SPECIFIC DISEASE ENTITIES AND PLACEMENT

Certain clinical states will be discussed separately, for over the years they have led to considerable disagreement and misunderstanding when entered into the employing process.

DIABETES MELLITUS

Periodically, knowledgeable concerned groups have published guidelines on the employment of persons with diabetes [30–33]. The pith of such recommendations has been that the individual with controlled diabetes can be employed, and it has been seen that most adults with diabetes, insulin-dependent or not, are gainfully at work.

More recently, the guidelines have been updated by Mastbaum, Tetrick, and Alexander [34] in light of contemporary knowledge to provide guidance for the employment and job placement of diabetic persons and to aid in ensuring a safe work environment for both individuals with diabetes and persons free from the disease. Based on conclusions of the National Diabetes Data Group of the National Institutes of Health (NIH), certain standards were established for the definitive diagnosis of the disorder, and emphasis was given to the fact that "a definitive diagnosis of diabetes cannot be made on the basis of random blood or urine sugar test results" [34].

A person with diabetes that is controlled can be employed, and control involves congruence with these minimum standards:

1. Only infrequent insulin reactions and none that is sufficiently severe to require assistance from other persons. The more remote these reactions, the less need for job limitations or modification.
2. Only infrequent occurrence of symptomatic hyperglycemia or hyperglycemia with marked acetonuria.
3. Continuing satisfactory supervision by personal physician.
4. No complications that would impair job performance or limit attendance.

The new guidelines, as before, divide individuals with diabetes into four categories in accordance with their treatment status:

1. Treatment by diet alone, thus rendering the individual capable of undertaking any job for which he or she is qualified.
2. Treatment by oral blood sugar–lowering agents, thus rendering the individual capable of undertaking any job for which he or she is qualified.
3. Treatment by use of insulin:
   a. The worker should be restricted from jobs where it would be difficult and/or hazardous to stop an operation to treat a reaction. Such individuals should not be at work where an unexpected insulin reaction would cause injury to themselves or other workers.
   b. Whether work restrictions are needed in hazardous operations that can be stopped for treatment of reactions should be determined by the frequency and severity of such reactions and the length of time since a reaction of this type was experienced. Driving a passenger vehicle is permitted if there has been no alteration in the state of consciousness in the past year.
   c. Undergoing frequent shift changes, or working split shifts, is undesirable if it interferes with the control of the disease.
   d. The individual is capable of performing any job for which he or she is qualified, if not coming within the above restrictive categories.
4. Presence of significant complications irrespective of treatment group: some limitations as applicable to workers with cardiovascular, visual, renal, nervous, or other system disease without the presence of diabetes.

In substance, the person with controlled diabetes is employable, and such absences as might be anticipated because of late-onset complications can be shortened or eliminated by good and continuing occupational medical oversight, meaning strict control of blood sugar levels and early and expert attention to impending complications.* In addition, no person

*It must be noted that under Federal Aviation Administration (FAA) regulations [35] a medical certificate of any class will be denied if an applicant for airman status has an established medical history or clinical diagnosis of diabetes requiring insulin or any other hypoglycemic drug. In a more recent review by the American Medical Association of the medical standards for civilian airmen [36], it was recommended that strict guidelines be followed concerning the appropriate administrative management of pilots with non-insulin-dependent diabetes. There should be trials of diet therapy only or diet therapy with oral hypoglycemic agents for at least 3 months, during which time the airman must be educated about his or her diabetes.

with diabetes should be assigned a task that would either preclude eating a regular meal or make the meal late. Problems of alcoholism should be identified early and treatment and counseling instituted. Also, the presence of diabetes cannot be blamed as a cause of even a minor accident with the erroneous notion that such attribution would obviate legal penalty.

Although much has been written regarding the work attendance patterns of diabetic individuals, no consistency existed among the conclusions. In a study involving employees at the Hanford Operations in Richland, Washington [37], the records of 108 employees out of 8,000 (prevalence of diabetes of 1.4 percent) were reviewed for absences over one-half day. The group had an average annual sickness absentee rate of 6.3 days, and in every age group the rate was less than that for workers free from diabetes.

Another concern regarding the employed diabetic person has been the risk of skeletal fracture. Heath and coworkers [37] studied 1,000 individuals with diabetes, matched with appropriate controls, and found that the risk ratios were not significantly greater than 1.0. Considered were both osteoporotic and nonosteoporotic fracture sites.

It should be pointed out that for appropriate medical designation of employed persons with diabetes, the new standards for classification should be used and old terms discarded. The work of the National Diabetes Data Group of the NIH included the development of a new classification for the purposes of a uniform framework for use in research and the production of more meaningful and comparative data [39,40]. The essential changes are as follows:

Class	*Former Terminology*
Diabetes mellitus (DM) type (IDDM), type I	Juvenile diabetes, juvenile-onset diabetes, brittle diabetes
Non-insulin-dependent types (NIDDM), type II Nonobese NIDDM Obese NIDDM	Adult-onset diabetes, maturity-onset diabetes, stable diabetes
Other types, including DM associated with certain conditions and syndromes	Secondary diabetes
Impaired glucose tolerance (IGT) Nonobese IGT Obese IGT IGT associated with certain conditions and syndromes	Asymptomatic diabetes, chemical diabetes, latent diabetes
Gestational diabetes	Gestational diabetes

The use of this classification will allow comparison of data derived from a work population with national epidemiologic or research findings.

One additional point should be included. It was once expressed in connection with the work of the individual with diabetes that peaks of emotional excitement should not be inherent in the position. With the employment of such a person, there should be frequent, possibly quarterly, visits to the occupational health service for a general review and counseling, with an occupational health nurse or a physician, regarding the employee's disease status as it relates to work stressors, change of assignment, and the like. Preventive intervention is indicated whenever therapeutic balance seems threatened.

A brief questionnaire can be devised for completion by the applicant's (or employee's) family physician. The information resulting will be useful in both placement and follow-up of the new employee. The queries should concern the status of control, the understanding of the disease by the individual, the insulin dosage, weight, adverse reactions (insulin reaction or acidosis), complications, and any additional areas relative to work assignments.

CONVULSIVE DISORDERS

Applicants with epilepsy have fared poorly in the labor market and most often have had to meet their needs for employment in sheltered workshops where the wages may not be proportionate to their skills. Those persons with an early onset of the disease may have been educated inadequately, may have suffered some social isolation, and subsequently may have developed certain personality deficits that would make interpersonal relationships difficult. Many individuals with epilepsy, however, have completed college and have entered into jobs, assuming responsible positions, particularly when the employer proved to be understanding of the problem. In recent years, acceptance of the individual with epilepsy, as a person, has been given reinforcement by the successful acting career in television and films of David Carradine, a young man who has publicized his own condition, as has Congressman Tony Coelho of California.

It is with epilepsy that most denials of chronic illness appear among applicants' medical histories. Through experience, they have learned of their low level of acceptance, so that the presence of a convulsive disorder is disclaimed. Such individuals, if hired, come to work with the added concern that, given sufficient stressors, they will have a seizure, and thus their disease will become known. Embarrassment ensues bilaterally, and the employee may be discharged for falsification of records—even though work performance to date might have been excellent and lengthy. It is best for applicants to declare the condition, even though there may be many rejections before they are successful in obtaining employment. Riley [41] has pointed out that lying about the disorder when seeking either employment or insurance leaves both the patient and the physician vulnerable to ethical and legal charges. No physician should advise a patient to disclaim a convulsive disorder, nor should the physician employ diagnostic euphemisms to avoid facing the patient with the word *epilepsy.* It is to be noted that a woman who lied on her job application about having epilepsy was subsequently terminated when a trace of an anticonvulsive medication was found on laboratory testing. The applicant admitted to the falsehood, for she believed she had no physical disability, having been free of seizures since the age of 14. Hired in September 1977 and fired 9 days later, the woman appealed, and in May 1980, General Motors was ordered to offer her the job with back pay and benefits. The employer refused the order, a referee upheld General Motors, but the Civil Rights Committee of Michigan ruled in favor of the appellant. The issue involved entitlement to be in response to an illegal question [42].

When there is concurrence that an applicant with a convulsive disorder can be employed, the immediate work-group leader must be apprised of the condition so that if a seizure takes place, the worker's peers will be able to assist intelligently and without panic. Rarely does an applicant or employee object to planning of this type, and most fellow workers wish to be and are helpful. At no time should there be a change in assignment without agreement by the medical authority, even if a temporary change only is planned.

Some occupational health personnel have established time criteria for employment of the person with epilepsy. For example, an applicant who has been seizure-free for 2 years will be employed. This type of yardstick is believed to be spurious because a person under good control with anticonvulsive medication may still have a seizure when subjected to a stressor sufficient to cause a safety-valve release. To be sure, if an applicant's immediate history reveals that there have been frequent severe seizures, then it is assumed that the candidate either is inadequately controlled or is under severe emotional tension; with either situation, the applicant is not employable until there is a cessation of the seizures. When the seizures cease for 6 months, employment should be considered but restrictions would be placed on the individual including no work at heights (over 5 feet), no work in or near pits or open tanks, no driving of motor vehicles or other mobile equipment, no work involving open containers of caustic or other toxic chemicals, no work around hazardous motorized equipment, and the like.

While anticonvulsant medications decrease or abolish the seizures characteristic of the disorder and optimize the employment outcome for innumerable individuals, there is the possibility of untoward side effects. Needing research, as indicated by Blank and Anderson [43] is the one important dimension of drug therapy, namely evaluation of the differential effects of these agents in regard to the psychological, cognitive, and performance factors. With the work applicant in question, contact must be maintained with the private physician so that the seizures remain controlled without the damaging psychopharmacologic effects. The employee must remain seizure-free and, at the same time, not be subjected to the toxicity of the medication.

Halen [44] has highlighted a significant issue in the employment of persons with epilepsy. He suggests that those individuals should be counseled relative to entry work where reasonable advancement might occur. It is possible that there could be progression to work with hazards inappropriate for such a person. It would be most prudent for the individual to make a career judgment at the time of initial or early employment so that the problem can be averted before a career is too solidly established.

As indicated, the knowledgeable assistance of a supervisor may be required at the time of seizure of one of the group's employees. The following instructions can be issued to the supervisor at the time of placement so that if the individual has a seizure, the usual distress among fellow workers can be avoided.

First aid for a person with an epileptic seizure:

Keep calm. The person is usually not suffering or in danger.

Help the employee to a safe place but DO NOT restrain movements. Loosen tight clothing.

After the jerking of the seizure has subsided, and if the individual is still unconscious, *turn the person on his or her side* with the face gently turned downward.

DO NOT PUT ANYTHING BETWEEN THE TEETH.

DO NOT give anything to drink.

Stand by until the person has recovered consciousness and from the confusion that sometimes follows a seizure.

Let the person rest if tired, then encourage him or her to resume regular activities.

It is rarely necessary to call public authorities, a physician, or an ambulance. However, in cases of prolonged seizures, or if a person injures himself by falling, it may be wise to secure professional help.

CANCER

To most employers, the question of hiring an applicant who has had surgical extirpation of a malignant growth will not loom large. In the occupational health service (OHS) with which the author was associated previously, where an extremely large number of preplacement medical examinations was done each day, there were only a few persons who applied for positions who had experienced recent surgery. Candidates who have reached a 5-year cure normally present no difficulty in acceptance for employment. Even if prosthetic appliances are used—for an extremity, breast, or ear—placement is not made more complex. Occasionally, in an older worker, the problem of mobility will require study if a lower-extremity prosthesis is involved. Postlaryngectomy patients and persons with colostomies can be employed, being able to perform effectively physically, psychologically, and aesthetically. Difficulties in persons of this group may be emotional disorders rather than primary problems in physical readjustment.

The term "cure" in this connection implies that the patient remains free of disease and has the same life expectancy as a person who has never had cancer. The problem of employment is a continuing one, for millions of Americans now living will eventually have cancer; many, therefore, will be persons available to the labor market, a large number of whom will be seeking work or a return to their former jobs. Two fears have been expressed—that subsequent industrial injury will bring about large workers' compensation awards, and that death sometime after employment will affect a group insurance plan adversely. No documentation has been encountered to support these beliefs.

It has been the author's practice to study each applicant individually rather than to apply a rigid "5-year-cure rule" to all. Complete documentation of the case history is obtained, with particular concern that copies are received of the surgical report and of the histopathologic findings of the excised tissue. It is known that when regional disease is present, the 5-year survival status is significantly impaired. Regionalization, age, site, type of cancer, and other variables are considered, and a decision is made as to the risk of employability. In most instances, post-surgical patients have been accepted. Again, judging from personal experience, without substantive data, it seems that less difficulty as to recurrence and early lethality has been experienced among applicants than among employees in whom malignant growths were encountered during the work career.

Wheatley and associates [45] at the Metropolitan Life Insurance Company reported on a 14-year study concerned with the employment of persons treated for cancer. Between 1959 and 1972, 74 men and women with a history of malignant disease were accepted for employment, representing about 1 in 1,600 applicants. The shortest interval between treatment and employment was 1 month, and nearly three-fifths of the candidates entered service within 5 years following therapy. The time was determined by the applicant and was not a prerequisite of the company. During the study, because of experience, the acceptance rate increased. The turnover rate of the study group was about the same as that of comparable employees of the same age, and work performance was satisfactory. Further, cost was not noticeably increased by excessive absences, reduced productivity, or increased mortality. It was concluded that selective employment of such applicants in positions for which they were physically qualified was sound industrial practice.

In a second report from essentially the same group [46], the roles of the personal and occupational physicians are detailed in the referral and evaluation for employment of the cancer-treated patient. The essence of the described program involving 74 individuals was stabilization of the lesion so that there could be a reasonable expectation of continuous service. While this program was centered around selective employment, it was found that the attrition rate was similar to that of noncancer employees—it did not exceed the usual "turnover" rate. Given emphasis was the need for good cooperation from the primary care physician and knowledgeable decisions regarding employment.

With the conditions of the Rehabilitation Act of 1973 still in effect, most likely every applicant with a history of treated malignant disease will be employed. Survival and mortality rates are reviewed in recent writings [47–50].

In most post–cancer surgery patients, few problems present themselves in placement, but some precautions are to be noted. The ostomy patient must be certain that the stoma is sufficiently covered or sealed so as to avoid mucosal absorption of toxic materials if a spill of liquids occurs. In postlaryngectomy patients, it was learned through query of 3,000 members of Lost Chord Clubs [50] that certain industrial processes cause irritation to breathing. The industrial activities are numerous, and the noxious contactants comprise earth, dust, fibers, particles of brick, lime silica, wood, metal, a variety of chemicals, and their resultant fumes, vapors and mists. See Gardner [50a] for a complete list of sources and "incidental dispersoids, vapors, and gases."

The laryngectomized individual presents no difficulty in placement apart from the potentially noxious exposures noted above. The person whose larynx has been removed surgically can communicate either through learned esophageal speech or through the use of a hand-held artificial larynx or the new "hands-free" stoma-insertable prosthesis [51]. Laryngectomized individuals have been employed in all positions, from plant manager to heavy equipment operator to waitress [52].

That considerable education still is required at the worksite has emerged from two classic studies by Feldman [53–54] involving cancer patients. Of 127 white-collar workers interviewed, 54 percent had work-connected problems that they attributed to cancer. A fourth of the sample met discriminatory action through job loss, refusal of promotion or another job, or changes in working conditions, hours, salaries, or insurance coverage. Of the blue-collar workers studied, 84 percent of 120 individuals associated work problems with their medical history. A third of the respondents had been demoted or denied cost-of-living increases that were received by others. Most striking, though, was the experience of a man who had lost his job—"You'll be absent too much now"—when he applied for other work. The employment interviewer asked him to complete his application with a pencil instead of the office pen, for pencils were cheaper to discard [53].

CEREBRAL PALSY

One of the most perplexing problems in placement is that offered by the person with severe spasticity who applies for employment. The difficulty is not one of less intelligence on the part of the applicant, but in the inability to compete in most areas of communication. Because of spasticity, and as determined by the degree of involvement, there is great difficulty in writing legibly, typing with any speed, using the telephone, or conversing understandably. The picture is further clouded by the impatience and embarrassment manifested by the listener. The person with cerebral palsy with only mild involvement can communicate, particularly after having lost much of the stress experienced with the new job. A new situation, with people unfamiliar to the individual, accentuates every problem the spastic person has—speech, coordination, gait, grasp, and tremor. Once the individual is comfortable with the new scene and is accepted, much of the exaggeration of the basic problem clears.

Without question, there is considerable prejudice against the person whose appearance, motions, and oral sounds are abnormal and who may show, in addition, some drooling. Placement should involve related disciplines such as social case work, vocational rehabilitation counseling, psychiatric or psychological counseling, and speech therapy, in addition to medicine. As in the case of the applicant with epilepsy, an understanding, helpful, and challenged supervisor should aid in the placement. Frequently encountered is the "over-rehabilitated" client who has been educated to a level beyond that which he or she can use in the work scene. The employee becomes disenchanted with the work assigned, yet the employer cannot provide the communicative aids (or aides) that will allow full expression of the capacity to contribute.

Finally, certain orthotic or assistive devices can be fabricated that will provide some control of involuntary movement so that machine operation might become possible.

HEART DISEASE

The growth of the concept in workers' compensation administration that work can cause heart disease has made employers extraordinarily wary about hiring the cardiac applicant. The resistance has increased particularly with the greater utilization of saphenous or arterial bypass grafts in the correction of coronary artery insufficiency, where the costs can become overwhelming. The high awards that have been given, plus the actions undertaken in California in keeping with the presumptive clause indicated earlier, have led employers to reject almost every applicant with a history of cardiovascular disease, whether it was static or progressive, old or recent, or incapacitating or unimpairing. Certain factors should be considered in the employability of persons with heart disease, including the clinical nature of the disorder, the therapeutic regimen, such personal characteristics as age, education, and work experience, the type of work to be undertaken, and specific environmental factors concerning the emotional climate at home and on the job, commuting demands, and even the idiosyncrasies of the weather.

There is need, therefore, for an individual, well-honed, and studied evaluation of the candidate presenting with a positive history. Of greatest need for consideration is the type of job being sought. Positions requiring arduous labor rule out most cardiac applicants, and many unskilled and semiskilled candidates are not trained for less-demanding work activity.

A special cardiac appraisal should be conducted, which includes, in addition to the complete history and physical examination, a resting electrocardiogram (ECG), and if hypertension is present, renal function studies should be added. If conditions warrant—no evidence of ischemia and medically controlled, lowered blood pressure—one might consider dynamic electrocardiography utilizing a stationary bicycle ergometer or the treadmill. Particularly emphasized is the need to confirm the diagnosis of a cardiac disorder. Early work by Dr. Leonard Goldwater and the work classification units revealed the great number of erroneously labelled cardiac patients.

Of particular concern in placement of the individual with heart disease is the applicant presenting with a history of ischemic heart disease who has had surgical intervention by means of coronary artery bypass grafts (CABG). Several studies have been conducted of the return-to-work and employability of such persons. In one organization it was estimated that there were 100 CABG operations in a 6-year span within a work force of 15,000 [54a]. All but two of the employees returned to work. The initial reduced work schedule following release by the private physician and the medical director's approval consisted of 4 hours a day, 5 days a week for the first 1 or 2 weeks. This limitation was raised to 6 hours per day, 5 days a week for the next 1 to 2 weeks, and finally there was a return to a regular 8-hour daily schedule. If the employee had a strenuous job assignment presurgery, he was given a "light" or sedentary job on return. In no case was any returnee permitted to climb stairs or ladders, bend or stoop frequently, or lift items over 25 pounds in weight. All followed a prudent regimen—close attention to weight, diet, smoking, and exercise. The belief was expressed that the workers who had cardiac surgery were "better employees" because of improved morale and greater dedication.

In an investigation by Stanton and coworkers [55], preoperative predictors of postoperative employment status were studied in 228 patients undergoing either CABG or cardiac valve surgery. Of the 150 persons employed in the year before surgery, 73 percent returned within 6 months. Of those patients not working previously, 18 percent began working. Those individuals expecting preoperatively to return to work did so at a rate of 82 percent, in contrast to a rate of 39 percent for the others. Educational level and family income were stronger predictors of return than occupation or required level of physical exertion. The authors concluded that determinants of resumption of work activity are largely present before surgery and that patients' attitudes and expectations play a significant role. These findings are in parallel with observations of the comeback made by persons with serious disablement following other acute illness or trauma.

A later study involving most of the same investigators [56] revealed that 75 percent of employed persons returned to work after CABG surgery, suggesting that the great majority of patients were able to resume normal economic and social functioning within 6 months following intervention.

It was pointed out by Dimsdale and colleagues [57] that, following their first myocardial infarction (MI), 40 to 60 percent of patients failed to return to work within 6 months in spite of their physical ability to resume normal activity.* A 1-year follow-up showed that of 42 percent of 182 men were either persistently unemployed or working at a lower level, 40 percent were at their same jobs, and 19 percent were in more demanding jobs. The most important variables predictive of work status—in diminishing importance—were age, subsequent morbid cardiac events, past MI, and mood during the follow-up year. It is of interest that the extent of vessel involvement was important as a work-prognostic variable. The factor of age was seen in the finding that the older the patient, the less likely the resumption of work, irrespective of symptoms or rectifying surgery.

The essence of this research is that persons who have had an MI or CABG surgery, or both, will return to work and that none need be rejected provided job demands and physical and emotional capacities are matched for good placement.

Some jurisdictions have issued standards for motor vehicle operators, with particular reference to drivers with cardiac difficulties. Such regulations should be sought from all local or appropriate sources [58].

In the placement of an applicant with a heart disorder, it might be useful to classify the individual in keeping with *Nomenclature and Criteria for Diagnosis of Diseases of the Heart and Great Vessels,* as promulgated by the New York Heart Association [59]. In this schema, the etiology of the heart disease, the anatomic lesions identified, and the physiologic disturbances are noted, to which two other categories are added, specifically the cardiac status and prognosis.

Complete nomenclature is provided for the etiologic, anatomic, and physiologic diagnoses, and the cardiac status and prognosis are derived from this classification [59]:

Cardiac Status	*Prognosis*
1. Uncompromised	1. Good
2. Slightly compromised	2. Good with therapy
3. Moderately compromised	3. Fair with therapy
4. Severely compromised	4. Guarded despite therapy

*The failure to return to work was accredited to smouldering depression, lack of understanding of the implications of the heart disease, employer discrimination, and secondary gain from insurance benefits [57].

An example is the following for a patient with rheumatic heart disease [59]:

Etiologic	Rheumatic fever, inactive
Anatomic	Enlarged heart (left atrium, pulmonary artery, right ventricle), mitral valvular deformity
Physiologic	Atrial fibrillation, mitral obstruction, pulmonary hypertension
Cardiac status and prognosis	3.2

Through discussion with the applicant's treating physician, such a set of diagnoses should be obtained and updated periodically as an aid in both initial and continuing placement. Through use of these various mechanisms, placement can be effected without hazard to the applicant or his fellow workers.

As more and more exercise testing may be used in placement, particularly in stress-intensive positions, rational decisions must be made in keeping with significant ECG findings. A complete guide for placement, insofar as ECG abnormalities are concerned in clinically normal persons, will be found in Barret [60].

EMOTIONAL AND MENTAL ILLNESS

As psychological counseling and psychotherapy have become more commonplace in society, the job applicants presenting a history of this type of care will be in greater number than ever before. With divorce rates rising, an additional number of persons will have consulted marriage counselors. With the increased emphasis given behavioral science and psychiatry in the medical schools, there are fewer physicians in the occupational scene who bear prejudicial intolerance for anyone with a history of emotional or psychiatric illness.

If a consultant in clinical psychology or psychiatry is available, certain factors may be used as bases warranting referral for a professional evaluation. These include (1) history of emotional problems; (2) history of substance abuse; (3) atypical behavior (during preplacement examination); (4) presence of physical disorders with a possible behavioral etiology, such as duodenal ulcer or hypertension; (5) related emotional difficulties, as determined by responses on a health questionnaire; (6) applicant seeking a "high-stress" or critical position; and (7) history of unstable work career or numerous, frequent job changes.

Applicants so referred may be qualified for employment, disqualified if placement would put the candidate's or fellow worker's health status in jeopardy, or conditionally qualified, which would allow periodic evaluation during a probationary period. It may be that, with concurrent counseling or therapy from an outside specialist, the applicant could meet the demands of the job. Further, supportive counseling could be provided by the OHS. The seeking of needed treatment may be made a condition of employment.

It must be stressed that observations or the development of an opinion in this area may not be the exclusive role of the physician or the consultant. It was pointed out many years ago by Fulton [61] that any member of the OHS team can make critical observations of applicants, and the custodian, receptionist, clerk, and technologist can all add worthy comments regarding a candidate's behavior.

Although the determination of a person's emotional status can become a lengthy and highly complicated procedure in certain settings, Pies [62], in a plea actually for medical evaluations of patients prior to calling in a psychiatric consultant, offers a simple procedure for the identification of a disturbed individual. In 3 minutes, "a confused and bizarre patient" can be asked, "Where are you now?" "What is today's date?" "Are you hearing voices when nobody is around?" "Are you seeing things that nobody else sees?" and "Are you feeling that you might hurt yourself?" The seasoned occupational physician will not question the need for such a brief questioning, for both psychotic applicants and employees do appear in the OHS. One candidate for work recalled by the author laid claim to the fact that he was the son of the late President and Mrs. Kennedy, had spent most of his youth in the White House, and suddenly and inexplicably had been forced to leave that domicile a few years ago.

The principles of employing the physically handicapped apply with equal impact here. If applicants can meet the demands of the particular job being sought, then they should be viewed positively, and considered judgment should override unscientific, biased thought. Prediction is difficult in this area for, as an experienced British psychiatric evaluator has written [63], "The art of prognosis is unlikely to become a science for a long time."

It must not be forgotten that job applicants may not offer a history of emotional illness, particularly if they have been encouraged to disclaim such an experience. Quoting directly from one writing, Melchiode and Jacobson [64] have commented, "Our advice to an employee in therapy is, 'don't tell your boss.' Clearly dishonesty may be the best policy."

WEIGHT

In a nation seemingly dedicated to thinness and modestly concerned with the prevention of degenerative disease, there should be little difficulty in the employment of all applicants if weight is a factor. However, after 1965, with programs emphasizing the utilization of the hard-core unemployed and affirmative action in hiring and other personnel actions, the matter of weight standards assumed a new dimension. Most companies have used no standards involving height-weight-age levels. There may be contraindications to employment in certain jobs when *gross obesity,* undefined, is an issue. Governing factors would include narrow work areas, use of ladders, or small portals for ingress. Another explanatory element offered by some employers is the lack of protective clothing in extraordinarily large sizes.

Henschel [65] has pointed out the occupational hazards of obesity in heat stroke and heat exhaustion, hard physical work, respiratory distress, accidents, decompression, attitude tolerance, and pesticide toxicity. He concluded that the obese person is at a disadvantage in several occupational situations and that obesity must be considered a significant work hazard.

Certain employers, however, did use height and weight standards in the evaluation of job applicants. The requirements of the Rehabilitation Act of 1973, as indicated previously, have nullified discrimination against applicants with handicapping conditions, and if obesity became the basis for medical rejection, then that particular state made the candidate handicapped by definition. Although it has been believed that the obese individual is much more likely to develop cardiovascular disease, hypertension, and diabetes mellitus, as determined by actuarial experience, the principle of "future risk" cannot be applied. Even though the presenting clinical disorder may lead to more serious entities that might affect the employer's economy through an untoward drain on the health insurance, life insurance, and disability retirement programs, the obesity itself, except in rare instances, is not immediately job-related. In addition, job rejection on the basis of overweight or underheight has been questioned in the courts, and in nearly every case, the plaintiff has had a favorable ruling. In some instances, back pay was ordered for the period the appellant could have been working.

In actuality, although no data have been offered to substantiate the belief, the dilution factor—adding a handful of overweight applicants to a labor force of thousands—would show little tilting of the cost-benefit relationship. One must determine, however, the subscriber population base, because the number of employees taking advantage of a company-offered policy frequently is much lower than planned or believed.

Many investigators have instituted the use of body mass index* as a criterion by which to judge the relationship between weight and health. Such an index has been favored by Keys and associates [66] and by Bray and colleagues [67]. Prior to the development of this measure and other indices, various tables developed by insurance companies (in 1911, 1929, and 1959) were based on actuarial experience, showing the body weights at which the lowest mortality was observed. At the time of their preparation, little was known of risk factors other than hypertension. For example, information derived from epidemiologic data regarding the relationship of heavy cigarette smoking to lung cancer and other serious disorders was not available in the early years. Only in the 1950s was the role of cholesterol clarified and a rapid method of measurement of blood cholesterol developed.

The tables used for years had the defect of oversimplification because the risk was assumed to be that of obesity, while actually diabetes mellitus, hypertension, and heavy smoking interacting with the obesity were the conditions that increased the level of risk. As Bray [68] has described it, an obese person who is not hypertensive, diabetic, or a smoker is often not at greater risk than the general population and actually has a better health prognosis than an individual of normal weight who is a moderate to heavy smoker and has elevated blood pressure or diabetes. The former disqualification of a person for employment on the basis of obesity alone was being done, therefore, through use of a risk factor that by itself was of lesser importance than several others that would not cause rejection of an applicant.

In connection with the use of weight standards in employment, an opinion was sought of the County Counsel, County of Los Angeles, who stated, "The County may not impose a maximum weight standard which acts to disqualify applicants who exceed it unless such standard is sufficiently supported by sound, current and relevant data which establishes [sic] that obesity significantly contributes to poor health and that the poor health of its employees would substantially limit or prevent the County from providing services to the public or that obesity would prevent adequate performance of a particular function" [69]. This opinion is consistent with comments made earlier regarding the job-relatedness of certain health deficits.

As most weight or height-weight standards have been invalidated by the courts, even for applicants aspiring to positions in law enforcement, it would be

*The body mass index is derived as follows:

$$\frac{\text{weight}}{\text{height}^2} = \frac{\text{kilograms}}{\text{meters}^2}.$$

extremely difficult to justify rejection for work except for the conditions indicated previously, as noted by Henschel [65]. It is desirable, however, that obesity or extreme underweight be corrected, and the current tables developed by the Metropolitan Life Insurance Company (MLIC) can be used as a gross baseline in a health counseling program.

In 1983, the new tables were announced and were derived from data developed in the Build Study conducted by the Societies of Actuaries and the Association of Life Insurance Medical Directors of America. The study, using data from 25 insurance companies, traced the mortality experience of approximately 4,200,000 persons for up to 22 years. Those individuals with such major diseases as cancer, diabetes, or heart disease were excluded to isolate the effect of weight on longevity [70].

The weights given are the levels associated with the lowest mortality and are higher than the weights published in 1959. The new tables do not carry the previous labels of "ideal" or "desirable" weights for "these adjectives mean different things to different people" [70]. They can serve, however, as sound guidelines in weight control. The new values are available in MLIC publications [70].

Although the weights show an increase over the 1959 levels, they still indicate, with the change, the weights manifest with the lowest mortality. The tables are not used for underwriting purposes, and they do not indicate the weights that reduce the likelihood of disease. Also, they are not the weights that optimize job performance or necessarily allow the individual to look his or her best [70]. The MLIC has provided the following suggestions in the determination of body frame by elbow breadth. To make a simple approximation of one's frame size:*

Extend the arm, and bend the forearm upward at a 90-degree angle. Keep the fingers straight, and turn the inside of the wrist away from the body. Place the thumb and index finger of the other hand on the two prominent bones on *either side* of the elbow. Measure the space between the fingers against a ruler or a tape measure, or have it measured by a health professional using calipers. Compare the measurements with those in Table 5-3, which lists the elbow measurements for medium-framed men and women of various heights. Measurements lower than those listed indicate a small frame, and higher measurements indicate a large frame.

TABLE 5-3. *Elbow Measurements for Medium-Framed Men and Women*

Height in 1-inch heels	*Elbow breadth*
Men	
5′2″–5′3″	2½″–2⅞″
5′4″–5′7″	2⅝″–2⅞″
5′8″–5′11″	2¾″–3″
6′0″–6′3″	2⅞″–3¼″
Women	
4′10″–4′11″	2¼″–2½″
5′0″–5′3″	2¼″–2½″
5′4″–5′7″	2⅜″–2⅝″
5′8″–5′11″	2⅜″–2⅝″
6′0″	2½″–2¾″

The MLIC has pointed out that the concepts of obesity and overweight often are confused. Obesity indicates excess body fat, while overweight connotes excess weight [70,71]. The difference in meaning is exemplified by weightlifters who, because of extreme muscular hypertrophy or muscle mass, exceed the weights given in the tables. Although there are complex methods of determining body density, they are impracticable in the OHS setting. A measure used for this purpose—one of several indices—is the body mass index, as indicated earlier. Such an index, to be of value, should be highly correlated with weight or other measures of adiposity and independent of height. The MLIC has used its tables to develop the body mass index values for men and women, which may be found in another MLIC publication [71].

A second method of differentiation, although an indirect correlate of obesity, may be used, employing skinfold thickness measurements, as derived from the work of Durnin and Womersley [72]. A small percentage of body fat is essential for normal function—in men 3 percent, in women 12 percent. Men with more than 25 percent fat are considered obese, as are women with more than 33 percent. The Lange or Harpenden skinfold calipers may be used for this purpose.

The issue of weight is of interest because former disqualification of an obese candidate was based, in the main and as mentioned previously, on an anticipated health change in the future. In comparable

*In a somewhat less exact method of measure, it has been suggested that to determine frame size one wrap the thumb and index finger around the wrist. If the thumb extends past the finger, one has a small frame; if the two digits just meet, the frame is average (medium?); and if the fingers do not meet, the frame is large. (Hayward, T. In T. Parker, *Rules of Thumb*. Boston: Houghton Mifflin, 1983. P. 108.) A convenient estimate of the writers' term "ideal body weight" is shown in this equation: for women, ideal body weight = 100 pounds + 5 pounds for each inch over 5 feet; for men, 106 pounds + 6 pounds for each inch over 5 feet. (Pohl, S. L., and Clarke, W. L. Diabetes update: Some new thoughts about an old disease. *Occup Health Nurs* 30:15, Dec 1982.)

vein, should applicants with a history of many years of heavy cigarette smoking be rejected because of possible lung disease in the future? Should the *controlled* insulin-dependent diabetic person be disqualified because of the known abbreviated longevity in persons with early onset of the disease? Is the candidate with hypercholesterolemia, borderline hypertension, and borderline obesity to be turned down because of the expected cardiac future? Or, are applicants with a poor family history of heart or vascular disease to be rejected because statistically they will undergo detrimental cardiac or vascular changes? Are we justified in acting on known epidemiologic or actuarial data when pathologic change has not, *as yet,* manifested itself? These questions have been given response initially by the writers of the Rehabilitation Act of 1973 and its interpreting jurists. To reiterate two issues, the ability to work is judged on job-related factors solely, and future risk cannot be used in the measure of work capacity.

HEARING

Efforts have been made to establish scientifically based hearing criteria for employment, but such trials have been difficult because of many related factors. As communication is carried on not only with one's ears but with one's eyes, previous experience, and level of intelligence, rigid demands for hearing acuity may render unemployable great numbers of persons who have developed adjunctive communicative skills. Further, as many systems of sound transmittance depend solely on the spoken word, defects in speech discrimination may nullify an acuity level that appears high on audiometric testing.

Individuals learn to adapt to a certain amount of hearing loss, and in accordance with otologic opinion, if a person is born with a hearing loss of 40 decibels, this decriment may present no problem when the individual is an adult. However, if one were to lose suddenly 40 decibels of hearing bilaterally, one would not be able to compensate for such a loss. The use, therefore, of inflexible standards would be unfair to an applicant who already has a limiting condition.

It is the belief of otologists concerned with the problems of noise in industry that hearing may be considered within "normal" limits from a 0 to a 25-decibel loss, and in questions of placement, this level would represent a reasonable cutoff point. A 35-decibel unilateral loss could be considered equivalent.

Some employers are governed in their selection of personnel by workers' compensation rulings regarding noise-induced hearing loss. If a mean of the loss in decibels of the four frequencies of 500, 1000, 2000, and 3000 Hz is greater than 25 decibels, using the International Standards Organization (ISO) level, then that loss is ratable were the measurements to be made on a worker who had been exposed to noise. When such a loss is presented by an applicant at the time of hire, because of workers' compensation experience, the candidate might not be employed for fear that the loss would be aggravated by the usual work exposures. However, it has been observed by otologists that the greatest risk in developing a hearing loss when subjected to untoward ambient noise is in the person with normal acuity. If an individual has a loss, there is much less risk of further loss.

Special tests can be used for speech discrimination. In jobs where this skill is important, as in the radio communication involved in law enforcement or in vehicle dispatch and operation, training will improve a deficit. Acquiring familiarity with certain speech patterns and learning a particular "shop talk" or jargon of an occupation will increase the capacity to understand speech.

There are certain extremely noisy jobs where total hearing loss is of advantage. The author visited a cordage plant at one time, and in the area where window sash cord was being made, the entire workforce was deaf, and lipreading was the mode of communication. The noise created by the constant hitting of cams against solid steel rods fixed into the floor and the ceiling precluded all conversation. One could not hear one's own voice. Visitors were warned not to speak because of the workers' speech-reading ability.

In view of the requirements of the Rehabilitation Act of 1973—reasonable accommodation on the part of the employer—certain facilities may have to be made available to allow the worker to function effectively. Visual hazard alarm systems may be substituted for sound systems, and certain communications aids may be required such as teletypewriter (TTY) via phone lines, video phone, or computer-based messaging networks. If necessary, employees in strategic, related work assignments might find it helpful to learn to sign with the nonverbal deaf employee.

If a hearing aid is required and the job demands protective eyewear, it is possible to build the device, either air conduction or bone conduction, into the eyeglass frame.

When doubt exists regarding an applicant's hearing, special study and evaluation by an otologist will allow consideration of such entities as the etiology, duration of loss, progression of the impairment, potential remediability, prognosis of defect, demonstrable pathologic or physiologic change, and the like.

The following additional information would be helpful in placement:

Description of disability and age at onset.
Method of applicant's communication with others.
Comprehension of applicant's speech.
Applicant's ability to read lips.
Use of hearing aid.
Ease or difficulty with which interview is conducted.
Significant working conditions and physical activities.
Applicant's adjustment to the impairment.
Applicant's ability in written expression.
Applicant's reading ability.
Applicant's tolerance for loud noises and vibrations.
Applicant's sense of balance.
Relation of any job loss to hearing impairment.

Needless to add, periodic audiometry should be performed after placement at yearly intervals, unless certain factors indicate briefer intervals between tests.

A standard that may be applied in positions requiring "job-related" good-to-peak hearing is the following: Uncorrected hearing in each ear at 500, 1000, 2000, and 3000 Hz must show an average loss of not over 30 decibels and a single peak loss of not over 40 decibels (ISO). Candidates whose hearing does not meet this standard, and whose uncorrected hearing in each ear at 500, 1000, 2000, and 3000 Hz shows an average loss of not over 40 decibels and a single peak loss of not over 45 decibels, with an average loss of not more than 10 decibels between the two ears, may be qualified for employment after individual study and evaluation.

HERNIA

The point to be emphasized regarding hernia is the need for ridding the occupational medical literature of the term "potential hernia" when discussing an inguinal defect. A hernia is present or absent. In keeping with a sharpened nomenclature is the requirement of examiners to define what is meant by a "relaxed ring," an "enlarged ring," or a "potential hernia" insofar as any of the three designations relates to an actual hernia. Is an enlarged ring that anatomic body encountered by a small examining finger? Is a relaxed ring a nosologic ambiguity? When does a "potential hernia" become a true hernia? Further, it is suggested that the examiner might be better able to detect a protruding hernial sac if the subject is asked to strain and hold the pressure rather than cough intermittently; the former procedure places the sac in position for a longer period of palpation than the short-duration cough in its production of a tussal impulse.

Ponka [73] has expressed this concern in another way, in that he warns against diagnosing a "pre-hernia." He states that "it is a hernia or it isn't. . . . Some patients have a large dilated ring; they have a rotund abdomen; and if you get your finger through the ring, you can palpate the floor of Hesselbach's triangle. That, in my opinion, is not a hernia, and I don't recommend repair of it. Furthermore I don't make a diagnosis of pre-hernia because once you use the word hernia in the presence of a patient or in one of those industrial cases, you've had it. The patient becomes totally incapacitated. . . . If it doesn't come through the external ring, I do not call it a hernia; and in my practice, I do not recognize the so-called pre-hernia."

Applicants with a definite inguinal, umbilical, or femoral hernia should not be placed in positions requiring excessive lifting or extremely strenuous physical exertion. Candidates for clerical or sedentary work may be employed with a single hernia, but presence of multiple herniations should defer acceptance. With the change in surgical corrective procedures—almost total ambulation throughout a brief hospital stay or repair in an ambulatory surgical unit—it would be most advisable to recommend that the applicant have the lesion(s) operated on and then reapply for employment.

An early study by the U.S. Department of Labor showed that the job applicants experiencing difficulty at work, in regard to hernia, were those individuals in whom the hernias were not detected at entry, but who subsequently presented the defect as an occupational injury. Candidates who were employed with recognized herniations were able to work without hazard to themselves, and in a 1948 study of 3,544 workers with hernia, only one individual developed a disabling injury from "abdominal strain" [74].

Berliner [75], speaking from an experience of surgical repair of more than 2,000 inguinal hernias, indicates that over a 10-year period of observation, many asymptomatic small to moderate-sized hernias on the side that was not operated on remain stationary in size and continue to be asymptomatic, despite the fact that the individual may be engaged in heavy manual labor. He deplores the extraordinary costs entailed in the third most common surgical operative procedure. In essence, he states that an inguinal hernia does not necessarily signify a handicapping condition. It will be a long period before physicians in industry, employers, and surgeons acquire this philosophy.

BLOOD PRESSURE

In light of the current large-scale screening programs for hypertension, there has been need for a new look at hiring standards as they relate to blood pressure findings. The World Health Organization [76] established the criteria for referral to a secondary screening as a systolic pressure of 160 mm Hg or greater or a diastolic pressure of 95 mm Hg or greater, irrespective of age. These subjects on recheck showed 20 percent to be normotensive. For practical purposes, referral should be made definitely at 165 mm Hg for the systolic blood pressure and at 95 mm Hg for the diastolic, although present trends point to referral at much lower levels of hypertension. Subjects with a diastolic pressure greater than 120 mm Hg should be referred immediately to a source of medical care, while individuals with a recording of less than 140/90 mm Hg would receive no further attention other than eventual reevaluation.

The criteria that have been followed in the OHSs with which the author has been associated have permitted employment of any applicant over age 35 years with a recording not exceeding 160/100. For candidates less than 35 years of age, the level of acceptance is 150/90. These applicants and persons manifesting variations from these levels required referral to the individual's private physician for examination and treatment. A subsequent examination would be conducted within 6 weeks to determine if the employment standard had been met, and a written report from the applicant's physician, concerning treatment, is required. Any job candidate whose diastolic pressure exceeds 110 mm Hg is not qualified for work until adequate observation confirms that the individual's hypertension is under control.

Some organizations are more liberal; for example, a pressure of 170/104 mm Hg is acceptable in one company, provided there is "no evidence of cardiovascular or renal disease." The same firm will accept applicants with a pressure not in excess of 200/110 mm Hg but will place job restrictions such as no heavy lifting (above 25 pounds for men, over 10 pounds for women) and no work at an unguarded elevation. If the same person presents evidence of significant cardiac or renal disease, he or she is rejected for employment. Recordings over 200/110 mm Hg disqualify the applicant.

It must be emphasized that referral to a primary care physician does not necessarily guarantee long-term follow-up or even adequacy of the antihypertensive medication plan or dietary regimen. The physician or occupational nurse must make reappointments with family physicians for employees when blood pressure rechecks indicate a cessation of medication or other infraction of the control protocol.

VISION

For most jobs, workers should have a near and distance visual acuity of at least 20/40 in each eye, with or without correction. When vision is poorer than 20/40 but is correctable to 20/40, corrective lenses must be worn at work.

Certain positions will require maximal skill in color discrimination, and these jobs should be known to the examining physician. Of concern to many examiners is the potential hazard in motor vehicle operation of color-blind drivers. A Swiss study is cited [77] in which the behavior in traffic of 160 color-blind drivers was compared with a normal-vision control group, on the basis of offense and accident statistics. Each group drove about 80 million kilometers, and 40 percent drove taxicabs, motorcoaches, or trucks. No statistically significant differences were found between the study and control groups, and no difference was encountered in traffic performance between subjects with slight and drivers with severe color blindness. The conclusion was that, if otherwise qualified, color-blind persons could safely be allowed to drive any type of vehicle.

The blind may be employed, and this type of placement will be discussed under the utilization of the handicapped.

The use of contact lenses in industry has been reviewed, and although the subject will be treated under vision conservation programs, it should be mentioned that such lenses, in general, should be prohibited in the industrial setting, with certain exceptions. It is the belief of ophthalmologists that only with a general prohibition can the wearers be identified and evaluated. If certain users are permitted to wear these lenses, the fit should be evaluated, and it is mandatory that the wearer carry both a spare pair and a pair of standard spectacles on his person at all times. Safety glasses must be provided and must be worn when necessary.

Hard lenses are used in workers with aphakia, and soft lenses cannot be worn in areas where chemical irritants are present, for the soft material absorbs the chemicals. Also, hard lenses are used occasionally in high myopia, in keratoconus, and for the irregular corneal astigmatism that may follow trauma. It is imperative that wearers of contact lenses understand the care that is required (for example, to avoid the use of saliva as a lens lubricant) because of the possibility of infection.

In a study of law enforcement personnel [78], it was found that the wearing of contact lenses had no adverse effect on marksmanship, and in training sessions with tear gas, the subjects felt that they were able to perform their duties effectively. In fact, it was believed that the lenses acted as a barrier, preventing the dramatic irritation that usually followed such exposure. Contrary to belief, officers reported that over a 9-month period not one police wearer had a lens dislodge or "pop out." In contradistinction to corrective glasses, the contact lenses presumably could not be dislodged in a scuffle.

TUBERCULOSIS

Probably the most noticeable turnabout in ill employees has been evidenced in those persons in the workforce who developed tuberculosis or, more likely, underwent a reactivation. Prior to the introduction of chemotherapy, the absence from work was long, and the patient and family frequently were impoverished by the disease.

A new view exists today in that the most important requirement in the interruption of the transmission of tubercle bacilli and the cure of the disease is that the tuberculosis patient receive an adequate course of chemotherapy. It is the opinion of the American Thoracic Society, as expressed in its "Guidelines for Work for Patients with Tuberculosis" [79], that what the patients do or where they are has no influence on the course of the disease, provided that they take their medication. Because of this fact, patients are encouraged to continue with or return to their previous activity as soon as they are physically able.

Today, short-term drug therapy, using a combination of isoniazid and rifampin for a minimum of 9 months, is the simplest regimen for adults with uncomplicated pulmonary tuberculosis and is the recommendation of the American Thoracic Society and the Centers for Disease Control (CDC) [80]. The statement gives emphasis to the joint use of the two drugs to avoid emergence of resistant organisms. In many studies, ethambutol or streptomycin was added during the initial 2 to 8 weeks. Some patients may require extension of the customary regimen. Patients have been told that they need not stop work with the institution of the regimen. They must, however, take the medication each day; when they begin to feel better, they often forget to take their capsules. Further, some patients who are on other medication, for heart disease or hypertension for example, will overlook their antituberculosis drugs in favor of the other therapeutic agents.

The guidelines [79] stated that "if drugs are self-administered, adherence to the regimen should be carefully monitored by such indicators as clinic attendance, pill counts, urine tests, and bacteriologic examinations of the sputum."

It must be remembered when placing applicants in health service agencies or in hospitals that a treatment program confers no immunity against exogenous tuberculosis infection from reexposure to an "open case." The therapy only reduces the risk of disease developing endogenously from a past infection. It is the primary tuberculous infection that effectively stimulates cellular immunity against the infection [81].

In a work setting there is usually great concern manifested over contagion in communicable (or other) disease. The American Thoracic Society's ad hoc committee that prepared the guidelines believed that there is rendered a disservice to the patient, the patient's family, and the community if absolute proof is required that the transmission of tuberculosis is impossible. Currently, there are no incontrovertible data pointing to the moment when patients, once started on treatment, no longer excrete particles capable of transmitting tuberculosis. The risk of infection is low when patients are on adequate chemotherapy, even though there may be limited numbers of bacilli in the sputum.

In the guidelines [79] it is concluded that an otherwise healthy tuberculosis patient may continue his usual work activity when adequate treatment has been initiated and the sputum is free of bacilli or the number of bacilli present in sputum smears is declining; hospitalization is not required; and contacts, liable to severe consequences, in a closed environment, are not anticipated.

In accepting for employment a person who is on medication, there should be individual study conducted of the applicant, the work environment, and the factors of contact. Placement would be poor were the candidate to be given work in a closed environment such as a ship or an institution where the ventilation is inadequate as a result of recirculation in an air-conditioning system. As in all problems of selective placement, consideration must be given such determinants as stamina, exercise tolerance, and the specific demands of the job being sought. Houk [82] has observed that in all but the most severe cases of pulmonary tuberculosis and in special instances of extrapulmonary disease, physical capacity returns rapidly to the predisease level and, in many instances, is never impaired. It is to be emphasized that the patient should not be deprived of work because of "well-intentioned, but unproven, concepts of the past." Communicability in tuberculosis is limited to the period prior to diagnosis and treatment.

A current classification of tuberculosis and other mycobacterial diseases is available from the American Thoracic Society [83].

SKIN ALLERGIES AND SKIN TESTING

Frequently an examining physician on learning of an applicant's sensitivity to a chemical will feel the need to prove the allergic state as an aid in placement. The conducting of patch testing at the time of the preplacement medical examination is contraindicated. As Birmingham [84] has expressed it, "Other than history, there is no practical way of predicting sensitivity in a new employee. To perform a predictive patch test on an individual with a negative history

. . . and then have that individual subsequently develop contact dermatitis might be taken as inducing sensitivity via the patch test. Further, a negative patch test on a new employee in no way precludes that he is immune and, therefore, will not develop contact dermatitis. . . ."

The reaction that may be produced as a result of preemployment patch testing will be considered an occupationally induced illness, even though the applicant is yet to be placed on the payroll.

ARTHRITIS

Although the term *arthritis* includes a large group of soft-tissue and joint disorders with differing symptoms resulting, some observations can be made regarding placement. The individual with acute rheumatoid arthritis in one or multiple joints usually will be too uncomfortable to accept employment until the pain, swelling, and dysfunction subside. As more total joint replacements are being carried out, a greater number of workers will be able to return to gainful employment. Obviously, the convalescence should be complete, and placement should be in parallel with the abilities of the applicant to perform in the position. Cold and dusty work environments should be avoided.

Applicants with stable or so-called burned-out rheumatoid spondylitis even in light of the resultant flexion deformity and limited rotation of the spine present little difficulty in placement, as many such persons have worked well in a variety of supervisorial, managerial, and professional positions. Destructive osteoarthritis, common to nearly all employees aging in the later years of service, can cause severe pain in the large joints such as the hips, but with restorative surgery, a full return to work can be anticipated.

Many craft workers who have had years of heavy industry employment will experience the effects of traumatic wear and tear and frequently will no longer be able to function effectively in jobs demanding great physical activity in crowded work settings.

In essence, each person with arthritis requires individual evaluation. Most affected candidates prove to be excellent workers, particularly if the work setting is one of hospitable understanding, free from the stressors that would have adverse effects on the worker. The introduction of altered work schedules and flex time has been helpful in the cases of flare-up among employees with rheumatoid arthritis. Initial and frequent measurements of joint motion with use of a goniometer or a special finger arthrograph should be made.

Classifications have been developed by the Arthritis Foundation in Atlanta, Georgia for use in patients with rheumatoid arthritis, indicating levels of disease progression and functional capacity.

PARAPLEGIA

Innumerable persons with paraplegia, incurred traumatically or after poliomyelitis, have been effectively employed, particularly as exemplified by the multi-term American president of the 1930s and 1940s. The only special arrangements that need consideration concern a parking area adjacent to the worksite and the availability of a wide cubicle in a nearby restroom with the appropriate grab bars on the walls to allow chair-to-toilet transfer and back. If great distances are involved for the wheelchair-bound worker, a battery-operated chair can be maintained at the building entrance, where exchange with the lighter folding chair customarily in use can be carried out. In addition, a plan, with appropriate rehearsals, should be developed for direct evacuation from the worksite in the event of fire or other disaster.

Individuals with triplegia or quadriplegia should be adjudged individually both as to ability and needs in reasonable accommodation.

END-STAGE RENAL DISEASE

As facilities have become more readily available for patients on dialysis for end-stage renal disease (E-SRD), the potential for employment has increased. Bryan [85] has reported that home-dialysis patients are more frequently employed than patients coming to dialysis facilities. Of the first group, 10 percent were employed part-time and 21 percent full-time. In the facility-dependent group, 7 percent were employed part-time, and 6 percent were on a full-time work basis. In another study [86], 25 percent of the patients—irrespective of the type or location of the dialysis facility—worked outside the home, and one-third worked at home. For those individuals receiving such therapy, work schedules should be structured to fit the dialysis time frames. With flex time and altered work frequencies being used currently, such as the 10-hour day, 4-day week, a work calendar could be designed that would both allow such a patient to be socially useful and provide the employer with a set of employable skills.

With the passage of time, several studies have brought new information concerning the survival and quality of life of patients with E-SRD. Vollmer and associates [87], in an examination of the survival experience of over 1,000 patients with E-SRD, learned that there was significantly better survival following transplantation with a graft from a living related donor than with either transplantation with a cadaveric graft or dialysis. No significant difference was encountered in survival between treatment by dialysis and cadaveric transplantation. The writers concluded that an integrated program of dialysis and transplantation provides the greatest opportunity for optimal treatment, with particular reference to the effects on general lifestyle, opportunity for rehabilitation, and family and social responsibilities.

In a 4-year study of nearly all persons with E-SRD* [88,89], it was found that among patients receiving transplants in successive years between 1977 and 1980, the rates of graft retention showed progressive and substantial increases. The survival rates for patients either on dialysis or who were recipients of transplants remained stable. The group receiving dialysis experienced a nearly constant death rate, which was generally higher than the stable late-mortality rate of transplant recipients.

Johnson and his colleagues [90] studied nearly 500 patients at the Mayo Clinic who were maintained on outpatient dialysis between 1963 and 1977. Of the group, 24 had had previous untoward cardiovascular events. Subsequently, 30 persons experienced myocardial infarction, and 45 had cerebrovascular accidents. More importantly, 183 patients (38 percent) were employed, 124 remained active at home or at school, and 115 were totally disabled. The survival of patients maintained solely by dialysis was 52 percent at 5 years. For the total group—including patients with their first allograft—the rate of survival was 65 percent. Of 2,728 patients with E-SRD, including both persons on dialysis and patients receiving transplants, it was found by Hellerstedt and coworkers studying survival rates [91] that general survival rates were lower for patients with diabetes than for nondiabetic persons, except for subjects over age 60. The highest survival rates were seen among patients with systemic lupus erythematosus, focal glomerulonephrosis, or glomerulonephritis. Patients with primary renal malignant lesions, primary hypertensive disease, or diabetes mellitus as the cause of the renal failure displayed the lowest. Other disorders also affected the survival rate adversely. Persons with cadaveric grafts had lower survival rates than all other groups.

As an aid in judging illness—or therapy-associated absenteeism—further data from the Mayo Clinic are helpful. In a report by Carlson and associates [92] covering 946 patients maintained by dialysis, it was learned that 558 patients were hospitalized 1,207 times (mean of 1.8 stays/year and 15 days/year), mainly because of dialysis access problems or gastrointestinal or cardiac complications. The two rates increased with age, and the rates were higher for patients maintained by peritoneal dialysis than for persons receiving hemodialysis.

Evans and his group [93] reviewed the quality of life of patients with E-SRD and found that nearly 75 percent of transplant recipients were able to work, in contrast to 24.7 percent of patients undergoing continuous ambulatory peritoneal dialysis and 59.3 percent maintained by home hemodialysis. Only 37.2 percent receiving in-center hemodialysis were employed. Although the quality of life of transplant recipients compared well with the general population despite favorable subjective assessments, patients undergoing dialysis did not work or function at the same level as persons in the general population.

The studies reviewed briefly here are cited to apprise the physicians concerned with placement recommendations with the anticipated morbidity and mortality outcomes. Applicants presenting with E-SRD will be accepted for employment under the aegis of the Rehabilitation Act of 1973 provided they are able to function in expected job-related activities. It might be that a high illness-absence rate may eventually prove excessive, but only experience will indicate the time lost from work. In essence, both the person maintained on dialysis and the transplant recipient are employable with special, careful placement. It is obvious that there can be no exposure to nephrotoxic materials or environments. Each candidate must be assessed individually and followed assiduously.

It must be remembered, in placing a worker who is on dialysis, that the treatment may have an energy-reducing effect and that the time involved in the recovery from participation in dialysis may further reduce the number of available work hours [94].

SICKLE CELL TRAIT AND DISEASE

Some OHSs may include testing for sickle cell trait and disease. Even now, among many lay groups, the two states are confused. The heterozygous sickle cell trait bears no significance to employment, and even with an exposure to benzene and carbon monoxide, the risk is no greater than for an individual with normal hemoglobin.

There are limitations, however, in the work setting for persons with homozygous sickle cell *disease*. As provided by the Occupational Medical Practice Committee of AOMA [95], they are as follows:

> A variety of clinical problems must be considered when determining the employability of workers with the homozygous sickle cell disease, as follows:
>
> Heavy manual labor in a hot environment with result-

*The data for study were collected by the Medical Information System of the Health Care Financing Administration, which covers nearly all patients with this disease state.

ing dehydration can precipitate a sickle cell crisis. Special precautions should be taken against dehydration and the employee should be educated on the subject of adequate hydration.

Any work in a cold environment can precipitate a sickle cell crisis.

Anatomic and functional change can be present in any tissue, owing to the cumulative effect of recurrent vaso-occlusive episodes, and these changes can be severe enough to preclude manual labor. They can also predispose the employee to ulceration of the lower extremities from minor trauma.

Hemolytic anemia is present to a variable degree, and if severe can preclude physical activity.

Carbon monoxide exposure can produce carboxyhemoglobin and would add to the physiologic effects of the anemia with respect to oxygen transport. However, carboxyhemoglobin is more resistant to sickling than normal hemoglobin.

If the benzene exposure levels are safe and acceptable for normal employment, there is no increased risk for employees with sickle cell anemia.

Workers with appropriately confirmed sickle cell anemia, in general, can be expected to be more sensitive than most people to occupational or environmental insults that involve their genetically impaired RBCs. However, it would be inappropriate to recommend a placement policy without regard for the work and medical histories of an individual employee. It seems evident that the proper disposition of any particular individual rests with the informed clinical judgment of the responsible physician. Persons with sickle cell disease should receive personal evaluation and appropriate job placement.

MISCELLANEOUS DISORDERS

Innumerable conditions* remain for consideration, but the examiners' general knowledge of the natural history of various disease processes must guide them in their certification of applicants for employment. Acute processes require treatment and recovery, and the candidate should return at a later date for reexamination. Persons with orthopedic defects must be studied individually in relation to the demands of the position being sought, the injury potential, the possibility of spontaneous or nonoccupational recurrence, the need for consistent conditioning, and the like.

At best, each candidate who presents an unusual disorder—congenital anomaly, post-traumatic disability, postillness residua, post-surgical status, a progressive clinical entity—should be studied individually and not matched coldly to rigid criteria that may make the preplacement procedure easier, but employment for the candidate and human progress more difficult.

*Some of the many disorders or disease states presenting need for accurate matching of the physical and environmental demands of the job with the physical and emotional capacities of the applicant that have not yet been considered are alcoholism, amputations, developmental disabilities, drug abuse, Hansen's disease, hemophilia, mental retardation, parkinsonism, and speech impairments.

CLASSIFICATION SYSTEMS

Once the examination is complete, it is necessary to classify the applicant so that the needs of placement, follow-up, personal safety, and medical surveillance may be met.

Probably in most common use is a five-point scale, as follows:

A. Medically qualified for position applied for.
B. Medically qualified for position applied for, but has minor deficits.
C. Medically qualified for position applied for, with certain job restrictions (the appropriate ones to be checked or completed):
  1. Must wear protective eyewear.
  2. No back bending.
  3. No climbing of stairs or ladder.
  4. No dust exposure.
  5. No inside work.
  6. No lifting over ________pounds.
  7. No outside work.
  8. No second, third, or rotating shift work.
  9. No sudden temperature changes.
  10. No work around hazardous machinery.
  11. No work around moving objects.
  12. No work around toxic materials, specifically, ________, ________, and ________.
  13. No work in high places.
  14. No work in cold quarters.
  15. No work in hot quarters.
  16. No work in noisy quarters.
  17. No work in wet quarters.
  18. No work productive of excessive emotional stress.
  19. No work other than sedentary.
  20. No work involving the operation of automotive equipment or mobile power equipment.
  21. No work in areas with infectious disease.
  22. No work in unpressurized aircraft in flight.
  23. To be rechecked periodically by OHS.
  24. Other limitations:
  ____
  ____

D. Not medically qualified for position applied for.
E. Classification deferred.

CLASSIFICATION A

Classification A means that the medical or health examination has been passed successfully and that the applicant is medically qualified for employment in the position that was sought. The results of all laboratory procedures and the findings of all related examinations have been received and are within normal limits.

CLASSIFICATION B

Classification B is given to an applicant who has minor clinical findings, such as small varices, hypertrophied tonsils, large healed thermal burn scars, or seborrheic dermatitis, that do not relate to employment and that require no modifications, restrictions, or limitations of the work assignment.

CLASSIFICATION C

Implicit in classification C is the applicant's medical qualification for employment, but certain clinical findings have been encountered that require a limitation or restriction in the work to be undertaken. For example, an applicant with grand mal epilepsy could be employed, but specific restrictions would be placed on his or her job, such as No. 10—No work around hazardous machinery; No. 11—No work around moving objects; No. 13—No work in high places (above 5 feet); and No. 18—No work productive of excessive emotional stress. These restrictions are made known to the employee's supervisor so that the precautions can be observed.

CLASSIFICATION D

Classification D means medical disqualification and that the individual is not considered employable. There may be untreated hypertensive heart disease, acute polyarticular rheumatoid arthritis, or a progressive disease incompatible with the safety and health of the applicant or that of fellow workers, the needs of which cannot be met by any means of reasonable accommodation.

CLASSIFICATION E

Classification E usually is a temporary one, given to an applicant while recovering from an acute disease process, while certain special test results are being awaited, or until helpful past medical information is obtained from previous sources of health care.

CHANGES IN CLASSIFICATION

A classification need not be a permanent designation. For example, an employee who develops a nonoccupationally incurred inguinal hernia will be changed from classification A to B if the hernia is compatible with the person's job. If a person with insulin-dependent diabetes, for example, loses a great deal of weight, which cancels the need for daily injections, it is conceivable that certain restrictions would be lifted, changing the C to a B classification.

Changes can be effected as a result of periodic medical examinations, as a product of a release-to-work examination, or when the goal of an intensive physical conditioning program is reached. Normally, the C classification is reserved for the so-called handicapped workers, and a count of such classifications can serve as a measure of the extent of the organization's employment of physically or emotionally limited persons.

On completion of the examination, the classification assigned to the applicant is transmitted to the personnel department. This action is all that is needed to indicate that a preplacement medical assessment has been completed. No diagnostic information need be forwarded, thus retaining the privileged information accruing from the medical history and examination or from the psychological evaluation.

THE CASE AGAINST EXAMINATIONS

A discussion of industrial placement procedures should not be closed without indicating that a minority opinion exists in opposition. Nearly two decades ago a debate was held at a professional meeting, and subsequently the papers appeared in print. Hanks [96,97] argued against the procedure, while Luongo [98] upheld its worth. It was Hanks's belief that the use of a restricted examination (use of a questionnaire) can effect significant savings, which can be applied to a considerably broader occupational health program. Workers' compensation claims seemed to be unaffected by utilizing a medical examination. He pointed out also that the true handicap of workers is not physical disability, but lack of skill, and that it is indefensible to impose unrealistic physical standards on the physically marginal applicant.

Further, Hanks indicated that examinations are no better than health questionnaires in detecting epilepsy, angina pectoris, or controlled diabetes *if* the applicant wished to withhold information. At best, the "routine physical examination" is nothing more than a gross screening device, whose chief findings can be duplicated by the use of the questionnaire. He pointed wisely to the fact that "the injury done to a man and his family through ill considered and improperly administered physical standards may extend far beyond that potentially arising from a work-aggravation of a disability"; and in these matters, the physician may be "the only source of a company conscience." In substance, Hanks pointed out that the examination is subordinate to selection based on skill, adaptability, and motivation, all manifested after the time of hire, and inferior also to environmental control measures and safety training.

The use of a questionnaire has endured in the same organization once headed by Hanks. Dr. M. N. Cooper [99] employs a modified form of the original questionnaire in keeping with the requirements of both the Occupational Safety and Health Administration (OSHA) and Fair Employment/Equal Opportunity Agency. He feels that the questionnaire saves the time-consuming cost and effort of the prehire examination. In some instances, where the work applicant is to be assigned to a potentially hazardous job, a baseline evaluation will be performed. If an individual is hired into a "general job" category and later is to be transferred to a department with potentially hazardous materials, a preassignment physical examination will be completed. The supervisors are cognizant of the jobs that require medical review.

It was made clear, Dr. Cooper reports, both to the applicant and the government agencies, that information from the health questionnaire is needed to effect good placement and to protect health. In this manner the issue has been freed of any charge of discrimination advice, and the wording of the questions was provided by company counsel and persons connected with the equal employment opportunity (EEO) activity of the organization. In essence the use of the prehire questionnaire and limited examination has proved to be not only cost-effective but also medically effective in providing information about the health problems of an employed population. The examinations mandated of employees exposed to hazardous materials are repeated at the needed intervals after the first employment evaluation.

The experience of the Massachusetts Institute of Technology (MIT) has been reviewed by Rodman [100]. A 2-year period provided 2,833 examinations for study. The yield of discovered abnormalities was low—65 persons, or 2.3 percent of the number seen. The findings in applicants under age 30 was even lower at 1 percent. In keeping with the industrial concern over turnover, Rodman pointed out that of 150 women under 30 years of age, 47 percent left within 1 year, the majority terminating within 6 months. These short-term employees were followed for medical-clinic utilization, and it was found that this group used the facilities infrequently. Rodman believed, then, that preemployment examinations served little purpose in women under age 30 and, on the basis of the study findings, converted the procedure for women under 30 years of age who were not to be employed in hazardous occupations from a complete preemployment examination to a three-point screening of chest film, hematocrit, and urinalysis. After 1 year of employment, an examination was offered on a voluntary basis.

Leckey [101], in a beautifully expressed paper, studied a group of men—men with known good work records—examined at the time of transfer to a new plant. He hoped that he could present a correlation between examination results and the person's ability to work. Among 73 men in the group of 104 examinees, there were 84 positive findings, ranging from hypertension to hernia, commonly disqualifying disorders. Leckey stated the findings simply: ". . . 1) on pre-employment examinations the physical findings may exclude many excellent employees as well as the incapacitated; 2) the medical history obtained during such examinations is next to worthless; 3) any record of previous minor accidents at work is of no use in predicting a man's future worth; and 4) the only information of use in foreseeing a man's potential contribution to the company are his age and marital status, which information can be obtained by the personnel department." In summary, Leckey cautions that before the procedure is jettisoned by cost-conscious managers, it does serve as a significant introduction of the new employee to the OHS, and at times of medical need in the future, he or she will seek counsel from the medical department. Secondly, it is emphasized to the organization that, while costly and possibly nonproductive, the preplacement examination process allows the discerning physician to identify "qualities and attributes, and detriments as well, which might not be apparent to the interviewing member of the personnel department, but which might affect significantly the candidate's potential contribution to the company." He concluded insightfully with these words: "Just as in many other aspects of this particular medical discipline, the greatest challenge to the industrial physician's talents is the need to bring understanding to an area in which misunderstanding prevails. This is, to a considerable extent, the vocation of the industrial physician."

The use of a questionnaire in place of the actual physical examination conducted at time of hire has been undertaken at a few installations. Schneider and McDonagh [102] utilized a preemployment questionnaire to evaluate university graduates, and subsequently the subjects were examined a short time after accepting job offers. The conclusions were that the questionnaire effectively evaluated the graduates' fitness for work, and the authors suggested that it might be of use with middle class, young applicants seeking white-collar jobs.

Other observers have commented on the lessening

need for medical examinations before beginning new employment. The contemporary viewpoint of the federal government was offered by Siegel [103] when he stated the current employment philosophy of a tax-spending rather than a profit-making enterprise:

1. To require only the minimal physical and mental capacities consistent with safe and efficient performance of the job sought.
2. To place emphasis on current physical and mental capacities, rather than an assessment of future capacities.
3. To endeavor particularly to place handicapped applicants.
4. To place relatively light weight on any estimated future period of probably total employment or productivity, and
5. As a mammoth self-insurer not to be overly or unduly concerned with compensation and insurance liability potential.

In light of this philosophy, medical examinations currently are not required for most white-collar appointments, with appropriate exceptions such as motor vehicle operations and food handlers (for example, dietitians) and on applicants for jobs involving considerable stress, such as air traffic controllers. This change in policy was based on the desire to employ greater numbers of handicapped persons, to economize in government operations, to recognize the high turnover in many occupations, and to take greatest advantage of the shortage of medical talent. Siegel felt that even a greater number of jobs would be considered as not in need of preemployment medical examination of applicants and, further, that the examination should be reserved for the applicant for the exceptional job.

The successful use a questionnaire has been described also by Voelz and Spickard [104] in a nuclear energy facility. But the longest experience was that of Williamson [105], who reviewed 18 years of the use of such a document without the performance of preemployment medical examinations. During that period, 470,000 persons were hired, while 324,000 exited from the payroll. Had examinations been done, the cost would have reached $5,640,000. It was believed that an examination program would have avoided only five or six industrial injury claims. Examinations are done, however, on drivers, firefighters, guards, and test pilots, and employees who are on the job and are to be assigned to potentially hazardous work are given a preassignment physical examination. Workers so covered include toxic-fuel and chemical handlers, beryllium workers, employees in unusual atmospheric-pressure settings, workers with radiation, and the like. The emphasis is given to protection of the individual in the work environment, obtained through environmental control and training in safe work practices.

A further questioning of the worth of the prehire medical examination was offered by Thomson [106], speaking from the point of view of British Civil Service. Because of difficulties attendant upon conducting the program, evaluations were carried out only on those prospective employees who were seeking positions that demanded considerably above average physical fitness. These classes included members of the diplomatic service who may have to serve overseas for long periods in trying conditions and climates with limited medical facilities; officers of customs and excise; coast guards; driving and traffic examiners; persons serving in weather ships; and air flight and accident inspectors. In addition, for certain groups, only color vision tests were carried out, for example, illustrators, printing operators, and draftsmen.

It is reasonable now to ask about a rationale for the conducting of examinations before hire. There are many factors to consider:

1. The characteristics of the population from which applicants are drawn.
   Issue: Presence of high-risk characteristics, in isolation or as co-morbid states—hypertension, venereal disease, post-hepatitis state, glaucoma, diabetes, substance abuse, emotional disorders. (Examples of populations: disadvantaged, chronically unemployed persons; adolescents; veterans.)
2. The cost.
   Issue: Cost-benefit analysis reveals savings when examination costs are balanced against workers' compensation losses or against narrow profit margins on marketing of product.
3. The quality of the medical examination conducted.
   Issue: Many preemployment examinations are desultory systems reviews, hastily done, frequently unrevealing of significant defects, not helpful in the employing process.
4. The availability of postemployment medical care.
   Issue: The assumption by the employer of clinical risk in isolated or hostile work environments, domestic or foreign.
5. The philosophy of employers regarding their social role.
   Issue: This role as it relates to affirmative action, employment of the handicapped, or broadening of the available talent base.
6. The relationship of health to work longevity.

Issue: Financial protection of the investment in human resources.

7. The relationship of health to use/abuse of health insurance programs supported by employers.
   Issue: Excessive drain on hospital benefits by segments of the labor force.
8. The need for a time-of-hire health-status base for use in future comparisons.
   Issue: Scope of a preventive medicine program.
9. Image of the organization.
   Issue: Appearance or skill of employees in interaction with customers, the public, or foreign hosts if abroad.
10. Realities of legal codes.
    Issue: Statutes that presume named diseases to be work-caused among certain employees (for example, heart disease or cancer among police officers and firefighters in California).
11. The level of turnover.
    Issue: The cost versus durability of a transient labor force (includes state of pregnancy).

It is the employer's need to decide with the consultative assistance of the medical director certain elements concerning the preplacement medical examinations; their performance by physicians or as assessments by nurses under supervision; their selective use in conjunction with questionnaires; their level of sophistication, for example "heart-lungs-blood pressure" versus sophisticated dynamic electrocardiography under stress challenge; and their worth in merit employment where the appeal process increases all operating costs. These decisions can be made on the basis of cost experience, desire for peak image, sense of community, and the like. It is in this situation that the medical director becomes a true interpreter and guide to managers in the formulation of operating policy.

LEGAL ASPECTS

It is important that certain cases be cited because of the relevance of the opinions to preplacement physical examinations. In *Laeng* v. *Workmen's Compensation Appeals Board,* it was argued that Laeng, while participating in the "obstacle course" phase of a physical agility test conducted by a city in California as part of a "tryout" competition for the position of "refuse crew worker," fractured a foot and was therefore entitled to benefits under the Workers' Compensation Act. The city claimed he was only trying out for the job and therefore was not an employee. The board denied benefits.

Laeng took the case to the California Supreme Court, where the decision was reversed. The court used the broad definition of "employee" as set out for purposes of the act in the state labor code, as "every person in the service of an employer under any appointment or contract or hire or apprenticeship, express or implied, oral or written. . . ." The tryout was, the court reasoned, for the benefit of both the employer and the applicant, and the agility test was the equivalent of an on-the-job trial performance, during which Laeng was under the employer's control. If the test proved hazardous, the court reasoned further, there was no reason why the applicant should not be entitled to the protection of the law [107].

In another case, a patient who had radiographs taken in the course of a preplacement medical examination brought suit against the radiologist, claiming that the interpretation of the x-ray film was erroneous. It was held by the Superior Court of New Jersey that the roentgenologist had to defend this suit even though the report had been prepared for the prospective employer of the plaintiff and not at the request of the plaintiff for purposes of treating him.

The court stated that "where physical health is a factor in the determination of qualifications, the worker has a right to have the state of his health diagnosed with reasonable care and reported with reasonable accuracy and correctness." It was further held by the court that "the relationship of physician and patient is readily implied and did exist between the defendant and the plaintiff, with consequent duty on the part of the defendant to exercise reasonable care in the examination and diagnosis he was called upon to make." It was pointed out by reviewers of the case that there seems to be a trend toward the view that a contract between an examining physician and the examinee is not necessary to give rise to a cause of action for malpractice in cases arising from such examinations. A physician has a responsibility to be as careful when examining a job applicant as with any other examination, to be as thorough in such a procedure as the circumstances reasonably warrant, and *to report to the applicant any condition that is disclosed for which treatment or a course of action appears advisable.* The fact that there is third-party payment by a prospective employer does not exempt the physician from this responsibility. It is suggested that practitioners conducting preplacement examinations retain in their files complete records of patients encountered in their regular practice [108].

From these cases, it can be shown that any untoward event, or misadventure, incident to a preplacement medical examination would result in assumption of liability by the employer. In the Laeng case, further, a signed waiver of injury was disregarded by the court. The legal consequences of complications or untoward results stemming from immunizing injections given on conclusion of a preplacement physical examination will be discussed in Chapter 8.

In a case heard on behalf of the California State Fair Employment and Housing Commission, the complainant alleged that a municipal police department had discriminated against him, by rejecting his application for employment following the examination on the basis of physical handicap, in violation of the Fair Employment and Housing Act (Gov. Code, §12900 et seq.). The city had required preemployment spine radiographs since 1975 on all police officer applicants. The complainant had bilateral spondylolysis and spondylolisthesis grade I of the fifth lumbar vertebra at the lumbosacral joint. He had a history of several years of police work in other jurisdictions. The court ordered that the complainant be hired and be accorded all benefits and seniority status as of the date that initial employment would have taken place. The interval approximated 6 months [109]. Such decisions give further credence to the intent of antidiscrimination legislation and its interpretations as applied to the rejection of job applicants on the basis of medical findings.

Although presumably not tested legally, as yet, in the examination setting, an interesting method of obtaining a medical history has been noted. Because of the prior existence of workers' compensation claims for back injuries or because of aggravations of previous injuries, many companies carry out special examinations of the neck and back or may obtain preplacement films of the cervical or lumbosacral spine. One cargo flying company [110] has given lie detector tests to applicants for jobs in its air cargo facilities, some of the questions referring to workers' compensation claims and existing injuries. Whether the procedure will see more universal use or will be tested in the courts following objection remains to be determined.

REFUSAL OF EXAMINATION

Infrequently an individual will refuse to submit to a medical examination. If this action is based on religious beliefs, there may be misinterpretation on the part of the applicant of the examination as medical treatment. There may also be fear of the procedures involved. The question was submitted to the Committee on Occupational Medical Practice of the AOMA, and its reply is given in its entirety [111]:

> The members of the occupational medical practice committee believe that OSHA cannot require an employee to take tests or examinations but can require the employer to offer them. The employer can make certain required tests or examinations mandatory for job placement either as part of the pre-placement agreement or as part of any periodic health evaluation. When employees exercise their prerogative not to take such evaluations, the employer then has the right to transfer these employees to another area where examinations of this type are not required. OSHA does not have the authority to require an employer to permit an employee to work a job for which the employee is not qualified because of some medical reason. Refusal on the part of the employee to submit to a required medical examination for a specific job, in essence, disqualifies the employee for that particular position for medical reasons.

DISCUSSION

DIAGNOSTIC RADIOGRAPHY

Certain precautions must be exercised in the conduct of examinations for work. The inclusion of radiographic studies on asymptomatic patients (job applicants) has been questioned. Ashenburg, Medical Director of Eastman Kodak Company, observed at the 1981 American Occupational Health Conference that chest roentgenograms on candidates for employment may not be justified, and only employees exposed to substances causing pulmonary difficulties should have such examinations on a regularly recurring basis. The frequency was to be determined by the natural histories of the diseases associated with the specific exposures.

An 11-year study conducted by the Kaiser-Permanente Group in San Francisco on Kaiser Foundation Health Plan Members [112] demonstrated few benefits, so the examination was stopped as a "routine" procedure. In comparable vein, the Food and Drug Administration (FDA) [113], in keeping with the report of a special study group, recommended that such chest radiographic screening be discontinued, as the yield has been insufficient to justify the cost, the added radiation exposure, and the patient inconvenience. In short, the examination was considered unnecessary and unproductive, especially for job applicants. When specific items in the history or findings on medical examination indicate the radiographic study, then it should be conducted. Also, employees exposed to substances affecting lung function or causing disease should receive periodic chest roentgenograms. In 1983, the FDA issued its report as the second in a series of publications presenting panel-developed recommendations on selected x-ray examinations, the first having covered pelvimetry. The panel recognized that there have been many instances where freestanding screening chest x-ray examinations have been performed on asymptomatic persons solely because of administrative mandate or protocol. The productivity of such examinations depends on the prevalence of disease in those populations and whether its detection actually reduced morbidity and mortality [114].

The yield of unsuspected disease, such as pulmonary cancer, heart disease, and tuberculosis, from these examinations, not based on history, physical examination findings, or specific diagnostic testing, has been shown not to be of sufficient clinical value to justify the monetary cost and, as indicated, the added radiation and inconvenience to the subject. The recommendation did not preclude radiography in selected populations shown to have significant yields of previously undiagnosed disease [114].

Insofar as preplacement chest radiography was concerned in industry, the panel recommended that occupational medical departments evaluate critically the current use of routine chest x-ray examination programs in their companies [114]. However, in its referral criteria statement in this connection, it was stated that preplacement chest films should be done selectively, based on pertinent factors in the occupational and medical history, the results of clinical examinations, and the proposed work assignment [114].

Other groups have voiced similar opinions. The AOMA has articulated its guidelines concerning preplacement chest radiography in parallel with the statement of the FDA [115,116]. The World Health Organization has indicated that in subjects occupationally exposed to respiratory hazards, there is justification for preemployment chest radiographic screening [117]. The American College of Radiology has adopted similar guidelines [118].

In connection with preplacement spine radiography, there are no indications for completing this kind of examination on employment applicants, for there is no relationship between the findings—usually congenital anomalies—and either the development of symptoms or the incurring of back injuries [119]. Insurance underwriters are also cautioning their assureds that this exposure to unnecessary ionizing radiation may initiate lawsuits. A few resistant medical advisers believe that radiographic studies of the lumbosacral spine can identify workers who will develop back injuries. There is no evidence to support this contention. The World Health Organization [117] put it bluntly: ". . . pre-employment lumbosacral radiography is of no clear medical benefit to the individual and should not be performed."

Certainly, job aspirants who are pregnant should not be examined radiographically, and as suggested by Saenger and Kereiakes [120] and as is fairly common practice now, a sign should be posted in the radiology section reading, "If there is any possibility you could be pregnant, notify the technologist or physician before your exam."

The "routine preemployment radiography for insurance purposes of some foodhandlers" is also mentioned by the National Research Council [121] as a procedure not productive of sufficient diagnostic health rewards for the costs incurred. An exception is made in the case of applicants for employment in skilled nursing facilities. Barclay [122] advises that such persons should receive both a tuberculin test and a chest radiographic examination for the protection of the patients they serve and for their own future protection should there be exposure to a patient with an open case of tuberculosis; a medical follow-up is indicated for determination of the presence of infection.

USE OF QUESTIONNAIRES

The issue of cultural bias in test procedures emerged strongly with the civil rights movement of the 1960s and 1970s. In design of a health history form, consideration should be given the fact that many immigrants will be completing the questions and either the queries may not be clear or they may not embody familiar, idiomatic expressions in the language native to the applicant when prepared by professionals.

In a study by Berkanovic [123], it was demonstrated through back-translation of a questionnaire that there were several instances in which the Spanish version was unidiomatic. There proved to be lower reliabilities and lower bivariate correlations among Hispanics interviewed in Spanish than among Hispanics interviewed in English. In essence, the writer pointed out that considerable care needs to be taken to ensure that a translation achieves a level of language usage equivalent to the original source.

LABORATORY TEST PROCEDURES

Although the conducting of clinical laboratory tests as part of the preplacement examination is different from the completion of such examinations during the diagnostic or follow-up phases of an illness, it should be understood that such procedures can be stressful. Kaplan [124] pointed out many years ago that patients being subjected to such testing, who were either uninformed or misinformed regarding these diagnostic aids, manifested considerable reaction to them, either fearing the apparatus or drawing unwarranted inferences as to the nature and gravity of their illness.

While such tests are included glibly in the prehire medical protocol, every procedure should be explained as to its purpose, its relevance to the job, and its side effects, if any. The applicants should be assured, in addition, that any tests resulting in abnormal findings will be repeated, and if consistently aberrant, will be followed with explanations and definitive study.

GYNECOLOGIC EXAMINATIONS

Normally, pelvic examinations are not included in the preplacement medical review. There may be rare occasions when such a procedure is indicated because of recent symptoms, findings on palpation of the abdomen, and the like and where the employer provides complete medical care. Is the presence of a woman necessary? The question has been asked [125] and the response is quoted in its entirety, for it depicts something of the changing ethos in American practice:

> If this question were asked 30 years ago, the answer would have been yes, with possible exceptions. Today the answer is no.
>
> In deciding whether to have an attendant present, one should determine first the desires of the patient. Many patients are extremely uncomfortable with a third person in the room. It is most appropriate for the attendant who prepares the patient for examination to inquire as to her wishes. In general, at the first visit, particularly with a teenager, an attendant may be desirable. This holds true even if the physician is a woman. The teenager may wish to have a hand to hold. One other consideration is the comfort index of the physician. If he is anxious—have an attendant during the examination.

The response may be extrapolated to the examination of any woman applicant for employment, without consideration of the pelvic aspect of the review.

A survey was conducted of British family physicians, and of 171 respondents, 23, or 13 percent, claimed they always used a chaperone during examination of female patients, while 42, or 25 percent, said they never did. Most of the practitioners had a third person present as a medicolegal protection [126].

SPECIAL ISSUES

Two issues warrant brief discussion: drug testing and genetic screening. Some companies have conducted urine screening for the evidence of drug use by both applicants and employees. Usually it has been interpreted as another urinalytic procedure and no more invasive of privacy than the testing for sugar or protein. In certain work populations, where the applicants may be drawn from a group known for, or suspected of, high chemical abuse, and where aberrant behavior or impaired judgment would be hazardous to the health of the tested subject and co-workers or would preclude completion in an orderly manner of job assignments, testing would be indicated. Screening would be appropriate in such sensitive positions as law enforcement or fire suppression, in work in health care facilities where the individual might have access to prescription medications, or merely to halt on-the-job drug abuse [127]. If on-site drug detection is indicated, systems are commercially available for this purpose. At the time of writing, the arguments for and against continue between corporate officers and civil libertarians, let alone between governmental units and civil servants. One precaution is indicated, though. While screening may be introduced at the time of hire, it should not be used as a basis for discharge of an incumbent employee. If the analysis is positive, referral should be effected for counseling, as it would be for a newly identified problem drinker.

Genetic testing conducted by certain companies* has met with nearly explosive reactions and has been investigated by the Congress [128]. Implicit is the potential of discrimination because of inherent inequalities in people as revealed by such screening when included in the preplacement evaluation. When used, the screening was conducted on a one-time basis to detect certain acquired chromosomal abnormalities or inherited genetic traits. Although there is no evidence to date, the monitoring for acquired chromosomal aberrations was conceived as aiding in the identification of a population at risk for future development of cancer. The screening for inherited genetic traits was based on the rationale that a particular trait might result in increased susceptibility to certain exposures (for example, glucose 6-phosphate dehydrogenase enzyme deficiency resulting in hemolytic anemia after exposure to certain oxidizing chemicals). The American Public Health Association (APHA), in a policy statement, urged industry to cease such testing for the purpose of job exclusion and urged the formation of a qualified panel to develop ethical and scientific guidelines for the workplace use of genetic testing [129].

Omenn [130], in a presentation to the AOMA, pointed out that the Office of Technology Assessment panel on which he served concluded that no genetic screening should be conducted *routinely* at this time. There was consensus that several areas show promise for research on potential genetic predispositions and warrant careful study. Further, there was considerable caution expressed concerning the difficulty of interpreting results of monitoring for mutagenic activity and chromosomal effects. The panel did endorse further development of these mon-

*As cited from *Fortune* (Strasser, A. L. Genetic screening can be a useful tool to promote safety. *Occ Health Saf* 53:29, 1984), 6 companies were doing the testing, and 17 had conducted some tests in the past.

itoring tools as indicators of exposure and as guides to efforts to reduce exposures and presumed health risks.

The emphasis still has to be given to engineering control of toxic exposures and not to highly discriminatory selection of a workforce that will nullify participation by *all* in a wage-earning society.

SPECIAL PARKING

Operating as the OHS must, under the beneficial constraints of the Rehabilitation Act of 1973, its physicians will be examining many persons with moderate to severe physical impairments. A question attendant upon such employment is the issue of special parking. As many organizations have parking facilities at some distance from the worksites, efforts are made by certain employees to have special parking privileges granted to preclude extended walking to and from their regular work areas.

In an effort to meet the need of this limited personnel and to counter when necessary the ill-based requests submitted by private physicians on behalf of their patients, a set of criteria was developed for use at one of the installations with which the writer was connected. The standards may serve as a guide for others who have been presented with this vexing problem. The criteria, in the form of a memorandum from the chief executive officer, follow:

1. "Handicapped" parking is a *privilege* that may be granted when the employee has certain debilitating physical disorders, subject to the needs of the company.
2. The medical conditions that *may* be considered for handicapped parking are:
   a. Blindness, total or with best corrected vision of 20/200 in both eyes.
   b. Malignant growths, other than of the skin, that require chemotherapy or radiation treatment.
   c. The presence of one lung only, secondary to surgical removal of the other lung.
   d. Angina pectoris, supported by a report of treadmill or other ergometric testing, which reveals electrocardiographic abnormalities while running for up to 10 minutes on a 5% incline.
   e. Conditions requiring the use of crutches, walking casts, or wheelchairs, for a 6-week period only, except for a permanent use of a wheelchair.
   f. Amputation of a portion of a lower extremity exclusive of the toes.
   g. Severe rheumatoid arthritis involving the lower extremities, exclusive of other sites.
   h. Intermittent claudication supported by a statement from a Board-certified vascular surgeon stating that there is *significant* arterial occlusion of a lower extremity.
   i. Acute injury, moderate to severe, to a lower extremity, for a 2-week period only, subject to extension, if absolutely necessary.

   Adequate medical documentation must be supplied in all of the above conditions, subject to additional examination at the OHS.
3. Further, a memorandum must be obtained from the employee's supervisor stating that adequate company transportation is not available to the employee with one of these conditions, from the parking lot within 100 yards of his worksite, and back.
4. The medical conditions that are not considered handicapping from the standpoint of special parking are:
   a. Neck and back problems, including degenerative disc disease, old compression fractures, and low back strain with or without leg pain.
   b. Diabetes mellitus, with or without complications, except for those disorders mentioned above.
   c. Chronic obstructive pulmonary disease.
   d. Cardiac conditions, including post-myocardial infarction status, and coronary bypass surgery.
   e. Gastrointestinal diseases, including dumping syndrome and post-operative states.
   f. All forms of arthritis, other than severe rheumatoid arthritis.
   g. Thrombophlebitis of a lower extremity.
   h. Varicose veins.
   i. Flat feet.
   j. Plantar warts.

Employees whose conditions do not fit into any of the above categories will be evaluated on a case-by-case basis.

The difficulty to be anticipated is that of employees who have been able to walk from their regular parking areas and back suddenly applying for the special privilege. Such individuals should be examined to determine the status of their claimed clinical deficits.

THE ESSENCE

Whatever the extent of the examination or its site of operation, the constellation of procedures can be developed into "a worthwhile and intellectual pursuit" by having the practitioner ask himself the questions propounded by the late Dr. L. G. Norman [131], former medical director of London Transport: "Why am I doing this?" "How can the results of this physical examination be usefully applied?" and "How should it be modified to serve a more useful purpose?" Perhaps a beginning will have been made when productive responses emerge.

REFERENCES

1. *Guiding Principles for Medical Examinations in Industry* (rev.). Chicago: American Medical Association, 1984. P. 1.
2. Blankenbacker, R., Hawkins, L., and Robbins, L. C. Overview of Health Hazard Appraisal. In *Into the Mainstream with Health Risk Reduction.* Proceedings in the Fifteenth Annual Meeting on Prospective Medicine and Health Hazard Appraisal, St. Petersburg, FL, October 3–6, 1979. Bethesda, MD: Health and Education Resources, 1979. Pp. 4–7.
3. Robbins, L. C., and Hall, J. H. *How to Practice Prospective Medicine.* Indianapolis: Methodist Hospital of Indiana, 1970.
4. Durfee, J. S., and De Grassi, A. Health Hazard Appraisal in the Workplace. In *Into the Mainstream with Health Risk Reduction.* Proceedings in the Fifteenth Annual Meeting on Prospective Medicine and Health Hazard Appraisal, St. Petersburg, FL, October 3–6, 1979. Bethesda, MD: Health and Education Resources, 1979.
5. Robbins, L. C. Overview: Health Hazard Appraisal. In *Heart Risk Estimation, Risk Reduction and Health Promotion.* A collection of papers presented at the 18th Annual Meeting of the Society of Prospective Medicine held in Quebec City, October 20–23, 1982. Ottawa: Canadian Public Health Association, 1983. Pp. 15–24.
6. Sacks, J. J., Krushat, W. M., and Newman, J. Reliability of the health hazard appraisal. *Am J Public Health* 70:730, 1980.
7. Wagner, E. H., Beery, W. L., Schoenbach, V. J., et al. An assessment of health hazard/health risk appraisal. *Am J Public Health* 72:347, 1982.
8. Schoenbach, V. J., Wagner, E. H., and Karon, J. M. The use of epidemiologic data for personal risk assessment in health hazard/health risk appraisal programs. *J Chronic Dis* 36:625, 1983.
9. Levinson, D. The physician and the medical history. *JAMA* 211:2158, 1970.
10. Meares, Source unidentified.
11. Liebman, J. Clothes make everybody more revealing. *Patient Care* 9:12, March 1, 1975. Copyright © 1975, Patient Care, Oradell, NJ. All rights reserved.
12. Friedman, E. To dilate or not to dilate. *JAMA* 205:928, 1968.
13. Benzinger, T. H. What is normal body temperature? *JAMA* 218:603, 1971.
14. Perlman, L. V., Chiang, B. N., Keller, J., et al. Accuracy of sphygmomanometers in hospital practice. *Arch Intern Med* 125:1000, 1970.
15. Nicholas, W. C. Cited in Wrong cuff size hampers sphygmomanometer reading. *Intern Med News* 17:23, Apr 1–14, 1984.
16. Mancia, G., Bertinieri, G., Grassi, G., et al. Effects of blood-pressure measurement by the doctor on patient's blood pressure and heart rate. *Lancet* 2:695, 1983.
17. Zanchetti, A. Cited in Iatrogenic factors may cause misleading blood pressure reading. *Intern Med News* 17:29, Nov 11–14, 1984.
18. Kroenke, K. Sphygmomanometry: The correct arm position. *West J Med* 140:459, 1984.
19. Hagelsten, J. O., Jessen, K., and Knudsen, J. B. Clinical application of bilateral blood pressure measurement with special regard to health examinations. *Scand J Work Environ Health* 8:94, 1971.
20. Seth, G. S. Original research into normal blood pressures. *Occup Health* 24:41, 1972.
21. Neumann, H. H. Blood pressure recording in the tense patient. *JAMA* 227:327, 1974.
22. *Kling* v. *County of Los Angeles et al.* Filed with U.S. Court of Appeals for the Ninth District, Dec. 8, 1980; Ramos, J. Appeals court rules against medical school: Aspiring nurse wins suit on admission. *Los Angeles Times* II:6, Aug 25, 1985.
23. "Obese" worker wins appeal against Xerox. *Los Angeles Times* IV:3, Aug 28, 1985.
24. *Federal Register* 42:22680, Section 84.12, 1977, Reasonable Accommodation. (Regulations to Sec. 504, Rehabilitation Act of 1973.)
25. Wen, C. P., Trai, S. P., and Gibson, R. L. Anatomy of the healthy worker effect: A critical review. *J Occup Med* 25:283, 1983.
26. Felton, J. S. Medical Examinations for Employment. In S. W. Nylander and J. Carmean, *Medical Standards Project—Final Report* (3rd rev. ed.). San Bernardino, CA: County of San Bernardino, Personnel Division, Oct 1984. Vol. I, pp. 1–5-I.
27. Nylander, S. W., and Carmean, G. *Medical Standards Project Final Report* (2nd rev. ed.), Vol. II. San Bernardino, CA: County of San Bernardino, Personnel Division, Jan 1983.
28. Carmean, G. Physical abilities analysis and job related medical standards. Presented at the First National Conference on Back Injury in the Workplace 85—Strategies for Prevention, Toronto, March 4–7, 1985.
29. Nylander, S. W., and Carmean, G. *Medical Standards Project Final Report* (3rd rev. ed.). San Bernardino, CA: County of San Bernardino, Personnel Division, Oct 1984. Vol. I.
30. Recommendations for determining the employability of job applicants with diabetes mellitus: Report of the Committee on Employment and Insurance of the New York Diabetes Association. *J Occup Med* 7:20, 1965.
31. Employment of diabetics: A statement of the Committee on Employment and Insurance, American Diabetes Association. *Diabetes* 21:834, 1972.
32. Lister, J. The employment of diabetics. *J Soc Occup Med* 32:153, 1982.

33. Lister, J. The employment of diabetics. *Br Med J* 2:1087, 1983.
34. Mastbaum, L., Tetrick, L., and Alexander, R. W. Physicians' guidelines for employment and placement of the diabetic in industry: An update. *J Occup Med* 22:601, 1980.
35. *Code of Federal Regulations.* Aeronautics and Space. Title 14, rev. Office of the Federal Register, National Archives and Records Service, Federal Services Administration, Jan 1, 1984, §67.13, §67.15, and §67.17.
36. Engelberg, A. L., Gibbons, W. L., and Doege, T. C. A review of the medical standards for civilian airmen: Synopsis of a two-year study. *JAMA* 255:1589, 1986.
37. Moore, R. H., and Buschbom, R. L. Work absenteeism in diabetics. *Diabetes* 23:957, 1974.
38. Health, H., III, Melton, L. J., III, and Chu, C-P. Diabetes mellitus and risk of skeletal fracture. *N Engl J Med* 303:567, 1980.
39. National Diabetes Data Group. Classification and diagnosis of diabetes mellitus and other categories of glucose intolerance. *Diabetes* 28:1039, 1979.
40. New standards for classification and diagnosis of diabetes. *JAMA* 243:2296, 1980.
41. Riley, T. L. Lying about epilepsy. *N Engl J Med* 303:644, 1980.
42. Woman who lied about epilepsy to get job back. *Stockton (CA) Record* 1:9, Aug 2, 1981.
43. Blank, J. R., and Anderson, R. J. The effects of anticonvulsant drugs on rehabilitation and employment of epileptics. *J Rehab* 49:61, Apr/May/June 1983.
44. Halen, R. J. Epileptics in mining. *J Occup Med* 25:356, 1983.
45. Wheatley, G. M., Cunnick, W. R., Wright, B. P., et al. The employment of persons with a history of treatment for cancer. *Cancer* 33:441, 1974.
46. Cunnick, W. R., Cromie, J. B., Cortell, R. E., et al. Employing the cancer patient: A mutual responsibility. *J Occup Med* 16:775, 1974.
47. Regional variations in mortality from cancer. *Stat Bull Metrop Life Insur Co* 54:3, Feb 1973.
48. Silverberg, E. Cancer statistics, 1981. *CA* 31:13, 1981.
49. Long term cancer survival among men. *Stat Bull Metrop Life Insur Co* 62:11, Jan–March 1981.
50. Cancer mortality—Tennessee, 1960–1980. *MMWR* 33:577, 1984.
50a. Gardner, W. H. Laryngectomees (neck breathers) in industry. *Arch Environ Health* 9:777, 1964.
51. Bullock, C. The "hands free" artificial larynx. *Med Trib* 25:6, June 27, 1984.
52. *Laryngectomees at Work.* New York: International Association of Laryngectomees, 1977. Pp. 6–7.
53. Feldman, F. L. *Work and Cancer Health Histories: A Study of the Experiences of Recovered Patients (White Collar Study).* San Francisco: American Cancer Society, California Division, 1976.
54. *Work and Cancer Health Histories: A Study of the Experiences of Recovered Blue Collar Workers.* San Francisco: American Cancer Society, California Division, 1978.
54a. Crowder, J. H. The Cardiac in the Workplace: Employment Aspects. In *The Cardiac in the Workplace.* Final Report and Recommendations of a Conference Held February 23, 1978, San Francisco, CA. Sacramento, CA: California Governor's Committee for Employment of the Handicapped, 1978. Pp. 29–33.
55. Stanton, B. A., Jenkins, D., Denlinger, P., et al. Predictors of employment status after cardiac surgery. *JAMA* 249:907, 1983.
56. Jenkins, C. D., Stanton, B.-A., Savageau, J. A., et al. Coronary artery bypass surgery: Physical, psychological, social, and economic outcomes six months later. *JAMA* 250:782, 1983.
57. Dimsdale, J. E., Hackett, T. P., Hutter, A. M., Jr., et al. The association of clinical, psychosocial, and angiographic variables with work status in patients with coronary artery disease. *J Psychosom Res* 26:215, 1982.
58. Placement of bus drivers who have had by-pass surgery. *J Occup Med* 26:800, 1984.
59. Criteria Committee of the New York Heart Association. *Nomenclature and Criteria for Diagnosis of Diseases of the Heart and Great Vessels* (8th ed.). Boston: Little, Brown, 1979.
60. Barrett, P. A., Peter, C. T., Swann, H. J. C., et al. The frequency and prognostic significance of electrocardiographic abnormalities in clinically normal individuals. *Prog Cardiovasc Dis* 23:299, 1981.
61. Fulton, W. J. How human relations problems are dealt with by medical directors, physicians, and nurses. *Indust Med Surg* 21:381, 1952.
62. Pies, R. A piece of my mind: A medical status exam. *JAMA* 245:2081, 1981.
63. Sergeant, H. Pre-employment psychiatric examinations. *Lancet* 2:212, 1984.
64. Melchiode, G. A., and Jacobson, M. Psychiatric treatment: A barrier to employment progress. *J Occup Med* 18:98, 1976.
65. Henschel, A. Obesity as an occupational hazard. *Can J Public Health* 58:491, 1967.
66. Keys, A., Fidanza, F., Karvonen, M. J., et al. Indices of relative weight and obesity. *J Chronic Dis* 25:329, 1972.
67. Bray, G. A., Jordan, H. A., and Sims, E. A. H. Evaluation of the obese patient: 1. An algorithm. *JAMA* 235:487, 1976.
68. Bray, G. A. Communication to County of Los Angeles Civil Service Commission, Jan 3, 1978.
69. Weight Standards. Communication from J. H. Larson to H. L. Hufford, July 25, 1979.
70. 1983 height and weight tables announced. *News from Metropolitan Life Insurance Company,* March 1, 1983. P. 4; Metropolitan height and weight tables. *Stat Bull Metrop Life Found* 64:3, Jan–June 1983.

71. Measurement of overweight. *Stat Bull Metrop Life Found* 65:20, Jan–March 1984.
72. Durnin, J. V. G. A., and Womersley, J. Body fat assessed from total body density and its estimation from skinfold thickness: Measurements on 481 men and women aged from 16 to 72 years. *Br J Nutr* 32:77, 1974; Siri, W. E. The gross compaction of the body. *Adv Biol Med Phys* 4:239, 1956.
73. Ponka, J. L. "Pre-hernia" in the pre-employment examination. *Calif Med* 114:105, 1971.
74. *Performance of Physically Impaired Workers in Manufacturing Industries*. Bull. No. 923. Washington, DC: U.S. Department of Labor, Bureau of Labor Statistics, 1948. P. 28.
75. Berliner, S. D. Inguinal hernia: A handicapping condition? *JAMA* 249:747, 1983.
76. Borhani, N. O. (ed.). *Medical Basis for Comprehensive Community Hypertension Control Programs*. Bethesda, MD: U.S. Department of Health, Education, and Welfare, Public Health Service, National Institutes of Health, National Heart and Lung Institute, National High Blood Pressure Education Program, July 1974. Pp. 46–47.
77. Zahnder, E. Performance of drivers with impaired color sense in traffic. *Schweiz Med Wschr* 101:530, 1971, abstracted in *JAMA* 216:1379, 1971.
78. Royall, W. W., III. Safe contacts and law enforcement. *Contact Lens Forum* 2:15, 1977.
79. Guidelines for work for patients with tuberculosis: A statement by the American Thoracic Society. *Am Rev Respir Dis* 108:160, 1973.
80. Treatment of tuberculosis and other mycobacterial diseases: A joint statement of the American Thoracic Society and the Centers for Disease Control. *Am Rev Respir Dis* 127:790, 1983.
81. Hsu, K., and Barclay, W. R. Reexposure to active tuberculosis after preventive treatment. *JAMA* 242:1543, 1979.
82. Houk. Source unidentified.
83. Weg, J. B. *Tuberculosis and Other Mycobacterial Diseases*. New York: American Lung Association, 1976. P. 3.
84. Birmingham, D. J. Predicting new employee sensitivity. *J Occup Med* 15:311, 1973.
85. Bryan, F. A., cited by Johnson, R. S. Social factors in dialysis. *JAMA* 245:1513, 1981.
86. Gutman, R. A., Stead, W. W., and Robinson, R. R. Physical activity and employment status of patients on maintenance dialysis. *N Engl J Med* 304:309, 1981.
87. Vollmer, W. M., Wahl, P. W., and Braff, C. R. Survival with dialysis and transplantation in patients with end-stage renal disease. *N Engl J Med* 308:1553, 1983.
88. Krakauer, H., Grauman, J. S., McMullan, M. R., et al. The recent U.S. experience in the treatment of end-stage renal disease by dialysis and transplantation. *N Engl J Med* 308:1558, 1983.
89. Johnson, J. P., and McCauley, C. Survival with end-stage renal disease. *N Engl J Med* 309:1519, 1983.
90. Johnson, W. J., Kurtz, S. B., Mitchell, J. C., III, et al. Results of treatment of center dialysis patients. *Mayo Clin Proc* 59:669, 1984.
91. Hellerstedt, W. L., Johnson, W. J., Ascher, N., et al. Survival ratio of 2,728 patients with end-stage renal disease. *Mayo Clin Proc* 59:776, 1984.
92. Carlson, D. M., Duncan, D. A., Naessens, J. M., et al. Hospitalization in dialysis patients. *Mayo Clin Proc* 59:769, 1984.
93. Evans, R. W., Manninin, D. L., Garrison, L. P., Jr., et al. The quality of life of patients with end-stage renal disease. *N Engl J Med* 312:553, 1985; Freeman, R. B. Treatment of chronic renal failure: An update. *N Engl J Med* 312:577, 1985.
94. Decker, R. S. Vocational Rehabilitation of the Renal Disabled. In S. B. Chyatte (ed.), *Rehabilitation in Chronic Renal Failure*. Baltimore: Williams & Wilkins, 1979. Pp. 86–114.
95. Fisher, T. F. Sickle cell anemia and occupational risks. *JAMA* 244:1987, 1980.
96. Hanks, T. G. The physical examination in industry: A critique. *Arch Environ Health* 5:365, 1962.
97. Hanks, T. G. The physical examination in industry. *Arch Environ Health* 12:267, 1966.
98. Luongo, E. P. The preplacement physical examination in industry—its values. *Arch Environ Health* 5:358, 1962.
99. Cooper, M. N. Personal communication, June 5, 1981.
100. Rodman, M. H. The pre-employment physical examination. *J Occup Med* 7:608, 1965.
101. Leckey, R. G. Pre-employment examinations: A pointed study. *J Occup Med* 8:532, 1966.
102. Schneider, R. F., and McDonagh, T. J. Experience data on university recruits hired without preemployment examinations. *J Occup Med* 13:363, 1971.
103. Seigel, G. S. Pre-Employment Examinations and the Federal Employee. Presented sometime during the 1960s at a society meeting relating to occupational health (typescript). P. 3.
104. Voelz, G. L., and Spickard, J. H. Preemployment medical evaluation by questionnaire. *J Occup Med* 14:18, 1972.
105. Williamson, S. M. Eighteen years' experience without pre-employment examinations. *J Occup Med* 13:465, 1971.
106. Thomson, D. Civil service experience of pre-employment examinations. *Proc R Soc Med* 67:182, 1974.
107. *Laeng* v. *Workmen's Comp*. Appeals Bd. 6C al. 3d 771; 100 Cal Rptr. 377, 494 P. 2d 1, March 1972.
108. Warshaw, L. J., and Thornton, J. V. Malpractice liability in pre-placement examinations. *J Occup Med* 6:353, 1964.
109. *DFEH* v. city of San Jose (Douglas R. Groshong) (1984). FEHC Dec. No. 83-14.

110. Pre-employment examinations. *Risk Management Notes,* No. 48, 1973.
111. Committee on Occupational Medical Practice of the AOMA. Legal implications regarding an employee's refusal to take medical examinations offered by a company. *J Occup Med* 23:460, 1981.
112. Chest x-rays administered routinely in job applicants, employees may not be justified. *Intern Med News* 14:17, Sept 1, 1981.
113. Many chest x-rays of asymptomatic patients held unnecessary. *Intern Med News* 14:1, Sept 1, 1981.
114. *The Selection of Patients for X-ray Examinations: Chest X-Ray Screening Examinations.* Rockville, MD: U.S. Department of Health and Human Services, Public Health Service, Food and Drug Administration, Aug 1983.
115. Chest x-ray examinations in occupational medicine. *J Occup Med* 25:773, 1983.
116. Hoops, D. L. Mistaken endorsement. *J Occup Med* 26:486, 1984.
117. *A Rational Approach to Radiodiagnostic Investigations.* Report of a WHO Scientific Group on the Indications for and Limitations of Major X-Ray Diagnostic Investigations. Geneva: World Health Organization, 1983.
118. Radiologists advise less use of routine x-ray screening. *Intern Med News* 16:3, Jan 15–31, 1983.
119. Felton, J. S. Unpublished data, 1974.
120. Saenger, E. L., and Kereiakes, J. G. Medical radiation exposure during pregnancy. *JAMA* 242:1669, 1979.
121. *Effects on Populations of Exposure to Low Levels of Ionizing Radiation.* Report of the National Advisory Committee on the Biological Effects of Ionizing Radiations, National Academy of Sciences, National Research Council 1972, cited in Brown, R. F., Shaver, J. W., and Lamel, D. A. *The Selection of Patients for X-ray Examinations.* Rockville, MD: U.S. Department of Health, Education, and Welfare, Public Health Service, Food and Drug Administration, Bureau of Radiological Health, Jan 1980. P. 15.
122. Barclay, W. R. Preemployment chest x-ray screening and prior BCG immunization. *JAMA* 244:2562, 1980.
123. Berkanovic, E. The effect of inadequate language translation on Hispanics' responses to health surveys. *Am J Public Health* 70:1273, 1980.
124. Kaplan, S. M. Laboratory procedures as an emotional stress. *JAMA* 161:677, 1956.
125. Nichols, E. E. Should a woman attendant be present at gynecologic examinations? *JAMA* 245:1165, 1981. Copyright 1981, American Medical Association.
126. Jones, R. H. The use of chaperones by general practitioners. *J R Coll Gen Pract* 33:25, 1983.
127. Jones, L. San Diego planning employee drug tests: New and current workers would be subject to screening. *Los Angeles Times* II:7, May 26, 1985.
128. Gore calls screening explosive. *Occup Health Saf* 52:8, Aug 1983.
129. Policy statements adopted by the Governing Council of the American Public Health Association, November 16, 1983. No. 8310, Guidelines for genetic testing in industry. *Am J Public Health* 74:281, 1984.
130. Omenn, G. S. The Roles of Genetics in Occupational Medicine. Keynote address, American Occupational Health Conference, Los Angeles, CA, May 2, 1984. P. 17.
131. Norman, L. G., cited by Chatterjee, B. B. The work of the factory medical officer: Some suggestions for reorganization. *Indian J Indust Med* 16:25, 1970.

549402

6. THE WORK ENVIRONMENT AND HEALTH EXAMINATIONS

The physician would be quick to admit that sometimes he has less certainty in certifying the normal than the abnormal state of organ or system. The early recognition of the transition from the healthy to the diseased condition may be difficult, if not impossible.

David Seegal, M.D.

As an occupational health service (OHS) is dedicated to the prevention of disease, many activities are devoted to the maintenance of the worker's health. If an employee's health suddenly changes, a constellation of events is precipitated:

Cessation from work—intermittent or continuous, brief or lengthy, temporary or permanent.

Emergency medical care in the plant health facility.

Definitive medical care from family physician, specialist, or both.

Temporary disruption of family life pattern.

Exposure of family members to possible contagion if the disease is infectious.

Notification of offices within the plant that relate to the illness: supervisor, payroll, insurance, and possibly employee assistance program.

Completion of report forms and statistical entries in the medical department, the employee's department, in the payroll office (to reflect altered work status during pay period), and the insurance office (to initiate any indicated benefit payments in the form of State or company disability pay, supplemental pay, and medical or hospital costs indemnification).

Shift of workforce to provide coverage of ill employee's job, if necessary.

If an injury, there are to be added the activities of accident investigation, reporting, and review by the safety committee; if a work-generated illness in a hospital, involvement of hospital epidemiologist and infection control committee; the initiation of reports to the insurance carrier and state labor authority, if required; and the anticipation or initiation of subsequent rehabilitative care, the initial modification of work on return, and final reclassification to preinjury status.

Sick visitation by the OHS physician or nurse, at the hospital or at home.

Communication between OHS physician and treating physician regarding progress of patient.

On return to work, closing of all medical and administrative records, filing of reports, readjustment of temporary substitute workers, updating of production schedules, and final payment of benefits.

Adjustment of worker to job in light of residual disability, asthenia, or impaired function or adjustment to alternative work; if unsuccessful, consideration of disability retirement.

In essence, the loss of a single person through illness or injury is upsetting to many co-workers, family members, and systems maintained as elements of production and community life. It is desirable through preventive, constructive, comprehensive medical practices to avert these irregularities; there are several opportunities for the physician and the OHS staff to exercise these measures.

MAINTENANCE OF A SAFE AND HEALTHFUL WORK ENVIRONMENT

The designation "safe and healthful" is used to imply the absence or control of factors, materials, processes, and equipment that in their operation, dissemination, assembly, or interaction could prove deleterious to the health or integrity of the worker. The maintenance of these controls is tripartite: the responsibility of the medical department; in part, that of the safety department—whose personnel usually concern themselves with potential physical environmental hazards; and finally that of the work team itself, the supervisor, *and* the employee. (Workers who rely on medical and safety authorities to prevent their becoming ill or injured are heading for personally acquired trauma. Control systems, perfect though they may be, when not utilized by the workers are totally ineffective. Accident or occupational-illness prevention is a form of work philosophy and behavior, the ultimate exercise of which rests with the employees themselves.)

Further, when complete environmental control is not possible through the addition of precautionary caging, railings, automatic devices that render equipment inoperable, or special structures that allow work to be conducted safely at great heights, over deep open areas, or on fast-moving vehicles, then personal protective devices are provided to the employee. Examples of these are leg protectors, fire-retardant suits, face shields, and impact-resistant hats.

The clinical area of concern, though, is with those elements on the work premises that are potentially productive of disease uncommon to the general population. There must be a control of dangerous materials that, through inhalation, ingestion, skin absorption, or entry through a break in the continuity of the skin, could be taken in by the body. These substances may cause untoward effects, may be metabolized to harmless end products and be excreted, may pass through the body unchanged, may be stored with or without danger to the host, or may cause clinical difficulty at a later period.

The illnesses resulting are the occupational diseases, which, through environmental control, can be obviated. Control, in another sense also, is a dual undertaking, accomplished in part by industrial hygiene surveys of the work areas (for identification of potentially hazardous work contacts), direct measurements of the level of contaminants, chemical analysis of samples of workroom air to determine the concentration of toxic materials present, comparison of the levels with the quantities permitted for safe human work activity,* and the installation of indicated exhaust ventilation systems, as well as, in part, by medical surveillance of the surveyed workers. Of course, in addition to the presence of harmful substances, there are various energies (for example, ionizing radiation, noise, vibration, and ultraviolet radiation) and such factors as illumination, temperature, ventilation, humidity, and extremes of atmospheric pressure, all of which can affect the worker adversely and which require measurement for the determination of safe or healthful levels.

Other elements of control are exercised over the sanitation of the plant, and the physician's opinion usually is sought regarding the health and morale-supporting or morale-limiting aspects of such installations as change rooms, washrooms, waste-disposal facilities, showers, food-service areas (cafeterias, snack bars, vending machines), and departmental bag lunchrooms. Sanitation includes the quality of the drinking water and appropriate separation of industrial and potable water sources.

It must be emphasized that if an occupational hygienist is not on the staff, and if the services of one are not available from the corporate level of the company, the physician must be able to conduct an informal survey of the work areas periodically. Assistance can be obtained from local health departments.

*Levels considered safe are termed Threshold Limit Values (TLVs) and are reviewed annually by the American Conference of Governmental Industrial Hygienists (ACGIH). They are updated as changes are indicated by research in toxicology involving human and animal studies, by clinical experience, by judgments based on knowledge of the biologic effects of related substances, or by a combination of these derived data. By publication in the *Federal Register,* vol. 36, no. 105, May 29, 1971, the TLVs became official federal standards for industrial air. Copies of *TLVs Threshold Limit Values for Chemical Substances and Physical Agents in the Workroom Environment and Biological Exposure Indices with Intended Changes* may be obtained from the Publications Office, ACGIH, 6500 Glenway Ave., Bldg. D5, Cincinnati, OH 45211. Alphabetically listed are the levels for chemical substances in the form of gases, vapors, toxic dusts, fumes, and mists, and various forms of physical energy, such as noise and lasers.

HAZARDS IN THE WORK ENVIRONMENT

The physician whose practice is full- or part-time in the work environment should be familiar with the potential hazards present in the industrial arena that may prove, under certain circumstances, to be inimical to health. It is this kind of knowledge that distinguishes the physician from the practitioner who has brought clinical skills into the OHS and exercises those skills in the more orthodox medical sense—in the examination of employees or in the treatment of ill or injured persons. The latter procedures may be executed with recognized expertise, but if they are performed with total disregard of the relationship of responsive tissue or behavioral change to work factors, the physician is providing a partial service only. Indeed, the service may be a disservice to both the patient and the employer and may, in the extreme, be viewed as negligence, in the legal sense.

The potential health hazards* that are present at work may be few or numerous. They may vary from plant to plant and industry to industry. They will

*A newer designation, in a slightly different sense, alludes to health-monitored occupations.

change as raw materials are converted to intermediate products to finished goods awaiting shipment for consumer use. New materials that are hazardous may result from misuse or through unduly lengthy storage, when dangerous substances may be generated within containers. Finally, workers may be exposed to products of pyrolysis or to residues long after a process has been shut down. It is the concept of the ubiquity of danger that must pervade every clinical action taken by the physician practicing occupational medicine. The picture is further clouded by such pathophysiologic phenomena as individual susceptibility (immunologic variance), delayed sensitivity response, and acquired toxicity resulting from increasing body burdens of hazardous substances.

Elements in the worksite that may prove hazardous to one employee or another, given the appropriate time-dose relationships or emotional climate, may be classified into chemical hazards, physical hazards, biologic hazards, and socio-emotional hazards.

CHEMICAL HAZARDS

Under the broad rubric of chemical hazards are included a host of materials, which may be elemental (mercury), inorganic (zinc chloride fume), or organic (methyl ethyl ketone) in structure; a mineral dust (diatomaceous earth), a vapor, a fume, a mist, a gas, an aerosol, or any one of these substances that is solely a skin irritant; a mixture; or a nuisance (inert) dust.

The materials, as implied from the classification given here, can be inhaled, ingested, imbedded in tissue, or absorbed by the intact skin or mucosa. The toxic reactions may involve a single bodily organ system, so that certain substances prove to be hemolytic, bone-marrow depressive, hepatotoxic, nephrotoxic, respiratory irritants, central nervous system poisons, or destructive of the integument. Many materials may be rendered more highly dermatogenic with a change in the vehicle. (Skin irritants usually are equally or more irritant to the mucous membranes or eyes.) Lastly, as given testimony by the catastrophic London and Donora air-pollution experiences, a preexisting organic change, cardiovascular or respiratory disease for example, may on exposure increase many fold the toxicity of a specific chemical compound. In any discussion of chemical hazards, the cautionary queries of Hatch [1] must be recalled when he asks, "Do prolonged contacts with hazardous agents, at levels of exposure below those necessary to produce specific occupational diseases, contribute in any way to the prevalence and severity of one or another of the chronic degenerative diseases that are common among aging individuals? In other words, do workers in certain hazardous occupations and industries show a poorer record of morbidity and mortality specific to these diseases than the experience in the general population?" Of course, only highly controlled studies, as Hatch suggests, might possibly substantiate the concern that a "unique excess of disease does exist in fact and is properly chargeable to particular conditions of work." One day, with extraordinarily advanced systems of inquiry, there may be an answer to the question of the extra health risks of certain occupations. Considered in this connotation are the diseases of aging or wear and tear, not necessarily the specific occupational diseases identified by sound epidemiologic study.

Finally, it must be remembered that certain substances may be carcinogenic, teratogenic, or mutagenic, may speed metabolism, may alter endocrine function, or may cause cosmetic disfigurement.

PHYSICAL HAZARDS

Potential physical hazards include such factors as heat and cold; abnormal (increased and decreased) atmospheric pressure; increased humidity and dampness; excessive or insufficient illumination; radiation, both ionizing and nonionizing; repeated motion, pressure, or shock (including vibration); odor (when excessive, socially unacceptable, or incapable of alteration or removal); and noise.

The physiologic responses to these stressors may range from heat exhaustion to fatal radiation illness, or from noise-induced hearing loss to depigmentation. In many instances, the consistent presence of one of these hazards in the work area may place extremely limited time constraints on the length of work permitted in an area or may require adjustments to preclude physiologic shock, such as moving from the interior of a walk-in freezer to an external temperature of 110°F (43.3°C) or vice versa.

BIOLOGIC HAZARDS

Biologic hazards go beyond the fibrogenic characteristics of the inhalable organic dusts to the field of microbiology. Workers in specialized settings such as service or research laboratories may be exposed to a broad variety of agents such as viruses, bacteria, and their spores, fungi, or rickettsiae, the invasion of which may produce occupationally incurred communicable disease. A different selection of pathogens will account for the zoonoses encountered among laboratory, curatorial, farm, and zoo or vivarium animal-caretaker personnel.

In a grosser sense, the infrequently presenting problems in injury versus illness classification are insect bites and stings, the bites of reptiles, rodents, and certain toxic forms of sea life, and the effects of contact with poisonous plants.

SOCIO-EMOTIONAL HAZARDS

Although most of the discussion of interpersonal difficulties at the work scene will be offered in the chapter on Employee Counseling, the presence of these hazards has been sufficient for Levinson [2] to entitle one of his writings "Emotional Toxicity of the Work Environment" and to state in that piece, "He who would be concerned with occupational health cannot avoid the impact of feelings on health. He must create for himself a psychological stethoscope to sense the feelings of his patients and must evolve means of keeping noxious feelings from inducing symptoms or even death."

An example of extreme social stress may be seen in the following:

A student nurse who was Catholic affiliated for a few months with a university school of nursing to obtain specialized training not available in her home school and lived in the school's residence hall. The university's facilities, although in a large city and representative of many faiths and creeds, did have in their nursing students nearly a pure culture of a single protestant, somewhat fundamentalist belief. The outside student was shunned by the city students in the university center almost to the point of ostracism. The student developed a classic picture of acute anxiety, and sought help from the student and employee health service. When the problem was presented to the student group and to her church for aid in social acceptance, attitudes were changed, and her symptoms disappeared.

ERGONOMIC HAZARDS

A possible fifth class of hazards might be considered, even though it is less obvious. Faults in ergonomics may be encountered, wherein there is a mismatching between operators and their equipment that can result in fatigue, tenosynovitis, or other soft tissue inflammatory response to bodily maneuvers that are physiologically or anatomically unsound, but nevertheless demanded by the job, such as pitching in baseball, prolonged overhead work (for example, plastering of ceilings), removing tile by hand from racks used in kilns, and the like.

Not all efforts in ergonomics are received positively, as retold here:

Judges have complained for many years about the uncomfortable chairs given them for use at the bench. An occupational environmentalist studied the high-backed, long-seated furniture piece and developed a design more in conformity with human anatomic demands and that provided comfort for long periods of use. The new chair was rejected for it did not portray adequately in size the authoritative "seat of justice."

Although the environmental hazards are described in this chapter and while they may seem more appropriate under a discussion of occupational illnesses, they are placed at this point in the text because the assessment of work hazards is an ongoing activity of a preventive nature, aimed at hazard control and thus obviation of job-caused illness.

ASSESSMENT OF THE WORK ENVIRONMENT

Physicians who wish to familiarize themselves with the hazards present in the institution where they have responsibility for occupational health should undertake a survey of the plant in the company of a person knowledgeable of the work processes and their possible effects on the health of the workers. Depending on the size of the plant, such a resource individual might be in management, in production, or in personnel or safety management. If there is an environmentalist* on the OHS staff, he or she would be the most logical person to conduct the walk-through, or preliminary, survey.

In such a survey, as provided in one of the early statements of the Council on Occupational Health of the American Medical Association (AMA) [3] and later indicated by the American Occupational Medical Association (AOMA) [4], the physician is cautioned that equal consideration to accident and health exposures should be given. For the small organization, where job descriptions may not be available through a formal personnel activity, the survey will provide the physician opportunity to view the workers, the jobs performed, the exposures involved, the equipment used, the general environment, and the socio-emotional factors attendant upon the performance of the assigned tasks. From the data derived, the physician should be able to establish a system of medical classification of jobs—based on their environmental and physical demands—that will aid in the selective placement of work applicants.

ASSESSMENT OF ACCIDENT HAZARDS

In most situations, the physician will serve as a member of a safety committee or occupational health and safety team so that there should be awareness of the general philosophy of accident prevention, the be-

*Other OHS personnel might include an engineer, an industrial hygiene chemist, a sanitarian, or a radiologic health or radiation safety specialist (health-physicist).

havioral elements operative in injury causation, the contribution of engineering to the design of safer equipment, and the methodology utilized in safety training in industry.

As observed in the council's statement, a safety checklist may be used—with full recognition of the faults and omissions of such a device—but must be prepared for each separate plant or facility. Such a list can be developed with the understanding that the items selected will be determined by the type of operation. The potential accident/injury hazards may include any or all of the following:

1. Housekeeping, control of waste, oil spills, etc.
2. Floors, stairs, platforms, railings, work surfaces
3. Aisles, walkways, exits, clearance, etc.
4. Ladders, stability, etc.
5. Material handling equipment, types, traffic control, etc.
6. Storage and material piling
7. Machinery—guards and maintenance
8. Tools—use and care of, etc.
9. Electrical and welding equipment, shielding
10. Pressure equipment, steam lines, tanks
11. Overhead pipes, valves, and superstructure
12. Hot materials and heat
13. Chemical hazards, estimate of employee exposure, availability of emergency showers and eyewash facilities
14. Flammable or explosive substances—storage and handling
15. Solvents used for maintenance and cleaning
16. Dusts, fumes, vapors, and gases
17. Fire-fighting equipment, drills and training (including rescue drills)
18. Smoking areas, regulations
19. Personal protective equipment—hard hats, safety glasses, goggles, safety shoes, respirators, when and where mandated for use
20. Washrooms and locker rooms—sanitation, towels, soap, etc.
21. First-aid equipment—availability, contents, training in its use
22. Ventilation
23. Noise
24. Illumination
25. Ionizing radiation—x-ray, alpha, beta, gamma, or neutron, personal monitoring devices
26. Electromagnetic radiation—infrared, laser, microwave, ultraviolet, etc.
27. Job permit procedures
28. Unauthorized job transfers
29. Food handling
30. Miscellaneous unsafe practices

While observing, the physician should attempt to understand the full cycle of a production operation, acquire knowledge of the lexicon peculiar to that operation, develop a feeling as to the stressors and satisfactions present in participation in the process, and lastly, look for and greet any worker who may have been seen as an applicant or patient.

In the council communication there are additional guidelines offered, credited to Solomayer [5], that suggest to the surveying physician the kinds of interrelationships that should be watched for between workers (or applicants) and jobs. For example, the following are cited:

1. Hazardous machinery or mobile equipment: Handicaps which increase the hazard when working with machinery such as rotary saws, punch presses, power trucks, cranes, etc., are serious visual defects, deafness, diabetes, inadequate height or reach, heart disease, hypertension, and epilepsy. Machine-paced procedures may become intolerable to workers who are aged, hypertensive, or who are convalescent from peptic ulcer, coronary artery disease, angina, or emotional stress.
2. Lifting, carrying, pulling, pushing, or reaching: Workers with various disabilities such as back injuries, bursitis, hernias, arthritis, heart disease, or emphysema may aggravate their existing condition or cause serious injury to fellow workers in their inability to carry out these functions.
3. Climbing: Restrictions should be placed on workers with dizziness or deformities or limitations of the extremities which prevent safe working on ladders, scaffolds, cranes, unit stairways, tank car platforms, etc.
4. Extensive walking or prolonged standing: Limitations should be placed on individuals with chronic arch disabilities, back lesions, varicose veins, muscular atrophies, heart disease, etc.
5. Twisting, stooping, squatting, kneeling, or bending: Restrictions may have to be placed on individuals having certain musculoskeletal disabilities which limit the extent to which such activities may be conducted.
6. Driving vehicles: Individuals with poor distant vision or conditions that decrease normal reaction time should be prevented from operating such vehicles as cranes, payloaders, trucks, etc., or working in areas in which there is an exposure to moving equipment and falling objects which involves the risk of bodily injury.

ASSESSMENT OF HEALTH HAZARDS

The type of survey that the physician might conduct can be termed the inspection survey, for it will include no precision of measurement in the appraisal of potential health hazards. Repeated plant tours by physicians will gradually orient them more solidly to the work performed by their employee-patients and will give them a base on which to build future, more informative visits into the plant.

In an inspection survey, these basic demographic data or an elementary knowledge of the plant's operations should be determined:

Type of industry (petroleum, electronics)
Type of plant (refinery, small parts assembly)
Number of workers by sex, age, length of service, ethnicity, gross job classification (craft, service, managerial), department, and location
History of plant (wartime conversion, diversification, mergers, ultimate ownership)
Products (canned fruit, research, power distribution, steel pipe)
Raw materials utilized
Absenteeism, by occupation, sex, age, marital status, ethnicity, department, work location
Accidental injury rates by occupation, sex, age, marital status, ethnicity, department, work location
Turnover rate by occupation, sex, age, marital status, ethnicity, department, work location
Chemical hazards by operation
Physical hazards by operation
Biologic hazards by operation
Socio-emotional hazards by operation (e.g., slaughtering cattle in a meatpacking plant, company pilot)

As the inspection is being made and the environment-worker interactions are being understood, the physician should formulate the type of clinical review that is indicated by the exposure encountered.

Further, one should note the improvements needed in the control systems, if such are lacking. Brandt [6] has outlined the methods of engineering control of air contaminants:

Elimination of the sources of contamination or reduction of the amount
- Building and equipment design, alteration, and maintenance
- Substitution of less toxic materials
- Changes in process or operation
- Housekeeping

Prevention of contaminant dispersion
- Segregation of hazardous processes
- Enclosure of hazardous processes
- Wet methods
- Local exhaust ventilation
- Equipment maintenance
- Worker education
- Housekeeping

Protection of the worker
- Equipment alteration
- General ventilation
- Respirators
- Education of the worker

Other control devices may be required, as determined by the hazard, such as noise-attenuating surfaces, ear muffs, shielding around radioactive sources, shielding with reflecting surfaces in areas of radiant heat, or protective eyewear against glare or laser sources.

The type of survey conducted by the environmentalist is given in greater detail in writings on industrial hygiene [7,8]. Additional AMA guides may prove helpful in relating survey findings to clinical procedures [9,10].

Not to be omitted from the survey by the physician is a review of sanitation in the plant. The sites to be inspected are the areas devoted to food preparation and serving, including cafeterias, snack bars, and vending machines; change rooms and restrooms; shower facilities; drinking water sources; garbage disposal facilities; solid waste management systems; laundries; shop hand-washing fixtures; gymnasium and exercise facilities; swimming pools; and systems of hand-cleanser dispensing. Evidence should be sought of rodent or insect infestation, and methods of foodstuff storage should be investigated.

Large food or beverage processing plants may have sanitary engineers as full-time staff members, but as a rule such personnel is rare. Consultative assistance may be obtained from local health departments.

Standards to be followed for toilet facilities, washing facilities, change rooms, and retiring rooms for women vary considerably by jurisdiction. In many instances they are provided in the state labor, health, or occupational safety and health codes or will be delineated in local building codes. The numbers are determined by the occupancy of the facility (numbers and sex of workers), distance from the work area, and the presence of food-displaying activities, among many other controlling factors. Local ordinances in addition to state codes should be consulted.

Examples of sanitary standards possibly not universally enforced are taken from the General Industry Safety Orders of California; Title 8, Industrial Relations; subchapter 7; article 9, Sanitation.

No. of Employees	*Minimum No. of Water Closets*
1–15	1
16–35	2

No. of Employees	*Minimum No. of Water Closets*
36–55	3
56–80	4
81–110	5
111–150	6
150+	1 additional for each additional 40 employees or fraction thereof

The equivalence of trough urinals and individual urinals is seen in the following:

Length of Trough Urinal	*Equivalent No. of Individual Urinals*
24 in. (61 cm)	1
36 in. (90 cm)	2
48 in. (122 cm)	2
60 in. (152 cm)	3
72 in. (183 cm)	4

Washing facilities (lavatories) are to be made available in these numbers:

Type of Employment	*No. of Employees*	*Minimum No. of Lavatories*
Nonindustrial: office buildings, public buildings, and similar establishments	1–15	1
	16–35	2
	36–60	3
	61–90	4
	91–125	5
	125+	1 additional for each additional 45 employees or fraction thereof
Industrial: factories, warehouses, loft buildings, and similar establishments	1–100	1 for each 10 employees
	100+	1 additional for each additional 15 employees or fraction thereof

Provision is made for multiple-use lavatories in this manner:

24 lineal inches (61 cm) of sink or 18 inches (45 cm) of circular basin—with individual faucet—will be considered the equivalent of one lavatory.

Most of the facilities in the state code are defined, and provision is made for maintenance, distances from worksites, cleansers, water temperature, and the like. For a lengthy discussion of industrial sanitation, see Shapiro [11].

HEALTH EXAMINATIONS

An examination performed at the time of a person's employment is of value as a reference point in time in the employee's natural history of health status. Usually, it does not reflect the changes to come,* so that periodically a review must be carried out. The opportunities for reevaluation are many, and partial or complete medical examinations can be performed. Nearly a dozen examinations make up the variety of evaluations feasible in an occupational health program.

PERIODIC GENERAL HEALTH EXAMINATION—THE CONVENTIONAL VIEW

To be stressed in this aspect of preventive or predictive medicine is the understanding that the examination should be used to determine whether the worker's health is remaining compatible with the job assignment and to detect any evidence of impaired health that may be attributed to the employment [12].

This review may be conducted at an interval to be determined by the factors of physician-time available, the number of employees, and the mean age of the workers. Roberts [13] has suggested the following frequencies for periodic health evaluations:

Age 40 and over: Examine annually.
Age 30–39: Examine biennially in detail, with multiphasic screening examinations midway between the thorough reviews.
Under age 30: Examine every third year in detail, with multiphasic screening between the lengthier appraisals.

Of significance in this kind of redo is a detailed interval history covering the events of medical significance occurring since the last examination. In some plants, employees are examined annually, in others biennially. In many others, histories are taken, symptoms or events of importance are discussed by the physician or nurse with the employee, and referrals for diagnosis and care are arranged. Because of important physiologic and functional alterations in

*This statement may not be altogether true. As an example, a job applicant may present with many significant findings at the maximal limits of so-called normal ranges. His weight may be excessive, possibly 20 percent over the ideal, or he may have recently undertaken a crash dieting program to meet weight standards. His blood pressure might read 138/88, elevated for his age of 25 years, but he is not yet alarmingly hypertensive. The serum cholesterol and triglycerides levels may be just slightly under the local laboratory's peak for normality. Further, he could have a history of 9 years of heavy smoking. To be sure, these findings are a measure of the man today, but they do portend difficulties in the future if nothing is done to reverse the obvious trend of his risk factors.

midlife and later, efforts are made to increase the frequency of physical assessments after age 40.

The laboratory procedures to be included are those replicative of the battery accomplished at the time of hiring, plus those tests that may be indicated by specific deviations from physiologic norms or as dictated by certain potentially hazardous work exposures.

In several medical units, the history and physical examination record forms used differ from the blanks associated with the preplacement medical appraisal. Emphasis is given to the interval history, and the questions that appear with frequency relate to changes in health, weight, smoking and drinking patterns, shift assignments, second employments, pregnancy, exercise, work stress, or marital dissolution.

For convenience in recording sequential examinations, some medical directors have devised special forms for inclusion in the clinical record that comprise several duplicate blank columns, each with its own list of body parts or organ systems and space for the entry of the examination findings. The columns, in parallel, allow easy comparison of evaluation results from year to year or examination to examination.

PERIODIC GENERAL HEALTH EXAMINATIONS—THE NEWER VIEW

In recent years, the worth of the periodic health appraisal has been subjected to rather stringent scrutiny. As there has been debate over the worth of the preplacement medical examination, there has been serious question given to the benefits accruing from this procedure, which has seen prominence in occupational medical practice and has been promoted by concerned practitioners since the early 1920s. Many of the examinations conducted within industry and outside have produced significant findings, some at considerable cost, while many have represented routinistic maneuvers carried out desultorily, productive of nothing.

Physicians, in the main, have been disinclined to perform such evaluations, as they are more interested in identifying pathologic change, an attitude fully in keeping with the educational ethos of early medical school days. Further, when examinations are performed in the number required among workers, they are done hurriedly and may not be carried out with the precision or care required for the isolation of significant changes. Certainly, such examinations do not give a measure of functional decrement, which is particularly important in the older worker and of special relevance in work that is demanding of great physical effort.

As long ago as 1966, Siegel [14] questioned the value of the periodic examination, feeling that there was no proof that persons receiving such attention lived longer or were healthier or happier because of the procedure, nor was there proof to the contrary. The basic premise usually alluded to was that discovering frank disease or disease propensity in the asymptomatic stage permitted favorable intervention. Siegel raised doubt about the validity of the premise as it applies to the significant diseases of adult Americans and to the status of our knowledge of prevention. Proposed as an effective and more practical health measure was the promotion of early sickness consultation coupled with the use of periodic selected disease-screening mass procedures. A study that Siegel had conducted 3 years before this writing [15] brought out an interesting national difference in that the British, on the whole, appeared less enthusiastic over the alleged values of the periodic health examination than did their American colleagues.*

Even in the lay press, the pros and cons of the periodic review have been discusssed [16], with many of the procedures that the examination comprises being considered extravagant. Certain procedures were recommended on a selective basis by age, sex, or work exposure.

A certain kind of "packaging" of examination protocols has been advocated for the primary care physician. Shires [17] has developed a schema for noncrisis visits, and Table 6-1 shows the advised groups, exclusive of immunizations.

DeFriese and Hetherington [18] have traced the history of the periodic health appraisal movement and expressed regrets that much of the early enthusiasm that has emerged in recent years seems to have bypassed the clinical practitioners of medicine. However, they do believe, in spite of the doubt being expressed by both the provider and consumer of medical care, that certain preventive procedures must continue to be exercised.

An extensive study was conducted by the Canadian Task Force on the Periodic Health Examination, which probably, as expressed by Morgan [19], is the most rigorous, detailed, and comprehensive evaluation of this convention undertaken to date. The task force reported its conclusions in 1979 [20–22], basing its recommendations on the type of evidence available to consider a specific maneuver either for inclusion in the periodic health examination or for

*That Siegel's comments have weathered well is seen in the fact that 16 years later, in an editorial, Siegel's writing was again referred to in a discussion of one of medicine's "sacred cows," the periodic health examination (A.S.J. selective periodic health examinations. *Med Trib* 23:23, Jan 27, 1982).

TABLE 6-1. *Recommended Examination Protocol for the Adult*

Interval	*Sex*	*Procedure*
17–38 Years (young adults)		
6 months, annual, or biennial as determined by risk	F	Pap smear; pelvic examination
		Breast examination
	M,F	Dental examination
Annual	F	Hemoglobin
	M,F	Health risk assessment and life-style counseling
		Blood pressure
5 years	M,F	Emotional assessments
39–55 Years (middle-aged)		
6 months, annual, or biennial as determined by risk	F	Pap smear; pelvic examination
	M,F	Hemoglobin
		Breast examination
Annual	F	Counseling—menopause
	M	Counseling—identity crisis
	M,F	Counseling—pre-retirement
		Health-risk assessment
		Selective physical examination including BP, tonometry, and rectal examination
		Dental examination
56 Years and over (senior)		
Annual	F	Pap smear; pelvic examination; breast examination
	M,F	Physical examination including nutrition and podiatry, social and health maintenance
		Counseling and anticipatory guidance
		Dental care

SOURCE: Shires, D. B. Life Protocols: A Schema for Health Maintenance. In D. B. Shires and B. K. Hennen, *Family Medicine: A Guidebook for Practitioners of the Art.* New York: McGraw-Hill, 1980.

exclusion. Evidence for inclusion was considered as "good," "fair," or "poor," and evidence for omitting a maneuver was classified as "fair" or "good." On these grounds, certain age- and sex-specific health protection packages were proposed. The packages are tied to, or based on, certain target conditions that in most instances are specific disease states (for example, iron-deficiency anemia, cancer of the cervix) or in some instances are behavioral entities (family dysfunction, progressive incapacity with aging, retirement distress). The adult age groups used are 16 to 44 years, 46 to 64 years, 65 to 74 years, and 75 years and over. All terms are defined, and the effectiveness of prevention and treatment is rated, as is the quality of the evidence.

Certain maneuvers—actually interventions from which more good than harm accrues in their application—are conducted, such as immunizations, urinalysis, history, funduscopy, and the like, for each age-sex category. Table 6-2 lists those of specific relevance to industry. This scheme can be adapted for use in industry because it provides a set of guidelines for the maneuvers to be included in the periodic health examination that are based on sound evidence, can be used to replace the annual health examination, and can be added to the procedures that are carried out in the medical surveillance protocols.

About the same time that different views were being taken of the components and frequency of the periodic health examination, the American Cancer Society published new guidelines [23] for cancer-related examinations. In view of pertinent information about the costs, risks, and effectiveness of various test procedures used for the early detection of cancer, a new schedule has been promulgated, which unfortunately gives no consideration to the special case of potential industrially incurred dust diseases of the lung. The guidelines for early detection of cases in asymptomatic persons are listed in Table 6-3.

Even though periodic chest radiographs and sputum cytologic examinations are not recommended, decisions must be made as to their inclusion in the periodic health examination as determined by the potential health risks inherent in workers' exposures. Considerable rebuttal of the original guidelines, prior to revision, has appeared in the medical literature [24–27].

Breslow and Somers [28], in 1977, prepared a lifetime health monitoring program that utilized clinical

TABLE 6-2. *Conditions and Maneuvers in Women and Men Ages 16 to 74*

Targent condition and recommendation	*Maneuver*	*Best current estimate of optimal frequency of maneuver*	*Remarks*
Tuberculosis	Tuberculine sensitivity testing; immunization with BCG vaccine and chemoprophylaxis as necessary	On the basis of clinical judgment	For persons exposed to the disease through their work, etc.
Cancer of the skin[a]	Inspection; counselling	At appropriate intervals on the basis of clinical judgment	High-risk groups; persons who work outdoors or are in contact with polycyclic hydrocarbons
Cancer of the bladder	Cytologic analysis of urine	On the basis of clinical judgment	High-risk groups, workers occupationally exposed to bladder carcinogens and smokers

[a]Excludes women and men ages 65 to 74.
SOURCE: Modified from Task force report: The periodic health examination. *Can. Med. Assoc. J.* 121:1193, 1979.

TABLE 6-3. *Guidelines for Cancer-Related Examinations*

Type of cancer	*Test or procedure*	*Sex*	*Age*	*Risk*	*Frequency*
Lung	Chest x-ray (not recommended) Sputum cytology (not recommended)				
Colorectal	Sigmoidoscopy	M & F	Over 50		Every 3–5 years after two initial negative examinations one year apart
	Stool guaiac slide test	M & F	Over 50		Every year
	Digital rectal examination	M & F	Over 40		Every year
Uterine	Pap test	F	20–65 and women under 20 who are sexually active		At least every 3 years, after two initial negative tests a year apart; more frequently in high-risk women[a]
	Pelvic examination	F	20–40 Over 40		Every 3 years Every year
	Endometrial tissue sample	F	At menopause	High[b]	At menopause
Breast	Breast self-examination	F	Over 20		Every month
	Breast physical examination	F	20–40 Over 40		Every 3 years Every year
	Mammography	F	Between 35–40 Under 50 Over 50		Baseline Consult personal physician Every year
Health counseling and cancer checkup[c]		M & F M & F	Over 20 Over 40		Every 3 years Every year

[a]Early age at first intercourse, multiple sex partners.
[b]High risk is defined as having a history of infertility, obesity, failure of ovulation, abnormal uterine bleeding, or estrogen therapy.
[c]To include examination for cancers of the thyroid, testes, prostate, ovaries, lymph nodes, oral region, and skin.
SOURCE: Guidelines for the cancer-related checkup: Recommendations and Rationale. *CA* 30:1, 1980.

and epidemiologic data to identify specific health goals and professional services appropriate for 10 different age groups. They matched certain health goals with professional services. The age segments germane to employment were young adulthood (18–24 years), young middle age (25–39 years), older middle age (40–59 years), and the elderly (60–74 years). Recommended for the various periods were certain examinations, counseling, health education, instruction in self-examination (breasts, skin, testes, neck, and mouth), immunizations, dental prophylaxes, and podiatric treatment. In the first and third of the age groups, health education and individual counseling, as needed, were advised for occupational hazards and problems.

The AMA, which since 1923 has advocated periodic health appraisal, reviewed the protocols for examination offered by other writers [20–23,28–30] and published a summary of the recommendations [31]. At one point or another throughout an individual's lifetime, nearly every examination element is indicated, as are a limited number of immunizations. It was agreed that medical examinations could be helpful in the early detection of some treatable conditions—amblyopia, diabetes mellitus, cervical cancer, hypertension, and glaucoma. Primary prevention, a role for the patient or the employee, is effective in aborting poliomyelitis, motor vehicle–related injuries, lung cancer, and chronic bronchitis. The general recommendations presented should be modified in terms of certain factors, and "occupation" is included. No other mention is made of work-relatedness in the review.

In substance, the concept of the periodic health examination is changing, and it is advised that for the *general* health examination, the wise premises of the Canadian study be adopted.

MANAGERS' HEALTH EVALUATION

Because of the great investment in managerial persons* and because of their unique worth in the progress, growth, and guidance of the company, many OHSs conduct special examinations of this group, special in the sense of greater frequency, more extensive evaluation, or a different site for examination. Such a site might be that of an outside clinic, either in the geographic area of the company or at a remote point where 2 or 3 days away from the demands of work can accompany the clinical study.

Other procedures that might be added to the examination include a full battery of blood chemistry determinations, proctosigmoidoscopy, resting and exercise electrocardiography, tonometry, pulmonary function studies, hematologic survey, or, possibly, radiographic studies† of the gastrointestinal tract, cholecystography, and a psychiatric interview.

At the Mayo Clinic, the examiners recommend adding annually at age 40 cytologic studies of the sputum if the subject is a heavy smoker, every 5 years if a nonsmoker. Also, these procedures are suggested at appropriate intervals, if indicated and desired: refraction, dental radiography and consultation, and immunization against tetanus, poliomyelitis, and other diseases as may be needed for travel abroad. They suggest for women cervical cytologic studies if married, or beginning at age 21, and annual mammography at age 50 and thereafter.

Of greatest importance in this special examination, though, is the prompt collation of all the findings with an unhurried clarification or interpretation of the results with the executive. This moment is ideal for a review of the individual's method of handling stressors, of the early findings indicative of trends toward ill health, and of the means of subsequent medical or psychiatric attention. In relation to these examinations, the role of the physician in industry is that of interpreter, not informer, to both the executive and to management—to the latter only when administrative or assignment decisions hang in balance

*The questions—who is an executive, who is a manager—have not been answered too well. The late Dr. Leo Wade attempted to differentiate the two. In his view, executives were those members of management whose function was primarily to establish policy and to coordinate the implementation of such policy in the interest of the shareholder, the employee, the consumer, and the public. In contrast, the other members of management were concerned with the implementation of existing policy and in varying degrees to the shaping of new policy. He pointed to "management health," rather than "executive health." (Wade, L. What is executive health and how should it be maintained? *Med Bull* [Standard Oil Co. of NJ] 18:154, 1958.)

Ranazzini commented on executives: "As a rule, then, men of great talent devote themselves wholly to the pursuit of learning only under stress of poverty and when fired by the hope of making a fortune; and they do secure handsome incomes and, besides, a great reputation with the nobility who thereafter knocks at their doors and ask advice. But though [they] reap a rich harvest of wealth and fame, their occupation too often begets thistles and a troublesome crop of calamities for its votaries to gather in." (Wright, W. C. *The Morbis Artificum Bernadini Ramazzini Diatriba*. The Latin text of 1713 (revised, with translation and notes). Chicago: University of Chicago Press, 1940. P. 379.)

†Diagnostic imaging involving ionizing radiation must be kept at a minimal level. It renders a disservice to the patient to study roentgenographically all available bodily organ systems. There should be solid indications for specific reviews in this modality.

and when knowledge of the status of health, in a generic sense only and free from diagnostic detail, may aid in formulating such decisions. Such intelligence is important, for it may accelerate or deter upward, lateral, downward, or distant moves. The role is that of the physician, irrespective of the focus of the examination. As to action that might be taken regarding the findings, Shepard [32] stated it well:

> The employer has a right to know, for example, whether there is medical evidence that a man is overloaded with responsibilities; whether his physical and mental condition is such that he may safely be given additional responsibilities or a foreign assignment; and whether the years are treating him well or poorly. Such inquiries are legitimate and can usually be answered tactfully and satisfactorily without divulging privileged information.

If the employee wishes his private physician to receive a copy of the examination report, this request should be met promptly, when an authorization is signed and retained in the medical record. In some organizations, the medical director may not receive the report, a copy going directly to the personal physician.

In the description of the executive examination program at the Mayo Clinic, the issue of confidentiality is covered in this manner [33]:

> In our experience these examinations prove to be of greatest benefit to patients, and therefore indirectly their companies, if the information gained is held in strict confidence. Executives are more likely to be frank and open in giving their medical history when it is known that there will be no divulgences except through our oral and written reports to the patient. Patients may then share these reports with their personal physician or the appropriate company officer, as they wish. Under this plan, examinees develop full appreciation of the examination and its aims and do not withhold symptoms or complaints for fear such disclosures might prove prejudicial to their careers. With each patient's authorization, we gladly provide letters of findings and recommendations to the company physician.
>
> If a company does not have a medical advisor, we urge patients to discuss with the appropriate company official those medical findings that may have potential for affecting their safety, efficiency or eligibility for promotion.

Although the yield on survey of executives has led to a vast literature that has provided endless lists of both clinically significant and medically unimportant entities, it is helpful to site the findings from one representative series. Carryer and his coworkers at the Mayo Clinic [34] analyzed 2,812 examinations conducted on 569 subjects who entered the program over a 13-year period, following referral by their companies. The mean number of examinations per subject was 4.9. There were 50 instances of malignant disease encountered among 46 subjects followed during the program of repetitive reviews. Some of the pathologic changes found in the group by percent of patients included obesity (29.5%), colon and rectal polyps (21.6%), musculoskeletal disorders (17.6%), hypertension (15.8%), inguinal hernia (12.3%), coronary artery disease (7.9%), and diabetes mellitus (6.5%), among others.

Not included here for discussion are the arguments offered by the antagonists of the special periodic health appraisal as applied to executives. Many researchers have pointed out the fact that the health of business leaders is no different from that of their subordinates or from persons in occupations lower in the socioeconomic scale. It is the author's belief that this contention is true but that we are more keenly sensitized to the morbidity and mortality of leaders because of their greater newsworthiness and exposure by the communications media. Much of the explanatory truth behind executive health difficulties lies in personality structure, and both Braceland [35] and Farnsworth [36] have attested to the close intermeshing of emotional health status, lifestyle, company mores, and the demands of the business life. As Braceland [35] has put it, "Man is a psychosomatic unity predisposed by constitution and temperament, but conditioned also through a long series of changing environments to react in a certain way to the daily vicissitudes of life." It is through the job, in great part, that executives, exercising creative and productive skills, can undergo self-realization. The job is integral to their personality, so what affects the job affects them, their methods of coping, and eventually their system responses, so that heart disease, anxiety, and conversion reactions soon appear. Again as Braceland [35] has observed, "The executive in industry, then, because of the stress of his position, but more so because of the psychologic equipment that tends to bring him to posts of responsibility, is often vulnerable to the development of psychosomatic disorders. . . ." Farnsworth [36] concluded his review of executive stress by commenting that change now characterizes the manager's life, so that there must be a different orientation of the medical personnel, more realism and self-discipline from the individual executive, and greater flexibility and imagination from the company. Implicit in this view is the need for periodic appraisal of the manager's health, and the medical evaluation is the portal of entry to counseling and effective psychotherapeutic action with the executive.

MEDICAL SURVEILLANCE

Medical surveillance is evaluation of the physical/emotional status of workers exposed to potential health hazards, irrespective of the duration of contact. Such employees are asked to come in for examination at regular intervals, the nature of the examination being determined by legislative mandate (Occupational Safety and Health Administration [OSHA] standards), by agency recommendation (National Institute for Occupational Safety and Health [NIOSH] criteria documents), the nature of the harmful chemical substance, the biologic material, or the physical energy to which they are exposed as part of their work assignment.

In the criteria documents mentioned, in most instances, the interval between examinations, the bodily organ system that should be the particular target of the clinical procedures, and the accompanying clinical laboratory bioassay measurements are specified. The Industrial Hygiene Guides, published by the American Industrial Hygiene Association, may be consulted for the recommended examinations and test procedures.

Various schemata for detailing the components of medical surveillance procedures in a broad variety of exposures have been devised. It is suggested that each OHS develop such a model in parallel with the potential health hazards present, in use, or produced at the installation. Such a tabulation will facilitate both the scheduling of the examinations and their completion. An excellent medical reference chart detailing the legal basis, timing of the examinations, and the recommended tests is available from Health Evaluation Programs, Inc. (HEP), 808 Busse Highway, Park Ridge, IL 60068, (312) 696-1824.

If the OHS includes environmentalists among its professional personnel, they should be involved in this special examination program, for they know the workers exposed, the contact materials or energies, and the intensity of the exposure as measured by environmental sampling. An occupational history obtained and noted in the health record by the occupational hygienist can be used as a standard against which to measure the clinical findings. A joint operation between the environmentalist and the physician can produce the most worthy and critical appraisal of the effect of potentially harmful exposure on the worker.

The physical examination, apart from certain emphases because of exposure, differs little procedurally or in content from most health evaluations conducted periodically.

While most medical surveillance procedures are conducted during work time, the question of pay rarely arises. In a case taken to a federal appeals court, workers had been exposed to inorganic arsenic. The Occupational Safety and Health Review Commission overruled the company and voted to carry out an OSHA citation against the employer for having violated the 1978 standard that limits worker exposure to that material. The company scheduled the initial examinations of exposed workers during the regular workday when the standard became effective and paid for the tests, provided transportation to and from the hospital, and paid the employees their wages. Participation by the workers was 100 percent. When follow-up examinations were required, they were scheduled after working hours, and although the company paid for the surveillance procedures, they paid neither the transportation costs nor the wages, and participation dropped to 58 percent. The local union filed a complaint with OSHA for the employer's failure to provide the examinations without cost to the workers. An OSHA administrative law judge agreed with the citation and levied a fine of $100. The Review Commission upheld the citation, and the company appealed, but the appeals court held that there was sufficient evidence to support the commission's contention that death or serious illness could result from the company's failure to provide examinations without cost [37].

For a definitive review of all aspects of medical screening and biologic monitoring, see "Conference on Medical Screening and Biological Monitoring for the Effects of Exposure in the Workplace, July 1984" [38].

JOB TRANSFER EXAMINATION

A job transfer examination is an extension, in a sense, of the preplacement physical examination in that its objective is to determine, at the time of proposed job change, that the employee will be as physically and emotionally fit to perform in the new position as in the one being vacated. In the initial placement of medically limited applicants, as indicated previously, an effort is made to match capacities against job demands. To ensure that workers who have bid on or are being promoted to a new job are capable of performing in that job, without harm to themselves or coworkers and without jeopardizing company equipment or property, they should be reexamined as soon as a transfer is being considered.

In many instances, notification of the OHS will be sufficient to permit a review of the health record, and approval can be granted for the move. However, the change provides an excellent opportunity for a sequential appraisal, so the employee should be examined and such health counsel rendered as indicating by the findings and the pertinent points in the interval history. In most industrial experience it is found that there may be greater physical demands made through job changes early in employment—labor pool to apprentice program, for example—than in later progression upward in established work ladders or from worker to first-line supervisory positions.

PHYSICAL FITNESS DETERMINATION

A department head or supervisor may request an examination to determine the physical fitness of an employee to complete the assigned tasks inherent in a particular job. Such a request is usually based on observed changes in the worker's performance, although other reasons for the evaluation may include excessive absence attributed to illness, personality change, repetitive injuries, or any behavior during the work period that might possibly be related to a medical cause. In a manner comparable to the conduct of the preplacement examination, the physician determines if the incumbent is physically and emotionally fit to carry out the elements of the job as either noted by the referring supervisor or as delineated in the job description.

When the medical conclusion is reached, it is added to other evidence obtained by the unit head, such as attendance records, production levels, or previous performance evaluations, and administrative action is taken, if needed. The examiner or medical director usually states that in his or her opinion the incumbent is fit or not fit to perform the expected duties. The examiner may recommend some action therapeutically if, in fact, there is a medical (physical, emotional, or mental) explanation for the change in work performance.

Frequently the examiner meets informally with the referring individual before the employee is seen and often after the examination is completed and before a recommendation is submitted. The worker may wish to have a representative with him or her during the interview or any other deliberation with the physician or supervisor. Such an arrangement presents no difficulty. The representative cannot be present during the examination, for that would invade the physician-worker relationship.

In referrals of this type, there is rarely a physical basis encountered for the change in work productivity, attitude, or mood. The aging employee with symptoms of vessel change, for example, will demonstrate an organic reason for the request made by the supervisor. But most individuals who are referred are undergoing some behavioral difficulty because of impaired relationships with the supervisor, coworkers, or possibly spouse or children. Counseling follows, ordinarily, in an effort to understand and heal the interpersonal fractures that have developed. Outside referral to a mental health specialist may be needed when the emotional problem, irrespective of etiology, requires longer professional assistance.

The sage words of the late Dr. Leo Wade [39] concerning the nonproductive employee must always be remembered: "If an employee suddenly fails to measure up to job requirements, he should be considered ill until proved otherwise."

POST-ILLNESS–ABSENCE REVIEW

Certain institutions have requirements that employees returning to work after an episode of illness or recovery from injury must be cleared by the OHS. This regulation may vary in the number of days of absence requiring clearance, that is, the factor of a waiting period; in the need for a signed statement from the employee's personal physician; or in the occupational or nonoccupational nature of the condition causing the absence. Further, the method of review in the OHS may differ, in that employees having undergone extremely brief illnesses may be interviewed only, by a physician or nurse, while persons having been away for longer periods may require complete examinations. At times it may be important to obtain authorization from the returning employee for transfer of information from the treating physician regarding the absence—diagnosis, operative surgical procedure, complications, convalescence, and prognosis.

No immutable law should be established regarding this method of review, for flexibility or fluidity should be maintained. It would be desirable to have records forwarded immediately by the treating physician or hospital, but an employee's return should not be delayed because of their temporary lack.

The essence of this type of review is that an excellent opportunity exists with the employee's return to work for a partial or complete medical examination, for pertinent health counseling, or for psychological counseling, if emotional factors were significant in the loss of work time.

EXAMINATION FOR OVERSEAS ASSIGNMENT

The growth of multinational corporations* and governmentally supported operations abroad and the appointment of embassy and consulate staff to new independent nations have led to an increased number of American nationals living in countries vastly different culturally from the United States. Companies with long experience in this form of short-duration expatriation have noted the costs of premature returns of American nationals. Because of their inability to survive the multiplicity of contrasts in climate, associates, living quarters, diminished sensory in-

*There are now approximately 45,000 multinational corporate families with one U.S. member as the ultimate parent or subsidiary in 25 free-world countries. (Pelton, L. L. Personal communications, July 8, 1985.)

puts, and educational opportunities, overseas personnel in many instances have failed to complete their contractual terms. Recent events, all too well-known, have highlighted a series of true life-endangering hazards in the form of kidnapping for ransom of American nationals and diplomats, the bombing of embassies, and the holding of hostages.

The problem of selection has been difficult, as Miller [40] has pointed out, for several reasons. The person given a foreign assignment is separated from headquarters, necessitating the making of decisions without the counsel of superiors. Sociocultural pressures may be intolerable not only to the worker but also to his or her family. Further, the managerial skills needed in an overseas facility may be greatly different from the skills utilized successfully in the United States. Also, there may be effects on the person making the appointment. The manager who has made a poor choice may have jeopardized his own standing with the company by so doing and may have to spend considerable time in "shoring up the ineffective performer." He may have to reassign the employee abroad, and in so doing, the workload of the remaining members of the foreign subsidiary will have to be increased. Lastly, poor performance by the incumbent abroad may hamper the success of the company in that particular area.

The medical director will most likely be involved in the physical examination of the proposed candidates, in their psychological evaluation, and probably most importantly, in an evaluation of the health and psychological needs of the candidate's spouse and family. Persons who have negative attitudes toward non-Americans and other cultures will have great difficulty abroad and will turn an enriching experiential opportunity into a period of nonlearning isolation shared with fellow Americans only. Children or other family members with chronic disorders in need of skilled medical surveillance should not be sequestered in countries where such care is not obtainable or where certain pharmaceuticals are not available.

In the guidelines for the examining physician issued previously by the U.S. Department of State and now obsolete but still pertinent [41], the purpose of the examination was well stated, as follows:

To preclude the employment of personnel with disabilities or physical disorders that make them an undue risk for appointment to the foreign service or service abroad.

To select individuals for a foreign service career or overseas service whose physical condition, past medical history, and general health disclose no factors that might constitute a potential risk to the individual or to the government under the environmental conditions encountered in foreign countries.

To advise personnel officers as to limitations of duty or assignments that should be imposed for medical reasons.

To sift out personnel who are unable to perform their duties because of physical or mental disabilities.

To gather data and information for improving the health program.

Further, the State Department described the employment factors present in foreign service [41]:

> Foreign Service personnel are subject to assignment on a worldwide basis and as a consequence are exposed to a large variety of health hazards. Although these risks vary in degree and type, they are extreme at about one-third of the posts operated by the Foreign Service. Examples of adverse factors include extremes in climate and altitude, unsafe water and milk supplies, limitations in varieties of food, exposure to exotic diseases, inadequate hospital and medical services, unavoidable anxiety and stress incident to crises and other hardships. Personnel assignments to each post are not ordinarily for less than two or more than four years. Personnel transfers may occur on short notice. Thus an average career involves several changes with respect to culture, language, and health and living conditions. To withstand these basic environmental changes personnel serving abroad must enjoy more than average health in physical, nervous and emotional makeup and stability. It is for these reasons that the high medical standards established herein must be applied with great care. Furthermore, organic changes or failures must be promptly identified in order that corrective measures may be taken.
>
> Other factors incident to employment in the Foreign Service must be considered by examining physicians. Duties range from formal diplomatic representation to routine clerical work. But the difference in duties and responsibilities of different groups is not sufficiently great to warrant different standards as far as health requirements are concerned. Some must operate office machines, but the demand for muscular dexterity is not great. No unusual physical strain is involved except sustained close visual effort over long periods of time. On the other hand, prolonged emotional strain is common. Routine and special duties must sometimes be carried out under strange, trying and shifting situations. On occasions the exigencies of the Service require overtime or work at night. An effective Foreign Service establishment requires teamwork of high degree and each member must not only be proficient at his own task but willing and able to cooperate with others.

The need for understanding the prospective assignee's psychological structuring is described in this manner [41]:

> Psychotic and mentally defective individuals are normally disqualified prior to the medical examination but other types of mental deviations are not. Some candidates appear normal and seem to progress well at home yet harbor deep-seated fears, anxiety, somatic and other reactions characteristic of psychoneuroses. They are unhappy and

hope to secure contentment and relief elsewhere. Others, afflicted with innate abnormal personalities are unduly suspicious, sensitive, moody, or inadequate. Such inner troubles are not left behind when they go abroad. On the contrary, they are often aggravated and many frank failures fall in these categories. The difficulty in detecting such defects without verified historical data is obvious but examiners should keep them constantly in mind. Such candidates should be carefully evaluated to determine the degree of emotional disturbance and be referred for psychiatric opinion where indicated or desirable in borderline cases.*

The components of the examination should be comparable to those in a complete preplacement medical examination, with additional procedures being carried out as indicated by significant medical historic data or current findings. The dependents should be examined, and a psychological or psychiatric evaluation should be conducted on all adult members of the family and on minors who can be interviewed.

In some organizations, selection for overseas tours of duty is made by company officers without referral to the medical director.† In these instances, candidates frequently are chosen for their technical skills, without inquiry into their ability in interpersonal relationships, and poor choices can be made. Particular emphasis is given the need to evaluate the spouse of candidates to determine the ability to undertake change.

That care must be exercised in the approval of personnel for service abroad is given affirmation by an American physician overseas who found, among recent arrivals, one person with uncontrolled diabetes, one in acute depression, and a third who shortly went into status asthmaticus. Such problems can be compounded by the lack of appropriate medications locally.

*It is not possible to forecast who will become a chronic alcoholic under a given set of stress factors, but it is feasible to identify individuals with personal problems. I had the opportunity to remain in contact with an astute department head of an organization with which I had been associated for a number of years. As the years went by, I learned that many of the workers whom we had seen for emotional difficulties, manifested both at home and at work, went on to problem drinking. In retrospect, it was not likely that chronic alcoholism would have been predicted.

†Schneider put it this way: ". . . It is very unusual, indeed rare, for the medical intervention to impact [itself] significantly on the transfer decision, once higher management and the assigned case come to a decision." (International Health Considerations for Multinational Companies, presented before the American Occupational Health Conference, Denver, CO, April 17, 1985. P. 3.)

EXAMINATION ON RETURN FROM OVERSEAS ASSIGNMENT

In a sense comparable to a debriefing, assignees returning from work abroad should be examined as completely as when they departed. There may be a real culture shock awaiting their reentry into the American lifestyle, where servants are unknown and value systems are totally at variance. Members of the Peace Corps have manifested this difficulty on return, as have persons away on construction projects for long periods.

In addition to the usual medical examination components, clinical laboratory tests as indicated by the area of sojourn should be performed. A period of residence in the tropics would require testing for evidence of any residua of tropical infections or infestations.

Wolfe [42] treated the subject well in a review of the medical management needs of persons and their dependents returning from overseas employment, whether they were tourists, short-term consultants, or longer-term residents in the developing countries.

The screening procedures recommended and the acquired diseases to be considered are the following:

- The asymptomatic returnee
  - Stool examinations for ova and parasites
  - Stool cultures
  - Blood examinations
  - Liver function tests
  - Urinalysis
  - Tuberculin testing (before, during, and on return from residence abroad), with chest radiograph on persons demonstrating preexisting tuberculin positivity
  - Serologic screening (schistosomiasis, filariasis)
- The symptomatic returnee
  - Diarrhea and other gastrointestinal complaints (enteric bacteria, protozoa, certain helminths)
  - Fever
    - Malaria
    - Amebic liver abscess
    - Enteric fever caused by *Salmonella typhi* or paratyphoid species
    - Hepatitis (type A more frequent in tropics)
    - Other infections (trypanosomiasis, visceral leishmaniasis, brucellosis, leptospirosis, tuberculosis, and infections with Lassa, Ebola, or Marburg viruses)
  - Eosinophilia
    - Intestinal helminths
    - Filariae

The point emphasized by Wolfe is that certain exotic infections may manifest themselves months or years after return, so that the possible relationship of symptoms to previous travel must be considered in all personnel who have been in "out-of-the-way places."

EXAMINATION OF DIVER PERSONNEL

With the increase in oceanographic exploration for petroleum and minerals, the spread of interest in recreational diving, the expanded undersea experiments of the Navy, and the renewed efforts at salvage of sunken vessels, the number of persons undertaking depth diving has multiplied extraordinarily. At present there are over 2 million divers in the United States using self-contained underwater breathing apparatus (SCUBA). There are approximately 1,000 commercial divers working offshore in the United Kingdom sector alone in the North Sea oil operation [43]. The hazards are multiple in the individual who is neither physically nor emotionally fit to undertake this kind of activity occupationally or as a sport. Spivack [44] states flatly that no sports diver has any business doing decompression diving, which should be left to the professional diver whose job requires such frequent underwater activities.

The hazards are numerous, as Spivack [44] and Egstrom [45] explain. The diver is made up of relatively noncompressible tissue (because of water content and bone) and breathing various gases or air that are compressible and are of varying solubility. Breathing air under pressure puts nitrogen into solution, and if there is too rapid release of pressure, the nitrogen returns to its gaseous state, and bubbles form in the blood or tissues. This action can lead to vascular obstruction, or if the bubbles collect around the bones or joints, there will be pain and, later, aseptic bone necrosis may result. If the bubbles settle in the skin, pruritus, a rash, or edema may follow.

The serious forms of decompression sickness affect the central nervous system (CNS), the heart, and the lungs. The "chokes" is a disorder of the lungs resulting when more than 10 percent of the pulmonary circulation is obstructed. Barotrauma comes also from the presence of the bubbles, in essence, the expansion or contraction of gases in confined spaces—in a dental cavity, the middle ear, a blocked sinus, or in obstructive lung disease. Other hazardous conditions mentioned by Spivack [44] include the high pressure nervous syndrome (a general excitation and irritability of the CNS), the shallow water blockout of breathhold diving (from hyperventilation before free diving), and cold water drowning.

Physicians who are in institutions where divers are employed (marine biology research, ship overhaul, marine exploration) will examine such personnel with extreme care, for certain, even minor, clinical disorders will assume great significance in the underwater work environment.

The physical and emotional requirements as summarized from several sources [45–50] follow:

General health	Good, free from chronic disabling disease or injury.
Age	Persons over 40 years old require special consideration because of the demands of heavy physical exertion and strenuous activity.
Cardiovascular system	No gross impairment of exercise tolerance or evidence of cardiovascular disease. Resting electrocardiogram (ECG) and exercise ECG are preferred to rule out coronary arteriosclerosis. Recent myocardial infarction, syncope or arrhythmia-proneness, and cardiac murmurs contraindicate diving. Peripheral vascular disease that might interfere with gas exchange in an extremity rules out participation; varicose veins or hemorrhoids should be minimal. There should be no evidence of "bleeding tendency."
Blood pressure	Elevated systolic or diastolic pressure contraindicates; systolic pressure should not exceed 145 mm Hg and diastolic 90 mm Hg on repeated recordings. A hypertensive person on therapy is contraindicated.
Obesity	General fitness for strenuous exercise is questioned.
Ears and sinuses	Person must be able to equalize pressures in middle ears and sinuses. Sinusitis, polyposis, or severe allergy contraindicates. Perforation of eardrum is considered an absolute contraindication. Residual or prior ear, nose, and throat (ENT) surgery contraindicates.
Lungs	Chronic respiratory disease such as tuberculosis, bronchitis, emphysema, asthma, or other obstructive airway disease contraindicates. Standard chest radiograph should be done to reveal possible cysts, adhesions, emphysema, or calcified nodes, as they may contribute to air embolism even when standard safe procedures of diving are followed. Vital capacity should be 80 percent of predicted value. Recurrent pneumonia, prior thoracotomy, and history of pneumothorax are contraindications.
Nervous system	History of seizure disorder or attacks of unconsciousness are absolute contraindications.

Emotional status	Recklessness or emotional instability is a serious liability to diver and companions, as is a history of repeated accidents, with or without injury. Claustrophobia is incompatible with diving, as are chronic alcoholism, drug abuse, unusual use of medications, and heavy smoking.
Teeth	Dental caries or periodontal infections are not absolute contraindications but may cause great discomfort.
Diabetes	Individual evaluation is required regarding severity and exertion involved. Unstable diabetes contraindicates.
Acute infections	Temporarily contraindicating, such as upper respiratory infection or middle ear infection.
Anemia—mild, stable, chronic (thalassemia)	Individuals who are mature, trained, aware of limitations, and self-disciplined may dive under these guidelines: (1) hemoglobin level greater than 10 gm/dl; (2) ability to swim 50 yards without fins, 100 yards with fins, mask, and snorkel; (3) ability to breath-hold dive and retrieve a small weight from a depth of 10 feet; and (4) no evidence of cardiopulmonary dysfunction. In addition, they may engage in nonstrenous diving at depths and for times keeping diver within no decompression limits and should adhere to the buddy system. They should use SCUBA apparatus with low breathing resistance, a well-fitted wet suit for thermal protection, and a high-quality inflatable vest. A buoyancy compensator on the vest would allow descent and ascent with minimal effort [47].
Pregnancy	Contraindicates because of sensitivity of developing fetus to increased oxygen tension or depressant effects of nitrogen.
Musculoskeletal system	Chronic disc disease contraindicates.
Gastrointestinal system	Any disease productive of symptoms contraindicates diving, including severe gastroesophageal reflux.
Vision	Because of changes in distant vision under water, low illumination, and refractive changes introduced by the water environment, the following criteria [49] may prove helpful in decision-making: 1. Individuals with uncorrected vision of 20/50 or better in one or both eyes and with no evidence of organic ocular disease are unrestricted. 2. Individuals with uncorrected visual acuity of 20/50 to 20/100 for distance and the equivalent of 20/50 or better for near in one or both eyes and with no evidence of organic ocular disease may dive if the examining physician and a diving official advise them of the risks associated with decreased vision. 3. Individuals with uncorrected vision of less than 20/100 for distance and less than 20/50 for near in one or both eyes and with no evidence of organic ocular disease should be restricted from diving unless optical correction worn underwater improves vision to 20/100 or better for distance and 20/50 or better for near in one or both eyes. The examining physician and a diving official should advise these individuals of the risks associated with decreased vision. 4. Individuals with significant organic ocular disease affecting both eyes should be restricted from diving.

The General Industry Safety Orders for California have been revised regarding diving operations. As certain employers within the state are modeling their examination requirements after the new code, it is suggested as a guide [50].

EXAMINATION OF MOTOR VEHICLE OPERATORS

Most states require physical examinations of motor vehicle operators who drive commercial vehicles. In California, for example, examinations are given class 1 drivers, who may drive any vehicle or bus, except two-wheel motorcycles, and who may tow any vehicle or combinations of vehicles. Class 2 drivers are examined also, and these operators are comparable to class 1 except that they may tow a vehicle weighing less than 6000 pounds gross. Medical standards are set forth in the state's administrative code, in the form of minimum physical requirements. In California, operators must be reexamined biennially. The OHS of an organization can conduct these examinations, thus saving work time. Forms are provided by the state agency (Department of Motor Vehicles) and usually contain a wallet-size certificate that can be completed and given to the drivers attesting to their having met the medical standards.

The U.S. Department of Transportation (DOT) has issued Motor Carrier Safety Regulations [51], which include the required physical qualifications applicable to drivers of common, contract, and private carriers subject to the Department of Transportation Act (49 U.S.C. 1951 et seq.).

The standards as given by the DOT are as follows [51]:

A person is physically qualified to drive a motor vehicle if that person

Has no loss of a foot, a leg, a hand, or an arm, or has been granted a waiver pursuant to Section 391.49;

Has no impairment of a hand or finger which interferes with prehension or power grasping, or of an arm, foot, or leg which interferes with the ability to perform normal tasks associated with operating a motor vehicle, or has been granted a waiver;

Has no established medical history or clinical diagnosis of diabetes mellitus currently requiring insulin for control;

Has no current clinical diagnosis of myocardial infarction, angina pectoris, coronary insufficiency, thrombosis, or any other cardiovascular disease of a variety known to be accompanied by syncope, dyspnea, collapse, or congestive cardiac failure;

Has no established medical history or clinical diagnosis of a respiratory dysfunction likely to interfere with the ability to control and drive a motor vehicle safely;

Has no current clinical diagnosis of high blood pressure likely to interfere with his ability to operate a motor vehicle safely;

Has no established medical history or clinical diagnosis of rheumatic, arthritic, orthopedic, muscular, neuromuscular, or vascular disease which interferes with his ability to control and operate a motor vehicle safely;

Has no established medical history or clinical diagnosis of epilepsy or any other condition which is likely to cause loss of consciousness or any loss of ability to control a motor vehicle;

Has no mental, nervous, organic, or functional disease or psychiatric disorder likely to interfere with the ability to drive a motor vehicle safely;

Has distant visual acuity of at least 20/40 (Snellen) in each eye without corrective lenses or visual acuity separately corrected to 20/40 (Snellen) or better with corrective lenses, distant binocular acuity of at least 20/40 (Snellen) in both eyes with or without corrective lenses, field of vision of at least 70° in the horizontal meridian in each eye, and the ability to recognize the colors of traffic signals and devices showing standard red, green, and amber;

First perceives a forced whispered voice in the better ear at not less than 5 feet with or without the use of a hearing aid, or, if tested by use of an audiometric device, does not have an average hearing loss in the better ear greater than 40 decibels at 500 Hz, 1000 Hz, and 2000 Hz with or without a hearing aid;

Has no current clinical diagnosis of a drug dependence of a Schedule I drug, an amphetamine, narcotic, or any other habit-forming drug; and

Has no current clinical diagnosis of alcoholism.

The regulations include instructions for the performing and recording of physical examinations and a form to be used as a medical examiner's certificate. Waivers of certain physical defects may be issued, as indicated. Drivers who must wear hearing aids must carry a spare power source, and operators who use contact lenses must have a spare lens or lenses on them when driving.

In the *Federal Register* for November 23, 1977, the Bureau of Motor Carrier Safety published rationales or bases for the disqualification of drivers with certain clinical disorders. The discussions are offered to clarify standards that are not totally explanatory and relate the disease state to the particular circumstances of driving.

The note regarding diabetes mellitus is an example, as it pertains to the criteria under Section 391.41 (b) (3) of the regulations [51]:

> A person is physically qualified to drive a motor vehicle if he has no established medical history or clinical diagnosis of diabetes mellitus currently requiring insulin for control.
>
> There is no provision for a waiver of the minimum physical requirements with respect to the insulin dependent diabetic in the Federal Motor Carrier Safety Regulations. Diabetes mellitus is a disease, which on occasion, can result in a loss of consciousness or orientation in time and space. Individuals who require insulin for control have conditions which can get out of control by the use of too much or too little insulin, or food intake not consistent with the insulin dosage. Incapacitation may occur from symptoms of hyperglycemic and hypoglycemic reactions (drowsiness, semiconsciousness, diabetic coma, or insulin shock). The administration of insulin is, within itself, a complicated process requiring insulin, syringe, needle, alcohol sponge and a sterile technique. Other factors related to the operation of an over-the-road commercial motor vehicle in interstate commerce, such as fatigue, lack of sleep, poor diet, emotional conditions, stress, and in addition concomitant illness, compound the diabetic problem. Thus, because of the inherent dangers generally outlined, the Bureau of Motor Carrier Safety has consistently held that a diabetic who depends upon insulin for control does not meet the minimum physical requirements of the Safety Regulations.
>
> Insulin cannot be taken in pill (oral) form because it is destroyed in the digestive tract. Certain drugs, known as hypoglycemic agents, are sometimes prescribed for diabetic individuals to help simulate natural body production of insulin. These individuals are suffering from a less severe form of diabetes mellitus than those requiring shots of insulin for control. If the condition can be con-

trolled by the use of oral medication and diet, then an individual may be qualified under the present rule.

The issue of returning bus and truck drivers to their jobs following coronary bypass surgery was presented to AOMA's Committee on Occupational Medical Practice [52]. In addition to consulting state regulations, it was thought important to undertake evaluation through use of both Holter monitoring and exercise testing. Sudden death may occur in persons who have developed bundle branch block during the infarction, and dynamic electrocardiography may help identify high-risk individuals. The worker should be angina-free and have a negative graded exercise test without evidence of significant ventricular dysrhythmia during the test protocol. Further, it was the belief of some specialists that a nuclide ventriculogram should show an ejection fraction of 50 percent or greater. In substance, drivers should be adequately tested prior to resumption of duties involving responsibility for the lives of others.

Employers are concerned with driver capability in other areas of vehicle operation. Some companies reimburse workers on a mileage-traveled basis when their personal cars are used for business. In other instances, executives may be issued automobiles for full-time use, for both business and personal use. The physician may be called on to render judgment as to the ability of an employee to operate a vehicle. Executives are subject to the degenerative tissue changes of aging, and young persons, although physically capable of meeting standards, may have poor driving records or may be injury repeaters in their jobs. Medical standards lend themselves easily to measurement, but many factors—judgment, drinking, impaired reaction time, faulty attitudes, emotional disturbances—are less well understood and less subject to clinical mensuration.

In *Physician's Guide for Determining Driver Limitation* produced by the American Medical Association [53], the examiner may refer to discussions of various diseases, drug use, emotional and psychiatric disturbances, and aging for counsel as to the relationship of physiologic change to driving skill.

The need for more stringent examination of drivers was brought to light by Rees [54], who examined the medical records of nearly 1,200 "ordinary drivers." Of the group, 109 or 9.2 percent were found to have significant physical or mental illness, and it was thought that these conditions would probably impair their skill as motorists, rendering them unsuitable for employment as drivers of public service vehicles. It was believed that less than 1 percent of all drivers declared their disability when applying for a driver's license.

Shlensky [55] has objected to the use of psychiatric diagnoses as contraindications to the licensing of drivers, suggesting that disease labels do not relate to function, in this instance, the operation of a motor vehicle. Shlensky admits that balancing individual rights against society's interests is difficult and has offered in place of the usual list of restricting disorders a set of criteria claimed to be objective and addressed to function rather than diagnosis. Included are (1) intellectual impairment, with the potentials of impaired consciousness, disorientation, impulsivity, emotional instability, impaired memory, interference with symbol recognition and response, and deterioration of judgment; (2) impaired reality testing involving delusions and hallucinations; (3) suicidal or homicidal inclinations, including the more subtle manifestations of self-destruction seen in accident repetition; and (4) alcohol and drug abuse.

An excellent publication has been produced in the United Kingdom for the guidance of physicians who examine motor vehicle operators: *Medical Aspects of Fitness to Drive,* edited by Dr. Andrew Raffle, Chief Medical Officer of London Transport [56].* Special discussions are devoted to cardiac disorders, diabetes, epilepsy, disorders of the nervous system, mental disorders, vision, head injury, drugs and medicines, aging, and fatigue. The appendices cover the standards of fitness required for drivers, the Employment Medical Advisory Service, the adaptation of cars for physically handicapped drivers, and the medical aspects of exemption from seat belt wearing. The individual contributors are all specialists in their fields, holding appropriate hospital or academic appointments. The work is the most current, and it is recommended particularly to those physicians involved in the certification of great numbers of drivers.

Because of the increased use of motorcycles in general and as a means of transportation to work in specific, there should be concern regarding the employee who cycles to work. The AMA Committee on Medical Aspects of Automotive Safety has extended its interest to the "two-wheeled motor-powered" vehicle and has published its suggestions [57].

EXAMINATION OF FLIGHT PERSONNEL

Many companies have their own aircraft for the transportation of executives, other staff members, or supplies. The equipment may be of the fixed-wing type, jet- or piston-propelled, or helicopters, and

*Available from the Medical Commission on Accident Prevention, 35–43 Lincoln's Inn Fields, London, WC2A3PN, England for approximately $6.00.

there may be one or many full-time pilots or support personnel.

The responsibility for the recurring physical examination of pilots rests with the Federal Aviation Administration (FAA), Department of Transportation, as executed through its medical representatives, designated as Aviation Medical Examiners (AME). Medical standards established by law are contained in the Federal Aviation Regulations [58], and the Federal Air Surgeon's interpretation of these regulations is to be found in *Guide for Aviation Medical Examiners* [59].

Over 99 percent of the examinations are conducted by private practitioners who are AMEs, and about 475,000 applications for airman medical certificates are filed and processed annually. The AME has the delegated authority to examine applicants and holders of the certificates for compliance with the medical standards and to issue, renew, or deny issuance or renewal of certificates, again as based on compliance or noncompliance with the applicable standards. Flight personnel on scheduled airlines are examined every 6 months, other commercial flyers on an annual basis, and private pilots every 2 years (all holders of first-class medical certificates).

Designations of AMEs are effective for 1 year and may be terminated earlier or renewed annually. The AME is authorized to issue only second- and third-class medical certificates, while senior AMEs may issue certificates of all classes.* An AME may be appointed to the senior level on request and on meeting certain criteria. If one or more of a company's physicians were to be designated AMEs, the issuance of medical certificates to the flight personnel of the organization might be facilitated.

In October 1965, an air traffic controller health program was initiated to provide health maintenance and preventive medicine measures for some 16,000 FAA air traffic control specialists (ATCS). Physical examinations of the ATCS are performed by those AMEs who have agreed to participate in the program. The annual medical examination includes certain additional procedures such as an ECG, chest radiograph, audiogram, and tonometric and psychological examinations. These ancillary procedures may be obtained at some Department of Defense, Veteran's Administration, and Public Health Service facilities. When geographic constraints exist, certain private clinics or hospitals may perform these added examinations. If the OHS is in the public sector, that is, in an agency of the federal government, the ATCS who are FAA employees may be examined at that facility. It is to be noted that many of the controllers are pilots or airmen, in addition to being ATCS, a fact that became more fully known during the strike begun in 1981. The guide cited previously [59] also provides information regarding this personnel group.

Denial of a medical certificate is mandatory if an applicant has an established medical history or clinical diagnosis of the following:

Acute or chronic pathologic condition of either eye or adnexa that might interfere with its proper function, might progress to that degree, or might be aggravated by flying.
Acute or chronic disease of the middle or internal ear; mastoid disease; unhealed perforation of the eardrum.
Disease or malformation of the nose or throat that might interfere with or be aggravated by flying.
A personality disorder that is severe enough to have repeatedly manifested itself by overt acts.
A psychosis.
Alcoholism, unless there has been a 2-year period of abstinence.
Drug dependence.
Epilepsy.
Disturbance of consciousness without satisfactory medical explanation of the cause.
Myocardial infarction.
Angina pectoris or coronary heart disease that has required treatment or, if untreated, has been symptomatic or clinically significant.*
Diabetes requiring insulin or oral hypoglycemic drugs for control.

In addition, an airman who is undergoing continuous treatment with antihistamine, narcotic, barbiturate, mood-ameliorating, tranquilizing, motion sickness, steroid, antihypertensive, or ataraxic drugs will be denied certification. Other conditions

*First-class certificates are issued to airline transport pilots. Holders of second-class certificates include air traffic control tower operators, commercial lighter-than-air pilots, commercial pilots, flight engineers, and flight navigators. The designation of third-class medical certificate is reserved for free balloon pilots, private lighter-than-air pilots, and student pilots. Glider pilots and student glider pilots require no medical certificate.

*Concern was expressed by Sands (Sands, M. J., Jr. aviator medical certification after coronary-artery surgery. *N Engl J Med* 307:52, 1982) regarding the return to active flying status of pilots who had undergone coronary artery bypass procedures. While current regulations preclude such action, it still is possible through the special discretionary issuance of a certificate (exemption) or the "special issuance procedure" allowing the post-surgical flyer to resume pilot activity.

that lead to denial or deferment are given in the guide [59].

Because of the numbers of employed persons undergoing coronary artery bypass grafting (CABG), it is realistic to include aircrew personnel as patients experiencing such surgical correction. Parker [60], reporting from England, has indicated that the prognosis following CABG is still being established in the long run. Graft-attrition occurs at a rate of 10 percent in the first year, dropping to 2 to 3 percent per annum in the second and following years. But 46 percent of individuals with symptoms who were treated surgically were symptom-free at 5 years. Time increases the risk of graft atheroma, as it does with the native circulation. However, in one group studied in Europe, sudden, late cardiac death was not observed in a 3- to 5-year follow-up period.

Parker suggests that a pilot may be considered for certification in a multicrew operation 12 months after CABG, provided there is a normal contrast ventriculogram, patent grafts free of other significant disease, a normal exercise ECG, and a normal exercise thallium 201 scan. There should be a 6-month follow-up with exercise ECG and an annual thallium scanning. Coronary angiography should be conducted not later than 5 years following certification. The intermediate and long-term prognosis following transluminal angioplasty is not known.

There are 11 Regional Offices of the FAA with medical personnel and general aviation district offices in nearly all of the states. Directories of the AMEs are available for each of the regions.

The medical evaluation of candidates in the astronaut selection process is conducted by National Aeronautics and Space Administration (NASA) personnel at NASA's Lyndon B. Johnson Space Center in Houston, Texas, and physicians extramural to that facility are not involved except as consultants. See Nicognossian and Parker [61] for information about the medical and psychological tests administered to the candidates.

MISCELLANEOUS HEALTH EVALUATIONS

As determined by medical and managerial policy, other examinations comparable in depth to the periodic general health examination may be conducted. In some organizations, medical evaluations are conducted on employees prior to their *promotion*, particularly if a medical history is positive for one of the several stress disorders. The question will be asked if the candidate would be able to handle the demands of the higher level post or if the new position might possibly cause a recrudescence of a quiescent clinical condition. The OHS of some companies will be asked to perform an examination as validation of claimed disability for *retirement* purposes.* *Termination* physical assessments are standard procedures in some institutions, and under the provisions of the Occupational Safety and Health Act, such examinations are required on workers who have been in contact with certain hazardous substances.

Many second- or third-level managerial members will undertake *teaching* at night and may request reports of chest radiographs or the completion of a full history and medical examination record form. In summer, there will be requests for health status reports for young workers who will serve as *camp* counselors. Employees who carry insurance to cover *disability* may request brief examinations and reports. In the federal or state programs in *rehabilitation,* a candidate for service will have arrangements made for a general medical examination. If the individual is a disqualified or rejected applicant for employment, the examination just completed may serve in this capacity, or if an employee is being referred for service to the official rehabilitation agency, the OHS may conduct the general medical examination. In organizations where *recreational programs* are sponsored, physical examinations may be required of participants. A medical guide for the evaluation of candidates for school sports might be helpful [62], as many of the players on company teams are young.

Most of these procedures are carried out as courtesies to the employee, and the type or number performed may be determined by certain case load, budget, or personnel considerations. In most instances it would be desirable to provide the service, for not only is work time conserved, but the examination may aid greatly in effecting solid relationships with the employees so that medical counsel could be sought more readily at times of need.

By way of summation of the discussion of health examinations, Figure 6-1 shows the possible actions

*These examinations are of extreme interest sociologically and psychologically because they always follow employees' requests for retirement as based on their perception of a physical disablement that precludes continuing at work. Such a retirement—in contradistinction to a standard service retirement—frequently follows the individual's inability to cope with changes. Such changes include an altered mission of the company, a new and usually younger supervisor, automation or computerization of a process, or the need for retraining or learning. In the applications, the words "stress," "strain," and "pressure" seem to stand out, when what is meant is dissatisfaction, unhappiness, or the discontent following an adverse action. Minor chronic physical disorders, such as sinusitis, arthritis, or residua of an old injury, suddenly loom large and are offered as the ostensible reason for needing discontinuance of work. Disagreement with the applicant often leads to acrimony, for the disability retirement carries a greater income.

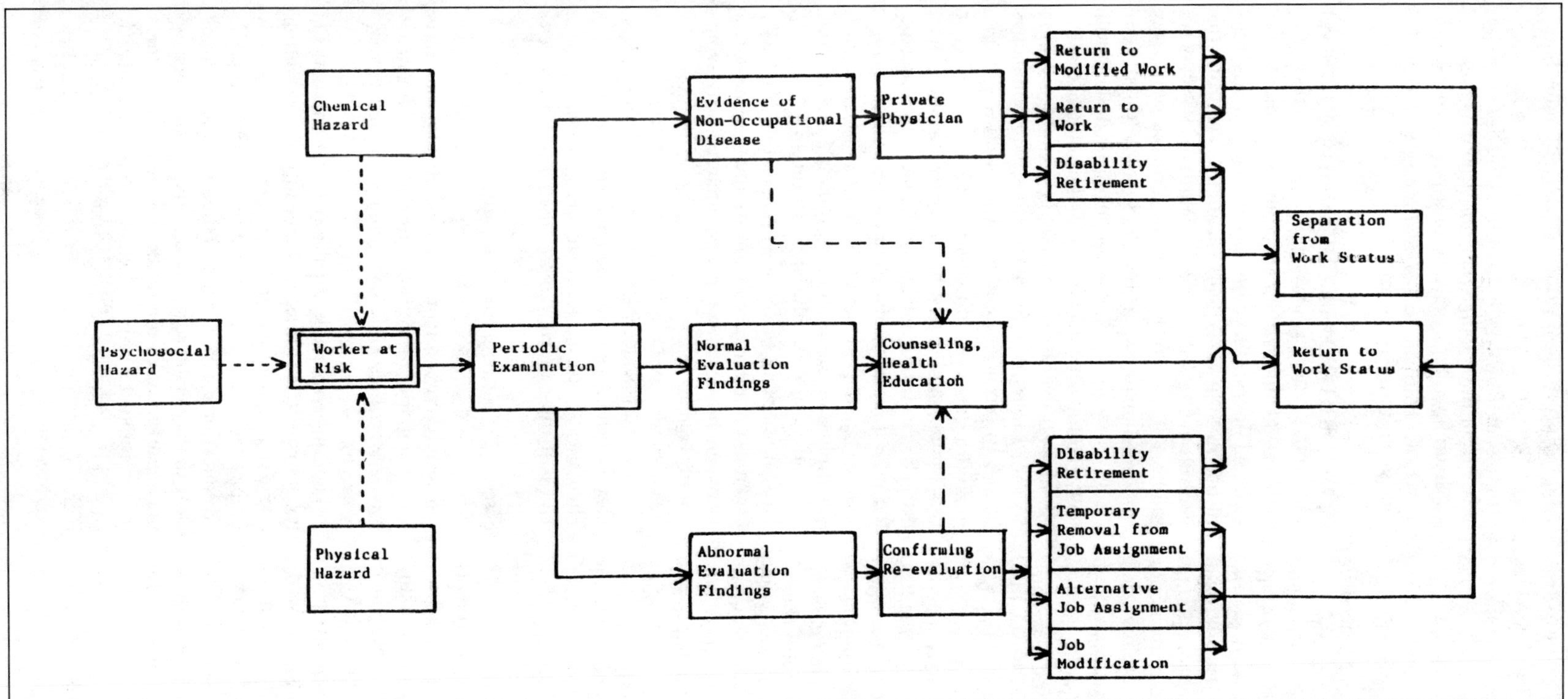

FIGURE 6-1. *Medical examination of the employee at risk.*

subsequent to the examination of the employee at risk. All of the choices, from retention in the same job to termination, are indicated.

HEALTH SCREENING

A benchmark in preventive medicine was placed in the 1950s by the early development of multiphasic testing or presymptom disease detection. In the beginning, standard instrumentation was utilized to measure an individual's functional capacities; in time, several other modalities were added, so that the status of a person's various physiologic systems could be measured without the immediate need of a physician.

The terminology might stand clarification, for a variety of terms have been used: multiphasic health testing, multiphasic testing, screening for disease, automated multiphasic screening, multiple screening for disease, automated multiphasic screening, multiple screening, and more recently and probably meeting with wider usage, automated multiphasic health testing (AMHT). The introduction of the modifier "automated" has implied the historic change from manually activated instruments like the audiometer to on-line equipment such as the automated clinical laboratory systems in hematology and blood chemistry, or the computer audiometer or spirometer. In occupational health today, there are several variations in use. Possibly most common are the dual employment of the time-honored vision and hearing testing equipment, coupled with an in-house or outside laboratory capability in the performance of complete blood counts or the analysis of a blood sample for a full battery of biochemical values.

ACCEPTANCE

Like all new programs in medicine, acceptance was slow. A procedure that seems invasive of the territorial imperative of the medical practitioner and that is promulgated by nonphysicians will experience much lengthier periods of adolescence. The methodology has proved itself though, and the concept has been accepted. The Judicial Council of the American Medical Association was asked to comment on the ethical aspects of the operation, on the use of automated programs, and on the use of the results [63]. The council pointed out that such programs have been used for the development of research in epidemiology in the following ways:

To test asymptomatic patients for occult or predisposing early signs of disease.

To establish medical priorities or case findings in a particular community.

To separate tested persons with certain characteristics from those individuals not showing them.

To determine the prevalence of a particular characteristic or group of characteristics in a particular segment of the population.

It was stressed that the testing consists solely of the collecting, recording, and reporting of factual observations and that the "testings are not diagnosis or interpretations." In relation to industrial programs, the council observed that they are directed primarily toward the prevention of occupational disease by selective job placement and the general preventive health maintenance for the employee, and that they are to be encouraged and commended. A statement issued by the American Medical Association through its Council on Medical Service and adapted by the House of Delegates [64] provided a set of guidelines for use by physicians and medical societies.

Wilson [65] early on enumerated the criteria for case finding, and they still, nearly two decades later, provide excellent guidelines for "clear thinking on the subject." His criteria were the following:

There must be an important problem (i.e., the condition must be worthy of detection).

There must be an acceptable treatment.

Facilities must exist for diagnosis and treatment.

There should be a recognizable latent or early symptom stage.

A suitable test or examination must exist.

The test must be acceptable to the population.

The natural history must be understood.

There must be an agreed policy on treatment.

The cost must be related to other medical care expenditures.

Screening must be a continuous process.

These 10 criteria represent the commonsense basis for the initiation or continuation of any of the many procedures or test protocols employed in multiphasic screening.

The American Public Health Association, in a policy statement [66], has recommended the extension and expansion of multiphasic screening programs. Emphasized was the point that the process should be an educational experience and that it should be made clear to the person screened that the tests are not definitive diagnostic procedures and are not substitutes for a complete physical examination. Further, it should be underscored that positive findings may be highly significant and must be followed up, that negative results do not ensure the absence of disease, and that the screening process should be repeated periodically.

Hearings were held before a Senate subcommittee in 1966 relative to the detection and prevention of chronic disease through use of multiphasic health screening. It was the opinion of the subcommittee that multiphasic health screening centers were greatly needed and that the program should go nationwide. Further, they cautioned that careful consideration should be given to follow-up programs to ensure that abnormalities found were brought to the attention of a physician for diagnosis and treatment [67].

Finally, acceptance by the patient must be considered. Soghikian and Collen [68] queried 1,754 subjects who had undergone automated multiphasic testing. It was learned that 77.05 percent found the procedures "worth the time," and only 0.5 percent believed the screening process to be "disturbing." About 20 percent classified the glucose ingestion and tonometry upsetting, as did 155 persons in relation to the blood tests. The majority, in spite of certain inconveniences, returned for repeat examinations.

OBJECTIVES

The goals of a testing program in occupational health have been delineated well by Collings and his coworkers [69], who have reduced the objectives to the following:

To improve the working efficiency of employees.
To reduce the impact and slow the progression of existing disease.
To prolong life and useful function.
To prevent the development of future disease.

The writers emphasized that programs of this type must be relevant to occupational health goals in particular and must not be instituted for the collection of data inapplicable to the effectiveness or health of the worker.

TEST COMPONENTS

Although screening programs vary as to their content, many of the elements are common to all. In companies with specific hazardous exposure or with populations in which a certain disease process is unduly prevalent, test procedures may be added to meet particular needs. The primary components, from which pertinent selections can be made, are the following: medical and occupational histories, personality or emotional status evaluation, anthropometry, vital signs, tonometry, visual acuity, audiometry, cardiovascular measurements, blood chemistry determinations, hematologic measurements, serodiagnostic testing for syphilis, urinalysis, spirometry, dental status determination, and exfoliative uterine cervical cytology.

Other procedures may be added in parallel with the program objectives, such as colon fiberscopy on employees aged 40 or over or a gynecologic examination. Immunizing injections, initial series or stimulating doses, may be given on conclusion of the testing, and a nurse may instruct women examinees in the technique of self-breast examination.

PRINCIPLES AND CRITERIA

The guidelines essential to the successful implementation of multiphasic testing have been given by Collen [70]. The testing:

Should be a multipurpose program for health and patient surveillance.
Must be an integrated component of the local medical care delivery system and closely coordinated with the care provided by the patient's physician.
Must provide a high quality of comprehensive health testing utilizing modern technology, with a high degree of accuracy, sensitivity, and specificity.
Must provide good service to patients and physicians so it will be accepted and the facility used as a referral center.
Should use computer data processing with a continuing patient record file so as promptly to provide the physician with a comprehensive profile of the patient's current status as compared with previous multiphasic examinations.
Must be economical; at a lower cost to the patient, its services should equal or exceed those offered by a traditional health review.

While all of these principles may not be applicable in the occupational health setting, the interrelationship between the private physician and the testing facility does hold.

Goroll, May, and Mulley [71] have indicated that whether a screening policy results in improved health outcomes depends on the characteristics of the diseases being screened, the characteristics of the tests used, and the characteristics of the patient population. They established the following criteria on these characteristics:

Characteristics of the disease
- Significant effect on the quality or length of life.
- Prevalence sufficiently high to justify costs.
- Acceptable methods of treatment available.
- Asymptomatic period during which detection and treatment significantly reduce morbidity and/or mortality.
- Treatment in the asymptomatic phase yields a bet-

ter therapeutic result than treatment delayed until symptoms appear.

Characteristics of the test

Sufficiently sensitive. (Sensitivity is considered as the probability that a person with the disease in question will have a positive test.)

Sufficiently specific. (Specificity is deemed the probability that a person without the disease will have a negative test.)

Acceptable to patients.

Characteristics of the population screened

Sufficiently high disease prevalence.

Accessibility.

Compliance with subsequent diagnostic tests and necessary therapy.

To be emphasized in these criteria are the desired characteristics of the ability to affect the life of the person in a positive way, of a cost-benefit relationship, and of an advantage of presymptom discovery of disease. Further, the point is made of screening groups at high risk or with high disease prevalence.

In a manner similar to the rationale employed in the Canadian study on the periodic health examination [19–22], Frame and Carlson [72] have examined critically the feasibility of screening procedures for 36 selected diseases of the respiratory, cardiovascular, central nervous, and genitourinary systems for certain endocrine, metabolic, and gastrointestinal diseases and for some miscellaneous disorders of rather rare prevalence. They formulated the justification for screening on the basis of six criteria, essentially the same as those indicated by Goroll, May, and Mulley [71]: (1) the disease must have a significant effect on the quality or quantity of life; (2) acceptable methods of treatment must be available; (3) the disease must have an asymptomatic period during which detection and treatment significantly reduce morbidity or mortality or both; (4) treatment in the asymptomatic phase must yield a therapeutic result superior to that obtained by delaying treatment until symptoms appear; (5) test must be available at reasonable cost to detect the condition in the asymptomatic period; and (6) the incidence of the condition must be sufficient to justify the cost of the screening.

A review of the disorders for which a screening procedure can be carried out in the asymptomatic stage will show few effective measures. Much of what can be done depends on patient or employee education. One difference between the use of these guidelines in a private office and at the worksite is that OHS personnel can conduct some of the screening methods with greater frequency, such as during visits for care for minor trauma or visits for medical surveillance because of specific, potentially hazardous work assignments.

A second difference must be considered, which relates to a rather intangible value attainable by an OHS. A health professional may offer a rather glib statement, based on good reasoning and the use of sound criteria, to the effect that screening is of no worth in certain clinical disorders.* What is heard and perceived by the workers, though, is disinterest, no matter how scientifically derived the conclusions might be. Therefore, it seems logical that certain procedures be carried out during visits to the OHS such as weight determination, blood pressure measurement, and the like. The workers know, then, that someone is concerned about their health and that "something is being done." One can forego the stringency of scientific guidelines periodically and substitute some personal, attentive warmth without sacrificing the principles of sound epidemiology. Wright and Bailey [73] introduced their discussion of screening with a brief but solid definition of the screening process as the identification of clinical vulnerability. Bailey [74] concluded wisely that health screening is still a controversial subject, although its benefit to people in certain occupations is beyond doubt. Further, screening may be a most powerful tool for disease prevention and health maintenance on a much broader front, and only through evaluation will it be possible to tell whether these expectations are fulfilled.

COST-EFFECTIVENESS

These points lead directly to much of the current thinking regarding screening. There has been opposition to large screening efforts because not only are the total efforts costly but also the cost per single positive result has been high. One of the largest and longest-lived screening programs has been conducted at a health maintenance organization (HMO) under the leadership of Dr. Morris F. Collen. The project was initiated at Kaiser Permanente in Oakland, California in 1964, and in 1980 a progress report was given at a national meeting. Friedman and associates [75,76] reviewed their controlled trial of urging middle-aged persons to have annual multiphasic health checkups, and recent follow-up experience con-

*Frame spells out, in another writing, the three major barriers to widespread implementation of periodic health screening: lack of physician motivation, patient resistance, and the fragmentation of primary care. If the physician is not motivated, he indicates, and does not initiate screening, the other two barriers are irrelevant. (Frame, P. S. Periodic health screening in a rural private practice. *J Fam Pract* 9:57, 1979.)

firmed their previous findings of a statistically significant reduction in mortality from "potentially hazardous" conditions, particularly hypertension and colorectal cancer, in the urged "study" group. There were unexpected excesses in deaths from suicide and lymphoma-leukemia noted in the group, but a review failed to substantiate responsibility in the checkups for this finding, except in one instance. With appropriate corrections made in the analysis, it was found that persons with four or more checkups by 1970 had a subsequent 5-year mortality rate about two-thirds as great as individuals with fewer multiphasic health screenings.

In an earlier study by the same group [77] of middle-aged men (45–54 years at entry), it was suggested that a net savings (preinflation) of more than $800 per man had been effected over a 7-year period.

Recent questions have appeared, as indicated, regarding the cost-effectiveness of mass screening. Vaisrub [78] asked in an editorial, recognizing that screening programs do find disease, especially when the efforts are directed toward high-risk groups, if the expense of mass screening, coupled with other costs created by methods of limited sensitivity and specifity, outweighs the benefits. Reiser [79] pointed out further that the problems of large numbers of false positives and false negatives, in addition to public apathy toward participation, still remain. Most important, though, Reiser adds, is the disinclination of the practicing physician to involve himself in health maintenance and disease prevention.

In a study conducted by the National Cancer Institute [80], 2,600 asymptomatic "high-risk" women were studied for endometrial cancer. In screening 1,280 such patients in the first phase of the study, 8 cases of cancer were identified, or about 6 per 1,000. The complete examination included breast and abdominal palpation, speculum examination, and cytologic sampling. Also found were three mammary cancers, two ovarian, one of a tube, and several precancerous lesions of the uterus. Although the project's total cost came to $800,000, the costs were not comparable to clinical practice, for part of the project incurred such expenses as recruitment through newspaper advertising and computer services. No accurate cost per positive finding was given. But who determines the true value of the discovery of a malignant lesion—the economist involved in health planning and cost containment, the social scientist who sees retention of the integrity of a family unit, or the patient who lives and remains productive? Perhaps it is the bioethicist who is the only one permitted to speculate in the framework of various value systems.

In keeping with this perplexing decision-choice is another perception. Garfield [81] proposed that the emphasis is wrong when it is stated that it cost $2,000 to detect one positive cancer of the breast by mammography in 500 women. It seemed more logical to him to underscore the health element and say that it costs $4 each to assure 499 women that they are free of breast cancer as demonstrated by mammography and $4 to detect one cancer, which, through early surgery, may allow the patient to experience a better prognosis.

In continuing a discussion of costs, the individual cost per test or test battery must be viewed in the overall perspective of the allocation of available resources. The OHS director must determine if the population for which he or she has responsibility has subsets of high-risk groups for one disease entity or another and if a certain segment of the budget should be devoted to health screening for the particular clinical disorder. Tests are priced in practice at different costs, obviously, and these figures are translatable into the cost per positive finding. Collen and his group [82] did just this exercise in 1970, but in light of inflation, the data are applicable only in comparing costs among a battery of test procedures. The cost per positive case did not necessarily follow the cost per individual test. For example, while the cost per individual tonometry was low, the cost per positive case was high, second only to mammography. They concluded that the prevalence of an abnormal test depends on the specific population examined, especially as related to its age-sex composition.

One other aspect of cost analysis involves the decision concerning the establishment of a laboratory facility within the OHS versus the use of an outside private laboratory. To aid in evaluation of the problem, a checklist of significant variables to be considered has been offered in a study of automated facilities [83].

Most important, of course, is the fact that there is no counterbalancing or offsetting income from patients, so that both the initial cost is high and no amortization is possible. With the competition encountered among the many commercial reference laboratories and the relatively low cost of many of the procedures clumped into batteries, it seems infeasible for an OHS to create and operate its own automated laboratory. But, again, this decision rests on the characteristics of the population served and the health risks inherent in the plant's operations and the resulting exposures.

NORMAL VALUES

With the onset of multiphasic screening, several organizations established their own ranges of normality. Reference is made to the individual sources, especially the Massachusetts General Hospital [84], the Metropolitan Life Insurance Company [85], and the New York Telephone Company [86] in addition to the publications available from the many commercial laboratories, for example, that of SmithKline Bio-Science Laboratories [87].

MISCELLANEOUS PRECAUTIONS IN HEALTH SCREENING

A few overall precautions in carrying out some of the multitest procedures may prove helpful.

Audiometry

As indicated previously, attention is directed to the removal of cerumen when an audiogram depicts an unanticipated hearing loss. In a series of 22 employee-patients who complained of hearing impairment, reported by Kawchak [88], 18 had definite objective audiometric evidence of improvement following correction of the ceruminosis.

Urinalysis

Even the simple urinalysis has been reviewed for possible sites of error. Townsend [89] warns that, in the use of multireagent dipstick, the rate of reaction on the impregnated chemicals is standard for each dipstick and color changes must be matched at the correct time after dipping for each stick. If the sticks are left too long in the urine, the chemicals impregnated on the cellulose may be dissolved out, and the results may be inaccurate.

Tablets, he points out, when used in urinalysis, are fashioned after the same principle, in most instances, as the dipstick. The reaction begins when the tablet is moistened with urine, so they will not function if they have been exposed to moisture before being used.

The urine specimen itself must meet certain specifications. A specimen that is over 2 hours old and improperly preserved will show a loss of formed elements such as casts, red cells, and white cells in the sediment. This fact holds true particularly if the urine is alkaline and of a low specific gravity. Further, old specimens may give a false-negative protein determination with the sulfosalicylic acid test and a false-positive protein test with the dipstick if a stale ammoniacal specimen is tested [90].

Metabolites may be produced in the urine by aspirin or L-dopa, which may give a false-negative urine glucose determination with the glucose oxidase reaction on the sticks. In addition, a high concentration of ascorbic acid added to a glucose-containing urine can give a false-negative reaction with both dipsticks and test tape [90].

If there need be a delay in delivery of the specimen to the laboratory, refrigeration or the use of preservatives will help. A tablet for specimen preservation, which has been used for many years by life insurance companies, is available commercially [91].*

Blood Chemistry Determinations

In the preparation of blood specimens for transport, if the analyses are not done on the premises, serum should be separated from a clotted blood specimen within 1 hour of collection. Glucose levels can drop as much as 24 mg/100 ml after 1½ hours of storage at 25°C. At the end of 3 hours, the concentration can diminish even more, for a total loss of 36 mg/100 ml. Other constituents that are vulnerable to loss are various electrolytes, pH, and inorganic phosphorus. If the specimen can be centrifuged and the red cells packed densely and transported quickly without disturbing the cell mass, the hazard might be lessened [92]. Under no circumstances should a whole blood specimen be frozen, thawed, and then refrozen. Once serum is separated from the cells, test results are reproducible for 4 to 10 days if the samples are refrigerated. Details concerning the transport of specimens for analysis may be obtained from any large commercial laboratory.

A moderate intake of alcohol between 1 hour before supper and 11 P.M. will lead to a slight decrease in blood glucose levels, an increase in urinary zinc level, and a slight increase in blood uric acid level, which will return to normal by 7 A.M. Carey and her coworkers [93] question the wisdom of removing the stressor—alcohol—with which the patient normally lives, thus altering the blood chemistry values, in a sense making the person more normal prior to testing. They conclude in their study that since the criteria for the diagnosis of some diseases are defined poorly, the practice of instructing a patient to abstain from alcohol for 24 hours prior to blood and urine tests may be questioned.

Innumerable medications can have a possible effect on laboratory test results, either increasing or decreasing the values of the elements being measured or actually interfering with the test procedure. Before a single or even a repeated test result is assumed to be valid, the employee's drug program should be reviewed in detail.

Erroneous laboratory results can be costly. Cavenaugh [94], in an intriguing analysis, has arranged sequentially the possible consequences of laboratory error, as shown in Table 6-4.

To each one of these events, Cavenaugh [94] as-

*One commercial source is the R. P. Cargille Laboratories, Inc., 55 Commerce Road, Cedar Grove, NJ 07009.

TABLE 6-4. *Possible Consequences of Laboratory Error*

Event	*Description of event*
1. Nothing	Medical management of the patient is not changed, test result is discarded, and no repeat test is ordered.
2. Repeat test is ordered	Original test result is questioned because of history and physical findings.
3. Battery of tests	A more detailed series of tests is ordered to determine validity of the original test. This could also occur if original test result indicated a disease condition not suspected from history and physical findings.
4. Extra appointments with physician	This includes hospital rounds and private office visits required for additional laboratory tests, therapy, and a more detailed diagnostic study.
5. Unnecessary drug therapy	Patient receives medication because of the original laboratory error.
6. Unnecessary medical or surgical procedures	It may or may not involve hospitalization. Examples include transfusions, biopsies, x-ray studies, appendectomy, etc.
7. Unnecessary hospitalization	Patient is continued in the hospital or admitted because of the erroneous laboratory result. Examples include time required for additional laboratory tests, time required to initiate or stabilize therapy, special facilities needed for diagnostic study, perform surgical or medical procedures judged necessary, etc.
8. Temporary disability	Impairment to the extent that the person is unable to carry out usual activity.
9. Permanent partial disability	Impairment of body function to the extent that the person cannot earn a livelihood but can care for self. Examples would include partial paralysis and mental impairment.
10. Permanent total disability	Impairment of body function to the extent that the individual is unable to earn a livelihood and is unable to perform routine personal care such as eating, bathing, using the bathroom, and dressing self.
11. Death	Death is attributable to the laboratory error. Examples include transfusion reactions, hemorrhage, and reactions to drug therapy, etc.

SOURCE: Cavenaugh, E. L. A method for determining costs associated with laboratory error. *Am. J. Public Health* 71:831, 1981.

signed costs derived from interviews with a panel of 40 judges. The cost per laboratory error (in 1981 dollars) ranged from $5.75 to $7,557.00.

In a case brought before the California Supreme Court [95], it was ruled that a plaintiff can file suit to recover for purely emotional injury unaccompanied by any physical harm. In point, the case was pressed by the husband of a woman who was misdiagnosed as having syphilis. She became suspicious that he might be engaged in extramarital sex relations, and ultimately the suspicion led to increased marital tension and breakup. When the error was discovered the husband sued the woman's physician and the laboratory. No laboratory test result can be taken lightly, nor should a single positive finding go unrepeated.

COLORECTAL CANCER SCREENING

Although the use of the Hemoccult screening method for the detection of cancer of the colon and rectum has been advised [96], Applegate and Spector [97] have pointed out serious weaknesses in its employment as a screening modality. When considering the usual criteria followed in screening, they believe that the method is at best 83-percent sensitive for cancer and considerably less for polyps. In an asymptomatic person with one or more positive slides for occult blood, there is only a 12-percent chance of there being cancer. Further, they question patient acceptance and indicate also that there is little current information on potential survival benefits. The procedure is expensive when one-fourth of all costs are incurred in follow-up diagnostic evaluation of false-positive results. They conclude that there is insufficient evidence to warrant the use of the procedure in asymptomatic persons as a cost-effective practice. In their review, the writers point to a comparable stand by the Canadian Task Force [20–22].

The test has been reviewed by Winawer and associates [98], who concluded that there have been no controlled studies demonstrating the value of the stool guaiac slide. Some investigators have shown that the test can detect cancers in an early stage, and when coupled with other study results, a reduction in mortality has been associated with earlier detection, making the procedure a reasonable one. They do point out, though, that the available data are as yet inconclusive and that the recommendations regarding its use should be considered only as guidelines to be tailored to the needs of individual people and programs. Before the tests become widely used, Winawer and his group felt that the evidence of benefits as well as potential risks and costs need further ascertainment [98].

A workshop consensus was presented by Gnauch and colleagues [99] stating that although fecal occult blood screening was not endorsed for use outside the health care system without information on mortality reduction as a result of that screening, it was considered desirable that the test recommendations be standardized. Although the recommendations offered may not be applicable to tests other than Hemoccult II, it was believed that the following represent the standards to be sought:

Testing should be done annually beginning between ages 40 and 50 years.
Subject should avoid rare red meat and high peroxidase foods for 3 days before and during testing.
Five samples of each of three consecutive stools should be tested, following the manufacturer's recommended procedure.
The delay between preparation and laboratory testing should not exceed 6 days.
Slides should not be rehydrated.
A single positive smear should be considered as a positive test and lead to appropriate investigation, even in the absence of dietary restriction. A positive result need not be repeated before diagnostic study.

A newer test procedure has been reported [100] in which blood loss in the stool is measured quantitatively, rather than qualitatively as it is in the guaiac-based screens. The HemoQuant test does not appear to produce chemical false-positive or false-negative results as do the qualitative tests with iron, cimetidine, or vegetable peroxidases (false-positive) or in the presence of substances like vitamin C (false-negative). The storage of fecal specimens does not affect the newer test, in which heme is converted to porphyrins, which are then measured fluorometrically. The test is read out as a number—an objective result—and is not subject to individual interpretation. In a study, 97 percent of patients found to have cancer of the colon had HemoQuant values greater than or equal to 2 mg of hemoglobin per gram of stool; 98 percent of the healthy controls had values less than 2 mg.

At present, there seems to be no strong confirmatory evidence for the reliability of the qualitative test, but it is still included in many multitest protocols in industry. If it is continued to be used, the standardized recommendations should be followed.

Greegor [101], the original proposer and strong supporter of this screening procedure, emphasizes the use of the pretest high-roughage diet and that, with a test period of 3 days, the Hemoccult slide testing is more than 90-percent reliable. In summary, the studies of Frank [102] are cited wherein he concluded that Hemoccult screening cannot be recommended for periodic health maintenance in any age group, as the procedure "represents premature enthusiasm rather than thoughtful medical practice."

Chest Radiography

While the debate slowly subsides regarding the worth of periodic examination of the chest radiographically, it must be admitted that, in industry, certain periodically recurring examinations have been mandated. In addition, the new immigration waves have brought applicants to the work scene who have increased the prevalence of pulmonary tuberculosis. In substance, there seems to be little indication for repetitive radiographic chest studies of employees, except in those persons at particular risk because of contact with fibrogenic work substances or materials that would adversely affect pulmonary function, in persons so exposed who are heavy smokers, or in heavy smokers alone. As long ago as 1968, even in steel foundries, Gregory [103] concluded that such a protocol, in the absence of a specific hazard, was not economically justifiable. He did suggest a plan for steel foundry workers, though, for chest films to be taken at time of entry, after 5 years in the hazardous environment, after 10 years, and then every 2 years thereafter.

While Ashenburg, medical director for one of the nation's largest chemical manufacturers, expressed comparable feelings in 1981, a majority of medical directors queried by him favored a periodic program of chest radiography even as an activity unrelated to job exposure [104].

Moving on from the point of disagreement to the issue of good radiography, certain caveats must be delineated. Many standard chest films from OHSs and industrial medical clinics are of such poor quality as to be uninterpretable by highly qualified radiologists. It is suggested that the consulting roentgenologist visit the OHS or clinic to review both the quality of the equipment being used and the technique employed by the x-ray technologist or person usually responsible for taking the films. The errors producing unacceptable radiographs can be corrected so that the finest quality films, capable of demonstrating subtle changes, can be offered to the radiologist. An excellent home study syllabus was prepared for NIOSH jointly by the American College of Radiology and the American Society of Radiologic Technologists [105] at the initiation of Public Law 91-173, relating to the examination program for the nation's coal miners. As stated by Sargent [105], the technique recommended is one that will produce roentgenograms of maximum detail and minimal variation in density and contrast so that the radiographs will be consistent in quality and the number of unsatisfactory examinations reduced.

An OHS that has responsibility for the surveillance of workers exposed to pneumoconiosis-producing hazards should utilize a so-called B reader for the interpretation of chest radiographs produced as part of the periodic examination protocol. A system of examination to determine the proficiency of physicians in the classification of pneumoconiosis chest films was developed to identify physicians qualified to serve in the national pneumoconiosis programs directed both to epidemiologic research and to the compensation of coal miners and others who suffer from dust-related chest disease [106].* B readers are qualified through examination.

Physicians who qualify utilize the ILO Classification of Radiographs of the Pneumoconioses, a system for classification created in 1930 and which subsequently underwent several generational changes until the current classification appeared in 1980. The complete classification has been published [107], and it is a system devoted to the categorization of technical quality of the radiographs, parenchymal abnormalities, and pleural abnormalities. The roentgenographic interpretation is recorded on a report form issued by NIOSH, which can be reproduced, with minor changes, for local use. The primary advantage in the universal use of such a scheme is the standardization of the designation of sites of change, nomenclature, degree or extent of change, and diagnosis or other findings. The ILO makes available a set of standard films of the pneumoconioses, which can be used both for preparation for the B reader examination and for teaching. The examination is given at intervals, and any physician, in addition to radiologists, may take it.

*An "A" reader is a physician who has completed an introductory 2-day course on the International Labor Organization (ILO) classification system given by the American College of Radiology. A "C" reader is usually a physician who is an experienced radiologist who serves as a referee or in research and is involved in devising and evaluating reading and classification methods.

Pulmonary Function Evaluation

As employer and worker awareness of industrially generated pulmonary disease has increased in recent years, it has become common practice for an OHS to perform pulmonary function screening on personnel exposed to potential health hazards in the form of respirable dusts, vapors, gases, mists, or aerosols. Technicians or nurses trained in pulmonary function testing carry out the protocol on one of many commercially available spirometers, some of which provide computed printouts of the findings. Further, such evaluation has been mandated in several of the standards promulgated by the U.S. Department of Labor.

Although many manuals are available for use and reference by the technician, the most important aspect is the coaching of the subject.* As many employees believe that they can simulate a chest disorder by inadequate performance on the test, they must be apprised that such action is readily detectable and only leads to an erroneous test.

A second caution relates to ethnic differences, and if so-called normal values are applied to all subjects, the interpreting pulmonologist may produce a strikingly abnormal result without full knowledge of the examinee.

It is suggested that certain writings [108–117] be obtained for reference in pulmonary function evaluation that will prove of worth in the testing of large disparate populations.

Genetic Screening

Probably no form of disease detection in asymptomatic populations has created greater public outcry than genetic screening in industry [118–121]. Objections have risen among women's groups, black organizations, and labor unions, all of whom have felt

*At the Snowbird Conference of the American Thoracic Society held in 1978, a series of standards was prepared for spirometry. In addition to instrument specifications and methods for the standardized measurement of forced expiratory volumes, an acceptable curve was to be defined through the technician's observation. The subject was to understand the instructions, perform the test with a smooth continuous exhalation, exert maximal effort with a good start and without coughing, premature termination, glottis closure, leak, or mouthpiece obstruction. Further, the participants recommended, as a minimum, three acceptable forced expiratory maneuvers. To ensure cooperation on the part of the subject and maximal efforts, it was proposed that the best two of three acceptable curves should not differ by more than 5 percent or 100 ml, whichever was the greater. (American Thoracic Society. ATS statement: Snowbird workshop on standardization of spirometry. *Am Rev Respir Dis* 119:831, 1979.)

that unjust discrimination would result from such testing. Actually, the objective is to identify the individual who is especially susceptible to certain chemicals or stressors encountered at the work scene. Initially, when testing was inaugurated for sickle cell trait and disease, there was overzealous action by unknowing personnel authorities against job applicants or employees with the trait, and the eventual mass objection in great part was legitimate.

There has been considerable state legislation aimed at the amelioration of the effects of genetic diseases, and most of the statutes relate to screening of the newborn, without reference to the industrially employed person [122]. The diseases covered usually include cystic fibrosis, hemophilia, sickle cell disease, hypothyroidism, phenylketonuria, galactosemia, homocystinuria, maple syrup urine disease, tyrosinemia, and other "allied" or handicapping genetic disorders. In some jurisdictions there is screening for Tay Sachs disease and Cooley's anemia. There are proscriptions against unfair insurance underwriting. The only immediate relationship to employment is in various state-assisted programs of therapy for the worker with hemophilia.

There has been acknowledgement of certain stigmatization of carriers identified through screening [123], and it has been the expressed opinion that there still are many unknown factors in human genetic monitoring. Few adequate studies have been performed on workers in well-defined industrial settings, it is claimed, and Dabney [124] believes that such testing is to be regarded as a research modality still undergoing development and that future studies should be carefully planned. Particularly, she feels that genetic monitoring should not be used to set standards for safe exposures or to establish conditions for the prevention of occupational disease.

While arguments continue, it is felt that with the increased number of chemicals being produced, and with the broadened knowledge of occupational carcinogenesis, a system of early determination of risk or susceptibility is in order. Eventually, there may be a willingness to be protected by highly sophisticated methods of identification, provided they are not used to discriminate against workers by rendering them unemployable. It must be remembered that it was only as recent as World War II that certain groups prevented their membership from undergoing preplacement medical examinations. Today, the same groups demand such beneficial procedures. Omenn [125] has commented that both sides must move toward cooperation so that technologic controls and personal practices can be mobilized to maximize health and safety on the job. Time will bring rational resolution.

Food Handler Examinations

For many years it was customary to conduct periodic examinations on persons working in industrial cafeterias. The ritual was performed usually on an annual basis, and infrequently a worker would be identified as infected or infested. Innumerable throat cultures were taken, and stools beyond count were studied.

The difficulty in the procedure was that while the food handler would be disease-free at the moment of the examination, he or she could be reinfected within hours, and this disease-carrying state would not be identified until another year had passed, if then. Most of the examination mandates have given way to food-handler education, which is strongly needed, without question, in light of the cultural and educational backgrounds of most workers of food preparation, serving, and cleanup.

In 1979, a World Health Organization (WHO) working group met to establish guidelines for this vexing problem of disease carriers in this particular sector of employees [126]. Objections to the well-known examination requirements were threefold: (1) It has not been established that most outbreaks of foodborne diseases are associated with food handlers; (2) medical examinations and laboratory analyses are costly; and (3) because of the turnover of workers in the food industry, it is difficult for administrators to be certain that all employees were checked.

Recognizing these problems, the following recommendations were made:

Train food handlers in hygienic work practices.

Have OHS personnel encourage food handlers to report staphylococcal skin infections and episodes of illness.

Examine food handlers promptly with outbreak of foodborne disease or when handlers have been ill.

Disallow food handlers to work when they could contaminate food through their gastrointestinal, skin, or respiratory infections.

Enforce frequent handwashing.

Conduct research to determine the efficiency and effectiveness of food-handler examinations.

These recommendations are the only logical and practical ones utilizable in the control of work-based foodborne disease.

Screening for Skin Lesions

In most industrial organizations, there is little concern for work-caused skin cancer, as the lesion, if it does appear, is usually nonoccupational in origin. However, in the county government with which the author was associated at one time, there was a large Department of Beaches whose personnel were responsible for lifeguarding on the many miles of beach on the Pacific Ocean coast of the County of Los Angeles. These men, lovers of the water and the outdoors, were moderately to deeply tanned and were not given to the use of sunscreening preparations for the skin. For several years a survey was conducted of the lifeguards at the two beach stations by a board-certified dermatologist and a health educator (Paul Smith, M.D., and Thomas F. Torpy, M.P.H.). Several cancerous skin lesions and many premalignant changes were found. Appropriate referrals for care were made, and the solar-induced cancers were eliminated. The use of protective hats and skin creams and lotions was introduced.

Tennant [127] has reported on a mass screening for skin cancer, and of 414 adults examined, 48 or 11.6 percent had lesions that were definitely cancerous or precancerous, while 89 or 21.5 percent had changes that possibly were cancer or precancerous.

If the organization has many workers exposed constantly to solar radiation, a screening for skin lesions with an accompanying educational activity would be in order.

Other Screening Procedures

As determined by the materials encountered at the worksite, other screening procedures will be carried out on personnel who have specific exposure. In keeping with suggested or mandated protocols, any of the following tests or measurements may be conducted: kidney function, sperm count, test for dermographism, nerve conduction velocity, electromyography, dental examination, neurologic examination, radiography of pelvis, follicle-stimulating or luteinizing hormone or total estrogen levels, erythrocyte cholinesterase activity, blood or urine trace metals, urine cytology, or other cytologic examinations.

A few companies test for the presence or use of marijuana or other drugs during working hours. The procedure may be done either as a safety measure in heavy industry or as part of a substance-abuse rehabilitation program. The custom is by no means universal.*

Tonometry may be performed using the Schiotz instrument or the non-contact applanation instruments, although the latter tonometers are costly. The addition of this screening procedure is determined by the age and other characteristics of the workforce.

Mammography ordinarily is not offered by an OHS as part of a screening program. Because of shifting opinion regarding its safety, the practice in this preventive procedure has flowed and ebbed. However, in one company, strongly health oriented, a mammography program was established at its general offices [128], being offered to all female employees aged 35 years and older. The examination was available at least every 4 years, as determined by risk factors, to women 35 through 49 years of age and at least every 2 years subsequently. Between August 1978 and February 1981, the radiography generated three "lumpectomies." Radiographically, two of the lesions were interpreted as "remotely, possibly malignant," and one was considered to be "almost certainly malignant." The first two proved to be benign, and the third was malignant, measuring only 3 mm in diameter. The population was estimated at about 120 women aged 50 or older and somewhat more in the 35- through 49-year group. The number receiving mammograms is not known.

It must be pointed out that the American Cancer Society in mid-1983, because of improvement in the quality and diagnostic accuracy of mammography in recent years, cojointly with the marked lowering of the radiated dose—one rad or lower at the midbreast, in a two-view examination—modified its guidelines concerning mammography. The society now recommends the following: Women in the age group 40 to 49 years should have a physical examination of the breast annually, and mammography should be performed at intervals of 1 to 2 years [129].

The mammography program mentioned above was accompanied by another effort in cancer prevention, that is sigmoidoscopy, and one in atherosclerosis prevention [128,130].

As a final note on screening of employees, it should be indicated that in most worker populations there will be some employees who present a family history that is remarkable for the occurrence of malignant growth among past and current generations and among other components of the nuclear family, such as aunts, uncles, cousins, nephews, and so on. It would be extremely beneficial to encourage such personnel to undergo frequent screening, for the statistical likelihood of their developing cancer is strong [131]. Often there is denial and the proferred examinations will be rejected.

The situation in industry is different from work elsewhere in the community where there may be no exposure to carcinogens. Counseling can bring to the attention of these members of known family clusters the great possibility of their manifesting a hereditary

*A helpful suggestion was offered during a recent conference. In biologic surveillance, if the need arises for blood specimens on former drug users, have them do their own venipunctures, for they will always be "on target."

cancer predisposition. In a joint effort with the family physician, secondary prevention should be practiced.

REFERENCES

1. Hatch, T. F. Criteria for hazardous exposure limits. *Arch Environ Health* 27:231, 1973.
2. Levinson, H. Emotional toxicity of the work environment. *Arch Environ Health* 19:239, 1969.
3. Surveying hazards in the occupational environment: The role of plant tours by physicians in the development of an occupational health and safety program. *Arch Environ Health* 10:115, 1965.
4. Occupational Medical Practice Committee, American Occupational Medical Association. Scope of occupational health programs and occupational medical practice. *J Occup Med* 21:497, 1979.
5. Solomayer, J. A. Place of physician in every plant's safety program. *Monitor* 3:78, 1963.
6. Brandt, A. D. *Maintaining a Healthful Working Environment.* New York: National Association of Manufacturers, Industrial Relations Department, 1967. Pp. 4–5.
7. Renes, L. E. The Industrial Hygiene Survey and Personnel. In D. Clayton and F. E. Clayton (Eds.), *Patty's Industrial Hygiene and Toxicology* (3rd ed. rev.). New York: Wiley, 1978. Vol. I, pp. 99–112.
8. Soule, R. D. Industrial Hygiene Sampling and Analysis. In D. Clayton and F. E. Clayton (Eds.), *Patty's Industrial Hygiene and Toxicology* (3rd ed. rev.). New York: Wiley, 1978. Vol. I, pp. 707–714.
9. Guide to diagnosis of occupational illness. *JAMA* 196:297, 1966.
10. Guide to the significance of occupational exposure limits, 1972 revision. *JAMA* 198:1126, 1966.
11. Shapiro, M. A. Industrial Sanitation. In G. D. Clayton and F. E. Clayton (Eds.), *Patty's Industrial Hygiene and Toxicology* (3rd ed. rev.). New York: Wiley, 1978. Vol. I, pp. 1333–1376.
12. Scope, Objectives, and Functions of Occupational Health Programs (rev. December 1971). Chicago: American Medical Association, 1971. P. 7.
13. Roberts, N. J. Periodic health evaluation: Some developments and practices. *J Occup Med* 8:581, 1966.
14. Siegel, G. S. An American dilemma: The periodic health examination. *Arch Environ Health* 13:292, 1966.
15. Siegel, G. S. *Periodic Health Examinations: Abstracts from the Literature.* Washington, DC: U.S. Department of Health, Education, and Welfare, Public Health Service, Division of Occupational Health, Division of Chronic Diseases, March 1963. P. v.
16. Those costly annual physicals. *Consumer Reports* 45:601, 1980.
17. Shires, D. B. Life Protocols: A Schema for Health Maintenance. In D. B. Shires and B. K. Hennen, *Family Medicine: A Guidebook for Practitioners of the Art.* New York: McGraw-Hill, 1980. Chap. 12, pp. 235–240.
18. De Friese, G. H., and Hetherington, J. S. The "periodic physical examination" as a strategy for prevention in clinical practice. *Mobius* 1:59, 1981.
19. Morgan, P. P. The periodic health examination. *Can Med Assoc J* 121:1161, 1979.
20. Task force report: The periodic health examination. *Can Med Assoc J* 121:1193, 1979.
21. Delbanco, T. L., and Taylor, W. C. The periodic health examination: 1980. *Ann Intern Med* 92:251, 1980.
22. Fletcher, S. W., and Spitzer, W. O. Approach of the Canadian task force to the periodic health examination. *Ann Intern Med* 92:253, 1980.
23. Guidelines for the cancer-related checkup: Recommendations and rationale. *CA* 30:1, 1980.
24. Fontana, R. S. Something old, something new, and something borrowed: The American Cancer Society's report on the cancer-related health checkup. *Mayo Clin Proc* 55:459, 1980.
25. Fontana, R. S. Screening for lung cancer. *Mayo Clin Proc* 55:654, 1980.
26. Fontana, R. S., and Sanderson, D. R. American Cancer Society's revised guidelines for annual chest Film: A Dissenting Opinion. *JAMA* 244:592, 1980.
27. Eddy, D. M. Screening for lung cancer. *Mayo Clin Proc* 55:653, 1980.
28. Breslow, L., and Somers, A. R. The lifetme health-monitoring program. *N. Engl J Med* 296:601, 1977.
29. Frame, P. S., and Carlson, S. J. A critical review of periodic health screening using specific screening criteria: Part 1. Selected diseases of respiratory, cardiovascular, and central nervous system. *J Fam Pract* 2:29, 1975; Part 2. Selected endocrine, metabolic, and gastrointestinal diseases. *J Fam Pract* 2:123, 1975; Part 3. Selected diseases of the genitourinary system. *J Fam Pract* 2:189, 1975; Part 4. Selected miscellaneous diseases. *J Fam Pract* 2:283, 1975.
30. Medical Practice Committee, American College of Physicians, Periodic Health Examination. A guide for designing individualized preventive health care in the asymptomatic patient. *Ann Intern Med* 95:729, 1981.
31. Council on Scientific Affairs, AMA. Medical evaluations of healthy persons. *JAMA* 249:1626, 1983.
32. Shepard, W. P. *The Physician in Industry.* New York: McGraw-Hill, 1961. P. 43.
33. *Executive Examination Program.* Rochester, MN: Division of Preventive Medicine, Mayo Clinic, [n.d.].
34. Carryer, H. M., Randall, R. V., and Mankin, H. T. Executive health examinations: Analysis of 2,812

examinations on 569 subjects at Mayo Clinic. *Mayo Clin Proc* 46:742, 1971.
35. Braceland, F. Emotional problems among executives. *Med Ann District Columbia* 24:219, 1955.
36. Farnsworth, D. L. Health under pressure. *Harvard Business Rev* 35:48, Nov–Dec 1957.
37. Phelps Dodge ordered to pay workers for time, costs in medical exams. *Occup Health Saf* 14:6, Feb 22, 1984.
38. Conference on Medical Screening and Biological Monitoring for the Effects of Exposure in the Workplace, July 1984. *J Occup Med* 28:543 (Part I), 901 (Part II), 1986.
39. Wade, L. J. Needed: A closer look at industrial medical programs. *Ind Med Surg* 25:167, 1956.
40. Miller, E. L. The overseas assignment: How managers determine who is to be selected. *Michigan Business Rev.* 24:12, May 1972.
41. *Instructions for Examining Physician.* Form FS-436. Washington, DC: Department of State, Foreign Service of the United States of America, Aug 25, 1955.
42. Wolfe, M. S. Management of the returnee from exotic places. *J Occup Med* 21:691, 1971.
43. Pearson, R. R. Occupational Health Problems in Diving. In A. W. Gardner (Ed.), *Current Approaches to Occupational Health.* Bristol, England: Wright-PSG, 1982. P. 107.
44. Spivack, A. P. Diving medicine. *Stanford MD* 19:6, Fall 1979–Winter 1980.
45. Egstrom, G. Diving Accidents. In R. H. Struass (Ed.), *Diving Medicine.* New York: Grune & Stratton, 1976. Pp. 303–308.
46. Huss, J. H. Scuba Diving. *JAMA* 193:166, 1965.
47. Richter, T., and Hoke, B. Hazard of scuba diving for patient with chronic anemia. *JAMA* 220:734, 1972.
48. Johnston, D. G. Risks of scuba diving during pregnancy. *JAMA* 220:734, 1972.
49. *UCLA Manual on Diving Safety.* Los Angeles: University of California, Los Angeles, 1968. P. 20.
50. General Industry Safety Orders (California), Title 8, Register 81, No. 12—3-21-81. Group 26. Diving Operations. Article 152, Diving Operations (Effective 1-1-81), Section 6053, Medical Requirements of Dive Team. Pp. 526.8.38–526.8.39.
51. *Motor Carrier Safety Regulations.* Title 49—Transportation, as amended, Section 391.41, Physical qualifications for drivers. Washington, DC: U.S. Department of Transportation, Federal Highway Administration, Bureau of Motor Carrier Safety, Oct 31, 1979.
52. Occupational Medical Practice Committee, AOMA. Driving ability following bypass surgery. *J Occup Med* 25:859, 1983.
53. American Medical Association: *Physician's Guide for Determining Driver Limitation.* Chicago: The Association, 1973.
54. Rees, W. D. Physical and mental disabilities of 1,190 ordinary motorists. *Br Med J* 1:593, March 11, 1967.
55. Shlensky, R. Psychiatric standards in driver licensing. *JAMA* 235:1993, 1976.
56. Raffle, A. (Ed.). *Medical Aspects of Fitness to Drive* (4th ed.). London: Medical Commission on Accident Prevention, 1985.
57. Committee on Medical Aspects of Automotive Safety, American Medical Association. Medical aspects of motorcycle safety. *JAMA* 204:290, 1968.
58. Medical Standards and Certification. In *Code of Federal Regulations,* Title 14, Aeronautics and Space, Part 67. Washington, DC: U.S. Department of Transportation, Federal Aviation Administration, 1985.
59. *Guide for Aviation Medical Examiners.* Washington, DC: U.S. Department of Transportation, Federal Aviation Administration, Office of Aviation Medicine, 1981.
60. Parker, D. J. The airline pilot after coronary artery bypass grafting. *Eur Heart J* 5:(Suppl A) 77, 1984.
61. Nicognossian, A. E., and Parker, J. F., Jr. *Space Physiology and Medicine.* NASA SP-447. Washington, DC: National Aeronautics and Space Administration, Scientific and Technical Information Branch, 1982. Pp. 235–241
62. Committee on Medical Aspects of Sports, American Medical Association. *A Guide for Medical Evaluation of Candidates for School Sports.* Chicago: The Association, 1972.
63. *Guidelines for Automated Multiphasic Health Testing Programs.* Chicago: American Medical Association, Judicial Council, 1971.
64. American Medical Association. *Statement on Multiphasic Health Testing.* Chicago: The Association, 1972. Pp. 10–11.
65. Wilson, J. M. G. Cited in D. F. Coulter and D. J. Llewellyn (Eds.), *The Practice of Family Medicine.* Edinburgh: Livingstone, 1971. P. 130.
66. Multiphasic screening. *Am J Public Health* 59:174, 1969.
67. *Detection and Prevention of Chronic Disease Utilizing Multiphasic Health Screening Techniques.* A Report of the Subcommittee on Health of the Elderly to the Special Committee on Aging, United States Senate (89th Congress, 2nd Session). Washington, DC: The Committee, 1966. Pp. 27–28.
68. Soghikian, K., and Collen, F. B. Acceptance of multiphasic screening examination by patients. *Bull NY Acad Med* 45:1366, 1969.
69. Collings, G. H., Jr., Fitzpatrick, M. M., and Stratton, K. L. Concepts, philosophy and general description (in multiphasic health screening in industry). *J Occup Med* 14:435, 1972.
70. Collen, M. F. Guidelines for multiphasic health checkups. *Arch Intern Med* 127:99, 1971.
71. Goroll, A. H., May, L. A., and Mulley, A. G. *Primary Care Medicine.* Philadelphia: Lippincott, 1981.
72. Frame, P. S., and Carlson, S. J. A critical review of periodic health screening using specific screening criteria: Part 1. Selected diseases of respiratory, car-

diovascular, and central nervous systems. *J Fam Pract* 2:29, 1975; Part 2. Selected endocrine, metabolic, and gastrointestinal diseases. *J Fam Pract* 2:123, 1975; Part 3. Selected diseases of the genitourinary system. *J Fam Pract* 2:189, 1975; Part 4. Selected miscellaneous diseases. *J Fam Pract* 2:283, 1975.
73. Wright, H. B., and Bailey, A. Screening Well People. In R. S. F. Schilling, (Ed.), *Occupational Health Practice* (2nd ed.). London: Butterworth, 1981. P. 204.
74. Bailey, A. Screening Organ Systems I: Cardiovascular System, Blood and Blood-forming Organs, Lung, Liver, Kidney and Bladder, and Central and Peripheral Nervous Systems. In R. S. F. Schilling (Ed.), *Occupational Health Practice* (2nd ed.). London: Butterworth, 1981. P. 239.
75. Friedman, G. D., Collen, M. F., Siegelaub, A. B., et al. Multiphasic Evaluation Study: Progress Report. Abstract of presentation for 108th Annual Meeting of the American Public Health Association, Detroit, Michigan, (Oct. 19) 1980.
76. Dales, L. G., Friedman, G. D., and Collen, M. F. Evaluating periodic multiphasic health checkups: A controlled trial. *J Chronic Dis* 32:385, 1979.
77. Collen, M. F., Dales, L. G., Friedman, G. D., et al. Multiphasic checkup evaluation study: 4. Preliminary cost benefit analysis for middle-aged men. *Prev Med* 2:236, 1973.
78. Vaisrub, S. Mass screening: Is it cost-effective? *JAMA* 243:2067, 1980.
79. Reiser, S. J. The emergence of the concept of screening for disease. *World Health Forum* 1:99, 1980.
80. Auersbacher, A. $800,000 to find 8 cases of endometrial Ca: "Worth it." *Med Trib* 23:3, Feb 24, 1982.
81. Garfield, S. R. Multiphasic health testing and medical care as a right. *N Engl J Med* 283:1087, 1970.
82. Collen, M. F., Feldman, R., Siegelaub, A. B., et al. Dollar cost per positive test for automated multiphasic screening. *N Engl J Med* 283:459, 1970.
83. Berkeley Scientific Laboratories, Inc. *A Study of Automated Clinical Laboratory Systems*. DHEW Publ. No. (HSM) 72-3004. Rockville, MD: U.S. Department of Health, Education, and Welfare, Public Health Service, 1971. Pp. 244–245.
84. Normal reference laboratory values. *N Engl J Med* 314:39, 1986.
85. More about biochemical profiles. *Stat Bull Metropol Life Insur Co* 52:3, Jan 1971.
86. Frederick, W. S., and Scott, M. R. Multiphasic health screening in industry: Medical statistics, system monitoring and provisional normals. *J Occup Med* 14:466, 1972.
87. *SmithKline Bio-Science Laboratory Service Manual*. Van Nuys, CA: SmithKline Bio-Science Laboratory, 1985.
88. Kawchak, J. Ceruminosis: A factor in audiometry. *J Occup Med* 3:21, 1961.
89. Townsend, F. Some Pitfalls of Urine Analysis. In *Proceedings of the Annual Conference of NASA Clinical Directors, Environmental Health Officials and Medical Program Advisors, Charleston, SC, Oct. 12–14, 1971*. Washington, DC: NASA, Office of Administration, Division of Occupational Medicine and Environmental Health, 1972. Pp. 151–161.
90. Feldman, J. M., Kelley, W. N., and Lebovitz, H. E. Inhibition of glucose oxidase paper tests by reducing metabolites. *Diabetes* 19:337, 1970.
91. Newell, J. E., and Duke, B. A. *The Routine Examination of Urine in the Laboratory*. Chicago: American Society of Clinical Pathologists, 1962.
92. Blume, P., and Benson, E. S. Time limits and storage form for blood shipped out for tests. *JAMA* 215:125, 1971.
93. Carey, M. A., Jones, J. D., and Gastineau, C. F. Effect of moderate alcohol intake on blood chemistry values. *JAMA* 216:1766, 1971.
94. Cavenaugh, E. L. A method for determining costs associated with laboratory error. *Am J Public Health* 71:831, 1981.
95. Calif. court permits suit for purely emotional injury. *Intern Med News* 13:3, Oct 15, 1980.
96. Consensus group does not recommend mass screening for colorectal cancer: Mortality reduction not shown. *JAMA* 240:2625, 1978.
97. Applegate, W. B., and Spector, M. H. Colorectal cancer screening. *J Community Health* 7:138, 1981.
98. Winawer, S. J., Fleisher, M., Baldwin, M., et al. Current status of fecal occult blood testing in screening for colorectal cancer. *CA* 32:10, 1982.
99. Gnauch, R., Macrol, F. A., and Fleisher, M. How to perform the fecal occult blood test. *CA* 34:134, 1984.
100. Ahtgust, D. Cited in Advantages are seen for new quantitative test of blood in stool. *Intern Med News* 17:29, Jan 1–14, 1984.
101. Greegor, D. H. Colorectal cancer detection. *JAMA* 245:571, 1981.
102. Frank, J. W. Occult-blood screening for colorectal carcinoma: The benefits. *Am J Prev Med* 1:3, 1985; The risks. *Am J Prev Med* 1:25, 1985; The yield and the costs. *Am J Prev Med* 1:18, 1985.
103. Gregory, J. Routine chest x-rays in industry. *Trans Soc Occup Med* 18:156, 1968.
104. Ashenburg, N. J. Routine chest x-ray examinations in occupational medicine. *J Occup Med* 24:18, 1982.
105. *Home Study Syllabus on Technic for Chest Radiography*. Prepared for the National Institute of Occupational Safety and Health, Department of Health, Education and Welfare, by the American College of Radiology and the American Society of Radiologic Technologists. Chicago: The College and the Society, [n.d.]. (The date of publication may possibly have been 1971.) P. 12.
106. Morgan, R. H. Proficiency examination of physicians for classifying pneumoconiosis chest films. *Am*

J Roentgenol 132:803, 1979.
107. Classification of radiographs of the pneumoconioses. *M Radiogr Photogr* 57(1):2, 1981.
108. Morris, J. F., Koski, A., and Johnson, L. C. Spirometric standards for healthy nonsmoking adults. *Am Rev Respir Dis* 103:57, 1971.
109. Weil, H. Pulmonary function testing in industry. *J Occup Med* 15:693, 1973.
110. Knudson, R. J., Slatin, R. C., Lebowitz, M. D., et al. The maximal expiratory flow-volume curve. *Am Rev Respir Dis* 113:587, 1976.
111. Cotes, J. E. When is a lung function result abnormal? *Proc R Soc Med* 70:166, 1977.
112. Corey, P. N., Ashley, M. J., and Chan-Yeung, M. Racial differences in lung function: Search for proportional relationships. *J Occup Med* 21:395, 1979.
113. Miller, A., Thornton, J. C., Smith, H., Jr., et al. Spirometric "abnormality" in a normal male reference population: Further analysis of the 1971 Oregon survey. *Am J Ind Med* 1:55, 1980.
114. Hamilton, T. E. Pulmonary function testing: Regulations and recommendations. *Occup Health Saf* 49:25, 1980.
115. Lewis, B. M. Pitfalls of spirometry. *J Occup Med* 23:35, 1981.
116. Component Committee on Disability Criteria of the American Lung Association Pediatric and Adult Lung Disease Committee. Evaluation of impairment/disability—secondary to respiratory disease. *ATS News* 7:20, 1981.
117. Glindmeyer, H. W., III. Predictable confusion. *J Occup Med* 23:845, 1981.
118. Severo, R. Genetic screening by industry: 1. Genetic tests by industry raise questions on rights of workers; 2. Screening of blacks by Du Pont sharpens debate on industry gene tests; 3. Dispute arises over Dow studies on genetic damage in workers; 4. Federal mandate for gene tests disturbs U.S. job safety official. *New York Times* Feb 3–6, 1980.
119. Holden, C. Looking at genes in the workplace. *Science* 217:336, 1982.
120. Uzych, L. Lack of research indicates genetic screening premature. *Occup Health Saf* 53:24, Apr 1984.
121. West, S. Genetic testing on the job. *Science* 53:16, Sept 1982.
122. *State Laws and Regulations on Genetic Disorders.* Rockville, MD: U.S. Department of Health and Human Services, Public Health Service, Health Services Administration, Bureau of Community Health Services, 1980.
123. Kenen, R. H., and Schmidt, R. M. Stigmatization of carrier status: Social implications of heterozygote genetic screening programs. *Am J Public Health* 68:1116, 1978.
124. Dabney, B. J. The role of human genetic monitoring in the workplace. *J Occup Med* 23:626, 1981.
125. Omenn, G. S. Predictive identification of hypersusceptible individuals. *J Occup Med* 24:369, 1982.
126. Health examination of food handlers—Europe. *MMWR* 30:267, 1981.
127. Tennant, F. S., Jr. Mass screening for skin cancer. *Am J Public Health* 71:1172, 1981.
128. Wear, R. F. Personal communication, Feb 25, 1981.
129. Mammography guidelines 1983: Background statement and update of cancer-related checkup guidelines for breast cancer detection in asymptomatic women age 40 to 49. *CA* 33:255, 1983.
130. Wear, R. F. An atherosclerosis prevention program. *J Occup Med* 17:295, 1975.
131. Lynch, H. T., Lynch, P. M., Albano, W. A., et al. Hereditary cancer: Ascertainment and management. *CA* 29:216, 1979.

7. WELLNESS AND HEALTH EDUCATION PROGRAMS

It is more advisable to pass a careful medical examination if one intends to be sedentary in order to establish whether one's state of health is good enough to stand the inactivity.

Per-Olof Astrand, M.D.

Let the purpose of this, our dialectic, be to discover and to use a method of instruction by which teachers teach less and learners learn more.

John Amos Comenius

With all the recent publicity about the risk factors involved in increasing morbidity and mortality from cardiovascular disease, there has been a great upsurge in the movement toward fitness. The jogger, the inside exerciser, the nutritionally prudent person, and the ex-smoker have replaced the former "physical culture" addicts in numbers greater than ever anticipated in the 1960s, '70s, and '80s. The move has so attained both speed and status that exercise clothing and footwear have become commonplace attire for both men and women in almost any setting.

A related factor that has involved the interest of employers has been the tremendous increase in the costs of medical care, directly reflected in the premiums required for group health (hospital and medical care) coverage, to which a company may contribute 50 to 100 percent of cost of the employee's insurance package. If there are means to control these accelerating costs, and the means are safe, then the employer will support efforts to effect such preventive action.

For years industry has sponsored various group activities as part of the total collection of benefits offered workers. Included were intra- and intercompany tournaments in softball, bowling, basketball, and tennis, and not too long after the inception of such organizationally sponsored activities, injuries sustained by participants were ruled as fitting under the company's workers' compensation umbrella.

But such fitness programs have changed in many areas from athletic contests targetted toward building morale to more scientifically and medically based undertakings geared toward health and wellness and the reversal of certain destructive lifestyles. While some companies have had gymnasiums for employee use, particularly in smaller communities, and industrial recreation directors for the planning and oversight of group programs, industry has begun to employ exercise physiologists and recreation therapists, among others, to assist the labor force in conquering the ill effects of the so-called lifestyle diseases of overweight, stress, alcoholism, and other chemical substance abuse disorders, including smoking and drug addiction. Lalonde [1] has listed the more destructive lifestyle habits:

Drugs
- Alcohol addiction: leading to cirrhosis of the liver, encephalopathy, and malnutrition.
- Social excess of alcohol: leading to motor vehicle accidents and obesity.
- Cigarette smoking: causing chronic bronchitis, emphysema, and cancer of the lung and aggravating coronary artery disease.
- Abuse of pharmaceuticals: leading to drug dependence and drug reactions.
- Addiction to psychotropic drugs: leading to suicide, homicide, malnutrition, and accidents.
- Social use of psychotropic drugs: leading to social withdrawal and acute anxiety attacks.

Diet and exercise
- Overeating: leading to obesity and its consequences.
- High-fat intake: possibly contributing to atherosclerosis and coronary artery disease.
- High carbohydrate intake: contributing to dental caries.
- Fad diets: leading to malnutrition.
- Lack of exercise: aggravating coronary artery disease, leading to obesity, and causing lack of physical fitness.
- Malnutrition: leading to numerous health problems.
- Lack of recreation and lack of relief from work and other pressures: associated with stress dis-

ease such as hypertension, coronary artery disease, and peptic ulcer.

Others

Careless driving and failure to wear seatbelts: leading to accidents and resultant deaths and injuries.

Promiscuity and carelessness: leading to syphilis, gonorrhea, and AIDS.

As indicated in a response to a query sent to the *Journal of Occupational Medicine* [2], the objectives of a program in industry will range from sports and clubs through fitness with or without health education to total fitness education and rehabilitation efforts. Variations of the primary theme may consider off-hours programs versus time-given involvement, off-plant resource utilization versus in-plant utilization of resources, availability to executives and supervisors versus involvement of all personnel, and absence of supervision versus medically supervised activities. The actual functions may include one or more of the following: club or class activities (basketball, bowling, karate, or dancing); fitness activities (jog-walk, calisthenics, or bicycling); fitness activities with medical involvement and health education (screening by medical personnel, exercise with nutritional, stress management and smoking-cessation education); total fitness/rehabilitation activities (same as the last item, but with alcoholism, musculoskeletal, and cardiac rehabilitation efforts added). These activities may follow or be concurrent with a complete physical examination, a health hazard appraisal, or both.

MEDICAL RESPONSIBILITY

In many companies, counseling that relates to alcoholism rehabilitation, behavioral problems, and other personal difficulties resulting in impaired job performance has been siphoned off into the euphemistically entitled employee assistance programs, to be discussed in Chapter 11. However, it is believed strongly that a comprehensive occupational health service (OHS), concerned with all aspects of a worker's health, physical or emotional, should be responsible for and offer guidance to the employees who are endeavoring to rectify some of their medical or behavioral shortfalls. Such a programmatic element as physical fitness improvement should be closely connected preliminarily to exercise- or stress-testing, medical approval, and medical supervision.

In large organizations where sophisticated cardiopulmonary laboratories are part of the OHS, such exercise testing is used as a segment of the preplacement protocol for applicants seeking energy-intensive positions such as assignments in law enforcement or fire suppression. Repeated testing is carried out regularly, and actual prescriptions for exercise programs are given the individual interested in a continuing fitness program. Appropriate interpretation of test results and counseling always accompany the wrap-up of the test effort [3,4,5]. In substance, the OHS should screen personnel for participation in a physical fitness program because of the more extensive knowledge of the individual's job demands, even though a written sanction may have been received from the worker's own physician. As Erb [6] has indicated, medical responsibility increases as one moves from the well population to the group at greatest risk, for example, from (1) competitive athletes in training, to (2) well subjects under age 35, to (3) well subjects over age 35, to (4) subjects any age with significant cardiovascular risk factors or associated diseases, and finally, to (5) subjects with proved cardiovascular disease. Examples of all five classes will be found in any industrial establishment.

Some years ago Haskell [7] observed that even though minimal medical approval for participation in a company-sponsored program can be provided by the employee's personal physician, frequently the worker will not have a family physician. Secondly, such consultation will cost the employee money he or she frequently will not spend, and thirdly, the type of examination provided would not serve as the ideal clearance procedure. He further suggested that the clearance examination should include the following: (1) medical history—family history, personal history, current habits; (2) physical examination; and (3) laboratory tests—blood, urine, radiography, resting electrocardiogram (ECG), exercise ECG. The purposes of such a protocol are to detect pathologic changes, that is, establish a diagnosis of overt or latent heart disease; to identify risk-precipitating factors; and to quantitate the fitness level (cardiovascular functional capacity, particularly to clear individuals for strenuous work or exercise programs) through prescription of the program, evaluation of change (response to conditioning program), and motivation of the participant (for entering and adhering to exercise programs).

EXERCISE (STRESS) TESTING

While the inclusion of an exercise test capability is desirable in an OHS—utilizing a treadmill or bicycle ergometer—not every facility will have a cardiologist to monitor the employees undergoing evaluation. However, if the health service of a company is considering the addition of this kind of laboratory, certain criteria must be met.

A special target activity group of the American Heart Association's (AHA) Subcommittee on Rehabilitation drew up a set of standards for adult exercise testing laboratories, under the chairmanship of Myrvin H. Ellestad, M.D. [8]. These guidelines should apply to all laboratories conducting graded exercise tolerance testing of adults at maximal or near-maximal levels. The objectives of these criteria are meaningful test results and patient (employee) safety. Table 7-1 illustrates the essence of the standards with some expansion [9,10].

A second target activity group of the AHA, with Herman K. Hellerstein, M.D., as chairman, developed specifications for exercise testing equipment, and the guidelines cover the testing devices—the treadmill, the bicycle ergometer, and the step ergometer—the monitoring equipment, other equipment, emergency equipment, and drugs [11].

A report emanating from the American Medical Association (AMA) Council on Scientific Affairs [12] points out that the procedure has come under attack because of the relatively high percentage of false-positive test results in the healthy population, as well as false-negative test results in patients with sympto-

TABLE 7-1. *Checklist for Operation of an Exercise Laboratory*

Physician immediately available in laboratory.*
Laboratory well-ventilated with comfortable temperature and humidity range.
Calibrated bicycle ergometer or treadmill or step ergometer with height stop.
Oscilloscope visible at working distance.
ECG recording instrument meets AHA standards.
Defibrillator present and tested before each day of use.
Procedures outlined for management of cardiopulmonary complication.
Medical kit fully stocked with drugs that are within the date for use.
Procedure for accepting patients.
Pre-exercise ECG.
Pre-exercise procedures for history-taking and examination by physician identified.
Exercise protocol established.
Initial and subsequent loads identified.
End point identified.
Indications for stopping test clearly understood by test operator.
ECG is interpreted by physician.
Exercise test interpretation is adequate.
Work capacity is entered in patient's record.
ST changes are entered in patient's record.
Dysrhythmias are entered in patient's record.
Format established for report of test results.

*While the responsibility for prescribing, supervising, interpreting, reporting, and recommending testing and training belongs to the physician, the American Heart Association (AHA) has pointed out that direct physician supervision of testing and training sessions, while desirable, is not always necessary *provided* the health service personnel involved are trained to the satisfaction of the responsible physician in cardiopulmonary resuscitation (CPR) and emergency cardiac care. This training must be in accordance with standards set by the AHA and the Committee on Emergency Medical Services of the National Academy of Sciences—National Research Council, Division of Medical Sciences. Such persons should have the capability and authorization to perform cardiopulmonary resuscitation, including electrical defibrillation. Such authorization may require changes in some state laws [9].

DeBusk [10], an experienced clinical and research cardiologist, has indicated that specially trained physician's assistants and nurses increasingly have assumed supervisory responsibility in exercise testing and with no increase in the occurrence of complications related to the test protocol. More important, he feels, is appropriate patient selection. Persons with known heart disease undergoing testing for the establishment of prognosis and functional status require special care—those patients manifesting left ventricular dysfunction or moderately severe angina pectoris and those within 10 days of a myocardial infarction. The decision to test such clinically fragile individuals is the prerogative of the attending physician, but most likely they would not be asked to undergo such procedures as part of the placement system. In DeBusk's operation, experienced physician's assistants and nurses have provided better test supervision than inexperienced physicians, even over high-risk patients. In that facility, a physician is available within 1 to 2 minutes. The commentary is concluded with the statement, "Medicolegal constraints on supervision of exercise tests by nonphysicians appear to have a stronger historic than medical basis."

SOURCE: Modified from American Heart Association, Subcommittee on Rehabilitation, Target Activity Group. Standards for adult exercise testing laboratories. *J Occup Med* 21:763, 1979.

matic coronary disease. When correlated with angiographic studies and with epidemiologic end points, the sensitivity has been found to be approximately 60 to 70 percent. The specificity—the percentage of patients without coronary disease who have normal exercise test results—has been about 90 percent.

The council, while speaking against the testing of healthy young asymptomatic subjects in the expectation of making a definitive diagnosis, does point out that in prospective epidemiologic studies of asymptomatic men, utilizing exercise tests, those subjects with abnormal test results had 10 to 15 times the chance of developing coronary artery disease manifestations than did those examinees with normal findings.

The pertinent issue at hand is whether all persons entering a company-sponsored physical fitness or wellness program that involves a strenuous physical expenditure of energy should have, on entry, dynamic electrocardiography. It is agreed that cardiac stress testing should not be used as a screening device in asymptomatic individuals *unless* specific variables or risk factors are known [13,14]. An AMA report [12] states, "Multistage exercise test[ing] . . . probably has little indication in the routine screening of the healthy population as a case finding device, but it may provide a useful indicator of coronary disease prevalence in the epidemiological studies of *middle aged men*."

Russek [15] does not recommend exercise testing of the general population to detect asymptomatic ischemia, for the test is neither sufficiently sensitive nor specific for mass screening. The procedure is indicated in post–myocardial infarction patients and those individuals who have been successfully treated for angina.

Finally, an opinion in parallel with the comments above has been expressed by McCunney [16], who feels that an exercise test prior to beginning a fitness program is unnecessary; it is not predictive, and it is costly.

While the observations made are cogent when applied to large groups strictly for screening purposes, they lose solidity in our contemporary litigious society, particularly in states where workers' compensation judges rule liberally in favor of the claimant. "Stress" as a claimed injury has increased in numbers, particularly among law-enforcement and firefighter personnel, in addition to executives filing for emotional damage. Further, it is these physically nonconditioned personnel who are being placed in fitness programs, and considering the unrelenting state of readiness required for police and firefighters, it is entirely conceivable that there will be ischemic vessels in need of challenge under near-maximal energy demands. It appears prudent to have candidates for the more intensive programs undergo treadmill or ergometric testing, particularly if they are over 40 years of age, have had a positive cardiac history, are cigarette smokers, have a high-risk family history, display significantly elevated blood chemistry values, and are borderline or clinically hypertensive. While most program participants will be younger, there will always be some who want "to get back in condition." The employer should exercise all precautions before attaching the company name to an activity that might prove to be a liability under workers' compensation coverage.

The choice of adding exercise testing to an OHS examination must be determined by a knowledge of the character of the jobs being filled, the known health characteristics of the population from which the work candidates are drawn, and the past experience of a stress response to the jobs being filled. With energy-demanding and stressor-surrounded jobs of the type indicated, and if in a political or governmental jurisdiction where heart disease is presumed by law to be job-caused, then exercise testing is indeed indicated. Further, it may be additionally indicated when an intensive fitness program is being planned by the parent organization.

PRECAUTIONS

Prior to the initiation of an exercise program for an individual employee, a signed "informed consent for exercise treatment" should be obtained. Such a form indicates the knowledge and prescription of the personal physician and conveys both the potential risks and precautions taken in carrying out the protocol. The content of such a form has been suggested by the AHA [9].

As indicated by Siegel [17], two elements are necessary for informed consent—knowledge and permission. This type of consent provides evidence that the employee has been made aware of the risks involved in the procedure, rather than just being asked for a signature on a blank consent form. Experience has indicated that with a good personal relationship with the employee (or patient) and with full disclosure of the facts, there is less likelihood of legal action. Siegel points out further that the employee who refuses to undergo a test after having been apprised of the potential risks is frequently the one most likely to have an untoward result and to initiate legal action.

There are certain physical and environmental states that temporarily contraindicate exercise. These factors [10], specific contraindications to exercise programs [18], the reasons for discontinuing an exercise program [9], the appropriate equipment and medications to allow treatment of a serious mishap [19], the abnormal responses to be watched for constantly in the test protocol [9] have been outlined by the AHA. The precautions to be taken in dynamic testing [20] are given in Appendix 7-1.

Lastly, there are some specific instructions to be given the test subject the day before the procedure. Smith [21] has suggested the following:

Get an adequate night's sleep before the test.
Eat a light meal 2 hours or more before the test.
Do not smoke or drink coffee, tea, or alcohol within 2 hours prior to the test.
Wear loose-fitting, comfortable clothes. Women should wear a bra.
Shoes must be comfortable, well-fitting, and supportive and have rubber or crepe soles. Women should not wear high heels.
Medications should be taken on their regular schedule if ordered.
Following the test, avoid any vigorous exercise for the rest of the day.
Avoid taking a hot or very warm shower within 2 hours of the test.

INDUSTRIAL OR CORPORATE FITNESS PROGRAMS

Certain companies or installations in both the public and private sectors have initiated fitness or wellness programs. These programs have been of three kinds: health hazard appraisal, directed fitness activities, or a combination of the two.

HEALTH HAZARD APPRAISAL

Although the health hazard appraisal has been discussed previously in Chapter 5, additional comments are in order.

At the Centers for Disease Control (CDC), Public Health Service, in Atlanta, as one example, an employee-directed lifestyle health education program was initiated through the employee organization. While not immediately providing a group-sponsored fitness improvement activity, it did lead to self-referrals to community resources. A health risk appraisal questionnaire was given to employees who wished to participate. The results were used to help the respondents identify potential health problems that might be related to modifiable behaviors. The questions related to sex, race, age; alcohol, tobacco and drug use; crime record and carrying of weapons; heart disease risk factors; anthropometry; exercise patterns; history of pulmonary disease; and gastrointestinal disorders and cancer.

After computerization of the completed questionnaire, the respondents received a printout that provided their chances of dying of certain diseases within the next 10 years, as based on the experience of other Americans of comparable age, race, and sex. In other words, they were provided with their "given age," their "appraised age," and their "compliance age," the last being a new figure were they to undertake certain activities directed toward changing their lifestyle. They were also given a complete directory of community resources for programs concerned with exercise, weight control, smoking cessation, stress management, and recreation.

The worth of such health hazard/health risk appraisal (HH/HRA) efforts has been studied by Wagner and associates [22], through a review of some 217 programs, discussions with and site-visits to users, and consultations not only with developers and users but also with experts in epidemiology, biostatistics, and behavioral science. Specifically investigated were the scientific basis for the assessment of individual risk and benefits of appropriate behavioral change, the methods of measurement, the settings where used, the supportive evidence of positive effects, the element of physical or psychological risk, the applicability to less-advantaged populations, and areas in need of further research. The procedures followed were fairly comparable to the protocol used by the CDC.

The criticism of the HH/HRA is harsh and devalues the worth of the undertaking. The reasons for interest in such a health educational activity are twofold. One-half of the programs were conducted at the workplace, and many are precedent to the physical fitness programs sponsored by industry. The findings of the study showed that nearly every step in the sequence described has been criticized and found to be wanting in terms of its effect on the accuracy of the prediction that results. In a short-term study of Lanzon cited by Wagner and associates [22], workers were divided into three groups, and follow-up information was obtained within 3 months. Multiple comparisons involving 11 dependent variables were made, and although several apparently positive effects of HH/HRA were noted, they were generally small and inconsistently distributed among the subgroups ("an attention control group" not receiving HH/HRA, one group receiving only HH/HRA results and interpretation, and a third receiving HH/HRA and personal health counseling).

Other findings pointed up certain adverse effects, such as anecdotal reports of depressive responses to life-expectancy predictions among older clients. Anxiety, depression, hypochondriasis, confusion, and unnecessary medical expenses could result.

Further, the procedure is one most relevant for white, middle-class clients. The mortality statistics used were total mortality statistics and were not specific for ethnicity, particularly important when certain causes of death were more prevalent among minority groups. Considerable additional research was recommended.

Because of its easy software packageability, the HH/HRA protocol has been taken up eagerly by the marketplace. Often, mass efforts that are offered to industry fail in adequate follow-up, and because, in the main, they do not interrelate an individual's efforts with his physician, there may not be appropriate attention given true health needs. HH/HRA awaits scientific verification for use by the OHS within a plant, even though Wagner and his associates indicated that programs integrated into an ongoing health or medical service, such as an employee health service, seemed to be the most stable and efficient.

Exxon, Rockwell International, Victoria Station (restaurant chain), Xerox Corporation, Excello Press, Phillips Petroleum Company, Kimberly-Clark, American Can, Johnson & Johnson, Pepsico, and Prudential Insurance, among others, have sponsored fitness programs [23,24].

A study was conducted at two large Canadian insurance companies [25] of the effects of fitness or wellness program participation. While there were small gains in productivity as judged by self-reports and supervisor evaluations following the 6-month period of trial, with some reduction of absenteeism at both the test and control sites, the results might have been traceable to sample attenuation, seasonal trends, and a "Hawthorne" effect.

The AHA conducted a survey, beginning in 1980, of the occupational medical activities of American companies offering programs to reduce the risk of heart attack and stroke and published a directory the following year [26]. The data base comprised responses from 405 companies, classified by number of employees from 1000 or fewer to over 25,000. As only 396 of the replying health services gave company size, it is not possible to determine the total percentage of the American labor force represented by the data. Queries concerned screening for hypertension, smoking, obesity, serum lipids, and lack of exercise.

Most programs were implemented after 1974, although there was some limited activity prior to 1960. The frequency with which risk factor detection was offered varied from daily to less than annually. While all risk factors were detected in 85 to 95 percent of the companies by their own health personnel, hypertension detection seemed to represent the greatest effort in the various programs. The employees in whom risk factor reduction was indicated were either referred to the company medical department, referred to an outside medical faculty, given information handouts, provided with individual counseling, or brought into group education sessions. Presumably, most of the intervention activity was carried on by occupational health physicians and nurses, although other personnel in some companies, such as licensed vocational nurses, physician assistants, medical technologists, exercise physiologists, psychologists/psychiatrists, health educators, and nutritionists participated in the detection programs. No evaluation of the worth of the effort was included in the survey.

Pertinent material has appeared in house organs distributed to employees [27–29], and packaged programs are being marketed [30].

PROGRAM CONTENT

In the 1980s, more firms are publicizing the wellness programs being made available to their employees. Most of the activity probably results from their desire to effect some control over the extraordinarily high health care costs, for few industrial benefit packages remain static from year to year. Either the premiums rise or the benefits lessen. In organizations where the employer contribution is at the 100-percent level, the increase is felt acutely. So, if it is the lifestyle diseases that lead to a greater need for medical and hospital care, then attempts are made in both primary and secondary prevention at the worksite.

Another motivation might be the desire to improve a company's image. Wellness can join readily the mother–flag–apple pie sanctity of the United States, and by offering wellness programs, the organization is perceived as a caring institution. The firm becomes a good neighbor as a sequela to its interest in workers' fitness.

Program Designation

Usually a catch phrase is selected and frequently a logo is designed to give identity and uniqueness to the program. At the Xerox Corporation, it was termed the Xerox Health Management Program [31], while one of the Honeywell plants called its plan Life Plus [32] and a back-care class, "Back on Trac." It was the Health Promotion Service at Blue Cross and Blue Shield of Indiana [33], while a segment of the wellness program at the Lockheed Missiles and Space Company [34] was termed "Take It Off 83." The Campbell Soup Company has a Turnaround Health and Fitness Center [35], and at the

S. C. Johnson & Son plant, the effort carries the title Johnson Mutual Benefit Association (HMBA) Fitness Program [36]. Aerobic Challenge is the designation given the program at the Nashville headquarters of the Hospital Corporation of America [37], and at the DuPont installations the health improvement program is termed Health Horizons [38]. Other efforts were termed Lifestyle Enhancement Program and WellWay Program [39]. With some of the undertakings, awards are made when specified goals are reached, or the program is structured so that certain publicity is given successful participants.

Program Elements

Many of the wellness programs are constituted similarly in that efforts are targeted toward the reduction of risk factors (change in lifestyle) and ultimately the lowering of morbidity, the lengthening of life, and even the possibility of better morale and improved job performance. The following are components of many of the contemporary worksite activities:

Examination	Questionnaire
	Screening ("mini-exam")
	Complete medical examination
	Exercise stress testing
	Clinical laboratory tests
	Health risk profile
Repetitive controls	Blood pressure measurement
	Weight measurement
	Blood chemistry levels
	Serum lipids levels
Counseling	Weight reduction
	Nutrition (general) counseling
	Smoking cessation
	Cancer risk reduction
	Alcoholism rehabilitation
	Chemical dependency
	Stress management
	Accident prevention
	Special chronic disease educational classes
	Seat-belt usage
Educational materials	Inserts or articles in plant publications
	Brochures
	Slides with soundtrack
	Tape cassettes or videotapes
	Publicity releases
	Food content lists (calorie charts)
	Special newsletters
Exercise	Treadmill use
	Ergometer use
	Ski simulation
	Weight lifting
	Walking
	Jogging
	Rowing machine use
	Stretching bars
	Other resistance devices
	Aerobic dance
	Jazzercise
Other activities	Breast self-examination
	Health-related seminars
	Health fairs
	Vocational rehabilitation
	Return-to-work programs
	Back-injury prevention programs
	Referrals
	Research
	Evaluation
	Brown-bag lunch presentations

The placement of the wellness/fitness program varies among companies. In some it has been an activity of the OHS, while in others it has been ancillary to the medical arm, functioning rather autonomously. Still other institutions have created a freestanding operation that has little tie to the OHS. In a conference held in 1985 in Los Angeles where many wellness program directors were convened, no consensus was reached as to the ideal placement. In organizations with strong medical leadership, it was advantageous to have the medical director voice the needs to the CEO.

Corporations selling their programs in the open marketplace usually had skilled professionals, frequently prepared at the master's level, to promulgate the concept and sell the product package. Health promotion directors were exercise physiologists or others dedicated to physical fitness and prudent, healthful lifestyles. It would seem logical that a wellness program—because of its counseling components and capability in exercise testing—be part of the total OHS, which in nearly every segment is, or certainly should be, devoted to preventive health care. Were the wellness offering split from the OHS, it would seem to be an unnatural splintering, for health monitoring is a continuing portion of any effort in lifestyle change. It might be that some of the self-felt deficits in oral and written communication preclude the more active participation of physicians in this special programming. Exemplary of skilled medical leadership was that provided by former Corporate Medical Director, Dr. Roland F. Wear, Jr., at the Campbell Soup Company of Camden, New Jersey, where innovative moves toward lifestyle reversal were initiated for employees years ago.

Dismuke and Miller have taken physicians to task for not being stronger participants in this kind of endeavor [40]. They offer this scenario in explanation: Keeping people in good health is important but "it is not the business of physicians. Physicians should stick to treating illness because that is what they have always done and what they do best." Health education by physicians, the plot continues, is downgraded as unenjoyable, unproductive, and financially unrewarding. They end their plea to the practitioners in this manner:

> Physicians must take a more active role in personal health promotion. Although multiple health professionals are needed for implementation of needed changes, the physician is an indispensable component. Physician support adds respectability and validity. It ensures changes based on scientific evidence and increases the vulnerability of health promotion to quackery and commercial exploitation. Physicians clearly have determined some pathways to better health. It is time that they share their secrets for good health and become active proponents of health promotion.

In industry, this kind of participation, leadership, and support is logical, reasonable, and an expected function in any position description of a physician. This aspect of the role should not be shunted off to others who are less knowing but more aggressive.

PREPARATION FOR FITNESS/ WELLNESS PROGRAMS

Seeds [41] has listed the key requirements of an ideal fitness program in the following:

A good program director to inform properly and help employees motivate themselves.
An employee education program.
Employee evaluation: Ideally part of an employee health program, but everyone participating in an exercise program needs basic evaluation, to include knowledge of
- Treadmill results.
- Presence of risk factors.
- Orthopedic problems.

Convenience: Employer-sponsored programs can be more convenient and successful than community agency programs because they are held in the workplace or with coworkers.
Variety: range should be broad.
Recognition for participation: It is important to recognize achievement, but most important to include all levels of achievement. Not everyone is a star, but most are trying. Recognition is a strong catalyst.
Family involvement: Some exercise or fitness activities should be planned with the family to maintain a cooperative home attitude.

Some of these points are repetitious of previous comments but give emphasis to the need for preprogram evaluation and for family participation to avoid the creation of the jogger's widow.

The objectives of a fitness program have been offered by Nast and McDonald [42] and epitomize the benefits of such an OHS effort:

To promote a preventive medicine approach to health through the use of regular physical activity.
To improve fitness needs of employees through participation in an exercise conditioning program.
To provide a means of screening for possible coronary heart disease risk factors and to establish appropriate referral patterns for risk factor intervention.
To identify employees for whom exercise without supervision may be contraindicated.
To perform fitness tests and establish acceptable fitness standards.
To provide an individualized exercise counseling service.
To educate employees about exercise prescription, the principles of conditioning, and the various ways of monitoring the response to exercise.
To supervise directly conditioning programs for those employees with a low tolerance to exercise or associated medical problems.
To reassess periodically fitness levels of employees.
To make resources available to direct employees into community physical activity programs.
To coordinate employee referrals to supportive services such as nutrition and weight-control counseling.

Shephard and his colleagues [43] studied the factors that influence recruitment of participants in a fitness program of the headquarters office of a large corporation. The rate of participation was 20 percent of eligible staff with convenient access to the health fitness center. Interest was equal among men and women, and typical recruits were middle-aged nonsmokers who previously had been active elsewhere. Factors of acceptability such as travel time, hours of work, and cost had little effect on participation. The male subjects perceived that they were active for health, fitness, and competition, and the women for appearance. It was concluded that general and specific health beliefs were well developed but bore little relationship to health practices and outcomes. It was felt that the shaping of attitudes by trial of an exercise program might be a more effective tactic for increasing exercise participation than general efforts designed to change attitudes and values.

HAZARDS

That there are certain hazards attendant upon exercise programs has been reported repeatedly. Stress fractures [44,45] are known among joggers, and runners have been injured and killed by motor vehicles and attacked by birds [46–49]. In an epidemiologic study reported by Kaplan and coworkers [50], who sent questionnaires to registrants for a 10-km road race, respondents reported dog bites, being struck by bicycles and motor vehicles, and being hit by a thrown object—cans, bottles, ice, liquids, and a rock-filled bag. Over a third of the runners sustained a musculoskeletal injury. These facts are mentioned because it must be remembered that company-sponsored programs entail risk for the organization if injuries occur as part of a recognized activity. If jogging or other exercise protocols are introduced, they are most likely to be interpreted exactly as have athletic injuries among company-league players, that is, such injured employees are eligible for all benefits under workers' compensation coverage. One recent decision [51] concerned a 54-year-old research department head who collapsed and died after jogging during his lunch hour. He was jogging on company time and in a company-furnished gym, in addition to the fact that the employer encouraged physical fitness of his workers. Further, users of the gym were given shirts bearing the employer's name, and the employer participated in an annual awards dinner for gym members for which he provided trophies. It was ruled that the decedent died in the course of his employment, and the award was upheld by the New York Supreme Court.

Several other decisions support the workers' compensation rule regarding injuries sustained during company-sponsored activities, but Larson [52] epitomized the rule by saying that recreational or social activities are within the course of employment when (1) they occur on the premises during a lunch or recreation period as a regular incident of the employment; or (2) the employer, by expressly or implicitly requiring participation, or by making the activity part of the services of an employee, brings the activity within the orbit of the employment; or (3) the employer derives substantial direct benefit from the activity beyond the intangible value of improvement in employee health and morale that is common to all kinds of recreation and social life.*

For a detailed listing of various sports/fitness activities and their accompanying potential injuries or risk, prevention of injuries (examples of equipment safety), and environmental risks and hazards, see Marks and associates [53].

*The rule is given further substance by such decisions as *Nazario v. N.Y. State Dept. of Corrections,* 441 N.Y.S. 2d 531; *Tocci v. Tessler & Weiss, Inc.,* 28 N.J. 582, 147 A. 2d 783 (1959); and *Wilson v. United Auto Workers International Union,* 441 S.W. 2d 475 (Ark. 1969).

RECORDS

All participant events entailed in a fitness program should be recorded in the health records maintained in the OHS. The exercise undertaken, the duration of the exercise, the workload attained if a stationary exercise bicycle or other equipment with a recorder is used, and any untoward effect should be entered in the record. An individual log should be maintained in the exercise facility so that statistical summaries can be produced indicating usage. If a system of notation is desired to indicate the type of exercise undergone, use can be made of a method described by Jokl and coworkers [54], which employs a variety of unique symbols.

MOTIVATION

The reasons for participating in an activity program are multiple. In 1981 the Canada Fitness Survey was conducted by Fitness Canada [55]. A lengthy questionnaire was completed by over 21,000 members, ages 10 to 97, of randomly selected households in all parts of Canada. Apart from obtaining a measure of the total daily energy expenditure of the respondents, the rationale for being active was determined. The overall findings indicated the following reasons and percent of respondents: feel better, 60 percent; fun, excitement, 44 percent; control weight, 42 percent; improve flexibility, 40 percent; relax, 34 percent; companionship, 24 percent; doctor's orders, 23 percent; challenge, 21 percent; learning, 20 percent; and fitness specialist advice, 19 percent.

There were not great differences among the age groups. More of the younger groups offered "fun, excitement" and "challenge" as reasons than did the older groups, and more of the 55-year-old persons checked "doctor's orders." Weight control was important to all [56].

PROGRAM BENEFITS

While individual participants may benefit from the various sectors of a wellness program, it must be remembered that a fitness activity is a benefit offered by employers and at their cost. Is the wellness package cost-effective, and do certain advantages accrue to the sponsoring company?

Possibly the most extensive evaluation that has been conducted has been that involving the "Go to Health" worksite health-promotion research project involving the Blue Cross and Blue Shield plans of Michigan [57]. The project was designed to measure the program's impact on economic and health-related outcomes. The rationale was that by encouraging lifestyle decision-making, the plan could enhance its predominantly provider- and administrative-oriented cost-containment programs. The objectives comprised (1) a measure of costs, changes in productivity, and utilization of health insurance benefits associated with comprehensive health promotion; (2) an assessment of changes in preventable risk factors that may contribute to disease; (3) a measure of change in attitude toward and knowledge of health promotion and disease prevention; and (4) conduct of a cost-benefit study.

Four groups, three experimental and one "no-treatment" control, were formed as follows:

Group A: Received all interventions—health risk appraisals, screening, group and individual counseling, and risk-reduction programs (stress management, exercise, smoking cessation, weight control, blood pressure measurement, medical self-care, and cancer awareness).
Group B: All interventions exclusive of individual counseling and risk-reduction programs.
Group C: Received health-risk appraisals only.
Group D: No interventions.

Over a 3-year period (1979–1981), 1,449 employees of the plan participated in various components of the wellness program. They were volunteers and tended to be older, more often male, less often minority, and more often managerial/administrative/technical personnel (rather than clerical) with less absenteeism and lower health insurance utilization than the nonparticipants. The results were reported as follows:

Productivity (Employee evaluations)
- Increases in hourly wage rate for each group.
- Group A received more promotions and transfers.
- Merit ratings: No change from 1979 through 1981, but in 1980 group A received higher scores.
- Efficiency ratings: No changes, but group A had higher ratings in 1980 than group B. No differences in 1981.
- Absenteeism: Declined 70 percent in group A, while increased in all others. Groups B, C, and D showed dramatic increase in severity of illness.
- Long-term disability: Increased in all groups between 1979 and 1980. Continued into 1981 for all but group A, which returned to 1979 level.

Health insurance utilization
- No change.* Group A had significantly lower drug charges and payments than group D in 1981.

Risk factors, morbidity, and mortality
- No changes over time in six risk indicator measures: blood pressure, weight, cholesterol levels, alcohol use, type-A personality, and physical activity.
- Smoking: Groups A and D significant rates of cessation. No changes in number of cigarettes among persisting smokers.
- Blood lipids: Lower levels of cholesterol and increased high-density lipoprotein (HDL) levels in groups A and B. Group A showed lower cholesterol/HDL ratios throughout the entire period.
- General well-being: All groups increased, with group A manifesting higher scores.

Health attitudes and knowledge
- No intergroup changes in summary measures of health beliefs, health barriers, or health knowledge.
- Group A was more likely to accept disease prevention efficacy than groups C and D in 1980 and all groups in 1981.

Cost-benefit analyses: Results unclear. Group A may have a theoretic extension of life expectancy, with impact on pension costs. In the short-term, costs outweighed measured benefits; therefore, further study is needed.

*Case finding usually leads to more health care.

Other observations of measurable benefits have been documented. Browne and colleagues [58] reported a reduction in major medical costs, disability days, and direct disability dollar costs, with a $353.38 saving per participant at a cost per cohort member of $120.60. Chenoweth [59] indicated a drop in absenteeism in a study group, and Bernacki and Baun [60] reported a positive although probably noncausal relationship between exercise adherence in a corporate fitness program and above average job performance. Aerobic reserve was increased among firefighters placed on an exercise program [61], suggesting that the postalarm tachycardia is dampened, which may lessen the risk of heart disease occurring in the postalarm period. Fielding [62] in a 1982 report felt that credible data concerning the cost-effectiveness of weight-management programs were not yet available, but smoking cessation and hypertension control programs are probably cost beneficial.

In the Coors Wellness Program [63], cost savings for 1983 are presented:

In-house treadmill testing saved	$ 46,472
Cardiac Rehabilitation Program saved	85,680
Reduction in return-to-work time saved	212,220
Well-Back Program saved	319,305
Total savings	$663,677

The savings exceeded the operating budget by over $107,500.

In summary, accurate cost-benefit data are still

being awaited in relation to company-sponsored wellness programs. O'Donnell and Ainsworth [64] discuss in a theoretical framework all the accruable benefits under the headings of (1) improvement of productivity, (2) reduction of benefit costs, (3) reduction of human resources development costs, and (4) image of the organization. A review of their analyses is encouraged.

COMMENT

Unquestionably there will be a continued growth of fitness and wellness programs, in spite of infrequent jocose anti-exercise commentaries [65]. Such activities may be included in programs of stress management, which will be discussed later, or related to specific efforts in individual- or group-relaxation techniques.

As a final note to those persons who believe such undertakings to be a product of the 1980s, attention is directed to classes offered to corporation employees in 1917, comprising folk dancing, swimming, social dancing, gymnastics, calisthenics, self-defense, and lectures on city government [66]. In the flowing prose of over six decades ago, the effect of the program was described: "The return of a healthy, ruddy color to cheeks which had been pale from confinement in the office, and the transformation of the careworn faces of the business women into fresh, radiant, buoyant girlish expressions, were rich compensation for the efforts expended in organizing this class [in dancing]."

Perhaps the effort was in response to a national malaise in health voiced in 1912 by the president of the Louisiana State Board of Health before the American Public Health Association (APHA): "It is conceded that as a nation, we have not valued health as a personal or national asset. We have been too busy tunnelling mountains, conquering space, boring for wealth, erecting skyscrapers, piling up vast fortunes to count the cost in terms of human vitality" [67].

HEALTH EDUCATION PROGRAMS

Until recent years, health education of the workers was a lately come, frequently tag end of a program in occupational health. Given positional primacy were the more conventional segments of employee care and environmental correction. If time permitted, and if the fiscal base allowed, minimal efforts were targeted toward bringing health knowledge to the worker.

The Occupational Safety and Health Act of 1970 brought new attention to the need of the industrial employee for information regarding the potential hazards present at his workplace. The legislation specifically charged the secretaries of labor and health, education, and welfare that they "provide for the establishment and supervision of programs for the education and training of employers and employees in the recognition, avoidance and prevention of unsafe or unhealthful working conditions in employments covered" by the act.* A second indicator of renewed concern is the expressed program goal, one of three, of the National Center for Health Education of "health education for employees" [68,69]. With these sharply delineated policy platforms, in addition to the federal and state "right-to-know" enactments (discussed in Chapter 14), it is the task of the occupational health professional to convert charges to commitments.

DEFINITIONS

Health

That health, as a concept, has been overdefined is accepted. But put succinctly, in the occupational sense, it can be thought of as a duality of effectiveness and happiness, a freedom from apprehension and anxiety, but not necessarily a freedom from tension or environmental adjustment or coping.

Health is well-being, it is comfort, it is, as Fishbein [70] once defined physical fitness, "bounce," meaning resiliency and elasticity, the ability to recover easily from a minor physical trauma or an emotional assault. These definitions in a generic sense are superficially satisfying, but do they fit in today's work scene, where, for example, an employee who has been well but has had long contact with material X, which recently has been found to be carcinogenic, and now has the added anxiety of belonging to the "walking wounded"—is he or she in good health? The sense of health as effectiveness should be retained, for it aids in the evaluation of the individual worker whose physical and emotional status is subject to the sway of innumerable variables.

Definitions vary widely. Wylie [71] altered a definition of Herbert Spencer's to read, "Health is the perfect, continuing adjustment of an organism to its environment." Is health possible in an industrial set-

*Occupational Safety and Health Act of 1970, Public Law 91-596, 91st congress, S. 2193, December 29, 1970, Sec. 21(c). To implement the generic directive, OSHA extracted all of the training or educational requirements from published standards—its own and those of others—and has assembled them in a single document: *Training Requirements in OSHA Standards* (rev.). Washington, DC: U.S. Department of Labor, OSHA, Nov 1979. See also OSHA Training Requirements. In *Best's Safety Directory—1983*. Oldwick, NJ: A.M. Best, 1983. Vol. I., pp. 53–57.

ting where the constant presence of certain uncontrolled exposures permit the gradual increase of the body's burden of toxic materials? In a study of a general population, Belloc, Breslow, and Hochstim [72] employed a gradient to measure health, coursing from a minimal state defined by inability to work and/or care for one's personal needs to an optimal state, expressed by no complaints and a level of energy. The latter can be equated with the effectiveness or productivity of the individual indicated previously.

Chapman [73] points up the confusion between health and abundant, readily available medical care. He indicates that no medical person can define health because the whole of medicine's structure rests on a foundation of a knowledge of disease. Even preventive medicine, he adds, constitutes a series of measures designed to avoid specific illness or injury. Continuing, he offers this wry definition: "Health can almost be defined as that condition of human biology in which medical men have received no training."

But in coming back to more positive views, one can turn to Goldsmith's [74] several citations of definitional attempts to understand health. In addition to Wylie's modification, he provides Hayman's definition of "optimal personal fitness for full, fruitful, creative living"; Lifson's perspective of "the degree to which a human's functions (sensing, data processing, motioning . . .) are performed and pain is absent"; Romano's inclination toward "the capacity of the organism to maintain a balance in which it may be reasonably free of undue pain, discomfort, disability or limitation of action including social capacity"; and lastly, Blum's modification of Romano's concept as "1. the capacity of the organism to maintain a balance appropriate to its age and social needs in which it is reasonably free of gross dissatisfaction, discomfort, disease, or disability, and 2. to behave in ways which promote the survival of the species as well as the self-fulfillment or enjoyment of the individual."

Talcott Parsons [75] sees health in its relationship to social role structure and social control when he defines it as "the state of optimum *capacity* of an individual for the effective performance of the roles and tasks for which he has been socialized." Such a view brings the meaning of health close to the work setting where members of a labor force have assigned roles, each with its own set of expectations for productivity—the product being a correctly packed carton of fruit, the completed transport of 300 airline passengers, the successful instillation of curiosity or a sense of inquiry in a student, or a new scientific truth. If effectiveness derives from health and is part of it, then the periodically dialyzed employee, the wheelchair-bound person with post-polio residuals, the well-controlled individual with diabetes, or the permanently flexed individual with the burned-out rheumatoid spondylitis are, in a sense, possessive of health as long as they can contribute to the mission of the group to which they belong. This contribution may be possible only through the use of orthotic devices, an insulin pump, a hip prosthesis, the daily injection of a compensating hormone, or the employment of a braille printing device, but the expected role *on the job* is being fulfilled.

Unfortunately, organizations tend to interpret health as presenteeism at work. If one were to ask a chief executive officer (CEO) what the health of the plant might be, or to ask a general officer what was the health of his or her command, both might be inclined to refer to the current attendance record or effective duty roster. Such action does not take into account all of the physically impaired persons at work, the individuals who should be at home because of acute respiratory illness, or the overconscientious workers who have returned prematurely following a surgical operative procedure. They are all present and working, meeting the specifics of their expected roles to a greater or lesser degree. So "health" as a rigidly defined concept is bent somewhat at the work scene, so that a person can contribute, in spite of the effects of chronic disease, aging, or congenital defects. Effective work, therefore, can be a measure of total health, irrespective of the presence of any one of the many socially considered indicators of ill health. As Cohen [76] put it, health is dynamic and flexible, takes account of normal age changes, and need not be impaired by physical defects if they can be artificially corrected.

The subject of precision in definition is one perhaps better left to the public health planners, the behavioral scientists, and the philosophers. But not to be left to members of these other disciplinary arenas is the effort to produce a better health behavior in those employees whose health is, in great part, the responsibility of the occupational health team. Health education at work is the expected and needed function of every participant in the health activity.

Health Education

While simplistic assumptions can be made regarding the transfer of health information in industry, there is little that is simple or easy in attempting to alter behavior that is lifelong, counterproductive to health, antithetic to cultural beliefs, or oppositional to deeply embedded perceptions of sex roles. The OHS has the greatest health education potential of any agency involved in the health care system because of the presence, ideally, of a known population, at fixed points, during a 40-hour work continuum. How well an individual OHS realizes its potential depends on many factors, such as the acceptance of health education as a primary function of an in-plant service; the willingness to insist that certain work time be released to this activity; the level of capability of the physician, the nurse, and the industrial hygienist, among other OHS personnel, to meet with and face workers who may be disinclined to separate the OHS from their hoary concept of the medical arm as "the tool of management"; the ability of the OHS team to translate technical jargon into understandable, even colloquial, but not vulgar, English; and most important, the sincere, dedicated desire to do something about the impaired health of certain employees, be it lifestyle generated, job nurtured, or family produced. Devoted health professionals can, with time, be identified for their sincerity, their concern, and their respect for the individual in need, regardless of the labor or managerial tag that individual may bear. The practitioner with bias is only a person whose transparency precludes the building of a solid relationship with the clientele being served.

As with the defining of *health*, lexicographers both professional and amateur have been at work with the interpretation of *health education*. Implicit in the activity are certain basic concepts. It is a process leading to behavioral change, going totally beyond the mere passage or transfer of information, irrespective of pleasant palatability. It involves the motivation of persons who may have had no knowledge of health values, who are resistant to change, and who are opposed culturally or psychologically to anyone's attempting to alter long-standing work or behavior patterns.

Kasl and Cobb [77], in an excellent, lengthy review, have offered a classification scheme for the health-illness continuum and opened with some definitions particularly pertinent in the industrial setting, where observations of workers can be conducted regularly. *Health behavior,* they define, is any activity undertaken by a person believing himself or herself to be healthy, for the purpose of preventing disease or detecting it in an asymptomatic stage. *Illness behavior,* they continue, is any activity, undertaken by a person who feels ill, to define the state of his or her health and to discover a suitable remedy. The last, *sick role behavior,* is the activity undertaken by those persons who consider themselves ill, for the purpose of getting well. Implicit in all of these definitions is the desire to remain functional or to return to a state of effectiveness. As someone once observed, the primary discommoding feature of illness is not necessarily the pain or discomfiture that arises with the disease or injury, but the inability to do what one wants to do. But in all of the three behaviors there are indications for professional, educative assistance.

Murray and Zentner [78], in their text for nurses, define health education as the learning process by which persons and groups learn to promote, maintain, or restore health. Emphasis is given here to all steps in the wellness-illness progression. Putting health education in the health maintenance organization (HMO) setting, Shapiro [79] has involved the staff jointly when he defines health education as an active process aimed at providing and strengthening influences and experiences for both staff and covered population that will encourage health maintenance and recovery from illness. A functionally useful meaning is Grout's view [80] that "health education is the translation of what is known about health into desirable individual and community behavior patterns by means of the educational forces." The definition is applicable, irrespective of the population involved, the issues of concern, or the site of health care.

Implied in the process are these sequential steps: (1) extracting a body of knowledge from research and practice; (2) preparing the material for palatable acceptance; (3) offering it, when asked or decided upon, in a meaningful manner; (4) making it a matter of personal significance, and thus motivating the learner to use this content when the time, the place, and the reason are appropriate; and (5) observing alterations in the recipient's health behavior.

And, lastly, is the clarification by Squyres [81] regarding patient education, which she does not equate with health education but interprets as planned combinations of learning activities designed to assist people who are having, or have had, experience with illness or disease in making changes in their behavior conducive to health.

OBJECTIVES

Although the goals of health education may be decanted from the definitions given, there are broader dimensions to the teaching/learning lineality. The health educator, as Steuart [82] has expressed it, must see "human motives and behavior as a thread in the seamless fabric of a total way of life, or culture," or the assessment of, and attempts to modify, that behavior are likely to be fragmented, partial, and in practice ineffective. The educator must be able not only to appreciate but also to canalize into practical channels of health education the dynamics of those sociocultural relationships that are the living context of habits, attitudes, interests, and motives of human beings.

The end point is not just an awareness of facts, but an emotional conviction and both attitudinal and behavioral changes. Providing a concrete knowledge of health is less important than imparting insight, rousing interest, and nurturing values that can achieve a healthful style of living. However, in modifying human thought, feeling, and behavior, one should not do so to the point of creating excessive anxiety or hypochrondriasis. Virgil expressed it well when he commented, "He destroys his health by laboring to preserve it."

INVOLVED PERSONNEL

All members of the occupational health team are, or should be, health educators. To carry out in the industrial setting the principles to be enumerated, one need not be profoundly educated in the large body of theory drawn upon for community teaching/learning. Although it might improve considerably the instruction in schools of medicine and public health, a degree in education is rarely possessed by medical or public health faculty members. Stallones [83] underscored this point when he observed, "A significant anomaly in the field of preventive medicine is the relative lack of attention or concern with health education in the preparation of specialists in this field. In the schools of public health, health education has generally been defined as the specific province of a group of people who seek identification as professional health educators and whose qualifications are in the process of education rather than disease prevention." He asked that preventive medicine specialists become much more involved with the methodology, uses, and evaluation of education and motivation. In essence, *all* professional members of the occupational health provider group serve as operational agents in changing the health-destructive behavior of employees to health-preserving and health-improving lifestyles.

The same point was expressed by McNerney [84], who wrote:

> Neither will the goal [of health education] be accomplished if we fall into the familiar trap of institutionalizing or professionalizing health education, as we have done with so many of our professional and technical functions in the health services, building walls of accreditation and credentials around them and guarding the gates against invasion by those without passports. There are already professionals in health education who have been trained for their jobs. They do useful work, and we need more of them. But we must guard against the erection of barriers that would permit this important function to become another little fiefdom run by the anointed for the anointed. More than most other health occupations, health education needs the strength and vigor of an innovative, imaginative drive that thrives on pluralism and is not smothered in the closed atmosphere of the fiefdom.

BELIEFS IN METHODOLOGY

The substratum on which all efforts at conversion are based is a strong adherence to the principles of sound mental health. There must be recognition of and respect for the dignity and worth of each human being entering into the professional-client interaction. There can be no humiliation of the less educated, the less sophisticated, the less physically or esthetically endowed, the less skilled in English, or the less urbanized or cultured worker.

One must avoid viewing all persons and all cultures through the glasses of middle-class standards so that one wonders why something as easily understood as this precept or that one is not immediately and graciously accepted as the thankful employee rides off into the sunset with this beautiful new set of health guidelines. Levine and associates [85] spoke similarly to this point when they discussed referrals, commenting that it is not sufficient to focus only on the deficiencies of the recipient, real and important as they may be. It is equally essential, they maintain, to realize the *dyadic* relationship between the culture of the professional on the one side, and the culture of the recipient on the other, and to focus on inappropriate approaches that stem from the culture of the professional as they are employed in meeting the problems of the recipient.

One must avoid any arousing of guilt through lofty warnings about behavior, and one must shun the role of the authoritarian person who demands submissive acceptance. Cohen [86] expressed it well when he wrote, "Experience with cigarette smokers quickly teaches that to know and indeed accept the evidence that cigarette smoking is a major cause of cancer of the lung, is not necessarily followed by prudent action; and intimidating exhortations however gruesome rarely achieve their aim." Statements such as "You should have come in sooner," or "You should have been more careful," or "You shouldn't have stayed up all night" usually lead to a negative, and not a positive response. Negativity or resistance results from anxiety and guilt. The situation is comparable to the parent's admonition to the child, "Don't let me catch you crossing the street!" being met with the unverbalized, "O.K., you won't catch me."

A second belief to be identified and, unfortunately, one that is not supported by hard data because they are not readily producible, is that most absenteeism is truly not caused by organic illness. Employees remain away because most work is anathematous, psychically unrewarding, and, to many, a deadly bore. Absenteeism statistics reflect socially popular medical reasons for the periods away; respiratory infections and "flu" usually go unquestioned, while almost never offered are statements containing diagnoses that would reflect negatively on the worker, such as sexually transmitted diseases or gynecologic disorders. Absences are most often withdrawals from a disliked workplace, so that a strong informative campaign against the common cold usually relates in no way to the worker's health status. A program of humanization of foremen might be singularly more productive in decreasing the amount of absence falsely attributed to illness.

One must know the employee as a human being. Fully logical is placement in the medical record of news clippings of the worker's activities or honors, notes of family health and interests, and questions asked of the health staff at sites away from the medical facility. Most employees are astonished when this author asks about the family constellation after health-related topics have been discussed. An insulator long exposed to asbestos was in to review the results of a periodic examination. When asked about his family (age, education, interests), his response concerning his daughter was followed almost sotto voce by "and is she a problem." This one-liner opened up the area of his real concern, which was total noncommunication with his 18-year-old. When the girl came in for an interview, instead of a preconceived mute, arrogant, asocial youngster, she turned out to be a creative young person who wrote poetry, composed music, played the guitar, and enjoyed serious drama. The parent and child were at psychological loggerheads because the daughter was exploring new concepts, entering new human interaction arenas, and foregoing family patterns and standards of worship and behavior. With referral of the daughter for therapy, and with counseling for the father, the true problem was attacked. The employee's chest condition, although meriting clinical attention, was entirely secondary. The parent's gratitude was considerable, for inroads had been made into the more major concern of his anxiety. A knowledge of the worker's home situation may allow a more effective health educational effort than a general approach to the reversals of a specific organic disorder.

Joint planning between plant personnel and the medical staff will allow true concerns in health to become apparent. Group review will lead to subsequent group decisions, which in turn will produce individual commitment to common group goals because the participants were personally involved.

In the work culture, one must understand the striving for masculinity, as indicated previously. The current machismo vogue brings to view the well-known locker room braggadocio, the swapping of lies by American men at stag gatherings, the topping out urination ritual of loggers, and the near pride of carpenters in their traumatically amputated digits or that of some stationary engineers who have extremely deficient hearing. This expression of supermasculinity is a standard component of heavy industry that has led to a disregard for personal protective devices because, "I'm tough!" In any educational effort, this characteristic of the male worker must be remembered. Every group has its informal opinion makers, and they must be identified, for their support in health education can be singularly important. In most communities they are not the ministers or social workers, but respected members who hold no formal position. In one production plant, the voice of the total union was expressed by a recognized leader who held no official designation except that of shop steward. Yet, he led, formulated opinion, and motivated his members to take appropriate action after he had studied a situation and had provided a direction.

The communication making up the health education message—written or oral—must avoid the complex. It would be redundant to say that it is no longer necessary to hide behind the lexicon of medicine, for in every medium there are simplified clarifications of medical problems given the eager reader, watcher, or listener. Even now, with such publications as *Expendable Americans, Peril on the Job, Muscle and Blood,* and *Work is Dangerous to Your Health,* the explanations of occupational disease, from etiology to ending, have reached workers not only in the United States, but elsewhere. (A British counterpart is *The Hazards of Work: How to Fight Them.*) In begging for the simple and straightforward, one is reminded of the nurse who, in her clinical records, always wrote "cephalgia" and never "headache." Other disciplines are equally guilty of obfuscating the story being told. An eminent psychologist discusses adolescence as ". . . a normative crisis characterized by increased conflict and a seeming fluctuation in ego strength and yet also by a high growth potential . . . producing an abundance of available energy . . . which supports new and expanded ego functions in the searchings for and engagement of new opportunities and associations." Tell that to a seasoned craftsman when he relates the problem he is having with his 13-year-old. Or try to understand a section from a book review: "Thus, social cultural linkage usually requires that the value orientation and the social structure of the change agent system and the target system are brought together in at least temporary closure" [87]. The eminent Richard Asher epitomized the practice as a "dislike of sharing words with the laity" [88].

The last credo involves the total omission of scare techniques in efforts to redesign human responses to threats to health. The old posters depicting amputation stumps, standard magazine covers printed in braille, or the demonstration or flipping of artificial eyes by a safety manager cruising through a shop are not only ineffective but may prove so distracting as to cause injury through preoccupation or inattention. Fright has no place in any form of communication intended for teaching.

THE WRITTEN WORD

The multiple forms of mass instructional media are mentioned first only to make known their availability and to move on to more productive means. It has long been one's feeling that the younger or less professionally sophisticated the educator, and possibly the younger the occupational health program, the greater will be the reliance on traditional printed materials. Further, the more distant, physically and emotionally, the educator is from the group he or she is hoping to interest, the broader will be the use of inanimate published pieces.

Too often a display of publications is thought to serve as a productive visibility, while, in actuality, much goes unread. Skills in reading may be limited, the brochure or article is perceived as the voice of management and therefore as biased, and the content often is threatening to long-established pleasurable, addictive life patterns. In a sense, the use of a publication purporting the virtues of health is comparable to writing a memorandum to a fellow staff member in the next office. Such action avoids a face-to-face confrontation, skirts one's being forced to think afresh on one's feet, and circumvents discussing an unpleasant subject.

However, if one does wish to reach thousands of employees, and one cannot meet with or address them all, the written word can be utilized to extend the message.

Pamphlets, brochures, and leaflets are readily obtained from a multiplicity of health agencies or commercial sources, or they can be produced locally. Articles can be placed in the company's annual report or in the house organ,* be it a slick monthly for joint distribution to employees and shareholders or a weekly paper in tabloid format. Do not fear the light touch, as exemplified in a Royal Air Force film [88a]:

> If you go out of your aircraft backwards, or dive with your knees drawn up, you will somersault. This is to be avoided, so keep your legs straight if you can, or straighten them as soon as you're clear, and BEFORE you pull the rip cord. Somersaulting may be great fun, and may make you feel young again, but it also means that when you pull the rip cord the lift webs will undoubtedly come up between your knees, and you'll make your descent upside down and with a certain amount of pain. A British pamphlet says, 'a very good view of the ground is at once obtained, but the position is extremely uncomfortable, definitely undignified, and you may even lose things out of your pockets.' If one of the things in your pockets happens to be your address book, you'll bewilder the farmer who picks it up and also leave yourself with nothing to do at night but go to the movies. That's hard on your eyes. So get your legs out straight before you pull the rip cord, and come on down right—this is no time for experimenting.

Posters should be kept simple and uncluttered, with the major point obtainable at a glance. Car cards can be prepared for company busses. Bulletin boards can be used for clippings or any printed materials but should have a schedule for regular change of postings. The bombing of Pearl Harbor or the prevention of poliomyelitis is no longer newsworthy. Payroll inserts have been produced but are considered a waste; a check of the payroll office floor on payday will give testimony. Exhibits are excellent and can be tied in with posters, the newspaper column, or a pamphlet. A lending library can be helpful in selected instances; films or video tapes can provoke group discussion; anatomic models and a book of illustrations back up a one-to-one counseling session; and lastly, comic books, although costly to produce, have been considered effective in public health educational efforts.

THE SPOKEN WORD

The best education in health is accomplished simply by talking with people, as the clinical psychologist does with one person or with a group. This mechanism allows a close relationship to be established between the teacher and the learner that is not possible with an intervening medium. It permits the employee to feel the warmth and concern of the occupational health professional. This kind of proximity lets a negative message (news of untoward clinical findings) be conveyed with considerable human feeling and compassion. Some medical directors have developed video cassettes* for use with new or current

*Outstanding examples of descriptive writings of a medical program are seen in Here's to your health, *Exxon Manhattan* for April 18, 1975; Tracking down health hazards, *Exxon Manhattan* for September 19, 1975; Medicine at work: People helping people, *Exxon Manhattan* for March 30, 1979; Exxon opens East Millstone facility [Environmental Health Science's facility], *Exxon Manhattan* for October 17, 1980; Locke, L., Paging Doctor Moore, *The Lamp* for Summer 1981; and N. J. Roberts, Medicine at work. *The Lamp* for Fall 1974. All publications cited are from Exxon Corporation, New York, NY.

*Examples of company-originated video presentations are the "Help Yourself Program" (counseling), "Medical Tests," and "Medical Record Confidentiality," prepared by the Allied Chemical Corporation, James A. Hathaway, M.D., former Medical Director.

employees offering descriptions of research findings in toxicology or serving as reviews of the examination program.

One-to-One

The most perfect milieu for understanding and behavioral change is that developed in one's office when an employee is asked to come in for a review of the results of periodic examination, as part of a medical surveillance or hazard control program. Attention is focused on one individual—at that moment the most important person in the plant because he or she is walking the treacherous path of apprehension and anxiety, nurtured by misunderstanding, folk beliefs, inadequate information, and fear.

Several years ago a high-level nuclear physicist called and, in an extremely agitated voice, requested an appointment. He knew, he stated, that personnel exposed to excessive ionizing radiation developed, as an undesired reaction, thinning of the eponychial folds. He presented his fingers and, almost shaking, sought confirmation of his fears. The core of his concern was immediately recognized, but under a good light and with a loupe, each finger and nail plate were examined carefully. On completion of this step it was explained that he had allowed his "cuticles" to adhere to the nail plates, which were advancing distally in their normal growth process, and that he had not pushed them proximally, a simple cosmetic procedure. The action was demonstrated, and he left, totally at ease, freed of visions of radiation-induced injury, malignant change, and amputation.

In recent years, considerably more experience has been had in meeting individually with pipe coverers-insulators who have had contact with asbestos of various types throughout work careers of 20 to 30 years' duration. With the publicity being given occupational disease, and with the educational programs of the parent unions, these workers were fully cognizant of their chances of developing asbestosis, a pleural or peritoneal mesothelioma, or a malignant growth of the lung or other organ.

These kinds of employees are the ones referred to earlier as the "walking wounded." They are carrying a time bomb whose exact moment of detonation is unknown. The lifetme smoker knows from group discussions of the relationship of his habit to the metaplastic potential of his asbestotic lung and bears considerable guilt because of this knowledge. Here is the *hora deverdad*—the time of truth. Reports from outside pulmonary disease specialists were gone over in detail, the medical lexicon was translated, and meaning was given to quantified laboratory test results. Following the interpretation, two areas were explored: recommendations regarding changes in work and lifestyles, and the issue of retirement versus continuation of employment. Men were seen who could not continue work because of pulmonary disability. Laggers were interviewed who, in spite of progressive dyspnea and pain, could not retire because of the lack of alternative work skills and minimal retirement incomes. Lastly, employees were encountered who knew they must retire but feared the emptiness of an unstructured, workless existence secondary to the absence of either interest or skills. As an example: A 59-year-old insulator, with three decades of his active trade behind him, had for years looked forward to stream fishing in California's Sierra Mountains. A recent vacation trip to that area by camper was aborted because it was impossible for him to stay at the 5,000- to 11,000-foot altitudes, and he was forced to return to sea level. Even there, he could not be comfortable because of cough and dyspnea. "What should I do, Doc?"

This type of expressed need for guidance requires the most compassionate, empathic kind of health counseling in the face of the stark reality of the chest radiograph, the impersonal numbers derived from the lung function studies, and the rigorous demands of insulating well below decks in the crowded spaces of a navy destroyer. A change in lifestyle? A slow death? Only in joint communion with such a beleagured human can a decision be made.

This point in a work life is the late stage for information and guidance. But early in the career of an asbestos worker, health education as to the use of personal protective devices, the employment of local exhaust ventilation, the use of wet methods in ripout and disposition of lagging, and cessation of smoking is imperative, by both legal and moral mandates. Needed are human feeling, strength without force or coercion, reason without exhortation, and above all, concern—concern for the welfare of the individual worker, above concern for management, the union, or even for medicine. The concern must extend to a total disclosure, as far as is known, of the clinical facts, the prognosis, and most importantly, the present and future levels of work capacity. We are in the era of frank discussions of worker health, irrespective of what is entailed in the way of workers' compensation costs, issues of product liability, or demands of process change or environmental control. The stories of kepone, vinyl chloride, and PCB presage more tales of occupational disease or mutagenesis yet to emerge. The beginnings of tremendously costly insulation ripout from relatively new public buildings are harbingers of the mass cleanups required in the future in the private sector. Such action will require considerable employee education in the construction industry, one almost untouched by occupational health programs. We cannot cause pulmonary asbestosis in one population as we eliminate hazardous fibers from exposure of a second population.

These situations exemplify the need for a close interaction between worker and health professional, which can only be effected in an unhurried, uninterrupted setting where two humans are in significant discourse involving the life, the career, and the future of one of them. As we learn more of the toxicity of currently used chemicals, the more will such sessions be needed to inform employees of their health status, to initiate appropriate referrals, and to allay an increasing quantum of job-provoked anxiety.

One-to-Many

In some employment jurisdictions and in some institutions governed by the specifics of labor-management contracts and right-to-know mandates, educational or training sessions are required. These meetings relate primarily to occupational health hazards but may be broadened to include issues in health that are unrelated to the job but where breaks in health may influence production.

The group conference is conducted by the occupational health staff, occasionally in concert with management's training arm. The speaker or discussion leader may be the medical director, the nursing director, the industrial hygienist, or members of their sections. Time has to be arranged with the managerial personnel concerned, for although training is accepted as an official activity, the actual time spent may be accounted for differently on work-time records.

The subjects for presentation may be mandated by law or by contract or may be selected through local medical experience or joint consultation with department heads, the plant manager, or heads of certain trade unions. The action can be initiated by any one of these sources, but the effectiveness is heightened if the topics are chosen in concert, preferably with the unions, or with the officials of a trades council, if one exists. Yankauer [89] has spoken to this issue in observing that enduring behavioral change must be self-imposed and cannot be administratively ordered and that the "learner" must be involved in defining his goals and actions and must evolve his own way of achieving them. He adds that these lessons are not new, but that the need constantly to relearn them reflects something pathologic in our social order.

A fused effort can result only if there has been consultation between the union and medical authorities throughout the year. If there is no ongoing contact between the two, a proposal to involve "their people" will usually meet with little reception. In one past experience, meetings were usually held twice weekly with the Metal Trades Council–designated liaison official, who handled medical matters; in addition, there were numerous telephone interchanges each week. With this kind of continuing conversation, the solicitation of assistance and the acceptance of a proposal were carried out with ease.

When a training conference was wanted, the completed staff work was presented to the manager, and approval was obtained. All union, professional health and safety personnel, and cognizant executives were apprised of the forthcoming session, and appropriate announcements were issued.

Such group meetings in the past have included presentations on injury prevention, skin decontamination, back injuries, personal hygiene, vacation first aid, mental health, alcoholism, psoriasis, mercury, asbestos-related disease, and chest radiography. At one installation, each meeting was opened and closed by the union secretary who, although not given to articulate oratory, provided a good sense of cooperative support.

On one occasion, a film on mental health was shown, and toward the end of the discussion that followed, an electrical engineer stated that he had a problem and went on to say, "I don't know how to keep my four-year-old away from my electric train." He was invited to review the question later, away from the group. The meeting of an employee with the health professional gives him or her a chance to see the physician or nurse as a human being concerned with the problems faced by the worker. Further, opening a matter for discussion provides the involved individual with a socially acceptable entry into the OHS, for the topic has already been introduced. Without the group meeting as an opener, needed conversations and counseling would not have been possible, for it was our belief that, spontaneously, he would not have come in specifically to discuss his problem.

A final modality of group education is the orientation program for new employees. The technique was reviewed many years ago [90,91], but in essence, the representative of the health service, preferably the medical director, meets with newly hired employees to discuss two subjects: the reasons for and the content of the preplacement medical examination recently completed, and the services available during the new worker's sojourn with the company. Again an opportunity is given to see the medical person in the flesh and to obtain some feeling of his or her interest in the employees. Pursuit of a health problem in the future will be effected more easily because of this initial introduction. The discussion group, further, is "in itself a new group to which the individual can feel he belongs and from which he can get courage and protection" [92].

In the conducting of group meetings for health educational purposes, it is desirable that a "sign-up" sheet be provided so that a person's attendance can be made a matter of record. The individual's participation is then entered into the health record, and the notation is signed by the staff member who conducted the session. In a series of meetings held to apprise workers of their findings on chest radiography, a rubber-stamped entry was made in chronologic order in the employee's record in the OHS indicating the worker's attendance, the content of the meeting, the recommendations made, and the materials distributed.

While some personnel may consider this form of record completion either time-consuming or unnecessary, it was the author's experience during a 6-day deposition to have each sign-up sheet of innumerable such meetings and his personal appointment book for one entire year photocopied and entered as exhibits to become part of the permanent record. In this litigious age, where many commonplace disease syndromes are alleged to be work-caused, all information is important and must be documented and readily available, preferably on an individual basis, in the employee's clinical folder in the OHS.

EVALUATION

The determination of worth of a health education program is difficult unless one designs the undertaking as a research project, with adequate controls, pre- and post-testing, and sequential follow-up at specified temporal increments. The chance to proceed in this fashion is not possible when the effort utilizes different formats, involves several teaching/learning individuals and groups, and covers a variety of health-related subjects.

There are yardsticks for informal judging, though. Additional sessions are requested. Individual employees, at one time angry unionists, express appreciation for the personal input into the resolution of their job-centered or family-connected problem.* Unsolicited notes of gratitude are sent to the OHS. Word-of-mouth travels, and other patients seek appointments. This activity is health education at a working level, targeted toward expressed needs and developed conjointly with anxious workers or groups. It is believed that, as Steuart [93] expresses it again, ". . . the more the system can elicit, listen to, and interpret such needs, and the more it can respond . . . the more it is likely to extend the base of its relations with its clients, reinforce its credibility and relevance, and assume greater power to affect social and behavioral change at the level of primary prevention." And further, "It is mainly through the advice and consent of consumers representative of a demonstrable community constituency that we can intervene in the daily life styles in the manner necessary for the maintenance of health."

*As one worker puts it, "Thanks for taking your time—a dumb old painter like me doesn't understand these things."

BROCHURES DESCRIPTIVE OF OCCUPATIONAL HEALTH SERVICE

Although not immediately fitting the usual concept of the educative process, certain brochures for distribution to employees have been published by various OHSs to describe the services offered. The booklets have carried such titles as *You and Your Medical Department* (Pacific Telephone Nevada Bell), *Your Health Center* (Equitable Life Assurance Society of the United States), *Health Division Services* (Texaco), and *Employee Medical Program* (Atlantic Richfield Company).

The essence of the publications is seen in brief descriptions of the services available, the confidentiality of medical records, the appointment system, cooperation with family physicians, Employee Assistance Programs (EAPs), frequency of periodic examinations, absence from work, procedures in the event of illness or injury both on and off the job, and locations of the company's medical facilities throughout the United States.

Such a brochure solidifies the significance of the health program which, during a lengthy preplacement examination, is not usually a deliverable message. The printed product can be given to new employees either after the initial examination has been completed or after an orientation program for recently hired personnel, or it can be made available at all times in the OHS. Its worth lies in its ability to describe the health program elements in understandable language and to provide answers to questions that the individual employee may be hesitant to ask.

COMMENT

One should not convey an impression erroneously that what has been done and what is proposed can be accomplished with the hope that all ills will be eradicated and all lifestyles will be converted so that our industrial workers will be vigorous, lean, nonsmoking, distainful of mood-altering medication, modest users of beverage alcohol, appropriate consumers of balanced foodstuffs, free from stress, and worshipful of balanced recreation and rest. The opposing forces in today's environment offer too strong a resistance to the development of such paragons of health virtues. Madison Avenue's continuum of commercial messages is matched only by the onslaught of untested chemicals that enter what we eat, breathe, or absorb through our skin. As the Special Commission on Internal Pollution [94] has concluded, our ecologic system has changed from a natural to a synthetic one, and the medical and social effects will not be known for perhaps two or more generations.

In spite of this overwhelming force of health-damaging stressors, one must continue to present to our labor force the elements of better living as we understand them medically. The selection will remain with them, but without a knowledge of the options, there will never be opportunity for the choice that might mean a more enriching, productive, and rewarding experience in living. As Etzwiler [95] put it, "The most important member of the medical team for health maintenance and chronic disease has been forgotten, i.e., *the patient himself*. Effective care of chronic disease and health maintenance cannot be carried out without the cooperation of an informed patient supported by an interested and knowledgeable professional health care group."

REFERENCES

1. Lalonde, M., cited in White, L. S. How to improve the public's health. *N Engl J Med* 293:773, 1975.
2. Wellness and fitness programs in industry. *J Occup Med* 22:712, 1980.
3. Felton, J. S., and Voss, H. R. Cardiopulmonary evaluation studies in an occupational health program. *J Occup Med* 14:552, 1972.
4. Felton, J. S. Conducting cardiopulmonary evaluations of County of Los Angeles safety personnel. *Health Services Rep* 88:515, 1973.
5. Felton, J. S. Exercise Testing in Preventive Medicine. In *Occupational Medicine Symposia*. Rockville, MD: U.S. Department of Health, Education, and Welfare, Public Health Service, Center for Disease Control, National Institute for Occupational Safety and Health, May 1975. Pp. IV-6–IV-12.
6. Erb, B. D. The Role of the Physician in Cardiovascular Health Programs. In R. M. Levenson, J. Maxon, and B. L. Alton (Eds.), *Conference Proceedings, Alternatives in Cardiac Care: Prevention and Rehabilitation*. Dallas, TX: American Heart Association National Center, Oct 9–10, 1979. Pp. 12–22.
7. Haskell, W. L. Physical fitness programs: Medical clearance, program design and operation. *J Occup Med* 14:306, 1972.
8. American Heart Association, Subcommittee on Rehabilitation, Target Activity Group. Standards for adult exercise testing laboratories. *J Occup Med* 21:763, 1979.
9. Committee on Exercise, American Heart Association. *Exercise Testing and Training of Individuals with Heart Disease or at High Risk for Its Development: A Handbook for Physicians*. Dallas, TX: The Association, 1975.
10. DeBusk, R. F. Exercise test supervision by nonphysicians. *JAMA* 252:3182, 1984.
11. American Heart Association, Subcommittee on Rehabilitation, Target Activity Group. Specifications for exercise testing equipment. *J Occup Med* 21:828, 1979.
12. American Medical Association, Council on Scientific Affairs. Indications and contraindications for exercise testing. *JAMA* 246:1015, 1981.
13. Committee on Occupational Medical Practice, AOMA. Cardiac stress testing in industry. *J Occup Med* 27:244, 1985.
14. Giagnoni, E., Secchi, M. B., Wu, S. C., et al. Prognostic value of exercise EKG testing in asymptomatic normotensive subjects. *N Engl J Med* 309:1085, 1983.
15. Russek, H. I. Cited in Mass screening for silent ischemia held unjustified. *Intern Med News* 17:66, 1984.
16. McCunney, R. J. Are exercise EKG's needed before a fitness program? *Occup Health Saf* 53:23, Oct 1984.
17. Siegel, G. H. Informed Consent in Exercise Testing and Training Programs. In Committee on Exercise, American Heart Association, *Exercise Testing and Training of Individuals with Heart Disease or at High Risk for Its Development: A Handbook for Physicians*. Dallas, TX: American Heart Association, 1975. Pp. 49–51.
18. Tennessee Heart Association Physical Exercise Committee. *Physician's Handbook for Evaluation of Cardiovascular and Physical Fitness* (2nd ed.). Nashville, TN: The Association, 1972. P. 4.
19. Committee on Exercise, American Heart Association. *Exercise Testing and Training of Apparently Healthy Individuals: A Handbook for Physicians*. Dallas, TX: The Association, 1972. P. 22.
20. Cady, L. Personal communication, 1974.
21. Smith, N. E. Exercise stress testing. *Occup Health Nurs* 32:89, Feb 1984.
22. Wagner, E. H., Beery, W. L., Schoenback, V. J., et al. An assessment of health hazard/health risk appraisal. *Am J Public Health* 72:347, 1982.
23. As companies jump on fitness bandwagon. *US News World Rep* 88:36, Jan 28, 1980.
24. Fitness fever: Everybody into the company gym. *Dun's Rev* 116:115, Nov 1980.
25. Shephard, R. J., Cox, M., and Corey, P. Fitness program participation: Its effect on worker performance. *J Occup Med* 23:359, 1981.
26. *Directory of Occupational Medical Programs to Reduce the Risk of Heart Attack and Stroke*. Dallas, TX: American Heart Association, 1981. (Obtainable from the Association at 7320 Greenville Avenue, Dallas, Texas 75231.)

27. Gadzik, C. How to keep your timber limber. *Resource* (Crown-Zellerbach Corp.) 9:22, Winter 1981.
28. PHS promotes wellness training. *The Reporter* (Newsletter of Federal Employee Health and Alcoholism/Drug Abuse Programs) 11:1, Sept 1980.
29. Group fitness program helps employees slim down, tone up and feel better. *Philnews* 5:7, Oct 1980.
30. Preventive maintenance for company employees. *JAMA* 245:1301, 1981.
31. Wright, C. C. Cost containment through health promotion programs. *J Occup Med* 24:965, 1982.
32. *Agenda* (Honeywell Corporate Human Resources Newsletter). Minneapolis, MN: The Corporation, March 1984.
33. Grove, D. A., Reed, R. W., and Miller, L. C. A Health promotion program in a corporate setting. *J Fam Pract* 9:83, 1979.
34. Seidman, L. S., Sevelino, G. G., and Ewald, P. A cost-effective weight loss program at the worksite. *J Occup Med* 26:725, 1984.
35. *Campbell's Turnaround Health and Fitness Center.* Camden, NJ: Campbell Soup Company, [n.d.].
36. Employees wax enthusiastically about their fitness program. *Natl Saf News* 129:59, Apr 1984.
37. Dionne, E. D. Corporate wellness programs can be cost-effective. *Natl Saf News* 129:70, March 1984.
38. DuPont introduces new voluntary health improvement program. *Occup Health Saf Letter* 14:3, July 22, 1984.
39. Smeetzly, J. Employee health promotion: The Hennepin WellWay Program. *Am J Public Health* 75:785, 1985.
40. Dismuke, S. E., and Miller, S. T. Why not share the secrets of good health? The physician's role in health promotion. *JAMA* 249:3181, 1983.
41. Seeds, R. An "exercise in fitness." *Occup Health Saf* 50:18, Oct 1981.
42. Nast, P. F., and McDonald, L. Planning the employee fitness program. *Occup Health Saf* 50:27, Oct 1981.
43. Shephard, R. J., Morgan, P., Finucane, R., et al. Factors influencing recruitment to an occupational fitness program. *J Occup Med* 22:389, 1980.
44. Increasing numbers of physical changes found in nation's runners. *JAMA* 245:547, 1981.
45. Daffner, R. N., Martinez, S., and Gehweiler, J. A. Stress fractures in runners. *JAMA* 247:1039, 1982.
46. Thompson, P. D., Funk, E. J., Carleton, R. A., et al. Incidence of death during jogging in Rhode Island from 1975 through 1980. *JAMA* 247:2535, 1982.
47. Virmani, R. Jogging, marathon running, and death. Primary Cardiology Supp. to *Hosp Physician* 18:A-28, 1982.
48. Williams, A. F. When motor vehicles hit joggers: An analysis of 60 cases. *Public Health Rep* 96:448, 1981.
49. Stin, P., Haenel, A., and Stadler, H. From the heavens, revenge on joggers. *N Engl J Med* 311:1703, 1984.
50. Kaplan, J. P., Powell, K. E., Sikes, A. K., et al. An epidemiologic study of the benefits and risks of running. *JAMA* 248:3118, 1982.
51. At issue: "Course of employment" rule. (Marion J. Vaccaro et al. vs Sperry Rand Corp. et al.). *Occup Haz* 44:66, March 1982.
52. Larson, A. *Workmen's Compensation Law.* New York, NY: Matthew Bender, Dec 1984, Vol. IA, Suppl., §22. Recreational and Social Activities. Pp. 137–144.
53. Marks, L. N., Martin, F. C., St. Clair, C., et al. Guidelines to a fitness program for previously sedentary employees. *Occup Health Saf* 53:34, 1984.
54. Jokl, E., Jokl-Ball, M., Jokl, P., et al. Notation of exercise. *Work Environ Health* 5:24, 1968.
55. *Canada's Fitness.* Preliminary Findings of the 1981 Survey. Ottawa: Canada Fitness Survey, June 1982.
56. What makes Canadians go? Canada fitness survey. *Highlights* No. 15, Oct 1983.
57. *"Go to Health" Executive Summary.* Detroit, MI: Michigan Health Care Education and Research Foundation, [n.d.].
58. Browne, D. W., Russell, M. L., Morgan, J. L., et al. Reduced disability and health care costs in an industrial fitness program. *J Occup Med* 26:809, 1984.
59. Chenoweth, D. Health promotion: Benefits vs. costs. *Occup Health Saf* 52:37, July 1983.
60. Bernacki, E. J., and Baun, W. B. The relationship of job performance to exercise adherence in a corporate fitness program. *J Occup Med* 26:529, 1984.
61. Puterbaugh, J. S., and Lawyer, C. H. Cardiovascular effects of an exercise program: A controlled study among firemen. *J Occup Med* 25:581, 1983.
62. Fielding, J. E. Effectiveness of employee health improvement programs. *J Occup Med* 24:907, 1982.
63. Wright, M. *Coors Wellness Program.* Golden, CO: Adolph Coors Company, [n.d.]. P. 10.
64. O'Donnell, M. P., and Ainsworth, T. H. *Health Promotion in the Workplace.* New York, NY: Wiley, 1984.
65. Grouse, L. D. A piece of my mind: Mesomorph metamorphosed. *JAMA* 247:2103, 1982.
66. Fuld, L. F. *Service Instruction of American Corporations.* Special Instruction in Physical Education. Bulletin, 1916, No. 34. Washington, DC: Department of the Interior, Bureau of Education, 1917. Pp. 70–73.
67. Dowling, O. Methods in educational hygiene. *Am J Public Health* 2:981, 1912.
68. Branchini, C. Broadening the Concept of Industrial Health. Presented at the Annual Meeting of the American Public Health Association, Chicago, Illinois, Nov. 18, 1975. P. 7.
69. Culliton, B. J. Preventive medicine: Legislation calls for health education. *Science* 189:1071, 1975.
70. Fishbein, M. Essential factors for health and fitness. *Occup Med* 2:566, 1946.
71. Wylie, C. M. The definition and measurement of health and disease. *Public Health Rep* 85:100, 1970.
72. Belloc, N. B., Breslow, L., and Hochstim, J. R. Measurement of physical health in a general population survey. *Am J Epidemiol* 93:328, 1971.
73. Chapman, J. S. A fractured figure of speech? *Arch Environ Health* 27:285, 1973.

74. Goldsmith, S. B. The status of health status indicators. *Health Services Rep* 87:212, 1972.
75. Parsons, T. Definitions of Health and Illness in the Light of American Values and Social Structure. In E. G. Jaco (Ed.), *Patients, Physicians and Illness.* Sourcebook in Behavioral Science and Medicine. Glencoe, IL: Free Press, 1958. P. 176.
76. Cohen, The Right Honorable Lord of Birkenhead. The pursuit of health. *R Soc Health J* 87:86, 1967.
77. Kasl, S. V., and Cobb, S. Health behavior, illness behavior, and sick role behavior. *Arch Environ Health* 12:246, 1966.
78. Murray, R. B., and Zentner, J. P. *Nursing Concepts for Health Promotion* (2nd ed.). Englewood Cliffs, NJ: Prentice-Hall, 1979. P. 21.
79. Shapiro, I. S. HMOs and health education. *Am J Public Health* 65:469, 1975.
80. Grout, R. Health teaching in schools. Philadelphia: Saunders, 1953. P. 2.
81. Squyres, W. D. (Ed.). *Patient Education: An Inquiry into the State of the Art.* New York: Springer, 1980. P. 1.
82. Steuart, G. W. The future of health education. *Health Educ J* 9:66, 1951.
83. Stallones, R. J. Health education in the preventive medicine curriculum. *Newsletter* (Am Coll Prev Med) 16(2):3, 1975.
84. McNerney, W. J. The missing link in health services. *J Med Educ* 50:11, 1975.
85. Levine, S., Scotch, N. A., and Vlasak, G. J. Unravelling technology and culture in public health. *Am J Public Health* 59:237, 1969.
86. Cohen, The Right Honorable Lord of Birkenhead. Problems of health education. *R Soc Health J* 84:293, 1964.
87. Kaufman, H. F. In review of C. P. Loomis, and J. A. Beegle, *Rural Sociology: The Strategy of Change.* Englewood Cliffs, NJ: Prentice-Hall, 1957, *Am J Sociol* 63:242, 1957.
88. Jones, F. A. (Ed.). *Richard Asher Talking Sense.* London: Pitman, 1972. P. 35.
88a. Ignatius, P. R. *The Film in Industrial Safety Training.* Boston: Division of Research, Harvard Business School, 1949.
89. Yankauer, A. Immunization and health education. *Am J Public Health* 65:1111, 1975.
90. Felton, J. S. Orienting the new employee in the services of the industrial health department. *Ind Med* 16:519, 1947.
91. Felton, J. S. Orientation of the new employee by the health division of an atomic energy research laboratory: A four-year review. *Ind Med Surg* 21:107, 1952.
92. Expert Committee on Health Education of the Public. *First Report.* Geneva: World Health Organization, 1954. P. 22.
93. Steuart, G. W. The people, motivation, education, and action. *Bull NY Acad Med* 51:174, 1975.
94. The Special Commission on Internal Pollution. Toward assessing the chemical age: Summary of deliberations, 1974. *JAMA* 234:507, 1975.
95. Etzwiler, D. D. Current status of patient education. *JAMA* 220:583, 1972.

APPENDIX 7-1
PRECAUTIONS IN EXERCISE TESTING

APPENDIX 7-1A. *Reasons for Temporarily Reducing or Deferring Physical Activity*

Intercurrent illness—febrile, injury, gastrointestinal	Environmental factors
Progression of cardiac disease	Weather—excessive heat or cold, humidity, or wind
Orthopedic problem	Air pollution—smog, carbon monoxide
Emotional turmoil	Overindulgence
Severe sunburn	Large, heavy meal within 2 hours
Alcoholic hangover	Coffee, tea, cola (xanthines and other stimulating beverages)
Cerebral dysfunction—dizziness, vertigo	Drugs—decongestants, bronchodilators, atropine, weight reducers (anorectics)
Sodium retention—edema, weight gain	
Dehydration	

Source: DeBusk, R. F. Exercise test supervision by nonphysicians. *JAMA 252*:3182, 1984.

APPENDIX 7-1B. *Safety Precautions in Exercise Testing*

Precautions	*Clinical features*
Pre-exercise criteria that contraindicate testing	Changes in the resting 12-lead ECG Congestive heart failure Third heart sounds Cardiac dysrhythmias such as second- or third-degree heart block, paroxysmal atrial tachycardia, atrial flutter, ventricular tachycardia, or multifocal premature beats Resting heart rate above 120, supine Resting systolic blood pressure above 200, supine Resting diastolic blood pressure above 100, supine Resting pulse pressure less than 20, supine
Exercise test criteria that contraindicate further testing	Systolic blood pressure above 220 Diastolic blood pressure above 120 Failure of the pulse pressure to increase with exercise Any development of light-headedness, chest pain, visual disturbances, nausea, or difficult, rapid breathing out of proportion to the degree of exercise Atrial dysrhythmias: more than one occurring in six beats Atrial flutter, atrial fibrillation Ventricular dysrhythmias: More than one occurring in six beats, maximum of six in a 1-minute period; coupled beats Any premature ventricular beat that originates in the T wave Second- or third-degree heart block
Exercise test criteria that require summoning of a physician	Ischemic changes in ST segment or T wave, for example: ST depression of 2 mm or more, lasting 0.08 second or longer T waves flattening or inverting Changes in the length of the PR interval or the QRS interval
Post-exercise precautions	Call a physician if any of the following occurs: Light-headedness, nausea, chest pain, visual disturbances, or dyspnea Sudden onset of bradycardia Pulse pressure less than 20 mm, supine
USE COMMON SENSE—IF IN DOUBT, STOP TEST.	

Source: Cady, L. Personal communication, 1974.

8. IMMUNIZATION, SKIN TESTING, AND BUSINESS TRAVEL

He is a better physician that keeps disease off us, than he that cures them being on us. Prevention is so much better than healing, because it saves the labour of being sick.

Thomas Adams

If we are continually guided in this enterprise by the spirit of genuine preventive medical science; if we utilize the experience gained in conflict with other pestilences, and aim, with clear recognition of the purpose and resolute avoidance of wrong roads, at striking the evil at its roots, then the battle against tuberculosis cannot fail to have a victorious issue.

Robert Koch

I am poured out like water, and all my bones are out of joint: my heart is like wax; it is melted in the midst of my bowels.

Psalms 22:14

IMMUNIZATION PROGRAMS

As industry has nearly a fixed population, it is an ideal setting for conducting an immunization program. An immunization program has the triple objective of protecting workers against (1) some of the diseases to which the general population is exposed, (2) the diseases that are unique to the operations of a particular worksite, and (3) the disease potentially sequential to trauma, specifically tetanus. As most occupational health services (OHSs) have the facilities needed for administering immunizing injections, the introduction of such a program would not represent a work overload or any great increase in cost, when compared with the losses incurred with absence attributable to disease or with the charges attendant upon a work-associated illness, particularly if death results from the acquisition of a rare laboratory-generated infection that defies current modes of therapy.

In a discussion of preventive inoculations it is important that the full spectrum of work locations be borne in mind, and not just the proverbial manufacturing plant, typical of heavy industry. Many workers in health service or research facilities are at risk, as are the personnel engaged in the production of biologic products used in immunization. Also, certain workers engaged in mineral exploration, animal husbandry, or activities involving contact with insects or mammals in the wild are subject to diseases far removed from the home offices of their parent organizations.

Further, there are some unusual considerations concerned with an immunization program, in that, for example, few workers' compensation authorities accept procedures in preventive medicine for coverage or reimbursement and reactions to inoculations may be productive of a work-related injury, iatrogenic absence, or both.

GENERAL RECOMMENDATIONS

It is reassuring to know that the Centers for Disease Control (CDC) in Atlanta, through its Immunization Practices Advisory Committee (ACIP), keeps the readership of its publication *MMWR* current as to advisable immunization protocols and practices, as determined by research and epidemiologic findings and experience.

In its "General Recommendations on Immunization" [1], attention was directed to a definition of terms; route, site, and technique of immunization; dosage; age of recipients; spacing of immunobiologics; hypersensitivity to vaccine components, altered immunocompetence; severe febrile illness, vaccination during pregnancy; adverse events following immunization; disease control through continuing programs; and sources of information. In a supplement [2], in addition to a discussion of specific immunobiologics, recommendations are offered for adults in various age groups and for persons with special requirements because of occupation, lifestyle, travel, environmental situations, and health status.

POLICY

To include an immunization program in an ongoing OHS effort, there should be a declared policy, in writing, based on the needs of that particular work population. Factors to be considered at domestic worksites include:

Contact with acute infectious disease patients.
Contact with large numbers of immigrants to the United States.
Work in laboratories involving contact with microorganisms, cultures, and so on, in a research, manufacturing, or diagnostic-service setting.
Work involving contact with children, as in nursery schools, foster homes, bus transport, day-care centers, or elementary education.
Work that subjects employees to trauma resulting in breaks of the intact skin.
Work in wilderness areas or in undeveloped areas adjacent to worksites where monitoring equipment is located.
Work in natural history museums, taxidermy, packing plants, archeologic diggings, or animal pounds.
Work requiring intermittent inspection of facilities enumerated above.
Work in municipal, hospital, or medical center morgues, blood collecting or banking facilities, dental clinics, dialysis units, or intensive care units.
Special populations at risk such as homosexual men or highly promiscuous women.

Factors to be considered at foreign worksites include:

Work involving travel in disease-endemic areas or high-risk areas.
Work involving contact with patients, wildlife, and other populations or settings as listed above under domestic worksites.
Work involving repeated short-duration activity in settings generative of communicable disease.
Work involving assignment as technical advisers or as supportive personnel in active combat zones.
Work with populations not in contact with health service personnel where acute infectious disease patients would remain unrecognized or sequestered in keeping with local belief systems.

The written policy should consider the personnel to be immunized, the targeted disease states, the procedures to be followed in the event of a serious reaction, and the procedures to be followed in the event of refusal as based on religious or philosophic beliefs.

The inclusion of a program segment involving immunizations should represent the thoughtful consideration given the scientific evidence of benefits and risks, so that optimal levels of protection can be achieved with the least harm and the greatest prophylactic accrual.

RECOMMENDATIONS

As indicated above, the ACIP has made certain recommendations pertinent to immunizing procedures.

MULTIPLE-DOSE VACCINES

Many vaccines require more than one dose for the development of clinical immunity. The ACIP believes that intervals between doses longer than the advised time spans are not usually productive of a reduction in final antibody levels. Hence, it is not necessary that an interrupted series of vaccinations be restarted or that extra doses be added [1].

SIMULTANEOUS ADMINISTRATION OF CERTAIN VACCINES

Consensus indicates that most of the widely used antigens can be administered simultaneously, an advantage in certain circumstances, such as the imminent exposure to several infectious diseases, the preparation for foreign travel, or the lack of surety that the subject will return for future injections.

Inactivated vaccines can be given simultaneously at separate sites, but those antigens commonly associated with local or systemic effects—cholera, typhoid, and plague vaccines, for example—when administered simultaneously could accentuate the side effects. When practicable, and for persons with a history of such reactions, the injections should be given on separate occasions [1].

An inactivated vaccine and a live, attenuated-virus vaccine can be injected simultaneously at separate sites with the same precautions as taken with the vaccines individually. It has been observed that the simultaneous administration of the most widely used live-virus vaccines has not resulted in impaired antibody response or increased rates of untoward reactions [1].

HYPERSENSITIVITY TO VACCINE COMPONENTS

Vaccine derived through use of embryonated chicken or duck eggs may provoke hypersensitivity reactions, including anaphylaxis. Yellow fever is representative of this type of agent. Although these preparations are usually avoided in persons with known sensitivity to components of the substrate, influenza vaccine antigens, although similarly prepared, are so highly purified that reactions are extremely rare. A prospective recipient of such a vaccine should be queried as to a dietetic tolerance of eggs. Individuals who respond to the ingestion of eggs with lip or tongue urticaria or swelling, acute respiratory distress, hypotension, or shock should not receive egg-grown vaccines.

Live-virus vaccines prepared by use of cell cultures—measles, mumps, or rubella vaccines—are without hypersensitivity responses. Vaccines derived from organisms grown in simple media may produce local or occasionally systemic side effects and should not be given to persons who previously have reacted badly to them.

ALTERED IMMUNITY

Persons with immunodeficiency diseases and individuals with suppressed capability for immune response, as with leukemia, lymphoma, generalized malignancy, or therapy with steroid preparations, alkylating agents, antimetabolites, or irradiation, should not receive live, attenuated-virus vaccines. In the same sense, other residents in the household of such a patient should not be given an oral polio vaccine, as vaccine viruses are excreted by the injectee and are transmissible [1].

SEVERE FEBRILE ILLNESSES

No vaccination should be administered to a person with such an illness.

LIVE VACCINES AND PREGNANCY

Live, attenuated-virus vaccines should not be given to pregnant women or to women likely to become pregnant within 3 months following immunization because of a theoretic risk to the developing fetus. Tetanus and diphtheria toxoid (Td) is advised, as it affords protection against neonatal tetanus.

REPORTING ADVERSE REACTIONS

All severe reactions should be reported after evaluation to the local or state health officials and to the manufacturer.

SMALLPOX VACCINATION

On September 30, 1971, the U.S. Public Health Service (USPHS) formally accepted the recommendation from the ACIP that a regular smallpox vaccination program be discontinued and a selective program be adopted for population groups exposed to smallpox [3]. The factors leading to the decision included (1) the absence of smallpox from the U.S. for the previous 22 years, (2) essential eradication of global smallpox, (3) decreasing probability of smallpox importation into the U.S., (4) risks of smallpox versus the risks of vaccination complications (postvaccinal encephalitis, eczema vaccinatum, and vaccinia necrosum), (5) failure of regular infant vaccination to produce effective population immunity, and (6) epidemiologic control of smallpox importations (isolation of cases, identification and surveillance of contacts, and selective, limited vaccination of persons at risk).

Needless to say, the declaration of the USPHS policy led to much published criticism [4–11], but the changes in state laws have remained. In May 1980, the World Health Organization (WHO) declared the world free of smallpox, and the indications for vaccination currently hold *only* for laboratory workers directly involved with orthopox viruses (such as monkeypox, variola, and vaccinia) [12]. Smallpox vaccine is no longer available to civilians [13] but can be obtained for the protection of occupationally exposed laboratory workers.*

Smallpox vaccination is no longer required for travel. Cases of vaccinia continue to be reported, primarily among recently vaccinated military personnel or their contacts, as military personnel, including members of the National Guard and Reserves, when entering into service and every 5 years thereafter receive the immunization [14–16]. The proscription against the therapeutic use of smallpox vaccine is being sounded again, as the antigen still is being employed erroneously in treating herpes infections [17].

RECORD OF VACCINATION

If used for laboratory personnel, entries in health records for smallpox vaccination should be recorded as "primary vaccination performed," "primary vaccination read as successful," or "revaccination," with appropriate dates, signature of person performing the vaccination, and the lot number of the vaccine.

ADDITIONAL NOTE

One cannot close a discussion of protection against smallpox without bringing forth an argument against the consideration of this once-dreaded disease as having undergone global eradication, as certified by the WHO, which recommended cessation of smallpox vaccination. Smith [18], in an attention-demanding communication, observed:

> It is a tragic commentary on our state of affairs that this recommendation is in fact inappropriate. On medical and

*Available from Drug Immunobiologic and Vaccine Service, Center for Infectious Diseases, Building 1, Room 1259, Centers for Disease Control, Atlanta, Georgia 30333, (404) 329-3356 [12].

epidemiologic grounds such a policy would be entirely defensible. This, however, is yet another instance in which the accomplishments of medical science have far outstripped those of social and political science. Such a recommendation fails to take into account the unfortunately very real possibility of biologic warfare. It is both impossible and inappropriate to ignore the chance that unscrupulous people may take advantage of an unvaccinated world population to threaten the use of smallpox virus for political or terrorist ends. Indeed, it is a paradoxical reality that the threat of smallpox is now much greater for the supposedly more developed nations of the world than for those considered less technically and socially advanced. At the very least, the real world of politics dictates that military personnel must still be subjected to the small risk associated with smallpox vaccination.

Suspected cases or rumors of cases are investigated. Between 1979 and 1984, 179 reports were received by the WHO, and none was found to be smallpox [19,20].

TETANUS IMMUNIZATION

Of special importance to industry is the protection of the workers against the acquisition of tetanus. Although the number of cases of tetanus has declined remarkably since the regular use of tetanus toxoid, there still are just under 100 cases reported annually, primarily among persons unimmunized, inadequately immunized, or whose history of protection was unknown.

Any applicant for employment who cannot present documented evidence of having been immunized within the past 10 years should be inoculated at the beginning of work and reimmunized at appropriate intervals. The spores of *Clostridium tetani* are ubiquitous, and there is no natural immunity to tetanus toxin. In a review of tetanus cases [21], no wound could be implicated in 6 percent of the patients. In 17 percent of the cases, nonacute skin lesions (decubitus ulcers) or medical disorders such as abscesses were involved [22].

BIOLOGIC PREPARATIONS

Although tetanus toxoid is available in both fluid and aluminum salt adsorbed forms, and recognizing that the rate of seroconversion is essentially equivalent with either form and that the adsorbed toxoids induce more persistent antitoxin titers, it is the adsorbed forms that are recommended for both primary and booster injections [2]. The preparation advised for adults is *tetanus and diphtheria toxoids adsorbed (for adult use) (Td)*. The amount of diphtheria antigen present is limited, not more than 2 LF per dose (the LF content is the quantity of toxoid as assessed by flocculation). Single-antigen products are available, such as *tetanus toxoid fluid* and *tetanus toxoid adsorbed (T)*, for use in situations contraindicating use of the combined forms.

USAGE

All products should be used in accordance with the recommendations provided in the manufacturers' package inserts. The adsorbed preparations should be given intramuscularly (IM). Administration by jet injection may result in more frequent local reactions.

Certain special considerations deserve attention. If a booster injection of Td is given sooner as part of wound management, the next booster injection need not be given until 10 years after that date. Booster injections given more frequently than decennially more often result in an increased incidence and severity of adverse reactions [23]. Actual tetanus or diphtheria infection does not confer immunity, so that active immunization should be initiated or completed during convalescence.

As some persons may be familiar with *diphtheria and tetanus toxoids and pertussis vaccine adsorbed (DTP)*, it should be pointed out that this preparation is for pediatric use only.

An Arthus-type hypersensitivity reaction consisting of several local reactions beginning 2 to 8 hours after an injection may occur, especially in persons who have received multiple prior booster doses. Such individuals have high serum tetanus antitoxin levels and should not be given further regular or emergency booster injections of Td more frequently than every 10 years.

The administration of immunosuppressive therapy measures may reduce the immune response to vaccines, so that regular vaccination should be deferred while individuals are receiving such therapy.

TETANUS PROPHYLAXIS IN WOUND MANAGEMENT

Chemoprophylaxis against tetanus should not enter into wound management. The need for active immunization (Td), with or without passive immunization (tetanus immune globulin [TIG]), is determined by the condition of the wound and the patient's history of immunization. Frank tetanus has rarely occurred when there has been a documented primary series of toxoid injections.

In individuals who have not completed a full primary series of injections, both tetanus toxoid and passive immunization may be required at the time of wound cleansing and debridement. The treating physician must determine if the patient has previously completed the full primary series and, if not, the number of doses received. In wound management, as indicated, *Td* is preferred, as some adults otherwise would remain susceptible to diphtheria.

If passive immunization is to be undertaken, *TIG* is the preparation of choice, as it gives longer protection than antitoxin of animal origin and causes few adverse reactions. Currently suggested for wound management is 250 units IM. If *Td* and *TIG* are given concurrently, one should use separate syringes and separate sites. In wound management the adsorbed toxoid is mandatory. The recommended protocol is available from the American College of Surgeons Committee on Trauma, Chicago, Illinois.

ADDITIONAL PUBLIC HEALTH AND LEGAL CONSIDERATIONS

A study was conducted in Los Angeles County of the level of tetanus immunity in the elderly [24]. Serologic levels were determined on a group of 363 volunteers from senior citizen centers and convalescent hospitals, and immunization histories were obtained. Of the group reviewed, 54 percent lacked immunity to tetanus, demonstrating a tetanus antitoxic titer less than 0.1 unit/ml. The point at issue is that, strictly as a public health measure, might it not be desirable to ensure tetanus immunity in all employees about to retire within the coming year—a period of time adequate to provide either a full primary series of injections or a booster inoculation? The cost is low, and such a measure would protect the elderly who are subject to trauma through gardening injuries, motor vehicle accidents, and falls while walking or exercising.

In connection with tetanus prophylaxis, the question arises of refusal by an injured worker to accept a booster injection of tetanus toxoid. The issue was discussed by Warshaw [25], who pointed out that the employee could not be forced to take the booster, nor would a signed waiver have any meaning, for it would not relieve the employer of workers' compensation liability. It was suggested that the physician prepare a statement for the employee's signature that would set forth the facts that he had been advised to have the injection in view of the nature of the wound and that, despite explanation of the rationale for it and the possible consequences of the failure to have it, the employee had refused consent for its administration. If, in turn, the worker refuses to sign a statement, the physician should enter into the record a signed note that relates all the details of the matter. The entry should be signed also by a nurse or other witness to the conversation.

Were the matter to become a litigated issue, in most jurisdictions the hazard of the offered treatment would be weighed, and if it were customary and of reasonable practice and not life-threatening or of undue risk, the fiscal responsibility for any untoward effects would most likely be assigned to the employee.

PLAGUE IMMUNIZATION

Of the cases of plague reported most recently in the United States, 31 occurred in 1984, indicating continued involvement with this rodent/flea disease [26]. The modes of infection included flea bite or direct contact with rabbits or were unknown. Many involving flea bites occurred in relation to epizootic plague among prairie dogs and rock squirrels. Explanations for the localized morbidity in the West may lie in the exposure of American Indians* to enzootic and epizootic plague foci through their hunting and food-gathering activities and the growth of non-Indian populations with expansion of their residential areas into regions that were previously uninhabited and that manifested enzootic plague. Some relationships may be traced to faulty environmental sanitation and management of premises that allow the harboring of rodents. Few laboratory-associated cases have been reported, and those persons developing the disease underwent unusual exposures. Although many of the nonprofessional cases occurred among children, true occupationally generated cases of plague have been incurred by veterinarians [27] and laboratory workers.

Nine cases of human plague encountered in past years involved interstate travel. For example, a patient exposed in Colorado was diagnosed in Texas, and one with exposure in New Mexico was identified in South Carolina [28]. Some precautions that should be taken if visiting plague-enzootic areas are the following [29]:

Leave pets at home; if they must be taken, keep them on leashes, and use flea collars and flea powder.
Do not handle sick or dead animals. Notify the nearest park ranger of such deaths.
Do not sit, place sleeping bags, or pitch tents on or near rodent burrows.
Do not feed the ground squirrels.
Use insect repellent and wear protective clothing on arms and legs. Spray socks and legs with insect repellent when hiking.

Residents of or visitors to plague-enzootic areas who develop fever along with swollen, painful lymph

*Of the 40 cases reported, 21 occurred among American Indians; 36 were noted in New Mexico and Arizona, the remaining 4 in other western states.

nodes should seek medical care immediately, and the treating physician should notify the state health authority promptly. Prompt diagnosis and early treatment can be lifesaving. These precautions are of particular importance to museum and university personnel engaged in anthropologic, archeologic, zoologic, or entymologic study.

To meet the need for a review of current practices in prevention and control, an ad hoc National Plague Prevention and Control Committee met in early 1984. The report of the meeting concerned funding for collaborative studies and the encouragement of plague research and consultation [30].

While plague vaccines have been used since the late nineteenth century, their effectiveness has not been measured with any precision. However, field experience seems to indicate that immunization does reduce the incidence and severity of the disease that results from the bite of infected fleas [2]. Persons exposed to pneumonic plague patients or to *Yersinia pestis* aerosols in the laboratory should receive a 7- to 10-day course of antimicrobic therapy irrespective of vaccination history.

Vaccination is recommended regularly for the following [2]:

All laboratory and field personnel who are working with *Y. pestis* organisms resistant to antimicrobics.
Persons engaged in aerosol experiments with *Y. pestis*.
Persons engaged in field operations in plague-enzootic areas where the prevention of exposure is impossible (as in some disaster areas).

Selective plague vaccination should be considered for these individuals:

Laboratory personnel working regularly with *Y. pestis* or plague-infected rodents.
Persons whose occupation brings them into regular contact with wild rodents or rabbits in plague-enzootic areas.
Travelers to areas known to have endemic plague in countries reporting plague, particularly if travel is not limited to urban areas with tourist-hotel accommodations.

ROCKY MOUNTAIN SPOTTED FEVER

Rocky Mountain spotted fever (RMSF), or tick-borne typhus fever, reached an incidence rate in 1983 of 0.48 cases per 100,000 population; 1,126 cases were reported. In 1984, there was a provisional total of 847 cases reported, a rate of 0.36 per 100,000 population [31]. The greatest number of the cases occurred in the South Atlantic states, and 56 percent of the total underwent laboratory confirmation. The number of cases had remained fairly steady between 1955 and 1970, at about a rate of 0.14 per 100,000, but in the last decade has risen to the level indicated. There were 30 deaths from this disease in 1981.

Prevention involves frequent inspection of personnel for ticks when exposure is likely. Removal of ticks is best accomplished by grasping the tick with forceps as close as possible to the skin at the point of attachment and pulling slowly and steadily. If no instrument is available, fingers protected by facial tissue may be used, but if bare hands touch the tick, they should be washed thoroughly with soap and water, as tick secretions can be infective.

The reason for inclusion of RMSF in this discussion is that employees are assigned to work in tick-infested areas, and care should be exercised. Although a RMSF vaccine had been used in the past, presently a vaccine against RMSF is in the developmental stage and is not expected to be available in the near future. None is currently produced commercially.

Although no indication was made of occupation in a 5-year epidemiologic study of 2,757 cases [32], it was observed that work-related exposures were few. However, there have been individual case reports of work-associated disease. A physician acquired his infection when he incurred an accidental puncture wound with a blood-contaminated needle while assisting in the care of a farmer who died of the disease [33]. The lack of efficacy of previous vaccines was indicated in the case of a laboratory worker, previously vaccinated, whose job was the inoculating and harvesting of *Rickettsia akari* and *Rickettsia rickettsii* in eggs, cultures, and animals. He presumably acquired his infection by the "aerogenic route," for there was no self-inoculation and there were no breaks in procedure [34]. Five years later, there was still a comment that "a vaccine is available, and two injections a month apart are believed to provide considerable protection" [35]. But by 1978 its effectiveness had been questioned [36,37]. The most recent *Physicians' Desk Reference* carries no reference to a RMSF vaccine.

Insect repellant must be used by workers in tick-infested areas, and it must be applied to socks, trouser cuffs, and any opening in clothing such as around the neck, top of the trousers, button areas, and the fly.

RABIES IMMUNIZATION

Changes in effective antigens for preexposure immunization against rabies have been recent and frequent. These efforts are significant even though the number of human cases of rabies has continued to decline. From 1946 to 1950, 22 cases per year were reported, while there have been but 2 to 4 cases per year since 1974. The cases in animals have undergone a similar numerical decline; in 1946, there were more than 8,000 reported, while in 1983, 5,878 appeared [38]. However, in the decade since 1974 there has been a striking upswing in animal cases. Wild animals represent the greatest current reservoir of the disease, especially coyotes, bobcats, skunks, foxes, raccoons, and bats, this source accounting for 85 percent of the animal cases since 1976 [2]. For travelers going to developing countries where rabies is endemic, the dog is the most likely disease focus.

PREEXPOSURE IMMUNIZATION

Certain workers in high-risk groups should be considered for preexposure immunization—veterinarians and their animal-handling personnel; zookeepers; workers in wildlife control programs; vivarium workers; laboratory workers whose contacts would rationalize such protection; and those other workers whose occupational demands would require possible exposure to wild, rabid animals. The reasons for immunization before actual infection have been laid down by the ACIP [39]: (1) it may provide protection to persons with inapparent exposure to rabies; (2) it may protect persons whose postexposure therapy might be delayed; and (3) although it does not eliminate the need for additional treatment after exposure, it simplifies that therapy by obviating the need for globulin and diminishing the number of vaccine doses needed. The ACIP has delineated the criteria for preexposure immunization [39].

It must be noted that after some 5 years and 400,000 doses of the human diploid cell rabies vaccine (HDCV) to about 100,000 persons in the United States, hypersensitivity reactions have been reported in about 6 percent, primarily in individuals receiving booster injections [40]. The revised recommendation coming from the CDC is that in preexposure immunization for persons scheduled to receive regular booster doses, the option should be given to have a measure of antibody titers before giving the vaccine. If it is shown that antibody titers are sufficient to neutralize the virus at a 1:5 serum dilution, then the 2-year booster can be skipped. The reactions have consisted of urticaria, angioedema, joint pain, and malaise—in essence, a serum sickness–like response, but not fatal. Currently manufacturers are attempting to produce an improved product [40].

Since the approval of HDCV, studies have been conducted of the effectiveness of the vaccine administered intradermally or subcutaneously [41–43]. In light of the success of the development of adequate antibody titers, the ACIP examined the data and agreed that the intradermal route offers an acceptable alternative to the previously approved intramuscular regimen [39,44,45], but only for the vaccine distributed by the Merieux Institute in Miami, Florida.

Some adverse reactions to the administration of HDCV have been reported and verified by physician statements [46]. The conclusion has been, though, that the vaccine is safe and effective and that physicians should be aware of the possible occasional adverse reaction.

INFLUENZA IMMUNIZATION

As influenza has occurred in all configurations from isolated cases to pandemics, there is always considerable concern expressed by members of employed groups as to the wisdom of obtaining influenza vaccine injections or the provision of such immunizations by the employer as part of the OHS program.

In the early post–World War II years, it was believed that because influenza resulted in considerable industrial-worker morbidity and some mortality, it would be desirable and feasible to conduct such protective programs on site. Influenza vaccine was administered in different work populations in the 1960s [47,48], and the effects were measured. The efforts continued into the 1970s [48–51] without there being a consensus as to the worth of the undertaking. Early on, the method of jet injection was introduced for the administration of influenza vaccine to large populations [52], with comparable demonstrable antibody responses between that protocol and the standard syringe and needle format.

Several issues are involved. First, it seems logical that immunization of a total work population with influenza vaccine should not be undertaken unless there is unquestioned epidemiologic evidence of oncoming morbid involvement of large masses of people in the United States or even abroad. The second issue, related to the first, concerns the etiologic identification of the causative agent with appropriate serologic studies because of the generic attribution to "the flu" of any variety of respiratory or gastrointestinal diseases, identifiable viral infections, or even psychogenic illnesses. It must be determined in affected populations that there is, in fact, an epidemic and that a particular community is likely to be attacked.

A third issue is one of cost and responsibility. Over the years, companies have offered injections at no charge to their employees, and the voluntary acceptance has not been high. In other situations, the immunizations were provided at actual cost. But the potential is always present of a serious, untoward reaction, which becomes, by definition, an occupational injury, the cost of which may nullify the total advantage being sought through the initiation and completion of the program. In addition, the medical community, while infrequently given to the practice of preventive medicine, may still consider the effort an infringement on private practice.

Whatever the perspective, there is no question that certain winters in the recent past have witnessed considerable absence of workers because of serious influenzal disease. A practical consideration is that of the demographic matrix of a plant's workforce. Turning again to the counsel of the ACIP [53], one encounters recommendations pertinent to recent winters. In general, annual vaccination is strongly advised for all persons who are at increased risk of adverse consequences from infections of the lower respiratory tract.

Studies among noninstitutionalized patients have demonstrated that chronic underlying diseases, especially disorders of the cardiovascular and pulmonary systems, may contribute more to the severity of influenza than age alone. These rather broad groups have been classified further on the basis of priority by the ACIP to allow the provision of vaccine to persons who may benefit the most. The groups for whom active vaccination efforts are most necessary follow* [53]:

Adults with chronic disorders of the cardiovascular or pulmonary systems severe enough to have needed medical care, follow-up or hospitalization during the preceding year.

Physicians, nurses, and other personnel having extensive contact with high-risk patients, who can transmit influenzal infections to such patients, should be vaccinated annually.

Otherwise healthy persons aged 65 years or older.

Persons with chronic metabolic diseases (including diabetes mellitus), renal dysfunction, anemia, immunosuppression, or asthma sufficiently severe as to have required medical care, follow-up, or hospitalization during the preceding year.

With the mandates in hiring laid down by the Rehabilitation Act of 1973, every plant will have employees with some of these disorders, for they may bear no relationship to performing a required set of functions. As determined by the mission of the company, there will be certain employees whose pulmonary capacity already will have been challenged by various occupationally induced fibrosing disorders, such as asbestosis, who are subject to severe complications from respiratory infections. Further, with the elevation of the retirement age to 70 years, and with the option that some workers may continue beyond that chronologic marker following annual review, there will be older employees in the labor force.

In parallel with the statements of the ACIP [53], a basic set of principles can be formulated, as determined by the mission of the company; the location of the facility with respect to climatic adversity, available medical care, and transportation capacity; the age and sex matrix of the population (considering working mothers with children subject to recurrent respiratory infections); the job assignments, fixed or engaged in interstate trucking or at work in the field; and, lastly, the general philosophy of the conduct of the health program. Not only should OHS personnel receive the vaccine but also those individuals who provide essential community services, such as law enforcement members and firefighters, to minimize the possible disruption of needed activities that can take place during severe epidemics [53].

Side effects usually attributed to the influenza virus itself, even though inactivated, consist of fever, malaise, and myalgia and may begin 6 to 12 hours postvaccination and last 1 to 2 days. Individuals with anaphylactic hypersensitivity to eggs should not be given influenza vaccine.

Persons who have had a recent viral infection can be given influenza vaccine, but it should not be administered to individuals symptomatically ill with an infectious disease, be it viral, bacterial, or other [54,55]. It might be wiser to conduct most of the immunization program on Fridays, obviating possible absence from work owing to postinjection reactions.

CHOLERA IMMUNIZATION

The need for cholera vaccination is rare. However, 17 cases were reported on a Gulf Coast oil rig off Texas in the late summer of 1981 [56–57], and there is concern among multinational corporations of outbreaks in cholera-endemic areas abroad where they have industrial facilities [58]. But one case was reported in the United States in 1983 [38], while as of April 1982 there were nearly 37,000 cases reported in 42 countries [59] in 1981 and approximately 55,000 the following year in 37 countries [60].

A complete primary series is suggested only for special high-risk groups working and living in extremely endemic areas with less than adequate sani-

*As children are usually outside the purview of an occupational health program, they are not included among target groups indicated in these discussions.

tation. The primary series need never be repeated for the booster doses to be effective.

The vaccine has been shown to be about 50-percent effective in the prevention of clinical illness for a period of 3 to 6 months [2]. The vaccine is indicated only for persons going to countries requiring evidence of vaccination for entry. A physician's statement concerning contraindication of administration may be issued. Pregnant women should not be vaccinated, as there is no specific information available on the safety of its use in pregnancy. Serious reactions, apart from local pain, erythema, and induration at the injection site, are rare. Infrequently there may be fever, malaise, and headache.

POLIOMYELITIS IMMUNIZATION

The success of the three decades of use of the poliomyelitis vaccine bespeaks the efficaciousness of strong community programs. Ideally, everyone should, by now, have been immunized against this extremely formidable disease. Whereas there were over 18,000 cases in 1954, there were but 15 in 1983, about twice the number of the 3 years before [38].

Certain workers will be at increased risk to poliomyelitis, if assigned to rural areas of developing countries or if engaged in the delivery of health services. Unvaccinated employees or job applicants who may be in contact with patients or specific biologic materials should be immunized.

Although the risk is extremely small in the United States today, epidemics are possible if the immunity of the population is not maintained by inoculating children in their first year. There have been small outbreaks in 1970, 1972, and 1979 as a result of virus introduction into susceptible populations where the communities presented low immunization levels [2].

Regular primary poliovirus vaccination of persons over 18 years of age living in the United States is not necessary, for most adults are immune and will almost never be at risk of exposure in this country. However, there are certain individuals who are at greater risk of exposure to wild polioviruses including (1) travelers to areas where poliomyelitis is epidemic or endemic; (2) members of communities or specific population groups with disease caused by wild polioviruses; (3) laboratory workers handling specimens likely to contain polioviruses; and (4) health care personnel in close contact with patients who may be excreting polioviruses.

Two poliovirus vaccines are licensed in the United States: oral polio vaccine (OPV) and inactivated polio vaccine (IPV). OPV bears the official name of "poliovirus vaccine, live, oral, trivalent," and the official designation of IPV is "poliomyelitis vaccine." OPV will produce long-lasting immunity to all three poliovirus types in over 95 percent of recipients, most being protected after a single dose. There has been infrequent association of OPV with paralytic disease in vaccinees or their close contacts—once in 3.2 million distributed doses. The occurrence of such a complication in the 12-year period of 1969 to 1980, when 290 million doses of OPV were distributed, as encountered among 92 cases, was as follows: 25 cases in otherwise healthy vaccine recipients; 55 cases in healthy close contacts of such recipients; and 12 cases in persons, either recipients or contacts, with immunodeficiency disorders [61].

IPV, used subcutaneously, has not been employed in the United States for more than a decade, and it is not known if the duration of immunity attained with IPV is equivalent to that obtained with OPV.

In spite of the lack of supporting evidence, on theoretic grounds pregnant women should not be given poliovirus vaccine. However, if immediate protection is needed, OPV, rather than IPV, is recommended [2].

RUBELLA IMMUNIZATION

As they are not directly related to employment, rubella immunizations have not been offered in most OHSs. However, were one to consider the many short- and long-term effects of fetal damage in a young, female labor force where most of its members would return to employment after delivery, one could readily decide that such a valued immunization protocol should be available at the worksite.

In New York State, the health code requires that all women of childbearing years who work in health institutions be screened for rubella and offered protective immunization [63]. A large urban hospital complied with this mandate, and all new female employees, 18 years and older, were tested for rubella antibody as part of their initial employment medical assessment. In addition, previously employed women were screened on the occasion of their annual medical examination or prior to receiving immune globulin (IG) for exposure to hepatitis. A third effort was seen in the issue of an exploratory memorandum announcing that rubella screening was available to any employee on request.

Those persons considered "susceptible"—individuals with titers of rubella hemagglutination inhibition (HI) of less than 1:8—were so informed by letter, and appointments for discussion of the matter were made. After informed consent was obtained, a brief medical history was developed, and if no contraindications surfaced, vaccine was given. Emphasis was given contraception during the ensuing weeks. The activity was carried out in the hospital's employee health service (EHS).

The screening was easily incorporated into the regular preplacement examination protocol, the EHS was "reasonably successful" in vaccinating the susceptible women, and side reactions were few.

Again, in light of the constant number—8.8 percent of the "ever-married women" of reproductive age in the current workforce—of pregnant women at the worksite, such a program is sound and indubitably cost-effective.

Whereas rubella, prior to the vaccine's becoming available in 1969, attacked primarily school-age children, it is now a disease of adolescents and young adults. Since 1976, more than 70 percent of persons with rubella have been 15 years old or older [64]. Of those age groups, 10 to 20 percent are susceptible. Even with the consistent community campaigns against the disease, rubella outbreaks continue in junior and senior high schools, colleges, the military, and places of employment, particularly hospitals. As recommended, "Ascertainment of rubella immune states and availability of rubella immunization should be components of the health-care program in places where women of child-bearing age congregate or represent a significant proportion of the workforce. Such settings include . . . companies, government offices, and industrial sites" [64]. With the passage of a "no immunization—no school" law in Wisconsin, the susceptibility rate dropped from 22 percent prior to the enactment of the statute to 5 percent following its enforcement [65]. Although such legislation is not intended for employed groups, it was demonstrated that rubella susceptibility can be lowered. It was suggested, however, that rubella immunity be made a condition for employment [2].

The emphasis currently is on (1) the elimination of serologic testing for females of childbearing age and (2) the vaccination of adult females, with the caution of not becoming pregnant for 3 months in the absence of a history of rubella vaccination (or serologic evidence of immunity), and if the employee is not pregnant, verbal assurance is acceptable. The County of Los Angeles Department of Health Services issued rubella screening guidelines for all health care agencies in Los Angeles [66], and those recommendations pertinent to employed persons follow:

As a first priority, in a high-risk setting (usually defined as clinics and service areas in which pregnant women constitute a significant number of patients), determine the rubella immunity status of all staff members (male and female) of all ages who have frequent and routine face-to-face contact with pregnant patients. Immunity should be documented either by (1) proof of immunization or (2) previous serology indicating immunity. Without either of these, a person should be considered susceptible and should be immunized (barring pregnancy or other medical contraindications). We suggest that this be required as a condition of new or continued employment in high-risk settings.

In outbreak situations, broader surveys of employees' immunity need to be done. Those employees, male or female of any age, not able to document immunity should be immunized.

Adopt a firm policy on prompt reporting of employee illness, and evaluate reports of any illness marked by rash and fever.

In substance, there should be premarital screening and vaccination, postpartum vaccination, patient vaccination in any medical setting, vaccination of medical personnel, vaccination of workers, and vaccination for college entry [64].

TYPHOID VACCINATION

Although typhoid vaccines have been used for decades, there are few indications for their stocking and administration by an OHS unless there are certain employees at high risk who are involved with the manufacture of specific biologic products or who are engaged in pertinent research. Otherwise, it is not recommended for use in the United States or in areas of natural disaster [2]. As the effectiveness of paratyphoid A and B vaccines has never been demonstrated, *typhoid vaccine* alone should be used if it is indicated.

ORAL VACCINE AGAINST TYPHOID

As parenteral vaccines frequently produce unwanted local and constitutional symptoms, thought has been given to oral, inactivated vaccines because of their nonreactogenicity. Wahdan and his associates [67] carried out a 3-year field trial in Egypt of oral typhoid vaccine (*Salmonella typhi* strain Ty 21a) involving nearly 33,000 children, one-half of whom received the vaccine, the remainder given a placebo. Each case suspected of being typhoid was investigated bacteriologically and serologically. In the vaccinated group, the incidence of typhoid was 0.2 cases per 10,000 children, while in the control group it was 4.9 cases per 10,000 children. It was concluded that with the three-dose schedule used, the vaccine was protective for at least 3 years, at an estimated protection rate of 95 percent. Adverse reactions were minimal and were comparable between the two groups. It is conceivable that the oral prophylaxis may replace the long-standing use of parenteral typhoid vaccine [68].

TYPHUS VACCINATION

As there has been no outbreak of louse-borne (epidemic) typhus in the United States since 1922 and no case reported in an American traveler since 1950, production of typhus vaccine in this country has been discontinued. Currently there are no plans for commercial production of a new vaccine.

MEASLES VACCINATION

Vaccination utilizing live measles virus vaccine relates nearly exclusively to infants and children. Most persons born before 1957 are likely to have been infected naturally and generally need not be considered susceptible [2]. As the risk is greater outside the United States of acquiring measles, travelers should be immunized before leaving.

YELLOW FEVER VACCINATION

As immunization for yellow fever is offered only at approved Yellow Fever Vaccination Centers, such injections are not germane to the inoculation program of an OHS.

PNEUMOCOCCAL POLYSACCHARIDE VACCINATION

In 1977 a polyvalent polysaccharide vaccine was licensed for use against disease caused by the pneumococcus *(Streptococcus pneumoniae)*. No occupational indications for its use appear at present, but the ACIP does recommend the use of the 27-valent vaccine in the following groups [2]:

Adults with chronic illness, especially cardiovascular and pulmonary disorders whose morbidity is increased with respiratory infections.

Adults with chronic illnesses especially associated with an increased risk of pneumococcal disease or its complications, such as multiple myeloma, cirrhosis, alcoholism, and renal failure.

Older adults, especially over age 65, who are healthy.

As indicated previously, persons of these classifications may be encountered in business and industry.

MENINGOCOCCAL POLYSACCHARIDE VACCINATION

Two polysaccharide vaccines against disease caused by *Neisseria meningitidis* serogroups are now licensed. It is the counsel of the ACIP that regular vaccination of U.S. civilians with meningococcal polysaccharide vaccine is not recommended because of the lack of availability of a good B vaccine (serogroup B strains cause most cases in the United States) and the low risk of infection in the United States [2,69].

COCCIDIOIDOMYCOSIS VACCINATION (TRIAL)

Persons providing occupational health services to natural history museum personnel such as archeologists—particularly in California where coccidioidomycosis (valley fever) has long been endemic in the San Joaquin Valley and in adjacent areas where spores of *Coccidioides immitis* reside in the topsoil—would be interested in an unsuccessful field trial of a vaccine. Under the direction of Hillell B. Levine, a multicentered, double-blind, clinical study was initiated [70,71].

The results of the vaccine trial, as reported by Pappagianis [72], in which the material used was formaldehyde-killed spherules of *C. immitis* grown in vitro, showed no significant difference in the incidence or intensity of disease between the vaccine and placebo groups.

Not only have scientific personnel acquired the disease in the field, but so have volunteers who have joined in the "digs." As Levine reported [70,71], about 60 percent of people who react to coccidioidin on skin testing have an asymptomatic disease without sequelae and without knowledge that they were infected. The remaining 40 percent will experience an influenzalike syndrome, and of that group, 32 percent will recover completely; 1.5 percent to 3.0 percent will go on to develop chronic pulmonary disease, and another 1 percent will have meningeal involvement. The disease, therefore, has broad public health implications, in addition to its occupational aspects.

HEPATITIS PREVENTION

The development by an employee of any disease that is known to be communicable usually stirs considerable concern among fellow workers, and the OHS will be queried regarding immediate protection of any possible contactant. Although such prophylaxis should be taken care of by personal physicians, workers will view the potential acquisition of the disease as job-related and, therefore, its prevention as the responsibility of the employer.

A difficulty that presents itself for consideration is the reality that under workers' compensation coverage there is little provision for preventive measures, for medical care is given only in the event of illness or injury actually diagnosed and accepted as arising in the course of, or out of, employment. So the costs of such prophylaxis, if decided upon, are directly chargeable to the OHS, and they can be high if sizeable quantities of injectable preparations are to be used, as determined by the number of employees claiming contact with the contagious disease source.

HEPATITIS A

"Viral hepatitis" is a generic term used for three diseases that are clinically similar but distinct etiologically and epidemiologically. Hepatitis A was formerly termed infectious hepatitis, and hepatitis B was called serum hepatitis. A third disease, currently known as non-A, non-B hepatitis, is caused probably by two different agents, and as there is no specific diagnostic test for its identification, it is diagnosed by exclusion. It is a significant form of hepatitis in adults and is responsible for most of the post-transfusion hepatitides in the United States.

Hepatitis A is caused by the hepatitis A virus (HAV). Transmission is by person-to-person contact, usually by fecal contamination, and it is facilitated by poor sanitation and close personal contact, which includes sexual exposures. There may be infections from contaminated food and water. The incubation period courses 15 to 50 days, with an average of 28 to 30 days. The greatest period of infectivity is in the 2 weeks prior to the onset of jaundice. A chronic carrier state, with HAV in the blood or feces, has not been shown [73].

Passive Immunization

Immune globulins as used today are sterile solutions of antibodies (immunoglobulins) obtained from human plasma. Immune globulin (IG)—formerly known as either "immune serum globulin" or "gamma globulin"—contains antibodies against the HAV (anti-HAV) and against the hepatitis B surface antigen (anti-HB_s). Hepatitis B immune globulin (HBIG), prepared from plasma, contains extremely high titers of anti-HB_s. Serologically it has been demonstrated that over half of the population aged 40 and older have been infected with HAV.

Preexposure Prophylaxis

There are no indications for the use of IG in any employed group in the United States, unless certain members will be traveling internationally and eating in areas of poor sanitation.

Postexposure Prophylaxis

Recommendations for the use of IG after exposure depend on the setting and the nature of the exposure [73]. Strongly urged, in light of the safety with its use, is that the IG be given as soon as possible after exposure, without waiting for antibody testing. If used, it must be given within 2 weeks after exposure.

Day-Care Centers. If there is evidence that HAV transmission is occurring in a center where care is given children in diapers, the staff and attendees should receive IG. Handwashing after changing diapers must be strictly enforced. In an outbreak, in addition to staff and attendees, household members of the diapered children attending should be given IG.*

Schools and Preschools. There is no indication for the use of IG in persons in close contact with patients. If epidemiologic evidence indicates an outbreak centered at that site, pupils and teachers can be given IG.

Institutions for Custodial Care. In such facilities as prisons or hospitals for the developmentally disabled, the transmission of hepatitis A is always favored. In the event of an outbreak, IG can be administered to residents and staff to reduce the spread of the disease. The extent of the prophylaxis—involving some or all contactants—should be determined locally.

Hospitals. The regular prophylactic use of IG for hospital personnel is not indicated. To be emphasized is intensive in-service staff education regarding precautions in patient contact and contact with potentially infective materials.

*This prophylaxis is important, for in several institutions the OHS has been given the responsibility of health oversight of the day-care center. If current thought continues, day-care centers either may become part of the school system or may be established more widely in industry.

Offices and Industrial Plants. IG is not indicated for employees exposed to a fellow worker with hepatitis A.

Common-Source Exposure. If recognized in time, IG might be effective in preventing hepatitis that is water-borne or food-borne. It is not recommended for individuals exposed to a common source of potential hepatitis infection once cases have begun to appear. If a food-handler has hepatitis A, a common-source transmission is possible, and IG should be given to other kitchen or dietary personnel. Patrons, who may be employees utilizing a plant cafeteria or snack bar, may receive IG if the involved food-handler works with foods that are not to be cooked or with cooked foods before they are eaten, if the hygienic practices of the food-handler are in question, or if the consumers can be identified and given IG within 2 weeks of exposure, the period within which IG is effective.

HEPATITIS B

Hepatitis B is caused by the hepatitis B virus (HBV). Hepatitis B surface antigen (HB_sAg), formerly termed either Australia antigen or hepatitis associated antigen, is an antigen found on the surface of the virus and can be identified 30 to 60 days after exposure to HBV. Antibody against HB_sAg (anti-HB_s) develops after a resolved infection and provides long-term immunity. Chronic carrier states follow 10 percent of infections and may be asymptomatic or infrequently associated with active liver disease [74]. If hepatitis B_e antigen (HB_eAg) is present in a carrier, it raises the potential infectivity, but it is lower if antibody against HB_eAg (anti-HB_eAg) is present.

Transmission takes place through percutaneous or permucosal routes. Blood or body fluids that are infective can be introduced by contaminated needles or through sexual contact. There can be infection in settings where there is continuous close personal contact—in households or among institutionalized mentally retarded children—presumably by inapparent contact of infectious secretions with skin lesions or mucosal surfaces. Previous transmission through transfusion of contaminated blood or blood products has been minimized since the introduction of regular screening with highly sensitive tests for HB_sAg. Hepatitis B is not transmitted either by the fecal-oral route or by contaminated food or water.

Persons at high risk are the following [73]:

Immigrants or refugees from areas of high HVB endemicity
Clients in institutions for the mentally retarded
Users of illicit parenteral drugs
Homosexually active men
Household contacts of HBV carriers
Patients of hemodialysis units

Those patients at intermediate risk are as follows:

Health care workers with frequent blood contact
Male prisoners
Staff in institutions for the mentally retarded

The low-risk group comprises these persons:

Health care workers with no or infrequent blood contact
Healthy adults (first-time volunteer blood donors)

The incubation period of hepatitis B is 45 to 160 days, with an average of 60 to 120 days. If the HBV infection is chronic, cirrhosis or primary liver carcinoma can be associated [70–72].

Passive Immunization

IG and HBIG differ in their amounts of anti-HB_s. IG is prepared from unselected plasma, while HBIG is especially selected for high-titer anti-HB_s, having a titer of less than 1:100,000 by radioimmunasssay (RIA). HBIG per dose is more than 20 times the cost of IG. These products offer temporary, passive protection and are useful only in certain postexposure settings.

Active Immunization

An inactivated hepatitis B vaccine has been tried in a high-risk group, and the preparation was found to be safe, with a low incidence of side effects [75]. Within 2 months, 77 percent of the vaccine recipients had high levels of anti-HB_s, the rate increasing to 96 percent following a booster dose, staying unchanged for the remaining period of trial. In 18 months of follow-up, hepatitis B or subclinical infection developed in 1.4 to 3.4 percent of those persons vaccinated, as compared with 18 to 27 percent of placebo recipients.

Recommended as recipients of the vaccine are homosexually active men, illicit injectable drug users, hospital personnel (especially surgeons and persons who work with blood products—medical, dental, laboratory, and other groups such as emergency room staff, operating room personnel, phlebotomists, intravenous therapy nurses, pathologists, and oncology staff persons), dialysis-center personnel, and transfusion recipients.

While hospital staff are at increased risk of HBV infection, the risk will vary among hospitals and within hospitals. To determine an institution's immunization policy or strategy, it is advised that published data be studied regarding the comparability between the two—or among more—bodies of experience with hepatitis B infections. Groups of exposees can be ranked at level of risk in accordance with the frequency of their blood/needle exposure. Other health workers, extramural to hospitals, who are at risk include blood-bank technicians, emergency medical technicians, and morticians.

For preexposure vaccination, other groups relevant to occupational health should be considered: clients and staff of institutions for the mentally retarded; homosexually active males, irrespective of age or duration of homosexual practices; users of illicit injectable drugs; classroom contacts of deinstitutionalized mentally retarded HBV carriers who behave aggressively or who have special medical problems that increase the risk of exposure to their blood or serous secretions; Alaskan Eskimos, and immigrants and refugees from areas with high endemic disease (especially eastern Asia and sub-Saharan Africa) who have high HBV infection rates; and inmates of long-term correctional facilities [73].

HBV vaccine, because of its inactivation, may be administered simultaneously with other vaccines. Side effects of the injections have included only soreness and redness at the inoculation site. Among 750,000 vaccinees, approximately 100 episodes of severe illness have been reported, including arthralgia, neurologic reactions, and others. Pregnancy is not a contraindication to the vaccination.

HBV carriers to whom the vaccine has been given have demonstrated neither therapeutic nor adverse effects. Active immunization need not be carried out in persons who have antibodies against HBV from a previous hepatitis; if the series is given, there will be no adverse effects, and the anti-HB_s level will increase. Passively acquired antibody will not interfere with active immunization [73].

The cost of immunization is high—approximately $100 for three injections. The determination of cost-effectiveness of screening depends on the cost of the vaccination, the cost of testing for susceptibility, and the prevalence of immune members in a group. The consideration of these factors will lead to a decision regarding screening of all, selective screening, or no screening.

Postexposure Vaccination

The only need for postexposure prophylaxis for hepatitis B in the work setting would be following accidental percutaneous or permucosal exposure to HB_sAg-positive blood.

Non-A, Non-B Hepatitis

As there are no specific test procedures, the worth of prophylaxis against non-A, non-B hepatitis cannot be determined. It is reasonable, however, to apply the counsel given for prophylaxis against hepatitis A [73]. Cases do occur, and in a 7-week period, four persons, participants in a plasmapheresis program, developed this form of hepatitis [76]. Laboratory tests confirmed the diagnosis. The disease is typically transmitted by blood transfusion, but there also have been occupational, nosocomial, venereal, and intrafamilial associations reported. The incubation period is 7 weeks with a range of 5 to 10 weeks. Chronic carriage is suspected. In nonepidemic hepatitis of this type, following percutaneous exposure to blood from a patient with non-A, non-B hepatitis, it might be reasonable to give IG as soon after exposure as possible [73].

ANTHRAX VACCINATION

Even though the number of human cases of anthrax in the United States is low—six cases in 1978, one in 1980, and one in 1984 [38,77]—there are certain workers at risk. Included are employees in contact with animal hair and hides and the products derived from these natural materials. For example, there was anthrax contamination of Haitian handicrafts made from goatskin that were collected at the Miami, New York, and San Juan quarantine stations in 1980 and 1981 [78]. This condition was encountered even though the importation of goatskin with attached hair has been prohibited since 1974.

As the risk of exposure in the general population is slight, no general immunization is advised. However, individuals who may come in contact with imported animal hides, furs, bone meal, wool, hair (especially goat hair), and bristles, workers in plants handling these materials, and laboratory personnel contemplating or involved in investigational studies utilizing *Bacillus anthracis* should receive the immunizing injections of the vaccine distributed by the CDC [2].

If the prospective recipient presents with an acute respiratory infection, the injection should be deferred. If the individual is receiving corticosteroid therapy or other agents tending to depress the immune response, an extra dose should be given once more after therapy is discontinued.

Local reactions to the injections occur in about 6 percent of injections, appearing within 24 hours and clearing after 48 to 72 hours. Severe systemic reactions are rare.

BCG VACCINE

Until recently, tuberculosis was considered one of the serious diseases of the past, but with the influx of immigrants from southeast Asia and elsewhere, the receiving communities have seen a recrudescence of the problem.

The use of vaccine prepared from bacillus Calmette-Guérin (BCG) has been more extensive abroad than in the United States, and the preparation has always met with considerable controversy in the cognizant medical community. In the United States, however, BCG has been used primarily among selected groups of uninfected persons who live or work where the risk of exposure to tuberculosis has been unavoidable [79].

There are many different forms of BCG vaccine, although all have been derived from the original strain—the first use in humans dates to 1921—and they vary in immunogenicity, efficacy, and reactogenicity. The protection afforded has ranged from 0 to 80 percent. The vaccine used in the United States has not demonstrated efficacy—only an inference of such worth. The Food and Drug Administration (FDA) standards of production have been rigid, and the vaccine must be capable of inducing tuberculin sensitivity in guinea pigs and humans. The product must be freeze-dried, reconstituted, protected from exposure to light, and used within 8 hours.

RECOMMENDATIONS REGARDING USE

Most tuberculosis encountered today can be eradicated through the accepted means of case detection, chemotherapy, and preventive treatment. The only situations in the United States where the use of BCG might be considered are the following [2]:

Persons in prolonged close contact with patients whose tuberculosis is untreated, ineffectually treated, or resistant to treatment.

Health care workers, such as hospital personnel, who have an annual new infection rate of 1 percent or higher in spite of other tuberculosis control measures.

Other groups in whom an excessive rate of new infection can be shown and the customary surveillance and treatment programs have either failed or are not feasible.

Even for the groups indicated above, the protection provided by isoniazid (INH) preventive therapy is much more predictable and reliable than BCG vaccination [79]. Although most work groups should be protected through adequate surveillance and control measures, some health personnel may be at increased risk of repeated exposure, especially individuals who work in institutions that provide care in large metropolitan centers where the endemicity of tuberculosis is relatively high. BCG vaccination might be considered when the frequency of conversion of skin-test results—the measure of new infections—is in excess of the percentage given above.

There have been adverse reactions among vaccine recipients, including prolonged ulceration at the injection site and lymphadenitis. Rarely, osteomyelitis, lupoid reactions, and disseminated BCG infection have been noted. Reactions depend on the particular vaccine used, the dosage, and the age of the vaccinees [80].

Individuals with impaired immune response or persons on therapy with steroids, alkylating agents, antimetabolites, or radiation should not receive BCG vaccine. The procedure should be avoided during pregnancy.

One difficulty presents itself, and that concerns postvaccination interpretation of the tuberculin skin test. It is usually not possible to distinguish between a tuberculin reaction from a virulent suprainfection and one resulting from a persisting sensitivity after vaccination. Great caution should be used in attributing a positive skin test to BCG—except in the immediate postvaccination period—particularly if the recipient has been exposed recently to infective tuberculosis. In substance, when deciding on the management of positive reactors, give no consideration to a history of BCG vaccination [79,80].

Full, lasting protection from BCG vaccination cannot be ensured, so that any tuberculosis-like illness in a vaccinee should call for consideration of tuberculosis in the differential diagnosis.

PRECAUTIONS DURING IMMUNIZATION

Because of the possibility of immediate adverse reaction to the administration of an immunizing injection, there must be available as part of the immunization equipment a tray or table with appropriate instruments and medications for instant use. Epinephrine, syringes, and needles must be at hand. Procedures include establishing airway potency, administration of oxygen, cardiac monitoring, and establishing an IV access for fluids and medications.

LEGAL ASPECTS OF IMMUNIZATION

An untoward response from any immunizing injection, whether in a person being examined for employment or in a current employee, should be considered an occupational injury and be so recorded. Even if the actual employment protocol has not been completed, the prospective employer is liable for the resulting illness or injury. Fortunately, the frequency of severe or unanticipated reactions is rare.

The standard question that is asked concerns the use of a waiver, signed by the vaccine recipient, by which the employer is freed of any liability for complications arising from any immunizing procedure. As in all workers' compensation considerations, an individual cannot waive his rights regarding compensation, medical care, or any other aspect of such coverage or benefits. Even if a waiver were to be signed, liability continues to exist [81].

The initiation of a third-party suit against the manufacturer of the vaccine in question is always a possibility [82]. Such issues underscore the need for the maintenance of detailed clinical *and* purchase records, the latter by the purchasing department of the employer.

Although it may seem to be an inappropriate use of valued time, it is suggested that, in a manner comparable to obtaining informed consent, the employee—or the parent of a child* who will receive immunizations—be told of possible adverse reactions, so that what proves to be a mild, customary response at the injection site is not misinterpreted as a gross misadventure. A note should be entered into the clinical record reflecting the fact that such information was given [83,84].

Because of the number of adverse reactions at the time of the effort toward nationwide immunization against the swine influenza virus in 1976 and following the use of polio vaccine previously, the question of physician, manufacturer, or agency liability was reviewed in many law, social science, and medical journals [85–94]. Arising from this dilemma of untoward results from the administration of preventive biologics, legislation has been proposed that would provide compensation for vaccine injury, particularly directed toward recipients of mandated immunizations. An ad hoc commission of the American Medical Association (AMA) addressed these issues, especially as they related to vaccines in pediatrics, because of the problem arising with pertussis vaccine in 1984 [95], and the Institute of Medicine has studied the problem in addition [96].

*Pertinent in cases of summer employees from high school or college.

Undoubtedly, society in general will develop a system of compensating the few who have sustained injury. In industry, the workers' compensation system will provide coverage for the misadventure occasioned by OHS-delivered immunizations. What third-party suits might result cannot be predicted.

RELIGIOUS OBJECTION TO IMMUNIZATION

Another question that arises is that of objection on religious grounds to employer-required immunizations. It is believed that, in light of the paucity of such persons in any particular plant, there should be forbearance. Schumacher [85] feels that there is little sense in forcing such ideologically bound individuals to comply by applying legal pressure or employment interdictions. The only difficulty is that this small group not only may refuse vaccination for themselves but also may attempt to counteract policy wherever they can. Tolerance should be practiced, as it is with conscientious objection.

IMMUNIZATION RECORD MAINTENANCE

It is extremely important that detailed records be maintained of all immunizations given to employees. Not only should such accurate notations be made for legal purposes, but also workers lose their own personal immunization cards or history of injections and a basic reference should be available for use in updating various vaccinations either for domestic use or for travel abroad.

CLINICAL RECORDS

The following information should be entered into the health record regarding each immunizing injection administered:

Date of injection
Type of vaccine or other prophylactic substance
Dose administered and route of administration
Manufacturer of vaccine
Product name, lot and batch number, and date of production*

*This information is of great worth in facilitating future epidemiologic studies regarding rare adverse reactions or failure of prophylaxis because of possible newly mutated viral strains or new strains that have been included. (See A. L. Fraikor, Adequate records for vaccination. *N Engl J Med* 293:201, 1975.)

Name of person ordering immunization
Signature, not initials, of person administering injection
Notation of untoward reaction, if any

INDIVIDUAL EMPLOYEE RECORDS
Each employee should have initiated at the time of hire or at the administration of the first immunizing injection, for personal retention, a wallet-size card that can serve as the record of all inoculations received. The card should contain the following information:

Name
Date of birth
Employee number
Type of immunization
Dates of all injections of basic series
Dates of all booster injections
Special sensitivities to vaccines, if any

REFERENCE POSTERS
To avoid having to consult several printed sources, an OHS required to maintain immunization schedules for its personnel engaging in travel to all parts of the globe, or for its representatives and their families undergoing assignment abroad, would do well to have posted in its immunization station two large documents. These information sheets will save considerable time and will offer ready reference to the details of the administration of any biologic preparation used in communicable disease prophylaxis and to the requirements for or recommendations regarding inoculations on a country-to-country basis.

OSHA COMPLIANCE OFFICERS

A variant of the many exposures discussed here that indicate prophylaxis is that inherent in the role of the OSHA compliance officer (CSHO). Pharmaceutical firms, medical research laboratories, and hospitals, as indicated, have areas where there is potential exposure to communicable diseases. In many such installations, the working personnel will undergo mandatory immunization. It is possible that the CSHO may be refused entry into these areas without current, valid proof of immunization. If immunizing injections are required, the OSHA area director shall determine that the inspecting CSHO has the proper immunizations and that the required incubation or waiting period (if any) is met prior to the inspection. All CSHOs potentially assignable to such inspection sites should be encouraged, if physically able, to be immunized against the communicable diseases they will encounter [97].

SKIN-TESTING PROGRAMS

As determined by local geography, epidemiologic findings in area studies, and job assignments, workers may be exposed to disease sources for which sensitivity testing would be appropriate.

In addition to serologic testing for the determination of specific antibody levels, certain immunobiologic products in the form of skin-test antigens can be used to establish sensitivity to latent or asymptomatic forms of diseases to which there may be exposure.

TUBERCULIN SKIN TESTING

The tuberculin skin test (TST) is used to diagnose infection with *Mycobacterium tuberculosis*. Such infection produces sensitivity to components of the organisms, or antigens, contained in culture extracts called tuberculins. Whereas different preparations of tuberculin were available in the past, today only two are licensed for use, old tuberculin (OT) and purified protein derivative (PPD). OT is available solely in multiple puncture devices, while PPD can be used for intracutaneous injection (Mantoux technique) or for percutaneous injection by multiple puncture. The use of tuberculin has become the primary method of understanding the pathogenesis and epidemiology of tuberculosis and the mechanism of delayed hypersensitivity and cellular immunity [98].

ADMINISTRATION OF TUBERCULIN SKIN TEST
Although the multiple-puncture method of testing seems to be favored in pediatic practice, the intracutaneous or Mantoux test is believed to be preferred for adult use.

The TST serves as a diagnostic skin test to detect delayed hypersensitivity in persons infected with *M. tuberculosis*. The test consists of the intracutaneous injection of 0.1 ml of PPD containing 5 tuberculin units (TU) into either the extensor or flexor surface of the forearm. An area should be selected that is clear of skin lesions and that does not overlie a superficial vein. A wheal, 6 to 10 mm in diameter, should result from the injection.

If the test was given improperly, a second can be given immediately at a site several centimeters removed from the first attempted injection site. Appropriate notation should be made indicating the location of the successful procedure.

The results should be read on the second or third day, the time when the induration produced is most evident. The criterion in interpretation is the presence or absence of induration at the point of injection, to be determined both visually—under direct light and by side-lighting—and by palpation. The diameter of the indurated area should be measured transversely to the long axis of the forearm and should be recorded in millimeters.

INTERPRETATION OF THE TUBERCULIN SKIN TEST

Individuals sensitive to tuberculin are "reactors," but not all reactors are infected by *M. tuberculosis,* for there are reactions throughout the world to infections with other mycobacteria, known as cross-reactions. There is no clear distinction between the two types of reaction, but ordinarily *M. tuberculosis* infection produces a larger reaction. The defining of a significant reaction has been rendered more difficult as the number of infections from nontuberculous mycobacterial infections has increased.

M. tuberculosis infections are likely to be more common in persons who have been in close contact with tuberculosis and in individuals with chest radiographic abnormalities consistent with tuberculosis. The distribution of reaction sizes is likely to be bimodal. By using a cutting point of 5 mm, significant reactions can be separated from nonsignificant reactions, without running a good risk of error in classification.

When considering persons who have had no contact with tuberculosis or who show no chest radiographic evidence of tuberculosis, a different cutting point must be used. Other considerations enter into the decision-making process, such as a greater prevalence of cross-reactions, the selection of reacting individuals for chest radiography—the factors of cost-effectiveness and exposure to radiation—and the expense of preventive therapy [98].

A reasonable compromise for the United States as a whole is a cutting point of 10 mm in Mantoux tests using 5 TU of PPD. It may be that ideally each locality should choose its own cutting point, as determined by the characteristics of the population being tested and the characteristics of the personnel administering and reading the tests.

When the TST is used in evaluating persons having a process that might be tuberculous, the main concern is with reactions falsely classified as nonsignificant. A nonsignificant reaction alone does not include the diagnosis of the tuberculosis. Conditions that may be responsible for impairing a delayed hypersensitivity, and thus causing nonsignificant tuberculin reactions in persons actually infected, include technical factors, age of the person tested, administration of immunosuppressive drugs, and coexisting diseases [98]. These factors, plus others unrecognized, combine to produce nonsignificant TSTs in patients in whom the presence of tuberculosis has been proved.

When reasonable cutting points cannot be established through use of applicable local data, the following interpretations are suggested [98]:

1. Significant reaction—a reaction of 10 mm or more in diameter; such reactions are likely to represent infection with *M. tuberculosis.*
2. Two groups may have small reactions to TST. One consists of individuals in close contact with someone with *M. tuberculosis*–positive sputum. The second group comprises those persons with radiographic or clinical evidence of "disease compatible with tuberculosis, or tuberculosis suspects" [98]. For these two groups, using 5 mm of induration to define a significant reaction will delineate more accurately individuals with and without *M. tuberculosis* infection.
3. Nonsignificant reaction—reactions of less than 10 mm in diameter in persons who are neither tuberculosis suspects nor contacts of sputum-positive individuals.

In substance, no longer are such test result descriptors as "positive" and "negative" used, and definitive millimeter readings are not considered as "negative," "doubtful," or "positive."

INDICATIONS FOR TESTING

There are several groups of people who should be tested, many of whom are employed in high-risk situations or have come into employment from situations at high risk of infection. These groups include (1) persons with suggestive signs or symptoms of current tuberculosis, (2) recent contacts of persons with known disease, (3) persons with abnormal chest radiographs compatible with past tuberculosis, (4) persons with disorders that increase the risk of tuberculosis (for example, silicosis, diabetes), and (5) groups at high risk of recent infection with *M. tuberculosis* such as Asian or African immigrants, some skid-row populations, and long-term residents of mental institutions, prisons, and so on.

TUBERCULIN SKIN TEST USE IN CONVERTERS

Occupational activities that bring tuberculin-negative persons into contact with persons likely to have tuberculosis call for the periodic use of the TST as a surveillance measure. As in any test, there are unavoidable errors, making small increases in reaction size not meaningful. When an individual undergoes a change in tuberculin reaction from less than 10 mm in diameter to 10 mm or more in diameter *and* an increase by at least 6 mm within 2 years, such a person should be viewed as newly infected. The cutting points (10 mm and 6 mm) may be subject to change; for example, when personnel in health care are in close contact with patients who have infectious tuberculosis, the cutting point should be dropped to 5 mm. For persons residing in areas where other mycobacterial infections are common and who are not exposed to tuberculosis, the cutting point could conceivably be raised to 15 mm, with an elevation of the 6 mm increase [99].

The booster phenomenon has been mentioned. Uninfected persons who undergo repeated skin testing do not become sensitized to tuberculin. Delayed hypersensitivity to tuberculin, whether established by actual myobacterial infection of any type or by BCG vaccination, as indicated previously, may wane slowly with aging. Testing at this point produces nonsignificant reactions. Subsequent tests may then boost the response, giving the impression of conversion or the development of sensitivity. The phenomenon is most frequent after age 50, and the effect may be discernible in a second test done within 1 week and may persist for a year or more.

The misinterpretation of a booster reaction as a recent infection can be obviated by using a two-step test. If the first TST is seen as producing a nonsignificant result, a second test should be given 1 week later. If that reaction is still below the cutting point, the subject is classified as having a nonsignificant reaction. If the latter test produces a significant reaction, that most likely is a boosted response and should be classified as significant, and the testee should be managed appropriately. A significant reaction to a third test, done within a few years, with a diameter increase of greater than 6 mm, represents an interval *M. tuberculosis* infection. Hospital employees in continuing surveillance programs should be tested not by means of a multiple-puncture device but should receive the Mantoux protocol.

As there is no reliable way to distinguish a reaction to BCG vaccine from a natural mycobacterial infection, it is wise to consider significant reactions in BCG vaccinees as representative of *M. tuberculosis* infections.

Untoward reactions to PPD are rare. An occasional extremely sensitive person may manifest vesiculation or ulcerative changes at the injection site, accompanied by lymphangitis, regional adenopathy, and fever. Such an infrequent response should not suggest the use of a 1-TU test, as the procedure has not been adequately standardized [99].

TUBERCULIN SKIN TESTING IN BCG VACCINEES

It has been recommended that immigrants coming to the United States from countries with high rates of tuberculosis be skin-tested with tuberculin. Making the procedure difficult in its interpretation is the history of vaccination with BCG [99]. As Snider [99] has indicated, vaccination with BCG leads to the development of tuberculin sensitivity; but the sensitivity is highly variable, as determined by the strain of vaccine used, the dosage, the method of administration, the age at the time of vaccination, the nutritional status of the vaccinee, in addition to a host of other influencing factors [99]. It is emphasized that there is no reliable manner of distinguishing BCG-caused tuberculin reactions from responses brought about by natural myobacterial infection. Further, tuberculin reactions resulting from infection with *M. tuberculosis* cannot be separated from those resulting from the sensitivity produced by nontuberculosis in mycobacterial antigens.

The history of a BCG vaccination must be confirmed. Merely because it is the policy of a country to vaccinate its citizens does not guarantee that a particular person has received the vaccine. Even with confirmation of the BCG protocol, a tuberculin skin test should still be conducted—the Mantoux test with 5 TU of polysorbate-stabilized PPD tuberculin [99]. To aid in interpretation of the test result, certain questions must be asked [99]: (1) How large is the reaction? (The larger the reaction, the more likely the possibility of *M. tuberculosis* infection.) (2) Is the subject a recent close contact of a patient with infectious tuberculosis? (Although BCG may reduce hematogenous spread, it will not prevent infection, so that preventive treatment with isoniazid will still be beneficial.) (3) If there was recent contact with infectious tuberculosis, was there evidence of transmission to unvaccinated contacts? (If so, it is most likely that the vaccinated contact was also infected recently.) (4) Is there a family history of the disease, or was the individual a recent immigrant from a country with a high tuberculosis rate? (With a positive response to either query, the probability of infection is heightened.) (5) How long ago was the BCG received? (The longer the interval, the less likely that the reaction is related to the BCG.)

A person vaccinated 10 years ago or more who has had recent contact with a patient transmitting infection to others should be considered infected with a skin-test response of 5 mm or greater. Immigrants from Southeast Asia with a history of BCG should be considered as having an *M. tuberculosis* infection if the reaction is 10 mm or greater. Snider [99] asks that one apply these questions rather than relying solely on skin-test size as the yardstick for a "significant reaction."

COCCIDIOIDIN SKIN TESTING

Coccidioidomycosis, by name a disease of fungal etiology, appears in many areas of endemicity. The causative organism, *Coccidioides immitis*, is found in the soil of California and the states that border Mexico and in certain Central and South American countries [100].

Because of today's extensive travel, both for business purposes and for pleasure, employees are at risk while en route or temporarily resident in the semiarid states and countries indicated. Further, considerable numbers of people are employed in California's agricultural industry in the San Joaquin Valley and, therefore, are constantly exposed to potential infection. Spore-laden products emanating from endemic areas spread the disease, more popularly known as valley fever. As land, heretofore strictly dedicated to the growing of fruit, vegetables, and cotton, is developed into housing tracts with such adjacent service facilities as shopping malls, access streets, public utilities, and small industry and is invaded by bulldozers and excavators, more of the arthrospores from *C. immitis* are freed to become airborne.

These spores can either reenter the soil and repeat the whole mycelial cycle, from septate mycelium to free arthrospores, or they can enter the human lung to develop into spherules, which in turn in a lesion will release endospores. The free endospores can then spread the infection by becoming blood-borne and lymph-borne. Such pathways allow nearly every organ or tissue to become involved.

Persons engaged in many occupations may be considered at risk when working in endemic areas. Mineral and oil exploration; experimental farming; archeologic digging; specimen collection in entomology, herpetology, zoology, and botany; highway construction; establishment of telecommunication and satellite tracking facilities; development of wilderness trails and ranger stations; conduct of military maneuvers; mapping; and geologic surveying, among many other occupational and avocational activities, can place workers at risk, so that the exposure is one of true occupational health concern. To all of these undertakings must be added the contact with *C. immitis* of laboratory personnel engaged in both diagnostic and research procedures.

Because 60 percent of patients experience asymptomatic or mild infections detected by coccidioidin sensitivity, the additional issues of illness absence and compensable occupational disease present themselves.

While the diagnosis of acute coccidioidomycosis is outside the purview of ambulatory occupational health care, it may be necessary to determine the diagnosis in a chronically or subclinically ill worker or patient or to differentiate the disease state from sarcoidosis, histoplasmosis, or other mycotic or bacterial infections.

Two types of spherule-derived coccidioidin are available*: usual skin-test strength (USTS) and high skin-test strength (HSTS).

USE OF COCCIDIOIDIN (SPHERULE DERIVED) USUAL STRENGTH

The usual skin test involves the intradermal injection of 0.1 ml of USTS coccidioidin on the flexor surface of the forearm. In the erythema nodosum patient, the first injection should utilize a 1 :100 dilution; if the reaction is negative, one can proceed to a 1 :10 dilution; and if again the response is negative, the USTS undiluted should be given. Dilutions can be made with sterile physiologic saline solution or buffered saline diluent and must be used immediately.

Interpretation

A positive reaction consists of an area of induration measuring 5 mm or more in diameter. Erythema without induration is a negative response. The test should be read at 24 hours and at 48 hours, as some test reactions may fade after 36 hours.

A positive test indicates a present or past infection with *C. immitis*. In a manner comparable to the tuberculin test, a negative reaction may indicate that the subject has never been sensitized or that the test subject has lost sensitivity. After an actual infection, though, skin sensitivity is long-lived.

If the reaction is negative, then HSTS coccidioidin (spherule derived) should be given, or the coccidioidin in lesser dilution, as it is 10 times the strength of USTS, which will prove conclusively that the patient is negative. The test material will not induce humoral antibodies in humans, and it will not cause skin sensitivity to develop in the nonsensitive individual. Spherule-derived coccidioidin will detect significantly more reactors than mycelia-derived coccidioidin.

*The coccidioidins are manufactured under the trade name of Spherulin by Berkeley Biologicals, Berkeley, California, and under the name of BIOCOX (Coccidioidin Bioproducts) by the Jatrix Corporation of Tempe, Arizona.

It should be noted that a positive reaction to mycelial coccidioidin may lead to a transitory rise in titer of complement fixation antibody to histoplasma antigens but not to coccidioidin. Spherule-derived coccidioidin, productive of positive test results, produces no change in the complement fixation titers for either histoplasmosis or coccidioidomycosis. The test material may cause skin-test cross-reactions in persons infected with *Histoplasma, Blastomyces,* and possibly other fungi. In already sensitive individuals, the test may raise the level of skin sensitivity to coccidioidin. Finally, in severe forms of the disease, the skin test may be negative (anergy), as it may be when long periods of time have elapsed since the initial infection.

USE OF COCCIDIOIDIN (SPHERULE DERIVED) HIGH STRENGTH

The HSTS is to be used only on test subjects who are negative to the USTS coccidioidin. The test protocol is identical to the one described for the lesser-strength preparation, and the precautions to be followed are the same. It should not be used on patients with erythema nodosum. The test dose is 0.1 ml given intradermally.

HISTOPLASMIN SKIN TESTING

Histoplasmosis is a disease acquired by the inhalation of dust particles bearing either the spores or infective mycelial fragments of *Histoplasma capsulatum,* with the primary focus being nearly always in the lung. This fungus-caused disease is both endemic and epidemic, and the classic study of Edwards and his colleagues [101] demonstrated that the epidemicity is fairly well localized to east-central United States. Positivity on skin testing was found with greater frequency among farmers (versus non-farmers), and among metropolitan populations (versus rural populations). The rates of reaction varied greatly within single geographic units. Other indices of epidemiologic concern involve cultures obtained from soil, the appearance of clinical cases, and the demonstration of calcified sequelae radiographically and by necropsy [102].

As with coccidioidomycosis, in histoplasmosis the response to the inhalation of the infective particles can vary from the asymptomatic appearance of hundreds of primary pulmonary foci on the roentgenogram to a violent, even lethal, reaction. Typical of granulomatous diseases, their development is slow, giving time for mobilization of the body's immune response, which in most individuals prevents overt disease, particularly progressive dissemination [102].

The occupational importance of the disease lies in the fact that workers come in contact with spore-containing soil—in caves, storm cellars, and silos—and are thus at risk. The bat has been a proven source of *H. capsulatum,* while there has been no recovery of the organism from chickens or other birds [102]. It is possible that radiographic changes may appear during the course of a worker's employment, and a workers' compensation claim could follow. The applicant would have a more justifiable claim to a work-associated disease if the preplacement chest film proved to be normal. If the worker were at specific risk through contact with suspect soil, the multiple calcified lesions seen on chest radiography could readily be supportive of an occupationally incurred illness—even though the claimant was asymptomatic and without disability. Adjudication would rest with the hearing officer, of course.

The role of the skin test is of significance in the workers at risk, particularly in laboratory personnel whose previously negative skin reaction upon change to positive may indicate recent infection.

ADMINISTRATION OF HISTOPLASMIN SKIN TEST

New disposable tuberculin syringes should be used, one for each subject. With a ½-inch 26-gauge needle, 0.1 ml of histoplasmin is injected intradermally on the alcohol-cleansed flexor surface of the forearm. The commercially available test material is the clinical equivalent of the U.S. Reference Standard Histoplasmin H-42, in a 1 :100 dilution. The injection produces a slightly painful bleb, which is followed within a few minutes by a nonspecific redness. Within a few hours—usually 24 hours—an area of redness with midpoint induration develops in the positive reactor, which may persist for 4 days or longer before fading.

INTERPRETATION OF THE HISTOPLASMIN SKIN TEST

A positive test consists of an induration of 5 mm or longer, read at 48 hours. The measure is made at the maximal transverse diameter. The peak reaction is reached in 48 to 72 hours.

A positive reaction indicates a past or present infection with *H. capsulatum* or related organisms such as *Blastomyces.* In critical illness or disseminated disease, the frequency of positives drops to about 50 percent. In epidemic situations, the rate of positivity is 100 percent.

A single skin test with histoplasmin is of limited worth in the diagnosis of early acute pulmonary infections because, as noted previously, a negative test frequently results. Repeat testing, however, may show the development of a positive skin test, which is significant. A negative result on repeated testing, in moderate illness, suggests the exclusion of histoplasmosis. In the evaluation of pulmonary nodules, a negative test in areas of high endemicity is strong evidence against *H. capsulatum* infection. A positive test, in association with a negative tuberculin test, in an area of low endemicity favors histoplasmosis.

OCCUPATIONAL HISTORY
Again, emphasis is given the history of work contacts. Suspicion of infection with *H. capsulatum* should be aroused with any work involving proximity to or the razing of abandoned chicken coops, cleaning of bridges prior to painting, spreading of topsoil in a garden, exposure to culture material in a laboratory, visits to caves or storm cellars (cave guides), digging in playgrounds (recreation directors), or major or minor excavation of soil [102].

BUSINESS TRAVEL

Since World War II contemporary commerce and international politics have made great demands for mobility on the part of executives, diplomats, and the personnel required in the establishment of new markets or the exploration for additional sites of natural resources. Travel has become an accepted way of life for innumerable employees in both the public and private sectors. From emergent diplomacy to the capping of a burning oil well, certain individuals are needed, usually with little notification and minimal time for preparation, to meet newly arisen situations.

CURRENT TRAVEL REQUIREMENTS

Travel takes a variety of modes, including flights by company, commercial, governmental, private, or chartered plane; the use of personal, government, or company automobiles; and less frequently, newly activated passenger runs by rail in the heavily trafficked East-West, North-South, or seaboard corridors or by ship. Apart from the usual demands for intracompany conferences, there are the needs for meetings and travel occasioned by the growth of conglomerates; the mergers of similar or hostile takeover of dissimilar firms; the development of new enterprises by multinational organizations; the support required of American specialists by military material and aircraft purchased by foreign powers; the establishment of sales offices worldwide; the search for sources of oil or valuable and rare minerals in undeveloped areas on land or at sea; the seeking of new customers in other countries; the growth of churches through the initiation of foreign missions; the cultural exchanges in the arts and sports; scientific expeditions in archeology, botany, entomology, zoology, and other natural science disciplines; the building of plants by American design-engineers and construction personnel; the dispatch, maintenance, and reassignment of foreign-service personnel; the replenishment of personnel in military bases and tracking stations abroad; the prolonged absence of workers in wilderness areas concerned with the extension of conduits for fuel, power, and telecommunications or with mining, forestry, weapon testing, or remote agriculture; and finally, the transport of persons who make the travel possible, such as airline crews, transcontinental truckline and busline operators, and the personnel staffing freighters and cruise ships.

Such activities have created the need for health service personnel abroad, for the international travel of occupational health specialists based in the United States, and for the knowledgeable clearance, support, and rehabilitation, when indicated, of staff persons in temporary or permanent travel status.

HEALTH CLEARANCE OF PERSONNEL

The health clearance of personnel has been covered in Chapter 7 in the discussion of the preplacement medical examination, but emphasis must be given to the careful evaluation required of persons being assigned to duty abroad. Current American education usually does not provide proficiency in foreign languages, and often assignments are made hurriedly to countries where the tongue spoken is totally strange and the time for preparation has precluded learning even commonly needed phrases. Further, there has been a certain downgrading of the so-called softer subjects in colleges and universities, so that cultural understandings of other peoples are given short shrift. Less preparation for life abroad is currently offered Peace Corps members than years back. One must be adequately grounded not only in knowledge but also in attitude.

Americans abroad tend to cluster in enclaves often provided by the multinational employer, and except for certain mandated intermixing required by the business at hand, there is little mingling or after-hours contact with the new country's nationals. The children go either to company-provided schools or to schools abroad in still different countries, and while other opportunities for personal growth arise, they do not share the experiences being gained by their parents.

Alcoholism becomes a common problem, and even the periodic vacations granted, with full travel back to the American home bases, are not sufficient to make life tolerable overseas for certain workers and their dependents. Emotional difficulties arise, and premature returns become necessary. The replacement cost is high and unquestionably disruptive to the parent organization.

Preparation for travel, though, even for short-term assignments or attendance at conferences, should include a health clearance to determine that the individual is not in the incipient stage of an illness or that there are circumstances in the worker's life that will be worsened by the absence. An examination by OHS personnel will be helpful, as will a review of the employee's immunization status. Further, the provision of a medical kit will allow self-care for most common illnesses, and counsel regarding sources of professional care will be invaluable.

AIR TRAVEL

As most travel is by air, it is germane to review first the medical criteria for passenger flying on scheduled commercial flights. In 1961, the American Medical Association and the Aerospace Medical Association published a statement jointly covering this area of need [103], and most of the material to follow is taken from that source, in addition to a more recent summary of the medical aspects of transportation aboard commercial aircraft, prepared by the American Medical Association Commission on Emergency Medical Services [104]. The criteria were to fulfill two main objectives: (1) to clarify, standardize, and establish medical measures that would expedite the transportation by air of properly selected and prepared patients and (2) to establish and clarify certain medical standards by which patients who would compromise the comfort of other passengers or who would be unable to tolerate the ordinary physiologic "stimuli" associated with flying could be disqualified from air travel.

The criteria would be equally applicable to the presumed well employee who has a history of past or chronic illness and to the company staff member who is taken ill overseas and should be returned for care and convalescence in the United States.

Much was learned during World War II and in successive actions abroad regarding air evacuation of ill and wounded service personnel. Death while in flight is a rare occurrence, and careful screening and preparation most likely would preclude this untoward event. Although airliners in flight usually are 30 to 40 minutes, at the most, from emergency landing facilities and modern centers for medical care, unscheduled landings are costly because of the need to dump thousands of gallons of fuel to permit landing within the prescribed weight limits for the plane during a normal landing.

An empiric principle followed years ago that appears still to be valid and to be of merit is that a person who looks normal, feels normal, smells normal, and can walk up the steps of a ramp can fly without likelihood of difficulty. Certain conditions associated with flight must be considered. The general disturbance caused by increased or decreased barometric pressure is termed dysbarism and includes such disorders as barotitis media, barosinusitis, aeroembolism, and aerodontalgia. Upper respiratory infections may predispose to the first two conditions, while the latter two states are not of great concern in commercial aviation. However, persons who have scuba dived should allow 12 hours to elapse between the last dive and boarding. If repeated deep diving has been undertaken, the interval should be extended to 24 hours. There may be some expansion of gases in the hollow viscera with certain gastrointestinal difficulties, and the presence of gases in the pleural cavity or mediastinum may prove serious through compression of pulmonary tissue or a mediastinal shift. Diagnostic air studies, if recent, may cause concern regarding the status of the nervous system, while hypoxia, because of the pressurization of contemporary aircraft, rarely will be a problem except in certain persons with severely impaired cardiopulmonary function or oxygen transport system.

MEDICAL CRITERIA

The medical criteria developed for passenger flying [103,104] have been divided by bodily organ system.

Cardiovascular System

Persons with minimal cardiac reserve should travel only if oxygen is immediately available. (Test: If one is able to walk 100 yards and climb 12 steps without symptoms, flight in pressurized aircraft is permissible.) Persons with a history of previous or current thrombotic or venous disease should not remain immobile for long periods during flight. Individuals should not fly until 4 weeks after a myocardial infarction or 2 weeks after a cerebrovascular accident. Severe hypertension and decompensated cardiovascular disease contraindicate flight.

Respiratory System

Asthma is not a problem. Ten days should elapse after an artificial or spontaneous pneumothorax. Pulmonary tuberculosis prior to initiation of therapy contraindicates flight because of the communicability of the disease. Individuals with a vital capacity of 50 percent or less must not fly. Persons with pulmonary secretions should be cautioned regarding the dry cabin air and hence the difficulty with coughing and expectoration. Congenital pulmonary cysts contraindicate flight.

Gastrointestinal System
A delay of 14 days is advised for air travel following a recent surgical procedure to avoid peritoneal soiling. Persons with colostomies should use larger bags during flight and carry an extra bag. Acute diverticulitis, ulcerative colitis, acute esophageal varices, and acute gastroenteritis contraindicate flight.

Neuropsychiatric Disorders
Persons with convulsive disorders are advised to use preflight sedative, have proper oxygenation during flight, and fly in pressurized craft, not to exceed a cabin altitude of 8,000 feet.

Nose and Throat Disorders
Passengers with acute respiratory infections, allergic rhinitis, or nasal polyposis should use a nasal vasoconstrictor or decongestant during flight, particularly before ascent and descent. Patients with postfracture mandibular fixation should refrain from flying unless equipped with a quick-release mechanism to avoid the possible effects of motion sickness, emesis, and aspiration. Acute sinusitis and acute otitis media contraindicate flight.

Hematologic Disorders
Hemoglobin values below 8.5 gm/100 ml and erythrocytes under 3 million contraindicate flight. Persons with sickle cell disease are advised not to fly, particularly at atmospheric altitudes above 22,500 feet, and persons with sickle cell trait may be subject to abdominal discomfort or pain and should have oxygen available during flight. Individuals with hemophilia should not fly.

Ophthalmic Conditions
Persons with recent eye injury or surgery* should not exceed 5,000-foot simulated altitude and would be advised to have oxygen available. Seeing-eye dogs appropriately muzzled and leashed are usually permitted in the passenger compartment. The blind person must be properly oriented to the aircraft to avoid confusion during an emergency.

Urinary System
Flying should be deferred 14 days after urologic surgery.

Pregnancy
There are no contraindications to flying during a normal pregnancy. If available, rear-facing seats are preferred to allow use of a loosely fastened seatbelt across the thighs, below the fetal bulge. Flight beyond 240 days into the pregnancy or during a threatened miscarriage should not be undertaken.*

Diabetes Mellitus
Diabetics have no problems with flying, provided control is good.

Communicable Disease
Persons with communicable disease are unacceptable for flight.

ALTITUDE LIMITS
Certain altitude limits have been recommended by the American College of Chest Physicians [105], and these criteria are particularly applicable to flights in unpressurized company planes, where the disease status may dictate specific limitations between 2,000 and 10,000 feet (see Welch [105]).

The following singular note relates not necessarily to health but certainly to one's perception of health as seen in anatomic perfection. An airline flight attendant who had undergone a bilateral breast augmentation recalled that prior to the operative procedure she had been involved in a decompression incident at 8,500 m, and now she was concerned about the effect of such an event on her augmentation devices. In response to a query regarding the problem [106], it was indicated that, assuming the silicone envelope was made at sea level, at 5,500 m the contained air would expand to twice its size in a flexible or elastic environment. At 9,100 m, the device would be three times its normal size. To determine the rupturability of the envelope, it would be necessary to know its strength. Even though the overlying skin is normally extremely elastic, some dis-

*Roper feels that the only contraindication to flying after eye surgery is the retention of an air bubble within the eye. As most intraocular air is dissipated by the time of hospital discharge, there should be no problem, he points out, even with rapid decompression. There should be ophthalmologic clearance before flight. (Roper, D. L., Air transportation after eye surgery. *JAMA* 247:3315, 1982.)

*Taylor (Should air hostesses continue duty during the first trimester? *Curr Med Dialog* 48:428, 1974) cautions merely against flights in unpressurized craft over 10,000 feet and advises that those women flying in pressurized commercial planes move about every 45 to 60 minutes to prevent venous stasis. (Taylor, E. S., Should air hostesses continue duty during the first trimester? *Curr Med Dialog* 48:428, 1974.)

comfort could be anticipated. It was suggested that the subject's tolerance could be determined by a carefully controlled gradual exposure in a decompression chamber. At normal cabin pressure, other flight attendants with breast augmentation had had no complaints.

FEAR OF FLYING

In all cases of illness or injury, there should be a medical evaluation before final consideration of travel by air. Mention must be made of the fear of flying. As programs have been successful in the elimination of such a phobia, referral should be effected for those persons whose business requires air travel.

TRAVELER'S KIT

A guide for physicians, *Travelers' Health Abroad,* has been published by the American Medical Association [107] in which a basic list of supplies, first-aid materials, and medications has been suggested for the traveler. It is recommended that all medicines be kept with the traveler in carry-on luggage or in a handbag and not packed with checked luggage. Medications specific to the person's needs—insulin, digitalis, antihypertensive drugs—are given particular emphasis. Adequate supplies should be taken, as the names and strengths of prescription drugs differ abroad, even in England, and there may be confusion or difficulty in obtaining refills. In fact, the same name may be used for different medications in different countries [108]. It is essential that travelers know the generic names of the medicines they use. The OHS can provide its personnel with a traveler's kit and instructions so that common symptoms or minor illnesses or injuries can be cared for by the individual.

Although travel is usually equated with an enteritis, many persons abroad, because of tension and time constraints, become constipated, so it would be wise to take along a laxative with which the traveler has had previous experience. The emphasis on American toilet paper cannot be too strong, for foreign facilities offer a variety of products from butcher paper to cut newspaper to tissue stamped "Government Property." An assaulted or protruding anal mucosa can make any trip distressful.

TRAVEL BY THE PHYSICALLY IMPAIRED

For years, commercial airlines refused to accept wheelchair-bound passengers. In the days before the use of jetways when, with insistence, plane personnel would allow such a mobility-limited person to board, the passenger would be placed on an open pallet and raised by a forklift to the doorway, with all the loss of dignity that such a maneuver could produce.

With changes in the regulations, physically impaired passengers are accepted, and considerable information is available as to areas of accessibility. In fact, special tours for the physically impaired are currently available. Airlines publish guidelines* that cover such subjects as early reservations, need for wheelchairs, preboarding, use of the *enclosed* "Handicapped *Lift,*" special orientation for persons who are blind, seat selection, special meals, oxygen requirements, and stretcher service. The new 767s being placed in service will have a complete system to meet the needs of the impaired traveler in the form of on-board aisle wheelchairs. Such passengers will be able to transfer from their own wheelchairs at the entry into the plane and use the aisle wheelchairs to get to their seats and to move to and from the lavatories. Four seats with movable armrests on the aisle will facilitate the chair-to-seat transfer. One oversized lavatory will allow easy accessibility through use of a large door and built-in convenience devices.

At the time of making flight reservations, hotels can be selected so that special accommodations can be arranged simultaneously for a nonslip bathtub, wheelchair-height toilet bowls, grab rails, or sliding bathroom doors.

To provide definitive information for impaired travelers, the Federal Aviation Administration of the Department of Transportation, has published *Guide to Accessibility of Terminals—Access Travel: Airports* [109], which provides design features, facilities, and services at 282 airport terminals in 40 countries. The same information is available commercially in the North American Edition of the *Travel Planner & Hotel/Motel Guide.*†

Many cities have published handbooks that provide similar but less detailed information regarding their facilities. One such example is *Access Washington—A Guide to Metropolitan Washington for the Physically Disabled.*‡ [110]. A special magazine, *The Itinerary,*§ is published specifically for "traveling with physical disabilities." It would be as helpful to

*An example is *Air Travel for the Handicapped,* published by TWA (Aug. 1981).

†Published by Official Airline Guides, 2000 Clearwater Drive, Oak Brook, IL 60521.

‡A single brochure, *International Directory of Access Guides,* published by Rehabilitation International USA Inc., of 20 West 40th Street, New York, NY 10018, lists several such handbooks from around the world.

§Published by Robert S. and Elizabeth C. Zyewicki, P.O. Box 1084, Bayonne, NJ 07002-1084.

the business traveler as it is to the person with a limitation who is undertaking recreational travel.

TRAVEL HAZARDS

It is not the intention here to discuss at length the extremely wide variety of diseases that one may acquire during travel abroad. Some disorders can be averted by specific immunizations, while others can be avoided through care in diet, sanitation, personal hygiene, or limitation of unnecessary exposure. But certain diseases have been acquired by travelers, some within the United States, including plague [111], cholera [112], amebiasis [113], cryptosporidiosis [114], malaria [115–117], hepatitis [118,119], shigellosis [120], diphyllobothriasis [121,122], giardiasis [123–126], brucellosis [127], dengue fever [128–130], typhoid fever [131–132], meningococcal meningitis [133], tungiasis [134], schistosomiasis [135–137], acquisition of cutaneous larva migrans [138], and ciquatera fish poisoning [139]. These diseases are entities separate from the disorders acquired while on cruise ships or from toxic sources traceable to air travel.

Accustomed as most business and industrial personnel are to the emphasis given safety as a way of doing business in the United States, these same expectations do not hold when in many foreign countries. Streets and sidewalks abound in potholes, rocky paths frequently are the only ingress to certain areas, handrails may be missing, if ever having been installed, native driving patterns course between armed warfare and total disregard of other users of public roadways, and irreparable breakdown of mobile equipment can be anticipated. Frequently, because of the absence of porters, one must carry heavy luggage or throw it out the windows of trains with the hope that it can be retrieved. Obviously, care should be exerted to avoid these common physical hazards.

Psychological pressures are everywhere. English is not spoken universally, and we are essentially a monolingual people. Too many travelers are victims of the "if-its-Tuesday-it-must-be-Belgium" syndrome* and endeavor to crowd an excessive number of activities into a time frame shrunken by innumerable hotel registrations, packings, and departures. Nighttime activities interfere with normal rest cycles. Strange cuisines are challenging at best and, although may not prove to be pathogenic, can be assaultive of otherwise well-tuned digestive tracts. In addition, there is usually more consumption of food and alcoholic beverages while traveling than is customary. Interactions with the concierge, the hotel clerk, the bus driver, the harried airline agent are not always pleasant, and it is not uncommon to be served after local residents' needs are met in restaurants. While we provide bi- or trilingual travel or shopping instructions in such places as Hawaii and the West Coast, important signs abroad usually are limited to the tongue of the country. But, then, if one wishes not to have the enriching experience of travel, one can stay home.

Food poisoning aboard aircraft is not unknown, *Staphylococcus aureus* being the causative pathogen in several reported episodes [140–143]. It is not passenger aircrafts solely that offer the enteric hazard to travelers. During the 1970s, many cruise ships had comparable problems. In late 1973, a survey was conducted by the CDC of cruise ships, and it was learned that 2 to 10 percent of passengers experienced a gastrointestinal illness [144].* Organisms identified as etiologic agents in various reports have included *Salmonella bareilly* and *Salmonella senftenberg*, [145], *Shigella flexneri* [146], *Vibrio parahaemolyticus* [147,148], and the Norwalk virus [149], and in one instance, trichinosis was confirmed [150].

Additional episodes have been reported [151–155] with *Salmonella heidelberg* and enterotoxigenic *Escherichia coli* as the offenders, and staphylococcal food poisoning on a cruise ship out of the United States was reported as late as 1983 [156].

TURISTA—ON LAND

Most disturbing to travelers is diarrheal disease acquired during visits to countries south of our border, particularly Mexico. That such terms as Delhi belly, Casablanca crud, Malta dog, the trotsky's (in Russia), Tokyo trots, gippy tummy, G.I.s, Poona pooks, tourist trots, squitters, Mexican two-step, rangoon runs, the Hong Kong dog, the Aztec two-step, and Montezuma's revenge [157], among others equally illiterative and more scatalogic and unprintable, have been coined has not been without cause. Opprobrious designations result usually from experiences common to many and lingering in memory. Nonvulgar terms have been used for this acute gastroenteritis—traveler's diarrhea, tourist's diarrhea, toxigenic

*A tour group was encountered in a funicular on Capri. A passenger was asked where he had been, and in order to respond, he turned to his wife, as he had lost track of yesterday's points of visitation.

*A case of gastrointestinal illness was defined as the onset of at least one of the following: (a) diarrhea, (b) cramps and one other gastrointestinal symptom, (c) gastrointestinal illness or disorder, (d) gastroenteritis, (e) enteritis, (f) enterocolitis, or (g) any illness for which antidiarrheal medication was prescribed.

turista, and emporiatric enteritis—the one title now used in most publications being traveler's diarrhea. "High-risk" areas include Central and South America, Africa, the Middle East, and southern Southeast Asia.

Travelers have acquired the disease either while en route abroad or have had symptoms delayed until returning home. It varies in intensity from mild to severe and may be markedly incapacitating for several days. The disease is given its accurate description in this paraphrased retelling of the early stages of the malady by a member of the research team involved in a study of traveler's diarrhea [158]:

> The following clinical description of a tourist was provided by a patient who was also a member of our team; on the day prior to the actual onset of illness he felt a slight malaise, but had 2 normal stools.
>
> At 4 a.m. he awakened with a start, desperately aware that he was about to move his bowels. He traversed the bed-to-bathroom distance in what must have been record time, and relieved himself of a totally watery bowel movement which was accompanied by slight "transverse colon" cramps. The patient returned to bed in a stunned state, only to discover that no sooner had he arrived that he was constrained to leave again, with uncustomary alacrity. This staccato ballet continued at 15-minute intervals with the patient exhibiting progressive weakness, profound malaise, increasingly severe cramps, almost constant nausea, and several episodes of vomiting.

It is now generally accepted that heat-labile toxigenic strains of *E. coli* are an important cause of turista [159–161]. *Shigella, Salmonella,* and *V. parahaemolyticus* are offenders still, comprising a group of multiple etiologies, pointing up the fact that the entity is not a single disease. Many medications have been advised prophylactically and therapeutically, but the success of each wanes with time. As most pretravel inquiries relate to prevention, it is suggested that the guidance given be current and the medications recommended be free of untoward complications.

The essence of prevention, however, lies in certain dietary and personal hygiene precautions, as follows [162]:

Eat only foods that have been cooked and that are served "piping" hot.
Eat only fruits that one must peel oneself, and avoid fresh salads and leafy green vegetables.
Avoid eating establishments that obviously lack good sanitary practices.
Drink only boiled water. Bottled water is not permitted, for it has been contaminated. Soft drinks and beer can be taken if bottled.
Use no ice in drinks.
Do not brush one's teeth with tap water.
Do not consume unpasteurized milk and milk products.
Never eat the food products offered by street vendors.
Avoid cream-containing desserts, fresh cheese, assorted cold meats, and foods including previously boiled, cold seafood.
Use no spicy sauces in an open container on the table.
Avoid meals aboard a plane leaving a high-risk area, for the food undoubtedly was obtained locally.
Eat only in establishments suggested by previous visitors who believed them to be safe.
Do not eat *any* meat, especially pork, unless it is well done.
Never eat raw shellfish or raw fish anywhere in the world.
Never eat crabs, snails, or crayfish in Asia, Africa, India or South America.

It must be pointed out that in an epidemiologic study [163–165] involving interviews with over 16,500 air passengers en route home, there seemed to be little difference in occurrence of traveler's diarrhea between those persons undergoing dietary self-restraint while abroad and the individuals exercising few or no restrictions in food or water intake/contact. As the authors [163] expressed it, ". . . diarrhea seemed to occur more frequently the more a person tried to elude it!" They concluded that the traditional nutritional recommendations for prophylaxis seemed to be unrealistic and usually unsuccessful.

Because of the ongoing debate concerning prophylaxis, early treatment, the risk of antimicrobial agents, the usefulness of currently employed treatment regimens, and whether certain groups of travelers should be advised selectively to follow certain regimens, the National Institutes of Health Office of Medical Applications of Research and the National Institute of Allergy convened a Consensus Development Conference on Traveler's Diarrhea from January 28 to 30, 1985. The panel involved a broad stripe of specialists and lay representatives [166]. An effort was made to answer specific questions, and the following statement summarizes the deliberations in relation to prevention: Meticulous attention must be given food and beverage preparation, and prophylactic antimicrobial agents are not recommended.

PRETRAVEL IMMUNIZATION AND PROPHYLAXIS

Ordinarily, no vaccinations are required for *direct* travel from the United States to most countries, but certain immunizations are required by some countries in Africa, Asia, and French Guinea in South America.

A service being used throughout the United States, Canada, and Europe is Immunization Alert,* which provides a computer-based information system for international travel. The material is updated weekly from information obtained from the WHO and CDC. The data base is available in both diskette and printed formats and provides the most current indications for immunizations by country and the sites of visitation where malaria prophylaxis is advised. Individual reports for travelers are available on a fee basis.

SMALLPOX

Many physicians believe that the risk of complications associated with smallpox vaccination is greater than the risk of smallpox, so that they will give their traveling patients a note stating that the procedure is medically contraindicated. Such a statement should be given on the physician's letterhead, dated and signed.

It is the belief of the Public Health Service [167] that there are no medical reasons for smallpox vaccination for international travel, and in fact the PHS ended that requirement August 14, 1978 [168]. Such precaution is indicated only for laboratory workers directly involved with smallpox or related viruses such as monkeypox and vaccinia.

CHOLERA

Vaccination against cholera is not recommended for travelers to countries not requiring an International Certificate of Vaccination Against Cholera as a condition for entry. Synder and Blake [169] have calculated that the chance of a United States citizen, who is returning to this country by a commercial air carrier from Asia, Africa, and Oceania, acquiring a reported case of cholera is less than 1 case per 500,000 returning travelers. Only 10 cases have occurred among United States returned travelers since the current pandemic (*Vibrio cholerae* 01 El Tor) began in 1961.

Vaccines are only about 50-percent effective in reducing clinical illness for 3 to 6 months, and they do not prevent transmission of infection. Avoidance of contaminated food and water is the best protection.

YELLOW FEVER

For purposes of international travel, the vaccine for yellow fever immunization must be WHO-approved and administered at a designated yellow fever vaccination center. Information regarding such centers can be obtained from local health departments.

Countries vary as to requirements for vaccination certification, but the immunization is recommended for travel to infected areas, usually limited to parts of Africa and South America, and for those persons traveling outside the urban areas of countries in the "yellow fever endemic zones." As the countries requiring yellow fever immunization differ so widely in their specifications, it is recommended that such sources as the CDC or WHO be consulted. The desiderata are at such variance as to the countries transited before arrival, the countries of origin, and so forth, that a listing would be both inadequate and dated. See particularly *Vaccination Certificate Requirements and Health Advice for International Travel,* published by the WHO.*

PLAGUE

Vaccination against plague is not required for entry by any country. Where plague has been reported, the cases have appeared in rural mountainous or upland areas. Immunization against plague should be considered only for persons who will have direct contact with wild rodents or rabbits in areas where plague is enzootic or for persons residing in such areas where avoidance of rodents and fleas is impossible. The vaccination is recommended for laboratory personnel working regularly with *Yersina pestis* organisms or plague-infected rodents.

OTHER DISEASES—NONQUARANTINABLE

The risk to international travelers of trypanosomiasis, dengue fever, giardiasis, and fassa fever is considered small, even though, as noted previously, infrequent cases are reported.

MALARIA

Because of the potential severity of malaria, all travelers, irrespective of age, who are going to risk areas should take prophylactic medication, even if the visit is as brief as one night. Additional precautions that should be taken include the use of mosquito netting during sleep, adequate clothing coverage outdoors, and the application of an effective insect repellent that should contain *N,N*-diethyltoluamide (deet) as the active ingredient [170]. Also, a pyrethrum-containing flying-insect spray is advised for use in living and sleeping areas during evening and nighttime hours.

*Immunization Alert, P.O. Box 406, Storrs, CT 06268, (203) 487-0422.

*Available from WHO Regional Office for the Americas, 525 23rd Street NW, Washington, DC, 20037, (202) 861-3200.

Areas of Risk
Specific information regarding areas of risk within countries, the months of risk, and other pertinent geographic data is available from Chief, Malaria Branch, Parasitic Diseases Division, Center for Infectious Diseases, CDC, Atlanta, Georgia 30333.

Prophylaxis
Irrespective of the prophylactic regimen used against malaria, travelers must be informed that malaria can still be contracted [171]. The symptoms of the disease—fever with chills and headache—demand immediate medical attention and should not be ascribed to a "flu-like" illness. In an endemic area, symptoms can appear early, even 8 days after initial exposure and can occur months after leaving a malarious area, even after chemoprophylaxis has ceased. Delays in treatment cannot be rationalized, for there can be serious or even fatal consequences [171].

For information concerning medications for use in the prevention of malaria, contact should be made with the CDC's Malaria Branch noted previously.

HEPATITIS
As the risk of hepatitis A may be greater for persons remaining 3 or more months in tropical areas or developing countries where the disease is prevalent, it is advised that some protection be obtained through the use of immune globulin (IG). Those individuals remaining abroad face a persisting risk and should have repeated injections, as needed.

OTHER IMMUNIZATIONS
Prophylaxis against other infectious diseases has been discussed earlier. However, Barrett-Connor [172] believes that additional, seldom mentioned vaccines should be given. She recommends oral polio vaccine for previously immunized persons and individuals under 18 years of age, particularly if they are headed for a developing country. Travelers over age 18 who have not been immunized previously against polio should receive parenteral polio vaccine. The same destination should indicate typhoid vaccination or a booster injection, using the preparation without the paratyphoid antigen that had such debilitating side effects. Finally, all travelers should have adequate protection against tetanus.

As many travelers allow their immunization status to lapse, there will often be the need to obtain multiple vaccinations simultaneously. One can give cholera and hepatitis B vaccines or influenza vaccine and combined tetanus and diphtheria toxoids at the same time at different injection sites. As Orenstein and Brink [173] expressed it, there is no good evidence that any inactivated vaccine or toxoid such as hepatitis, cholera, typhoid, rabies, plague, influenza, tetanus, diphtheria, pneumococcal polysaccharide, or inactivated polio will interfere with the immune response to another. However, because theoretically certain side effects might be accentuated, those vaccines associated with frequent local or systemic reactions—typhoid, plague, and cholera—should be administered on separated occasions if possible [173].

Generally live vaccines such as measles, mumps, rubella, oral polio, and yellow fever and an inactivated vaccine can be given simultaneously, except for cholera and yellow fever vaccines. These two should be separated by about 2 weeks.

Immune globulin should not interfere with the immune response to inactivated vaccines and toxoids or to yellow fever and oral polio given on the same day. There may be interference with the immune response to measles, mumps, or rubella, and these latter vaccines should be administered at least 2 weeks before or at least 6 weeks—preferably 3 months—after immune globulin [173].

MOTION SICKNESS

Some persons are troubled by transport in many common vehicles, including automobiles and elevators, or when descending a tight spiral driveway into an underground commercial parking garage. The DuPonts [174] advised these precautions while flying.

Avoid seats on the port side of the plane, as most turns seem to be made to the left.
Select or request an aisle seat at the base of the wing. This location will limit the view but will provide greater stability.
Take a light meal before departure.
Use some motion sickness medication to reduce the effects of turbulence.
Avoid the consumption of alcohol before and during flight, but do increase fluid before and during flight.
Do not read or watch the horizon.

While most medication used to prevent motion sickness is taken orally, to depress or reduce labyrinthine function or sensitivity, scopolamine is available currently as an adhesive unit, for use about 2 to 3 hours prior to travel.

When using oral preparations, it should be remembered that there may be a sedative or soporific effect, which should preclude vehicle operation immediately upon landing. Other precautions during flight have been mentioned such as avoidance of "gas-producing" foods and the wearing in flight of loose-fitting clothing.

JET LAG

The syndrome known as jet lag, the time-zone blahs, travel dysrhythmia, or as termed in a good health guide for travelers, circadian desynchronization [174] is a familiar phenomenon to travelers who have been crossing the time zones since the introduction of jet planes. Flight at 40,000 feet with an outside temperature of −55°F and a barometric pressure of less than 3 psi has become common experience. As indicated, pressurization has compensated for most of the potential hazards and physiologic disruptions, but disturbance of the several biologic clocks has seen no fast remedy. The rapid transit through the time belts has affected every flying person's decision-making, reaction time, and alertness. Other symptoms of the disorder include fatigue, headache, and dulled alertness, which can proceed to a true feeling of detachment from reality.

In an effort to conserve time and costs, executives, conference speakers, diplomats, and politicians are thrown into situations demanding of critical decisions following long flights east-west or west-east. Individuals on prescribed medications face problems because of the body's greater sensitivity to drugs at certain periods of the 24-hour cycle, partly because of different rates of excretion and cortical activity [175]. Medications to be considered are insulin, steroids, digitalis, diuretics, thyroid preparations, anticonvulsive drugs, and quinidine.

Certain precautions can be taken by the average traveler who, not being a delegated representative of his or her country, has no skilled planners preparing an itinerary that can account for appropriate departure and arrival times and judicious scheduling of important conferences with world leaders. While psychological adjustment may take place quickly, the body's functions such as the sleep-wake cycle, digestion, temperature regulation, pulse rate, renal function, hormone levels, alertness, and fatigue continue in a cycle—circadian rhythm—in parallel with the day-night change to which the traveler is accustomed. Any difference in the time of 4 hours or more will require a compensatory rest period.

Mohler, Dille, and Gibbons [176] concluded in a study of long-distance flights that the time-zone fatigue, or jet lag, cannot be prevented entirely but can be ameliorated. As rhythm rephasing will take several days, it was suggested that departure on an east-west or west-east trip be undertaken in as rested a physical state as possible and that a day following arrival be devoted to rephasing of cycles before beginning the demanding and often fatiguing activities involved in international travel. If such resting is not possible, flights should be scheduled to allow arrival before nightfall and a good night's sleep.

Long-distance travelers should pace themselves during asynchrony to reduce biologic and mental strain. Heavy increases in rich and noncustomary foods and alcohol, usual concomitants of travel abroad, should be avoided, as these are stressors in themselves and combined with the cycle disturbance are doubly tiring. Since physical fatigue is one of the best inducers of sleep, exercise would be beneficial in permitting sleep at local times before "normal" bedtimes. Nightclub tours should be avoided for 24 hours.

It has been recommended in recent years that one prepare several days in advance for rhythm disruptions, by going to bed 1 hour earlier for each hour to be lost going east or 1 hour later for each hour to be gained traveling west. Also, one can attempt this pattern change by going to bed earlier or later in increments of 1 hour each night prior to travel so that by the time of departure one is on the schedule of the travel destination.

HOTEL FIRE PRECAUTIONS

Because of the increased frequency of hotel fires in both urban and resort areas, it would be wise to familiarize business travelers with certain precautions to be taken that could be lifesaving. The procedures are given in Appendix 8-1 [177], How to Survive a Hotel Fire.

MEDICAL CARE ABROAD

An invaluable document for travelers that has been available for many years is the Medical Passport,* which is an individual medical record contained in a double-pocket plastic wallet, large enough to hold one's official passport and travel tickets [178–180]. In the loose-leaf booklet there is space for entry of the following data: identifying information, emergency information (diabetes, allergies, serum sensitivity), active immunizations, medical history and diagnostic summaries, findings on most recent physical examination, laboratory test results, radiographic

*The Medical Passport is available from the Medical Passport Foundation, Inc., P.O. Box 820, Whitehair Building, 104 East New York Avenue, Florida 32720.

findings, ECG results, most recent dental radiographs, eyeglass or contact lens prescription, current treatment, unfinished business, and some counsel for travelers.

Such a document will give pertinent medical information immediately to a health care provider in the event of illness or injury and will either obviate the need for duplicate and costly test procedures or provide a baseline of test results for comparison. Further, it highlights instantly certain allergic states so that the use of hazardous medications will be averted. The Medical Passport has been used by business executives in the United States, missionaries, representatives to the United Nations, and international corporation personnel.

To obtain information regarding sources of medical care throughout the world, one should make contact with the International Association for Medical Assistance to Travellers (IAMAT).* There is no charge for an IAMAT membership. IAMAT regularly publishes a directory that provides, by country and city, the names, addresses, and telephone numbers of medical institutions—hospitals, clinics, nursing homes, sanitaria—and the names of either the medical directors of such centers or the IAMAT coordinators. All personnel listed are English-speaking and have agreed to an established fee schedule, with charges varying for office calls, hotel calls, and night, Sunday, and local holiday calls. IAMAT also provides, in a large group of folders (World Climate Charts), information regarding altitude, monthly average high and low ambient temperatures, the sanitary condition of water, milk, and food, and advisable clothing for wear in nearly 1,500 parts of the world. Also, information can be obtained regarding malaria risk, several tropical diseases, and the immunizations required abroad.

In addition, IAMAT provides a four-page "Traveler Clinical Record" for entry of pertinent medical information, which can prove to be invaluable during emergent situations when traveling abroad. The blocks for recording include identifying information, photograph, emergency medical data, prescription for glasses, diagnostic summary, immunization record; if the person has diabetes, daily insulin requirements and urine-sugar-ketones analysis record; if the person is on anticoagulant medication, prothrombin time test and anticoagulant dosage record; and if the traveler has an allergic disorder, hyposensitization treatment record. A fairly comparable form, "Personal Health Record," is available from the Metropolitan Life Insurance Company.* Additional information includes names of the traveler's physicians, dentist, and pharmacist, company and number of health insurance policies, family history, record of periodic examinations, and travel outside the United States.

A worldwide directory of participating foreign physicians in over 200 cities is obtainable also from INTERMEDIC.† At no cost, the American Academy of Family Physicians‡ will provide a list of physicians in family practice in areas in the United States.

The Medical Advisory Services for Travelers Abroad (MASTA)§ provides an interesting service, using material from a data base validated by the London School of Hygiene and Tropical Medicine, Bureau of Hygiene and Tropical Diseases. For various fees, health briefs are provided at several levels (basic, concise, executive, updates, and families and groups) that give the information needed in the area of prevention—immunizations, medications, descriptions of relevant diseases, and the like. An application form provides space for entry of countries to be visited, immunization status, allergies, and other related information.

When executives travel abroad and become ill, corporate medical directors usually will be called, and arrangements for care or transport home will be made through known medical personnel in the cities where the company has either sales offices, plants, or representatives. Infrequently the physician will have to go abroad and accompany the ill person back to the United States.

Usually the larger hotels are familiar with local physicians and specialists and can arrange for professional visits. Other sources of information would be the United States embassies or consulates or installations of the armed services. It would be wise to obtain from the State Department the locations of such facilities if one will be staying in a foreign country beyond just a period of transit.

It should be determined before departure if one's health insurance is applicable in foreign countries. If so, the required forms should be taken along.

*IAMAT means "to cure," in Greek. IAMAT is located at 736 Center Street, Lewiston, New York 14092, (716) 754-4883.

*Metropolitan Life Insurance Company, 1 Madison Avenue, New York, NY 10010.

†INTERMEDIC, 777 Third Ave., New York, NY 10017, (212) 486-8900.

‡American Academy of Family Physicians, 1740 West 92nd Street, Kansas City, MO 64114, (816) 333-9700.

§The Medical Advisory Services for Travelers Abroad, Keppel St., London, England WCIE 7HT (01 631 4408).

Several commercial companies provide a variety of insurance packages covering medical care, transportation in the event of illness or death, and if necessary during medical evaluation, services of a health professional for travelers abroad. The benefits and costs vary. Most insurance agents can indicate the pertinent carriers.

COMPANY-PROVIDED INFORMATION

The International Division of Mobil Oil Corporation prepares for its personnel a series of "Location Data Questionnaires," some 47, one for each country or area where its personnel may be involved. Detailed information is sought and updated periodically, so that company representatives being transferred or in travel status for brief periods can be prepared for local customs, amenities, costs, and facilities. The information provided covers regulations, housing, household effects, shopping, clothing, automobiles, the community, climate, recreation, and other considerations. Such detail provided in advance will aid in coping with any culture shock and may obviate a premature return to the United States.

WORKING ABROAD

Business or related activities will take many American nationals abroad for periods of different duration, depending on the nature of the assignment, the mission of the parent organization, and the focus of the trip or stay. The frequency, intensity, or duration of contact with the personnel encountered in the foreign countries will test the individual's skill in adjusting to or coping with the mores and ethos encountered in strange lands.

Work overseas involves U.S. government employees, government contract personnel, private business enterprises, scholars on sabattical leave, students—exchange or for 1 year or more—and personnel of international organizations, voluntary agencies, and philanthropic foundations. Other individuals seek employment in foreign countries or are self-employed abroad. Besides these groups, members of various branches of the armed services are stationed throughout the globe.

As indicated by a Group for the Advancement of Psychiatry (GAP) study of some years ago [181], "... The mental health of the U.S. citizen working abroad has special significance. His individual state of well-being and the quality of his social relationships are most important. He must have a capacity for successful communication and collaboration with persons from widely differing cultures, as well a capacity to maintain his own emotional well-being for prolonged periods in conditions quite alien to him." While many persons fit well into the new areas of operations, other assignees may develop psychophysiologic problems, become substance abusers, or end suicidally. Symptoms of maladjustment are seen in frequent requests for transfer, premature return to the United States with the job unfinished, general dissatisfaction or disaffection, quarreling with colleagues, impaired job performance, increased and increasing absenteeism, disloyalty, or flouting of organizational regulations.

New stressors appear in the form of climatic extremes, totally different value systems, inequities among classes of foreign nationals, lack of knowledge of basic sanitary or health principles, and an inability to speak the language of the host country. The GAP study underscores the elements of a move [181]: "Even the well-integrated person sent overseas is likely, especially at first, to have a sense of geographical dislocation or isolation, a feeling of being 'out of things'; he often finds an intensified need for communication with home, a sense of frustration over the inevitable slowness of establishing the feeling of 'belonging' locally, and a feeling of boredom brought about by the monotony and limitations of social life." The individual destined for success abroad is one with the following qualities [181]: flexibility, personal stability, social maturity, a skill of social inventiveness, possession of fewer prejudices or a greater awareness of them, and the ability to tolerate the targets of their prejudice.

Many individuals go overseas expecting and believing all of the grandiose, colorful, idealized descriptions and potential rewards. True, they may have joined to "see the world," but they may see it from the insufferable cavern of the engine room. Much distance frequently exists between the promises of the new assignment and the realities of the equatorial life. Recruiters paint too wonderful a picture of the job abroad, often totally out of phase with the stark truths of life in the anticipated tropical paradise. When expectations are shattered, often the American national abroad ends up with deep feelings of hostility toward the foreign country, bitterness, and resentment of the parent company that failed to give the person transferred a fair picture of the new assignment.

When hostility or prejudice arises, it frequently is a recrudescence of feelings that the individual had in the home country, but because of social, geographic, political, or business constraints, they were kept under control or were unexpressed. The situation seems to resemble the course of events undergone during severe bodily injury or a serious illness that leaves the victim with a marked physical impairment. The person who weathers the trauma, survives with a wholesome outlook, and is able to cope with the newly acquired limitations usually is the one who was well integrated before the major derailment. Those patients unable to recover and who manifest debilitating personality deficits are those individuals who previously manifested serious behavioral problems. The GAP report mentioned previously points up the ideal method in adjustment [181]:

> It seems apparent that the ways in which the important work is done overseas and the quality of personal relationships developed by the people doing it, are bound to affect public relations between the United States and the host country. Ordinarily, patient exploration on both sides and mutual forebearance are required for good cross-cultural social relations. Gradually the image of each has of the other may become realistic instead of preformed and biased; gradually the personal experience may outweigh the stereotyped preconception, and mutually satisfying friendships may emerge.

Lastly, reference must be made to certain persons who are travel addicts, who seem to embark constantly on crisis flights. If there are employees who are ever "on the go," who attend an inordinate number of conferences away from home, one should determine if there are certain emotional situations at home from which they are escaping. The Travelers Aid Society became aware some years ago of chronic movers who could not tolerate "non-motion." These individuals, as explained by Schultz [182], are like the alcoholic or other substance abuser, who is trying to escape from reality, but instead take flight in space and time. This quality may be desirable in cross-country truck drivers, and may be afforded by the jet set, but when it afflicts an executive, it should be investigated so that some insight into the underlying personal problem can be obtained.

PHYSICIANS ON PROFESSIONAL TRAVEL

Many physicians or other personnel engaged in the practice of occupational health enjoy visiting medical directors or their disciplinary counterparts in the United States or abroad to undergo personal growth or to become apprised of new programmatic developments that could be adapted to their own activities at home. On the reverse side, many of us in this country have entertained visitors from abroad who were curious about certain aspects of either our in-plant programs or our training efforts for young physicians. No one has ever developed a particular protocol for visitations, but it has been expressed by some visitors to the United States that they had been given excessive amounts of hospitality whenever they had stopped and, as a consequence, were exhausted.

In a pointed writing, Gross [183] laid out some guidelines, and they are abstracted for those physicians who would like to visit colleagues overseas—or even in this country. In precis, the counsel was as follows:

Write a letter of personal introduction in advance, identifying the physician (or other person), giving some reference to his or her background, studies, present position, and sponsors of the visit.

Outline the purpose of the visit, and for future use, request the name, address, and telephone number of the person with whom one should make contact on arrival.

One should be familiar with the published works, the program in operation, or the project currently engaging the interest of the person or center to be visited.

It is helpful to have reviewed briefly the social customs, history, geography, and language of the country to be visited.

Appointments should be kept promptly, as considerable time is spent by the host in arranging itineraries, and if a change of plan is unavoidable, the host should be informed immediately.

Photographs should be taken only after seeking permission, particularly if one is in an industrial plant where production processes are in operation.

Do not request lodging or meals; if the host wishes to make accommodations available, the offer will be made.

The visitor should go to learn and not to teach, for he or she is the guest; advice should be offered only when requested, and no criticism should be offered, particularly of the kind that smacks of things "better at home."

As soon as possible, a letter of thanks should be written; the notes most appreciated are the ones sent at the end of the visit or from the next stopping point.

Finally, a single day's visit is productive; time after that initial stay may encroach on the host's schedule.

It frequently is advisable to seek counsel from one's hosts in foreign countries as to the sites or persons not to be missed. The opinions held abroad of certain practitioners may be at variance with the views of them held locally, and on-the-spot guidance may prove to be invaluable.

WORKERS' COMPENSATION

Frequently, the question of compensability arises when an employee on travel status is injured. Larson [184] summarizes the rules and pertinent decisions as follows: "Employees whose work entails travel away from the employer's premises are held in the majority of jurisdictions to be within the course of their employment continuously during the trip, except when a distinct departure on a personal errand is shown. Thus, injuries arising out of the necessity of sleeping in hotels or eating in restaurants away from home are usually held compensable."

REFERENCES

1. General recommendations on immunization. *MMWR* 32:1, 1983.
2. Adult immunization: Recommendations of the Immunization Practices Advisory Committee (ACIP). *MMWR* (Suppl 33):1S, 1984.
3. California Department of Public Health Ad Hoc Committee on Smallpox Vaccination. Change in smallpox vaccination policy. *Calif Med* 116:108, 1972.
4. Tizes, R. Discontinuance of routine smallpox vaccination. *JAMA* 219:908, 1972.
5. Huntley, A. C. Discontinuance of routine smallpox vaccination. *JAMA* 219:909, 1972.
6. Folge, W. H. Discontinuance of routine smallpox vaccination. *JAMA* 219:909, 1972.
7. Shaw, E. B. Discontinuation of routine smallpox vaccination. *Calif Med* 116:73, 1972.
8. Chin, J. Discontinuation of routine smallpox vaccination. *Calif Med* 116:68, 1972.
9. Tizes, R. Discontinuance of routine smallpox vaccination. *JAMA* 221:1521, 1972.
10. Piszczek, E. A., Lull, G. F., Stebbins, E. L., et al. Smallpox vaccination. *JAMA* 222:1185, 1972.
11. White, F. P. Vaccination at issue. *Med Trib* 7:5, July 9, 1973.
12. Smallpox vaccine. *MMWR* 34:341, 1985.
13. Smallpox vaccine no longer available for civilians—United States. *MMWR* 32:387, 1983.
14. Contact spread of vaccines from a recently vaccinated marine—Louisiana. *MMWR* 33:37, 1984.
15. Contact spread of vaccines from a National Guard vaccine—Wisconsin. *MMWR* 34:182, 1985.
16. Vaccinia outbreak—Nevada. *MMWR* 32:403, 1983.
17. Vaccinia necrosum after smallpox vaccination—Michigan. *MMWR* 31:501, 1982.
18. Smith, G. W. The eradication of smallpox. *N Engl J Med* 304:735, 1981.
19. Investigation of a smallpox rumor—Mexico. *MMWR* 34:343, 1985.
20. Khodakevich, L., and Arita, J. Investigating rumors of smallpox. *World Health Forum* 6:171, 1985.
21. Diphtheria, tetanus, and pertussis: Guidelines for vaccine prophylaxis and other preventive measures. *MMWR* 34:405, 1985.
22. Myers, K. J., Heppell, J., Bode, W. E., et al. Tetanus after anorectal abscess. *Mayo Clin Proc* 59:429, 1984.
23. Furste, W. Tetanus immunization booster intervals. *JAMA* 253:841, 1985.
24. Tetanus immunity in the elderly—A Los Angeles County Study. *Public Health Letter* (Los Angeles County Department of Health Services) 4:1, 1982.
25. Warshaw, L. J. Liability in refusal of tetanus toxoid booster injection. *J Occup Med* 11:689, 1969.
26. Barnes, A. M., Quan, T. J., and Poland, J. D. Plague in the United States, 1984. *CDC Surveill Summ* 34:955, 1985.
27. Plague pneumonia—California. *MMWR* 33:481, 1984.
28. Plague—South Carolina. *MMWR* 32:417, 1983.
29. Plague precautions. *Public Health Letter* (Los Angeles County Department of Health Services) 6:22, 1984.
30. Summary of First Meeting of Ad Hoc Committee, National Plague Prevention and Control, February 22–23, 1984, Santa Fe, New Mexico. Fort Collins, CO, Department of Health and Human Services, Public Health Service, Centers for Disease Control, 1984.
31. Rocky Mountain spotted fever—United States, 1984. *MMWR* 34:195, 1985.
32. Hattwick, M. A. W., O'Brien, R. J., and Hanson, B. F. Rocky Mountain spotted fever: Epidemiology of an increasing problem. *Ann Intern Med* 84:732, 1976.
33. Sexton, D. J., Gallis, H. A., McRae, J. R., et al. Possible needle-associated Rocky Mountain spotted fever. *N Engl J Med* 292:645, 1975.
34. Calia, F. M., Bartelloni, P. J., and McKinney, R. W. Rocky Mountain spotted fever: Laboratory infection in a vaccinated individual. *JAMA* 311:2012, 1970.
35. Massachusetts Department of Public Health. On the alert for Rocky Mountain spotted fever. *N Engl J Med* 292:1127, 1975.
36. D'Angelo, L. J. Rocky Mountain spotted fever tick control. *JAMA* 239:1661, 1978.
37. Weidhaas, D. E. Rocky Mountain Spotted Fever Vaccine. *JAMA* 239:1661, 1978.
38. Annual Summary 1983: Reported morbidity and mortality in the United States. *MMWR* 32:114, 1984.
39. Rabies Prevention—United States, 1984. *MMWR* 33:393, 1984.
40. Marwick, C. Changes recommended in use of human diploid cell rabies vaccine. *JAMA* 254:13, 1985.
41. Ajjan, N., Soulebot, J. P., Trian, R., et al. Intradermal immunization with rabies vaccine: Inactivated

Wistar strain cultivated in human diploid cells. *JAMA* 244:2528, 1980.
42. Bernard, K. W., Roberts, M. A., Sumner, J., et al. Human diploid cell rabies vaccine: Effectiveness of immunization with small intradermal or subcutaneous doses. *JAMA* 247:1138, 1982.
43. Burridge, M. J., Raer, G. M., Sumner, J. W., et al. Intradermal immunization with human diploid cell rabies vaccine. *JAMA* 248:1611, 1982.
44. Supplementary statement on pre-exposure rabies prophylaxis by the intradermal route. *MMWR* 31:279, 1982.
45. Rabies prevention: Supplementary statement on the preexposure use of human diploid cell rabies vaccine by the intradermal route. Leads from the *MMWR*. *JAMA* 257:1037, 1987.
46. Adverse reactions to human diploid cell rabies vaccine. *MMWR* 29:609, 1980.
47. Plummer, N. Essential industry and its role in an influenza epidemic. *Am Rev Respir Dis* 83:211, 1961. (Example of a program in a telecommunications company.)
48. Weaver, N. K., Lione, J. G., and Mogabgab, W. J. Recurrent Asian influenza in an industrial population. *Ann Intern Med* 54:843, 1961. (Example of a program in a petroleum-producing company.)
49. Brandon, F. B., Sadusk, J. F., and McLean, J. W., Jr. Influenza vaccines: The effect of chemical refinement on vaccine reactogenicity in an industrial population. *Ind Med* 40:44, 1971. (Example of use in a pharmaceutical manufacturing plant.)
50. Walker, D. D. Influenza immunization in industry. *Trans Soc Occup Med* 21:87, 1971.
51. Smith, J. W. G., Pollard, R., Fletcher, W. B., et al. Influenza vaccination: Acceptance in an industrial population. *Br J Ind Med* 31:292, 1974.
52. Anderson, E. A., Lindberg, R. B., and Hunter, D. H. Report of large-scale field trial of jet injection in immunization for influenza. *JAMA* 167:549, 1958.
53. Prevention and control of influenza. *MMWR* 35:317, 1986.
54. Eickhoff, T. C. Influenza vaccine and recent viral infection. *JAMA* 249:2834, 1983.
55. Polysaccharide vaccine for prevention of *Hemophilus influenza* type B disease. *MMWR* 34:201, 1985.
56. Cholera on a Gulf Coast oil rig. *MMWR* 30:589, 1981.
57. Johnston, J. M., Martin, D. L., Perdue, J., et al. Cholera on a Gulf Coast oil rig. *N Engl J Med 309:523, 1983.*
58. Khan, A. J. Savings in work-time loss to industry by intradermal vaccination against cholera in Pakistan. *Med Bull* (Exxon Corp) 33:129, 1973.
59. Cholera, 1981. *MMWR* 31:481, 1982.
60. Cholera in 1982. *WHO Chron* 37:214, 1983.
61. Poliomyelitis prevention. *MMWR* 31:22, 1982.
62. *Recommendations for Use and Storage of Common Immunobiologics and Other Prophylactic Agents.* Los Angeles: County of Los Angeles Department of Health Services, 1984. P. 7.
63. Weiss, K. E., Falvo, C. E., Buimovici-Klein, E., et al. Evaluation of an employee health service as a setting for a rubella screening and immunization program. *Am J Public Health* 69:281, 1979.
64. Rubella prevention. *MMWR* 33:302, 1984.
65. Nelson, D. B., Layde, M. M., and Chatton, T. B. Rubella susceptibility in inner-city adolescents: The effect of a school immunization law. *Am J Public Health* 72:710, 1982.
66. Rubella outbreaks in Los Angeles County: The need for a hospital screening policy. *Public Health Letter* (Los Angeles County Department of Health Services) 4:5, 1982.
67. Wahdan, M. H., Serie, C., Cerisier, Y., et al. A controlled field trial of live *Salmonella typhi* strain Ty 210 oral vaccine against typhoid: Three-year results. *J Infect Dis* 145:292, 1982.
68. Macek, C. New typhoid fever vaccine on international scene. *JAMA* 248:162, 1982.
69. Meningococcal vaccines. *MMWR* 34:255, 1985.
70. Gunby, P. Coccidioidomycosis vaccine trial planned with 3,000 volunteers. *JAMA* 245:1711, 1981.
71. Human trials of coccidioidomycosis vaccine begin. *Skin Allergy News* 9:5, Nov 1979.
72. Pappagianis, D. Evaluation of the Protective Efficacy of the Killed *Coccidioides immitis* Vaccine in Man. Abstract No. 784. *Program and Abstracts of the Twenty-Sixth Interscience Conference on Antimicrobial Agents and Chemotherapy.* 28 September–1 October 1986, Rivergate Convention Center, New Orleans, Louisiana. American Society of Microbiology, 1986. P. 240.
73. Recommendations for protection against viral hepatitis. *MMWR* 34:313, 1985.
74. Long, M. J., cited in Nelson, H. Hepatitis B virus linked to liver cancer in U.S. Asians. *Los Angeles Times* II:1, Aug 13, 1985.
75. Szmuness, W., Stevens, C. E., Harley, E. J., et al. Hepatitis B vaccine: Demonstration of efficacy in a controlled clinical trial in a high risk population in the United States. *N Engl J Med* 303:833, 1980.
76. An outbreak of non-A, non-B hepatitis associated with a plasmapheresis unit—Los Angeles County. *Public Health Letter* (Los Angeles County Department of Health Services) 3:25, 1981.
77. Summary of notifiable diseases, 1985. *MMWR* 34:15, 1987.
78. Anthrax contamination of Haitian goatskin products. *MMWR* 30:338, 1981.
79. *BCG (Baccile Calmette Guérin) Vaccination.* Los Angeles: American Lung Association of Los Angeles County, 1981.
80. *The Tuberculin Skin Test 1981.* New York: American Thoracic Society (Medical Section of the American Lung Association), 1981. P. 7.
81. Immunization program. *J Occup Med* 8:287, 1966.
82. Curran, W. J. Health department legal liability for injuries in vaccination programs. *Am J Public Health* 70:1215, 1980.

83. Curran, W. J. Public warnings of the risk in oral polio vaccine. *Am J Public Health* 65:501, 1975.
84. Cramblett, H. G. Important medical-legal aspects of immunization. *West J Med* 125:508, 1976.
85. Schumacher, W. Legal/ethical aspects of vaccination. *Dev Biol Stand* 43:435, 1979.
86. Franklin, M. A., and Mais, J. E., Jr. Tort law and mass immunization programs: Lessons from the polio and flu episode. *Calif Law Rev* 65:754, 1977.
87. Woolley, A. P. Informed consent to immunization: The risks and benefits of individual autonomy. *Calif Law Rev* 65:1286, 1977.
88. Trout, M. E. Immunization: A societal dilemma. *NY Law School Law Rev* 22:943, 1977.
89. Dover, J. E. An evaluation of immunization regulations in light of religious objections and the developing right of privacy. *Univ Dayton Law Rev* 4:401, 1979.
90. O'Brien, M. Legal implications of the use of vaccines. *Med Legal J* 47:152, 1979.
91. Wyatt, H. V. Vaccines and social responsibility: Here are some answers. What are the questions? *Monist* 60:81, 1977.
92. Nottebart, H. C., Jr. Immunizations: Risks and warnings about them. *Infect Control* 2:265, 1981.
93. Health and the law: Staff report. *Dimens Health Serv* 56:31, 1979.
94. Ladimer, J. Mass immunizations: Legal problems and a proposed solution. *J Community Health* 2:189, 1977.
95. Goldsmith, M. F. AMA offers recommendations for vaccine injury compensation. *JAMA* 252:2937, 1984.
96. Check, W. A. How to remedy possible harm to a few persons from vaccines that could benefit entire society? *JAMA* 252:2942, 1984.
97. *OSHA Field Operations Manual*. Chap. V—General Inspection Procedures (Amended by OSHA Instruction CPL 2.45, Sept. 15, 1980; OSHA Instruction CPL 2.45 CH-2, Aug. 19, 1981). B5 Immunization Requirements.
98. *The Tuberculin Skin Test—1981*. New York: American Lung Association, 1981.
99. Snider, D. E., Jr. Bacille-Guérin vaccinations and tuberculin skin tests. *JAMA* 253:3438, 1985.
100. Pappagianis, D., and Levine, H. B. *Focus on Coccidioidomycosis*. Park Ridge, IL: American College of Chest Physicians, 1978.
101. Edwards, L. B., Acquaviva, F. A., Livesay, T. V., et al. An atlas of sensitivity to tuberculin, PPD-B, and histoplasmin in the United States. *Am Rev Respir Dis* (Suppl 99):1, 1969.
102. Schwarz, J. *Histoplasmosis*. New York: Praeger, 1981.
103. Medical criteria for passenger flying: Scheduled commercial flights. *Arch Environ Health* 2:124, 1961.
104. AMA Commission on Emergency Medical Services. Medical aspects of transportation aboard commercial aircraft. *JAMA* 247:1007, 1982.
105. Welch, B. Some considerations before using the aerial ambulance. *JACEP* 6:155, 1977.
106. Gullett, C. C. Effect of decompression at high altitude on breast implants. *JAMA* 244:2209, 1980.
107. Dolge, J. C., and Bell, J. A. (Eds.). *Traveler's Health Abroad: A Guide for Physicians*. Chicago: American Medical Association, 1982. P. 29.
108. Eisenberg, N. H., Kitzes-Cohen, R., and Pitlik, S. Prescriptions for the traveler. *JAMA* 233:227, 1975.
109. *Guide to Accessibility of Terminals—Access Travel: Airports* (3rd ed.). Published in Cooperation with Airport Operators Council International, Inc., Architectural and Transportation Barriers Compliance Board. Washington, DC: U.S. Department of Transportation, Federal Aviation Administration, 1979.
110. *Access Washington: A Guide to Metropolitan Washington for the Physically Disabled*. Washington, DC: Information Center for Handicapped Individuals, 1976.
111. Mann, J. M., Schmid, G. P., Stolsz, P. A., et al. Peripatetic plague. *JAMA* 247:47, 1982.
112. Cholera in a tourist returning from Cancun, Mexico—New Jersey. *MMWR* 32:357, 1983.
113. Kean, B. H. The treatment of amebiasis: A recurrent agony. *JAMA* 235:501, 1976.
114. Ma, P., Kaufman, D. L., Helnick, E. G., et al. Cryptosporidiosis in tourists returning from the Caribbean. *N Engl J Med* 312:647, 1985.
115. Follow-up on malaria alert for travelers returning from Lagos, Nigeria. *MMWR* 26:93, 1977.
116. Reilly, P. C., Jr. Risk of malaria among travelers. *N Engl J Med* 303:587, 1980.
117. Increased incidence of malaria in U.S. said to be due to foreign travel, immigration. *Int Med News* 14:9, Oct 1, 1981.
118. Cline, A. L., Mosley, J. W., and Scovel, F. G. Viral hepatitis among American missionaries abroad. *JAMA* 199:119, 1967.
119. Hepatitis in overseas travelers. *Calif Morbid* 34:1, Sept 3, 1976.
120. Shigellosis among tourists—Union of Soviet Socialist Republics, 1983. *MMWR* 33:234, 1984.
121. Barclay, W. R. Diphyllobothriasis. *JAMA* 246:2483, 1981.
122. Dooley, J. R. Diphyllobothriasis in Americans and Asians. *JAMA* 247:2230, 1982.
123. Rabb, R. R., Peck, O. C., and Vescia, F. G. Giardiasis: A cause of traveler's diarrhea. *JAMA* 217:1359, 1971.
124. Schultz, M. G., and Giordano, J. F. *Giardiasis in Travelers Returning from the Soviet Union*. Advisory Memorandum No. 35. Atlanta: Centers for Disease Control, 1974.
125. Wolfe, M. S. Giardiasis. *JAMA* 233:1362, 1975.
126. Giardiasis—in Residents of Rome, New York, and in U.S. Travelers to the Soviet Union. *MMWR* 24:366, 1975.
127. Arnow, P. M., Smaron, M., and Ormiste, V. Brucellosis in a group of travelers to Spain. *JAMA* 251:505, 1984.

128. Dengue fever—Puerto Rico. *MMWR* 24:365, 1975.
129. Dengue in a traveler to the Virgin Islands. *Public Health Letter* (Los Angeles County) 3:23, 1981.
130. Lennon, J. L. Dengue in the Caribbean. *JAMA* 250:613, 1983.
131. Typhoid fever in American tourists to Europe. *MMWR* 20:428, 1971.
132. Typhoid fever in American tourists returning from Haiti—Connecticut. *MMWR* 23:433, 1974.
133. Epidemic meningococcal disease: Recommendations for travelers to Nepal. *MMWR* 34:119, 1985.
134. Goldman, L. Tungiasis in travelers from tropical Africa. *JAMA* 236:1386, 1976.
135. Most, H., and Levine, D. I. Schistosomiasis in American Tourists. *JAMA* 186:453, 1963.
136. Acute schistosomiasis with transverse myelitis in American students returning from Kenya. *MMWR* 33:445, 1984.
137. Istre, B. R., Fontaine, R. E., Jarr, J., et al. Acute schistosomiasis among Americans rafting the Omo River, Ethiopia. *JAMA* 251:508, 1984.
138. Cutaneous larva migrans in American tourists—Martinique and Mexico. *MMWR* 30:308, 1981.
139. Ciquatera fish poisoning in tourists to the British Virgin Islands. *MMWR* 27:39, 1978.
140. Staphylococcal food poisoning aloft—Pennsylvania, Puerto Rico, New York. *MMWR* 22:381, 1973.
141. Dakin, W. P. H., Howell, D. J., Sutton, R. G. A., et al. Gastroenteritis due to non-agglutinable (non-cholera) Vibrios. *Med J Aust* 2:487, 1974.
142. Outbreak of staphylococcal food poisoning aboard an aircraft. *MMWR* 24:57, 1975.
143. Outbreak of staphylococcal food poisoning aboard an aircraft. *MMWR* 25:317, 1976.
144. Survey of the incidence of gastrointestinal illness in cruise ship passengers. *MMWR* 23:65, 1974.
145. Salmonellosis on a Caribbean passenger cruise ship. *MMWR* 23:69, 1974.
146. Merson, M. H., Tenney, J. H., Meyers, J. D., et al. Shigellosis at sea: An outbreak aboard a passenger cruise ship. *Am J Epidemiol* 101:165, 1975.
147. *Vibrio parahaemolyticus* gastroenteritis on cruise ships. *MMWR* 24:109, 1975.
148. Gastroenteritis caused by *Vibrio parahaemolyticus* aboard a cruise ship. *MMWR* 27:65, 1978.
149. Gastroenteritis outbreaks on two Caribbean cruise ships. *MMWR* 35:383, 1986.
150. Trichinosis aboard a cruise ship. *MMWR* 24:319, 1975.
151. Diarrheal illness aboard a cruise ship. *MMWR* 24:419, 1975.
152. Diarrheal illness on a cruise ship caused by enterotoxigenic *Escherichia coli. MMWR* 25:229, 1976.
153. Gastrointestinal illness aboard a cruise ship. *MMWR* 25:309, 1976.
154. Gastrointestinal illness aboard the *T.s.s. Fairsea. MMWR* 26:176, 1977.
155. *Salmonella heidelberg* gastroenteritis aboard a cruise ship. *MMWR* 28:145, 1979.
156. Staphylococcal from poisoning on a cruise ship. *MMWR* 32:294, 1983.
157. Gorbach, S. L., Kean, B. H., Evans, D. G., et al. Traveler's diarrhea and toxigenic *Escherichia coli. N Engl J Med* 292:933, 1975.
158. Kean, B. H. The diarrhea of travelers to Mexico: Summary of five-year study. *Ann Intern Med* 59:605, 1963.
159. Merson, M. H. Toxigenic turista. *N Engl J Med* 292:969, 1975.
160. Merson, M. H., and Gangarosa, E. J. Traveler's diarrhea. *JAMA* 234:200, 1975.
161. Merson, M. H., Morris, G. K., Sack, D. A., et al. Traveler's diarrhea in Mexico. *N Engl J Med* 294:1299, 1976.
162. Scotti, F. A. Liberty in Mexico. *Prev Med Notes, PMU 5,* June-July 1980. P. 4.
163. Steffen, R., van der Linde, F., Gyr, K., et al. Epidemiology of diarrhea in travelers. *JAMA* 249:1176, 1983.
164. Du Pont, H. L., Ericsson, C. D., and Murray, E. E. Travelers' diarrhea: Can it be eluded? *JAMA* 249:1193, 1983.
165. Allard, R. Epidemiology of traveler's diarrhea. *JAMA* 251:1161, 1984.
166. Traveler's diarrhea: Consensus conference. *JAMA* 253:2700, 1985.
167. *Health Information for International Travel 1986.* Atlanta: U.S. Department of Health and Human Services, Public Health Services, Centers for Disease Control, 1986. Pp. 109–110.
168. United States ends smallpox vaccination requirement for international travel. *MMWR* 27:295, 1978.
169. Snyder, J. D., and Blake, P. A. Is cholera a problem for U.S. travelers? *JAMA* 247:2268, 1982.
170. Insect repellents. *Consumer Rep* 47:304, 1982.
171. Revised recommendations for preventing malaria in travelers to areas with chloroquine-resistant *Plasmodium falcifarum. MMWR* 34:185, 1985.
172. MD's office often a clinic for traveler's vaccinations. *Int Med News* 12:5, Nov 1, 1979.
173. Orenstein, W. A., and Brink, E. W. Combined immunizations for international travel. *JAMA* 252:278, 1984.
174. DuPont, H. L., and DuPont, M. W. *Travel with Health.* New York: Appleton-Century-Crofts, 1981.
175. Bateman, S. C. Physiological aspects of jet travel. *Occup Health* 24:3, 1972.
176. Mohler, S. R., Dille, J. R., and Gibbons, H. L. *Circadian Rhythms and the Effects of Long-Distance Flights.* Washington, DC: Office of Aviation Medicine/Federal Aviation Administration, U.S. Department of Transportation, 1968. P. 4.
177. How to survive a hotel fire. *Safety Flash,* Irvine, U.C. Irvine, Environmental Health and Safety Office, Bull. No. 56, Feb. 1981. Pp. 1–2.
178. Forkner, C. E. Virtues and sins of medical practice: Formula for better medical care. *NY State J Med* 78:1776, 1978.

179. Forkner, C. E. The Medical Passport: Its Concept, Development and Computerization. In H. E. Emlet, Jr. (Ed.), *Challenges and Prospects for Advanced Medical Systems.* Miami, FL: Symposia Specialists, 1978. Pp. 89–99.
180. Forkner, C. E. Young Health History at Your Fingertips. In K. Shenert, *How to Be Your Own Doctor—Sometimes.* New York: Grosset and Dunlap, 1975. Pp. 78–83.
181. Committee on International Relations. *Working Abroad: A Discussion of Psychological Attitudes and Adaptation in New Situations.* Report No. 41. New York: Group for the Advancement of Psychiatry, 1956.
182. Quoted in "Why Are They Always on the Go?" *Med World News* 10:182, 1969.
183. Gross, H. P. Physicians abroad: The medical scholars abroad. *JAMA* 192:251, 1965. Copyright 1965, American Medical Association.
184. Larson, A. *Worker's Compensation Law: Cases, Materials and Text.* New York: Bender, 1984. §25 Traveling Employees. P. 156.

APPENDIX 8-1
HOW TO SURVIVE A HOTEL FIRE*

Almost everyone stays in hotels during the course of their business or personal endeavors. We can greatly enhance our chances of survival in the event of a hotel fire by learning a few simple life-safety procedures.

PLAN FOR SURVIVAL WHEN ENTERING HOTEL ROOM

Plan your escape with *all* the members of your party or your family (including small children). Remember the fact that one or more members may be in another area of the hotel when the fire occurs and that independent escape routes should be agreed upon. *Decide upon a meeting place outside the hotel if you become separated.*

If you should all be together when the fire occurs, plan how you will stay together at all times. Decide how you will help each other with the tasks of survival.

1. Before entering your room check out possible escape routes and memorize them.
2. Walk along the corridor and find the closest exit in either direction from your room.
3. Check the exits and be sure that they are clear. If it is a stairway, are the doors propped open? If so, talk to the desk clerk or manager about closing them. Do not stay in a hotel that obviously has poor fire safety procedures.
4. Count the doors or other features between your room and the stairs. Orient yourself directionally. If there is smoke in the corridors, the exit signs above exit doors may not be seen.
5. Find the nearest fire alarm pull station.

PLAN FOR SURVIVAL WITHIN THE HOTEL ROOM

1. Always place the key where it can be easily found, and always keep it in the same place. Locate it near where you will sleep.
2. Check the windows. Will they open?
3. How far is it to the building or floor below? Is there a balcony? Jumping is a judgmental decision, but you should be aware that few survive a jump of 20 feet or more (two stories). Certainly, it should be a last resort decision.
4. Carry a smoke detector with you, and hang or place it on something near the ceiling of your room. Check batteries and operation before leaving home.

SURVIVAL WHEN A FIRE OCCURS IN YOUR ROOM

1. If fire starts in your room, call by telephone to the fire department **first**; then call the hotel operator.
2. Try to put fire out, but be sure you can handle it. If there is doubt, leave the room, closing the door behind you to keep fire out of the corridor.
3. Sound the fire alarm at the pull station location.

SURVIVAL AND ESCAPE WHEN FIRE OCCURS OUTSIDE YOUR ROOM

1. Grab your room key.
2. If there is smoke in the room, stay close to the floor and crawl to the door.
3. Feel the door knob, and if it is hot do not open the door. If it is not hot, open the door slowly so it can be quickly closed again if necessary.
4. If the corridor is clear, walk to exit, closing your room door as you leave.
5. If smoke occurs while you are leaving through the corridor, stay low and close to the wall, counting

*Source: Environmental Health and Safety office, University of California, Irvine. Reprinted with permission.

each doorway to the stairway. **Do not** use the elevators!

6. Use handrails since other panicky guests may knock you down in their flight.

SURVIVAL WHEN ESCAPE IS IMPOSSIBLE

1. Open window to ventilate room. If smoke enters from lower floors, close it again.
2. Signal that you are in your room—try the telephone or hang a sheet from your window. **Do not climb down makeshift ropes!**
3. Fill the bathtub, and turn on the fan. The fan can help ventilate, and the water can be used to fight fire or keep the door cool.
4. Soak towels or sheets and force them into heat registers and especially into door cracks. The ice bucket can be used to keep them wet or to fight fire.
5. If smoke gets into your room, make a tent out of a blanket over a slightly opened window to get fresh air. A wet cloth placed over your mouth and nose will help filter smoke particles.
6. If you are unable to stay in your room you may be forced to make the best exit possible. Use good judgment.

Stay calm! Fear is your greatest enemy!!

549404

9. EMERGENCY MEDICAL CARE

Let no one ever commit first aid.

Anon

One of the essential qualities of the clinician is interest in humanity, for the secret of the care of the patient is in caring for the patient.

Francis Weld Peabody, M.D.

Calamity is man's true touchstone.

Beaumont and Fletcher

FIRST AID IN INDUSTRY

Even though professional occupational health personnel are present and providing service in an organization, there will be occasional need for the application of first-aid measures to workers. Few companies have satellite facilities, except where distance demands such subdispensaries, so that physicians, nurses, or physician's assistants may not be readily available at critical times at the geographic site of injury or illness.

DEFINITION

First aid as defined by the American National Red Cross is "the immediate and temporary care given the victim of an accident or sudden illness until the services of a physician can be obtained" [1].

It must be borne in mind that not every demand for care is necessarily based on a major catastrophic episode, for some individuals are given to highly excited responses to minor events that are in no way life threatening. If persons trained in first-aid procedures care for the injured or ill individual, they usually can exercise judgment as to whether the services of a physician are needed and, if so, how quickly such professional attention is required.

LEGISLATIVE MANDATES

Included in the Occupational Safety and Health Act of 1970 rules and regulations are certain requirements for the provision of trained first-aid personnel. As many states pattern their safety orders or codes after the federal mandate, there is similarity among many of the regulations. The items covered at the national level are the following [2]:

> In the absence of an infirmary, clinic, or hospital in near proximity to the workplace which is used for the treatment of all injured employees, a person or persons shall be adequately trained—usually those persons holding a valid certificate in first aid training from the U.S. Bureau of Mines or the American Red Cross—to render first aid. First aid supplies approved by the consulting physician shall be readily available.
>
> The first aid kit shall consist of materials recommended by the consulting physician, maintained in a weatherproof container with individual sealed packages for each type of item. The contents of the kit shall be checked by the employer before being sent out on each job and at least weekly on each job to ensure that the expended items are replaced.
>
> Proper equipment for prompt transportation of the injured person to a physician or hospital, or a communication system for contacting necessary ambulance service, shall be provided. Where the eyes or body of any person may be exposed to injurious corrosive materials, suitable facilities for quick drenching or flushing of the eyes and body shall be provided within the work area for immediate emergency use.

A second mandate is encountered in the Federal Mine Safety and Health Act of 1977, which states that each operator of a coal or other mine shall have a health and safety training program [3].* New miners, without previous underground mining experience, are to receive 40 hours of training, which includes a segment on first aid. A shortened program of 24 hours of training is provided new miners who are to work on the surface who have had no previous

*The details of the training are spelled out in Code of Federal Regulations, Title 30—Mineral Resources, Chap. 1 Mine Safety and Health Administration, §48.5, §48.8, §48.25, and §48.28.

surface mining experience. All miners will be given refresher training—not less than 8 hours—once annually. The training programs are given during normal working hours, at the usual rate of compensation [3]. While federal regulations call for training in first aid, no specific details relating to the subject are given beyond, "The course shall include instruction in first aid methods acceptable to MSHA [Mine Safety and Health Administration]" [3].

Publications and visual aids for the program [4–8] are provided by the Mining Enforcement and Safety Administration (MESA),* as prepared by the National Mine Health and Safety Academy (NMHSA).

DECENTRALIZATION

It has been the experience over the years that several division heads or section chiefs will seek the placement of "first-aid boxes" in their areas so that personnel will have access to the usual supplies for application to the ill or injured. Also, many have requested that supplies of medical oxygen be placed in various offices or shops.

The decentralization of supplies rarely works well for several reasons. The cabinets are soon forgotten by the central health facility, and shortly they are soiled or covered or obscured by equipment or stock placed in front of them. If they are unlocked, the medications, dressings, and bandages soon disappear, not because of local indicated need, but because they are removed for personal stockpiling at the worksite or at home. If bottles of over-the-counter medications are included, the contents become soiled and repel the individual seeking medicine for either topical or oral use.

The only concession that can be made is to place a cabinet, appropriately identified, painted, and numbered, in a foreman's office, with such a person having sole responsibility for its safeguarding and for requesting replenishment of supplies, when required, from the central occupational health facility.

The deployment of oxygen tanks for emergency use is not indicated, as oxygen may actually be contraindicated in certain clinical states where a layman might believe it to be lifesaving. That certain strategically placed or located plant personnel should be trained in the administration of first-aid procedures is accepted practice and will be discussed.

It must be emphasized that the term *first aid* should be used correctly in the industrial setting. On many occasions while touring plant medical facilities one has encountered a sign reading "First Aid," accompanied by the usual green cross, only to find that the unit so labeled is staffed by professional nurses. Trained personnel provide *emergency medical care* and not "first aid," which has its own protocols and is to be conducted by trained laypersons. Physicians and nurses can offer first-aid services, but such an action is usually seen away from an equipped facility where surgical equipment, emergency medications, and monitoring instruments are at hand. First aid has a place in industry, and the term should be limited to the identification of supplies to be used by the trained first-aid attendant, such as blankets or litters for emergency transport. No nurse- or physician-staffed unit should be so tagged.

In substance, because of the potential for accidental injury, cerebrovascular accidents, myocardial infarctions, drownings, or accidental electrocutions, there will be situations warranting intelligent lay care until professional services are available. Also, certain workers may manifest insulin reactions or convulsive seizures, and supervisory personnel should be prepared to provide appropriate care and to defuse the usual group anxiety that leads to the needless calling of off-plant paramedics and ambulances. A knowing group leader can exercise great calm at such tense moments.

INDICATIONS FOR TRAINING IN FIRST AID

While it is a good policy to have personnel throughout a plant equipped to render first aid, certain factors should be considered when training is being planned. As all training is costly—downtime, instructors, supplies, utilities, and the like—the personnel selected for attendance at the course should be chosen in light of their need for such added skill. These elements should play a role in deciding on the trainees:

Members of a geographically isolated work group.

Work group members subject to adverse environmental health effects from exposure to excessive heat or cold, motion sickness, decompression illness, decreased atmospheric pressure, or explosive decompression in flight.

Supervisors of aged (or aging) work group.

Supervisors of work unit whose members may undergo acute exposure to a suddenly released toxin.

*MESA, originally the Bureau of Mines, has had changes in its governance, moving from the U.S. Department of the Interior to the U.S. Department of Labor, and back to the Department of the Interior.

Supervisors of a work group employed in or around fixed hazardous equipment.
Supervisors of a work group that has had a history of mass hysteria.
Firefighters.
Law enforcement officers.
Construction foremen.
Workers in operational areas with special hazards—formulation of pesticides, electroplating, operations requiring poorly contained boiling liquids, caustic solutions, acid baths, induction furnaces, work at heights, confined spaces, or the use of pavement breakers or power saws.
Workers around moving or motorized equipment—trucks, cranes, tractors, combines, earth-moving equipment, airplanes, military tanks, trapezes, railway rolling stock, mining equipment, presses, or road-race cars.
Athletes.
Animal handlers, vivarium personnel, animal trainers, zookeepers, zoologists.
Oil exploration crew leaders.

In essence, there should be one person in these types of work units who should undergo training in first aid. Such an individual should be able to handle emergent situations with dispatch and good judgment and be emotionally mature.

TRAINING PROGRAMS

GENERAL PROGRAMS

Although training can be conducted by members of a company's full-time staff-development personnel, it is desirable that the initial instruction be carried out by personnel who limit their activities exclusively to this form of teaching. Most commonly involved is the American National Red Cross (ARC), which has established guidelines at the national level for use by all of its chapters, usually there being one in each county. On request, the local chapter will send an instructor to conduct a 1-day program, the Multimedia System Standard First Aid course.

The standard 10-module course comprises the following subjects:

Emergency action principles
Respiratory emergencies
First aid for wounds
First aid for burns
Emergency rescue and transfer
Injuries to bones, muscles, and joints
Accident prevention
Bandaging
First aid for specific injuries
First aid for sudden illness

The required textbooks are *Standard First Aid and Personal Safety* [9] and a *workbook* [10], a looseleaf book that allows user interaction through questions and responses. Space is needed, and an area about 25 × 50 ft (1,250 square feet) will serve. A film is shown requiring a 16-mm projector. Certain supplies will be provided by the instructor.

If a company instructor is used, there is no charge made by the ARC, but if a volunteer instructor is provided, the cost would be on a per trainee basis. If no volunteer trainers are available and a paid instructor is used, the charge per student rises. The training program is aimed at teaching the students how to teach, so that they can train other personnel of the organization. Certifying cards of completion are distributed, and it is recommended that the course be repeated every 3 years.

DEFINITIVE PROGRAMS

Expertise at the first-aid level is required in other situations in an industrial plant. The first involves knowledge on the part of personnel who work consistently with certain physiologically hazardous substances or in areas where highly flammable or explosive materials are in use. The skill required may go beyond that produced through the standard first-aid training course, and a foreman or other responsible group leader should be equipped to provide the assistance needed at critical times. In addition to being prepared for the rendering of emergent care, this person should be familiar with the adjacent sources of definitive care and the available means of transport. It is the task of the physician or nurse at the plant to train the lead persons to meet the situation should it arise.

A considerable body of literature is currently available that provides the information for "first aid at the scene." Manufacturers of chemicals usually prepare Material Safety Data Sheets, in which are included discussions of the action required in the case of an area spill, skin contamination or burn, inadvertent inhalation or ingestion, wound absorption, or eye irritation. Comparable information appears in the Hygiene Guide Series published by the American Industrial Hygiene Association, and specific measures to be taken at the worksite following untoward contact with a dangerous substance can be learned from any of the many private consultants in occupational health and industrial hygiene who are listed periodically in the *American Industrial Hygiene Association Journal*.

The other area that calls for an extension of the generic training activity is knowledge of the care required if certain impaired workers suddenly present a need for assistance. Reference is made particularly to personnel with convulsive disorders, diabetes mellitus, or the habituating use of drugs. In these situations of stress in a work group—a colleague experiences a grand mal seizure, an insulin reaction, the high of an illicit or street drug, or even the breakage of a limb prosthesis or wheelchair—the group leader must be prepared to provide the indicated aid and to direct other members of the unit in conducting whatever ancillary help is indicated.

It is desirable, if possible, to have an area reserved for the provision of first aid that is readily assessible to the greatest number of employees and is close to an exit, quiet, clean (free of the usual shop debris, scrap, or stock), and adequately illuminated, heated, and ventilated. Hot and cold running water, soap, towels, and a chair should be at the selected site. The use of such an area is indicated only if the person in need can reach that site or can be transported there without incurring additional injury or aggravating the effects of an acute medical episode.

In this area, there should be a sign that provides the following information [11]:

Name of person in charge of first aid for each shift.
Instructions for calling a physician—name, office and home telephone numbers.
Instructions for calling an ambulance—name of company and telephone number.
Instructions for calling paramedics—fire station telephone number.
Name and telephone number of hospital to be notified that patient is en route.
Procedure for transport of ill or injured worker.
Manual (attached) containing written procedures provided by company's medical consultant.
First aid manual, attached.
Notebook or logbook for recording of name of patient, condition requiring care, treatment given or disposition, date, and name of first-aid attendant.

First-aid guides or ready reference posters frequently are provided by the casualty insurance companies that underwrite workers' compensation.

EQUIPMENT FOR FIRST AID

The stocked materials for use in first aid may be assembled locally and placed in specially designed portable containers or kept in permanently affixed wall cabinets. Commercial first-aid kits are readily available and may be obtained from any number of manufacturers of either medical/surgical supplies or safety devices and materials. Unstocked first-aid cabinets can be purchased for office or industrial use and can be filled in keeping with indicated needs. Most supplies are packaged in cellophane wrap or small standardized cartons holding items for one or two treatments; the cartons fit snugly into the kits.

Most commercial kits have first-aid items packed in color-coded packages, the color provided by the cellophane wrap. If the package appears white, one knows that a portion of the contents has been removed and replenishment is in order. The commonly used coding is as follows:

Blue—antiseptics
Red—burn medications
Yellow—dressings and bandages
Green—special items, such as eye irrigating solution, over-the-counter medication, ammonia inhalants, and the like

In certain areas where there is extremely high humidity or heavy rainfall, the first-aid kit must be rubber-sealed to keep out moisture.

A kit developed and standardized for a work group of 80,000 persons was one designed in the occupational health service (OHS) of the County of Los Angeles:

KITS, First Aid, complete, case of 20-gauge metal with handle and snaplock, and sealed proof from dust and water; holes to be on hinge so as to hang; approximate size 2¾″ × 9½″, enamel white, labelled "First Aid Kit," second line "County of Los Angeles," in ¼″ × 1″ red letters. Contents to consist only of materials approved by the Occupational Health Service as follows:

2 packages	BANDAGES, adhesive, plastic, Telfa[R] pad perforated, sterile, 1″ × 3¼″—16 to package
2 packages	BANDAGES, compress, sterile, offset, 2″
3 packages	BANDAGES, compress, sterile, offset, 3″
3 packages	BANDAGES, compress, sterile, offset, 4″
2 packages	BANDAGES, triangular, sterile, 4″, with 2 safety pins
1 package	BLANKET, rescue, 56″ × 84″
2 packages	COLD PAK, instant
1 package	EYE-DRESSING PACKET, containing 4 sets of adhesive strips and 4 sterile pads
1 each	FORCEPS, splinter, 3½″ in length, serrated inside, needle points
1 package	GAUZE COMPRESS, 3″ × 3″, 4 to package
1 package	PADS, wound cleansing and degreasing (alcohol prep pads), 10 pads per package, Webcol[R]
1 each	SCISSORS, bandage, 4″, blunt end, nickel plated
1 each	SPLINT, inflatable, G splint, Curity (Kendall), 15″ × 30″, with tube
1 package	SWABS for instant therapeutic relief from stings and bites of insects, ½ cc, sterile, 10 swabs per package, Sting/Kill
1 package	TINCTURE GREEN SOAP N.F., 10 ml vials, 3 vials, per container with 4 sterile gauze pads size 3″ × 3″ per container

CASE, only, First Aid, 2¾″ × 9½″ enamel, white, labelled "First Aid Kit," second line, "County of Los Angeles," ¼″ × 1″ red letters with handle and snap lock, sealed proof from dust and water, holes to be on hinge so as to hang. First Aid Guide instructions attached to inside lid of kit.

Special-purpose kits are supplied for the first-aid treatment of burns or snakebite and for mines, buses, fire departments, airplanes, the Coast Guard, railroads, welders, and food service workers, among others. Certain of these kits are stocked in compliance with Interstate Commerce Commission or Federal Aviation Administration requirements. The differences among the kits are seen in either the numbers of a certain item supplied or in the addition of a specific unit. None offers any item unique to the setting or the occupation; it is a matter solely of selection of standard, available contents. Refills are available to replace any used supply package or unit.

Larger pieces of equipment, as determined by local needs or potential hazards, can be purchased and placed at strategic sites. Such items would include the following:

Total body transport splint or spine board
Emergency stretcher (litter)
Basket stretcher (Stokes or modified Stokes)
Stretcher wall kit
Inflatable splints
Fire blanket
Wheeled stretcher
Stretcher chair
Disposable protective blanket

CARDIOPULMONARY RESUSCITATION

In addition to the training of designated employed persons in first aid, in the past decade or more there has been training offered to all citizens, whether in industry or elsewhere, in basic life support procedures, or cardiopulmonary resuscitation (CPR), the combination of mouth-to-mouth resuscitation and external cardiac compression. As cardiopulmonary failure (cardiac arrest) is most frequently associated with myocardial infarction, massive cerebrovascular accident, drowning, or electrocution, the opportunities for initiating cardiac life support procedures can present themselves at work or in the community.

Not only should professional persons be trained in CPR, that is, all members of an OHS, but certain individuals in a plant who are emotionally stable and who can respond intelligently and quickly to demand situations likewise should undergo the initial program and the annual recertification. Currently in certain jurisdictions, CPR training is required for the annual licensure of physicians. But to meet the problem of possible sudden death, which can and does take place in employed groups, a cadre of trained workers is essential.

As in first-aid training, the ARC offers courses of instruction that not only provide the technique for CPR but also increase the awareness of early warning signs, risk factors, and symptoms of heart disease. Both primary and review courses are available, and there are cost-recovery fees. In some communities the fire department paramedics may provide industry with CPR courses at no charge.

EMERGENCY HEALTH CARE

TREATMENT OF THE OCCUPATIONALLY ILL OR INJURED

PREMISE FOR OPERATION

Long before any in-plant medical program added some of today's sophisticated services to its list of professional activities, treatment of the person injured at work was an early and accepted benefit. While the inclusion of emergency care has been questioned by carpers external to industry, the provision of such a service is recognized as a needed on-site capability.

The American Medical Association (AMA) in *Scope, Objectives, and Functions of Occupational Health Programs* [12] lists the following as a basic objective of an occupational health program: "To assure adequate medical care and rehabilitation of the occupationally ill and injured . . ." and further, "Diagnosis and treatment in occupational injury and disease cases should be prompt and should be directed toward rehabilitation." Not only are these caveats repeated in other publications of the AMA [13,14], but further substance is provided by the Committee on Occupational Medical Practice of the American Occupational Medical Association (AOMA) [15] stating, "Occupational injuries and illnesses should be diagnosed as promptly as practical and treated as appropriate within the capabilities of the workplace medical facility."

The extent of the treatment provided will vary with the level of staff present in an OHS. If the service is represented by one occupational health nurse, the patient presenting with a serious traumatic injury may be given emergent care solely and be transported to a nearby hospital. If a physician is part of the occupational health team, a different level of care may be given, and finally, if by chance a surgeon visits on certain days, the injured worker may receive specialized care without having to be transported elsewhere.

It is accepted practice that if the injury involves certain tissues, such as nerves or tendons that have been sectioned in the course of the traumatic episode, if plastic or reconstructive repair of facial structures is indicated, or if there are multiple injuries, such as fractures or visceral ruptures, the patient will be transferred as rapidly as possible to a source of definitive, tertiary care, with such life support measures provided initially or en route, as necessary.

CHRONOLOGY OF TRAUMA

Notification and Transport

Employees who are injured on the job, as determined by the extent of the trauma sustained, may be

Retained at the site of the accident awaiting care, or
Transported by nearest available conveyance to the in-plant source of care, or
Transported by company (OHS) ambulance to the OHS, or
Transported by outside ambulance to a source of specialty care.

Infrequently, because of panic or ignorance during a first or second shift, an excited fellow worker may bypass the OHS and call the nearest paramedics. This procedure may be necessary during a third shift if no occupational health personnel are available.

If a call is received by the OHS requesting care for an emergent situation, complete information must be obtained so that either an ambulance can be dispatched or a car sent out from the OHS with an emergency medical technician (EMT), an occupational health nurse, or a physician, as warranted by the nature of the emergency. As the caller frequently is anxious, insufficient detail may be given as to the location or severity of the injury or illness. A form should be kept adjacent to the telephone designated exclusively for emergency calls and should provide pertinent information: date of call, number of caller, location of patient (building, floor), and name of person receiving the call. Sections for the name of the staff person dispatched and the ultimate disposition can be completed after the patient has received care. The options for disposition are the following:

1. Treated on site and returned to work.
2. Retained in OHS, treated, and sent home.
3. Sent home by company vehicle.
4. Treated in OHS and returned to work.
5. Sent to physician's office by company vehicle.
6. Sent to hospital by ambulance.
7. Family notified, disposition requested.

A system maintained in a facility with which the author was connected involved a limited communications network. A number reserved exclusively for medical emergency use was well posted in all areas of the plant and was displayed prominently in the company telephone directories. The ambulance was maintained in the fire department, and one of the firefighters was assigned as driver. A call placed to the OHS would be received simultaneously in the OHS and the fire department. The assigned firefighter would listen while the OHS representative noted the details of the emergency, and a decision would be made immediately if the ambulance were to stop at the OHS for an attendant (EMT, occupational health nurse, or physician) or go directly to the site of need. The system allowed a clear line and immediate communication between ambulance driver and the medical facility.

The procedures discussed relate to employees whose illness or injury precludes self-direction in obtaining care and represent, by far, a minimal number of patients. Most workers will be ambulatory and will come on their own for care at the medical facility. Many organizations, concerned that certain workers will wander from their assigned stations, require that an employee in need of care obtain a pass from his or her immediate supervisor before leaving for the OHS. It might be required further that the pass be signed, with the time of reporting and departure noted, by a dispensary receptionist, records clerk, or nurse. There is a need for such procedures, for many employees have claimed in various settings that the OHS "kept them" for 3 or 4 hours, which was a totally untrue statement made to cover up a period of dereliction of duty that may actually have included time away from the plant premises. If the pass system is used, it is advisable that the OHS employ a time stamp to authenticate the entries on the pass form.

Reception and Care

A special ambulance entrance similar to a loading dock is ideal for use, as it precludes transporting an extremely ill or injured worker through a busy dispensary, in view of applicants for employment, other workers who are less seriously ill or injured, or fellow employees awaiting medical surveillance procedures. Even though a surgically clean room may be used infrequently, it is desirable to retain such an area because of the privacy that can be provided. The viewing of an injured worker and the sensing of the professional concern can be extremely upsetting to the laity, particularly to emotionally labile persons who frequently attend an OHS.

Needless to say, all procedures indicated for care should be instituted immediately without awaiting extraction of the health record from the file or procurement of either identifying information or details of the circumstances of the injury or illness. Not every person seen for emergency care may be an employee, for visitors or vendors might become ill while on company premises, and no record would be at hand.

Records can be completed either after the treatment is finished and the patient is comfortable, on return of the OHS staff member accompanying the patient, or when the transport vehicle has departed with the patient. If fresh testimony is needed in regard to the particulars of an injury-producing accident, members of the safety department can be apprised of the event, and investigation can be initiated before recollection is altered by the passage of time.*

If the patient does not present as an emergency, he or she will be seen in the order of arrival, the record will be removed from the file and dated, the visit will be logged, the history will be obtained, care will be given, the entry into the record will be made, and in keeping with the requirements of the local statistical recording system, data will be noted, transferred, or forwarded for inclusion in the appropriate tabulation categories.

Documentation of Information

While medical records will be discussed later, certain recommendations are made regarding the notation of the patient's visit and treatment/disposition sequence.

If the patient can provide the history, the details should be recorded in the worker's own words, with full information regarding time, place, and his or her impression of the cause of the injury. The word "carelessness" is used with great frequency as a generic umbrella to cover a broad variety of behavioral causes for injury and should not be accepted without further inquiry as to the true etiology. It is wise to identify any possibly related events taking place prior to the injury or onset of symptoms, such as domestic problems occurring prior to or on departing for work, difficulties or misadventures while en route to work, or disagreements or altercations with supervisory personnel or coworkers preceding the medical event. Also, names of witnesses should be obtained if other persons were present at the time of injury.

If the visit involves treatment for an injury, a first report usually has to be completed, and it often is required that workers provide their view of the incident, in their own handwriting on a report form. If this documentation is not needed, the notes in the clinical record or "First Report of Injury" form should be shown to the patient for verification and co-signature. It cannot be stressed sufficiently that the first visit is the ideal time to obtain as factual a relating of significant details, before the history can be altered so as to have the patient appear either in a more favorable light or as the guiltless recipient of company-caused harm. Time will allow simulation of the truth if there is gain to be obtained.

One of the precautions to be heeded at this point in the rendering of emergency medical care is the fact that an employee presenting with an injury may have sustained the lesion at home, during recreational activity, or while working at a second job, where the medical benefits are either less attractive or where legitimate pursuit of such benefits would require time away from the primary job and thus wage loss. These comments are not made to imply that all employees are bent on deception. But many a seasoned occupational physician can attest to the constant presence of a few workers whose aim is to maximize an alleged disability or to remain away from work as long as possible. Such persons appear even in the most advantageous work settings and, in time, become known to both supervisory and occupational health personnel.

Every notation made in the patient's history should be signed, not with initials but with the full name followed by the degree or approved certification or registration letters used by state certifying, licensing, or quality-assurance bodies. In view of the number of years required before some claims are heard or adjudicated, the initials of the person providing care may no longer convey meaning to a reader of the record. Further, it is wise to stamp the name of the staff member below the signature, because the writing may defy all interpretive skills.

CHRONOLOGY OF OCCUPATIONAL ILLNESS

An occupationally generated disease follows, in part, a different course from an injury. Clinical responses to chemical exposure may be acute or chronic. Acute toxicity usually presents a true emergency, for there will have been prompt skin absorption of a hazardous substance, particularly if the formulation involves the use of a solvent as the vehicle. There may be a primary irritation or a corrosive effect on the skin, which will necessitate somewhat the same protocol as outlined for an injury. A splash of a chemical on an unprotected eye will result in an acute injury and a different treatment protocol. Every patient presenting with eye trauma should have an assessment

*J. J. Hutson, M.D., Corporate Medical Director of Eastern Airlines, Miami, FL, uses a special half-sheet "Medical Information Record," which he has the injured employee complete in his own handwriting, whenever possible, for this practice ". . . has saved much litigation in cases where the story changes to a more favorable statement for Workers' Compensation purposes" (personal communication, Jan. 5, 1981).

of visual acuity, whenever possible. A baseline determination will aid in estimating improvement or deterioration and can serve to prevent medicolegal problems [16]. Entry in the clinical record should indicate if the patient can see light and hand motion and can count fingers, not only with the affected eye but also with the uninjured contralateral eye.

A critical response may arise suddenly on exposure of a worker to an irritant gas, vapor, dust, mist, aerosol, or fume, and acute bronchospasm or pulmonary edema may follow on inhalation of the compromising material. Acute illness following accidental ingestion of a toxic substance is conceivable but less likely in the usual industrial setting.

Cohen [17] has suggested that a "Safety and Health Person (SHP)" be designated for the handling of toxic exposure emergencies. Such a designee might be a line supervisor, a personnel director (particularly in a small plant), or even an interested employee. Irrespective of position, the SHP should

- Be familiar with and capable of directing the emergency response procedure.
- Be familiar with the existing chemical and physical hazards.
- Be readily available.
- Be trained in basic first aid and safety skills.
- Be well-known to the employees. The SHP can direct fellow workers in the use, for example, of eyewash fountains for acid exposures or amyl nitrate pearls for acute cyanide intoxication.

In prolonged exposure to a chemical toxicant, however, there develops the element of chronicity, and pathophysiologic changes begin to be noticed subjectively or are detected clinically, after a lengthy period of continuing contact. Even at that time, both the worker and the practitioner may believe that the developing illness is common in the population at large, and no thought will be given to an occupational etiology. Such causation can be ferreted out only through the pursual of a detailed occupational history, which will be discussed later.

Medical Surveillance

There will be an awareness in nearly all industrial organizations of the presence of hazardous substances. Such agents can appear at any point in a manufacturing process and can effect workers and others at any of these steps:

- Extraction of basic resources (mining)
- Preparation for production (crushing, roasting)
- Reception of raw materials (transport and storage)
- Introduction into manufacturing process (unpacking, combination with other materials or reagents)
- Isolation of intermediate products
- Completion of manufacturing or formulation
- Packaging of finished product
- Transport of finished product
- Storage of finished product
- Distribution of finished product
- Use of finished product
- Deterioration of product
- Removal of deteriorated product from site of application or use
- Transport of scrap or waste
- Disposal of hazardous waste
- Residential contact with hazardous waste site or with imperfectly reclaimed or reconditioned material for second-time use

An example of a material that can have deleterious effects over a temporal continuum and can render pathologic change at any of the contact points indicated is asbestos. But the OHS of a company engaged in the use of health-hazardous substances will be conducting either mandated medical surveillance procedures or precautionary examination protocols so as to be aware of any possible ill effects from worker exposure. The sources of information fortunately are legion today and are available from official agencies, professional societies, and commercial sources.

Definitive Evaluation

An employee in whom an occupational illness is suspected can be studied preliminarily in an OHS, but usually the facilities for a total evaluation may not be available. Several resources for such investigation are frequently available in most large cities, and referral can be made to any of the following, provided discussion is held in advance to determine that the particular institution or individual will accept the patient for review: National Institute for Occupational Safety and Health (NIOSH)–supported educational resource centers; occupational medicine services of certain hospitals or group clinics; university departments of occupational medicine; and private consultants in occupational medicine, pulmonology, dermatology, neurology, ophthalmology, or toxicology.

Preparatory to referral of such a patient, the following documents should be forwarded:

- Complete occupational history
- Job description
- Container labels and data sheets for patient-contact substances
- Complete clinical history, including clinical laboratory and radiographic examination reports
- Authorization for examination(s) and purchase order or contract, if required by referring organization.

Information regarding previous submission or nonsubmission of "Doctor's First Report of Injury" to state workers' compensation authority
Radiographs that are pertinent to avoid duplicative studies

In some instances the medical director of the OHS will have attending privileges at a local hospital, and if hospitalization is indicated, he or she may have the employee-patient admitted. If the medical director serves as a consultant, it might be feasible to refer the patient to the appropriate specialist for care in the hospital, and the plant physician can serve as a consultant during the period of hospitalization. If no appointments are held, it still would be advisable to undertake frequent hospital visitation so as to assure employees of a continuing interest in their welfare and return to full employment.

TREATMENT OF THE NON-OCCUPATIONALLY ILL OR INJURED

There have been declared policies that sanction the provision of emergency medical care to an employee who presents either with an illness that bears no relationship to the job or has been injured and reports to work without having sought outside medical care. Early in its considerations, the Council on Occupational Health of the AMA documented its position as follows [12]:

> Treatment of nonoccupational injury and illness never has been and is not now ordinarily considered to be a routine responsibility of an occupational health program with these limited exceptions:
>
> In an emergency, of course, the employee should be given the attention required to prevent loss of life or limb or to relieve suffering until placed under the care of his personal physician. For minor disorders, first aid or palliative treatment may be given if the condition is one for which the employee would not reasonably be expected to seek the attention of his personal physician, or to enable the employee to complete his current work shift.

The council indicated further that in certain localities, either because of the lack of health care resources or because of the isolation of the industrial installation, the provision of definitive care may be undertaken in the OHS.

Other publications of the AMA [13,14] parallel the sense of the policy given above, and the stance of the AOMA committee cited earlier [15] is in keeping with the statements of the AMA, adding that treatment should be given workers presenting emotional crises.* In practice, an OHS will provide emergency care for such commonly incurred conditions as headache, dysmenorrhea, diarrhea, upper respiratory infections, small foreign bodies (splinters), household burns, or abrasions, including the provision of a small amount of oral or topical medication. There may even be a follow-up visit or two. Employees normally will not seek attention for these minor disorders from a personal physician because they would have to take sick leave, which they would like to reserve for more serious needs, or because they would lose part of a wage if there is no sick leave available. If the worksite is at a distance from the physician's office, additional time would be lost in travel. Further, the visit, if it would be possible to be seen on that particular day or be "worked in," would have to be paid for (in full or in part), and these disorders are normally cared for by the employee through use of over-the-counter medications.

If the physician or nurse believes that the individual is sufficiently ill as to preclude working, he or she will be sent home without completing the work shift. If it is suspected that the disorder will become worse or that a complication will develop, the employee will be advised to see a private physician as soon as possible, or, certainly, on finishing the work shift.

No OHS undertakes the prolonged care of a worker with a chronic disorder such as arthritis, coronary artery disease, hypertension, psoriasis, or chronic obstructive pulmonary disease (COPD), as examples. The OHS is involved with such affected employees only in relation to their placement or surveillance if there is a significant, potentially harmful exposure. On occasion, a laboratory test procedure may be carried out, particularly if sequential testing is desired by the treating physician and work time would be lost. An employee's blood pressure may be taken at intervals as part of an effort to ensure follow-up by the patient of a personal physician's prescribed regimen.

One other exception is seen in the employee whose private physician wants to conduct inhalant allergen immunotherapy, so as to lessen the response on natural reexposure to the offending allergen. As the treatment initially calls for once or twice weekly injections, which may with time be given every 2 or 6 weeks, considerable time is saved by having the employee receive these injections in the OHS, provided

*The committee summarized the position in a later note, saying that ". . . there are no fixed rules on how much non-occupational care will be rendered in the industrial setting. It is usually determined by the following: (1) company medical resources; (2) community medical resources (or lack of same); and (3) cost savings." (Clinical occupational inquiry. *J Occup Med* 22:780, 1980.)

that the private physician has given, in writing to the OHS, complete instructions regarding the allergen mix, the dosage, time intervals, and method of administration. Usually, if the physician agrees to have the patient receive the injections at work, the allergen mix will be brought in by the employee, for use and retention in the OHS. If such injections are undertaken, as with other forms of immunotherapy, there must be at hand appropriate medications for the treatment of systemic anaphylaxis [18].

It must be reiterated that emergencies do take place in a plant, and the OHS will be called when a worker sustains an acute asthmatic attack, a myocardial infarction, retinal detachment, renal colic, hemorrhage from the gastrointestinal tract, a cerebrovascular accident, or even an untoward emotional response to an inciting event. Whatever emergency care is indicated must be given, and contact is made with the worker's physician for instructions as to transport to a specific hospital or, rarely, to the physician's office.

Fortunately, there are exceptions even to this not too sharply dichotomized arena of care. In the forthright declaration of medical department policy by a large pharmaceutical manufacturer, one reads the following [19]:

> The Medical Department offers employees comprehensive medical care and consultation for medical problems, whether such problems are work-related or not. Since personal or family matters are frequently at the root of employee medical problems, family consultation is available. The Medical Department functions on the basis of employee trust, and all medical information is strictly confidential and made known only to the employee.

It is this kind of insightful dedication and purpose that makes for the best in occupational health service. The same company offers dental prophylaxis to its employees, a benefit exercised by others primarily during World War II and in a few years following, but almost absent in today's industries. Further care is provided third-party employees, a practice rare outside the hospital occupational medical department setting [19].

INDICATED CAVEATS

Though no specific treatment protocols are offered in this chapter, certain procedures or principles to be followed in the provision of care are indicated.

The most desirable policy to be established and followed is the provision of the best care as quickly as possible, which always proves to be the best for the patient, the company, the workers' compensation insurance underwriter, and the OHS. Efforts to obtain care at less cost or at the hands of less skilled practitioners is never advised, for frequently it proves to be more costly eventually and, in many cases, referral to a more qualified specialist eventuates anyway.

RADIOGRAPHIC STUDIES

While it has been traditional to order roentgenograms on all patients presenting with potential injuries to bone because of fear of medicolegal action alleging malpractice, there has been a movement away from unnecessary x-ray examinations, not only in light of the exposure to excessive radiation but also with a view toward greater cost-containment in medical care.

Cain [20] has stated that to protect the patient, x-rays should be taken whenever bony injuries or other conditions demonstrable roentgenographically are reasonably suspected, provided that moving and positioning the patient will not be harmful. Yet, he cautions that "the frivolous taking of x-rays" increases costs and radiation exposure and is time-consuming. He adds that the performance of such examinations for the purpose of providing answers to realistic clinical questions that are likely to be resolved by radiographic scrutiny, the use of radiology algorithms, and agreed-upon guidelines will lead to the most appropriate use of radiologic services.

Brand and his coworkers [21] have made an effort to meet the desiderata called for in the treatment of the injured. To curb the excessive use of radiography, they developed a protocol to select patients with injuries of the extremities who needed x-ray examinations. The strict application of the protocol—tested in 848 subjects—would have reduced x-ray usage by 12 percent for upper extremities and 19 percent for lower extremities. Because of patients' demands for radiographic examination, however, the actual reductions were 5 percent and 16 percent, respectively. Through nationwide elimination of superfluous radiography, the investigators believed that costs could be reduced between $79 million and $139 million, without compromising the quality of care or increasing malpractice liability. They admit, though, that even the best protocol cannot eliminate all negative roentgenographic studies.

The analysis of the patients studied allowed identification of a set of eight criteria that offered the best discrimination. They included

Three gross signs—bone deformity, bone instability, and crepitation
Point tenderness
Ecchymosis or severe swelling in an upper extremity

Moderate to severe pain with weight bearing, in a hip or thigh
Any positive finding in a knee

Once the patient has been examined for these eight critical signs, little additional insight would be gained from consideration of other indicators such as pain at rest, generalized tenderness, limitation of motion, moderate swelling, or pain on weight bearing for injuries distal to the knee.

It was admitted that all negative extremity films could not be eliminated, as there is "an irresolvable overlap in the clinical presentations of patients with and without bone injuries." The study is presented here in the hope that the protocol can be employed in the industrial setting where every injury represents a claim, and injury repeaters could be subjected to excessive amounts of diagnostic radiation.*

In keeping with radiography for trauma, Pitt and Speer [22] have offered a helpful discussion regarding the radiologist's report. Because of criticism of reports relating to skeletal trauma, they suggest a format that can be passed on to the radiologist(s) serving a particular OHS. The report should include the following items: impression or diagnosis; comments, including introductory remarks (technique, timing, presence of immobilization devices), general description (regarding fractures open or closed, complete or incomplete, simple or comminuted, direction of fracture line, location, length, angulation, displacement, rotational deformity, with subjective modifiers such as minimal, mild, moderate, or considerate), and additional statements, including follow-up studies, clinical remarks, and radiologist recommendations (additional views or other imaging technique).

It is cautioned that the recommendations be worded in a manner that will not pressure (often medicolegally) referring physicians to order a study that, in their judgment, is not necessary, for example, "Additional information might be gained by tomography," or "Follow-up views are suggested based on the clinical course."

Martin [23] has entered a plea for greater communication with the consultant radiologist than has been evidenced in the past. He asks for the inclusion of "a few words of pertinent clinical information [that] will permit a more reasoned analysis of roentgenograms." Although he addresses the hospital situation, he indicates that the radiographic request form is frequently filled out by a ward clerk with limited knowledge of the medical lexicon.* An example of misuse of such a form is seen in the request of a roentgenogram of the elbow in a patient with lupus erythematosus. Did she have migratory polyarthralgia? No, she fell out of bed. The sense of the message can be extrapolated to the OHS where frequent requests are made for studies of potential pneumoconioses because of certain dusty work exposures. The radiologist is helped when specific information is given concerning work contactants.

A final point regarding radiographs is that they be retained as long as possible, in keeping with legal mandates, available storage space, fiscal need for recovery of silver, or lack of microfilming capability.

Some jurisdictions require certification of radiology technologists by examination, permitting, if the applicant is successful, the use of the title certified radiologic technologist (CRT). It is advisable that the state regulations be explored regarding this assurance of professional qualification.

TREATMENT OF MINORS

There will be occasions when students under 18 years of age will be employed and treatment may be indicated because of injury. The state code should be consulted to determine the current interpretation of minority status.

A person under 18 years who is living separately and apart from parents or legal guardian, with or without consent, who is managing his or her own financial affairs, or who is married may in some jurisdictions give consent to treatment, radiographic study, or other diagnostic procedure. Advice of company counsel will govern the relationship of OHS action to a minor.

*Following the publication of the study of Brand and coworkers [21], there were arguments presented such as the possibility of a single successful medical malpractice judgment negating all savings accrued by the selection protocol. In the OHS, however, where there are the conflicting constraints of (1) every injured worker's reporting for treatment irrespective of the minor nature of the trauma and (2) the litigious trend under the workers' compensation system, extreme care has to be exercised in deciding that radiographic studies are needed or can be omitted. Unfortunately, in most instances, roentgenograms will be taken, for the specter of the courtroom interrogator always looms before the treating professional—"Doctor, you didn't take x-rays?" (See communications from D. O. Davis and M. T. Morgan, and response from D. A. Brand and W. H. Frazier, Protocol for selecting patients with injured extremities who need x-rays. *N Engl J Med* 307:256, 1982.)

*That some element of exactitude is needed in the completion of the request form is seen in examples of garbling offered by Martin [23]: Waldorf abscess (walled off); subdural hematemesis; insertion of Swan dance catheter; and fracture paroxysmal humerus (proximal).

ANIMAL BITES

In certain companies or public services, contact with animals may be part of the assigned duties or may be inadvertent. Animal bites may be sustained, and the affected worker will report to the OHS for care. In many states, such bites must be reported to the local health authority. The regulations extant in the jurisdiction should be studied for direction regarding compliance.

HANDWASHING

While it might seem totally unnecessary to introduce as elementary a subject as the washing of hands, a discussion is indicated by the consistent appearance of nosocomial infections. During the hurried moments of changing dressings on many employees, a good number of whom have been waiting an unreasonable length of time for care, the attendant may neglect the simple procedure of cleansing between patients.

In a study involving patients in intensive care units [24], it was found that handwashing occurred after only 41 percent of the direct contacts with either the patients or the support equipment. Physicians washed less frequently than did the nurses, and it was concluded that compliance with recommended practice was poor in that the basic concepts of infection control were frequently ignored. Not only do the hands of personnel transmit pathogens, but they may also become a reservoir for nosocomial organisms.

The most minor contact—taking the pulse, measuring blood pressure, or just touching the patient's hand—will allow transfer of organisms that are recoverable 2.5 hours later.

The same issue was given more evidence at the annual meeting of the American Thoracic Society, where Maki [25] indicated that transmission through medical personnel was found to be the major mode of spread of gram-negative bacteria in hospitals, particularly in critical care units. Although costly microbial surveillance methods can be conducted regularly at hospitals, the incidence of nosocomial infections can be cut by as much as half at some institutions "if staff would simply wash hands between patients." He continued by saying that he did not wish to be unkind and use the term *apathy*, but there was considerable apathy in this regard, and unfortunately the attitude was greatest for physicians.

Maki [25] noted that in any given hospital, half of the staff were likely to be carrying such gram-negative rods as *Klebsiella, Enterofactor, Serratia pseudomonas,* or *Acinetobacter,* and 10 percent can be exposed to carry *Staphylococcus aureus*. There is no need to duplicate some of the frightening nosocomial epidemics that appeared in the 1950s. OHS personnel, by virtue of the number of patients to be seen, may neglect this all-important step in personal hygiene. Occupational health is *preventive* medicine.

EMOTIONAL ASPECTS OF ILLNESS OR INJURY

Although the mental health aspects of work will be discussed in a later chapter, attention is directed to the fact that many injuries—and some illnesses—are direct results of the impact of certain stressors on the patient's life. Further, the event of an injury may trigger a response that will preclude the employee's return to work either after the expected period of convalescence or ever.

The attendant, whether it is the occupational health nurse, the physician, a physician's assistant, or an EMT, should, on obtaining the history and after caring for the acute lesion, explore the hours and days preceding the trauma in an effort to determine if the injury climaxes a period of stress response. The emotional etiologies of injury are numerous, and the causative setting and players may be at home, at work, or elsewhere. If the stressors are not identified and resolved, there is great likelihood that other injuries will follow, with the usual concomitants of pain, lost time, lost pay, and residual disability.

There must be concern about the individual, and in many situations caring for the trauma without caring for the patient is incomplete and disinterested professional attention. The initial contact with the caring person will frequently determine the course the injured employee will experience. The attitude of the treating individual, supportive and empathic, may mean an immediate return to work, while a cold, arrogant, impersonal response may lead to negative behavior on the patient's part that could course the complete path to litigation and settlement, in place of a pleased and prompt resumption of duties.

WAITING TIME

Most vexing to employees in need of care from an OHS is the time spent waiting for service. Perhaps more disturbing is the effect on the worker's supervisor who cannot spare the employee while the latter is awaiting attention. Most personnel will report promptly to the medical facility and after having their names recorded will find that a period of nonproductive time then begins.

One has been witness to OHS staff members engaged in personal telephone calls, reading the morning paper, or "out on break," while slowly angering patients remain witness to many of these frustrating scenes. In a series of small studies conducted among indigent patients [26], it was found that, even after improvement, 50 percent of the patients were still waiting for over 1 hour. As Foster and Lauria [26] commented succinctly, patients often equate quality of care with rapidity of services, and if we wish the public to continue to hold the professions in high regard, we should pay serious attention to their major complaint—waiting.

In some instances there seems to be a strange perception of employee-patients by professional staff, in that they are viewed as second-class citizens who are supposed to wait until those persons in the superordinate positions in the OHS are ready. It is difficult to convince some seasoned OHS staff members that they are engaged in providing a *service,* which implies the most immediate attention compatible with the caseload, accessible equipment, and available attendants and the fastest turnaround consistent with high-quality care. Every minute spent in an OHS not devoted to the rendering of care is downtime and is counterproductive in executing the mission of the organization.

Patients' records should be stamped to indicate times of arrival and departure so that data are available for review and deficiencies in performance can be rectified. There is time wasted by all levels of staff, and in many instances, it is this breach in good manners that solidifies a negative image of an otherwise capable therapeutic group.

One problem that has challenged resolution is the disruption in the sequence of patients when executives seek care at the health service. Frequently they are seen ahead of many who are waiting because a manager's time is "more valuable." Often such a person will be ushered into a consulting or examining room in full view of the more occupationally soiled workers whose arrival long antedated that of the manager. Such inequitable treatment further disenchants the workers awaiting call. If it is absolutely mandatory that the white-collar workers be seen in advance of those persons previously registered, there should be a separate entrance and examination area so that this differential selection process does not visibly flout custom.

EMERGENCY CARE FOR CHEMICAL INJURIES

Nearly every plant uses or produces chemicals in one form or another, which can prove injurious if they escape containment and are brought into accidental contact with workers. A systematic method of treating such burns or contamination should be documented and readily available in the OHS that is equipped to provide emergency care.

Attention is directed to a publication that can serve both as an information source and as a model for the addition of material not covered. The *Chemical Emergency Manual,* published by the American Lung Association of Western New York, Inc.,* provides coverage of 35 different chemical substances. The manual was prepared to aid occupational health personnel, among others, in protecting the rescuer and providing a continuum of preferred medical treatment to the victims of the chemicals described.

Through use of a "Hazardous Materials Classification" diamond, the characteristics of flammability, reactivity, specific hazard, and health hazard are given. On the obverse of the card devoted to each substance are outlined the health hazards and their severity under emergency conditions. On the reverse side of the card are the "Medical Instructions" for use in (1) the plant site, (2) during transportation, or (3) in the emergency room, with specific guidelines for treatment of the affected skin or eyes or the effects of ingestion or inhalation.

It is suggested that such a manual be available in the OHS of a plant where toxic substances are in use, and if there are materials not covered by the publication cited, additional guide cards can be prepared locally.

CONTINUITY OF CARE

One of the despiriting elements of health care in any group setting is the change of practitioners—be it physician, nurse or physician's assistant—on repeated visits to the facility. A patient values the rapport established with one treating professional and feels rejected on facing a different staff person on return. The thought is created that "he doesn't know my case," which is underscored by the usual scan of the record on the repeat visit.

Although involving a specific age group, the principle that is illuminated by Wasson and his coworkers [27] is applicable to any segment of an adult population. The question asked in the study was, "If an outpatient repeatedly sees the practitioner, is his care influenced?" In an 18-month period involving care of 776 men aged 55 years and older, a randomized double-blind trial demonstrated that continuity of outpatient provider care resulted in more patient satisfaction, shorter hospitalizations, and fewer emergent hospital admissions. It is conceivable that a comparable follow-up in the OHS will produce greater satisfaction with the program and possibly less loss of work time. A constant change in the treating personnel can alienate a worker. Continuity in care is the desirable goal for both the practitioner and the patient.

*Located at 766 Ellicott Street, Buffalo, NY 14203.

ALCOHOL AND TRAUMA

While the consumption of alcohol has long been associated with vehicular accidents and their resultant injuries, it usually is not thought of in relation to other accidental events. Maull [28] believes that the role of alcohol abuse is equally great or greater in falls, choking, and other major traumatic events and recommends that the blood alcohol concentration be measured in all patients, irrespective of cause. In several studies cited by Maull—analyses involving farm-machinery accidents, home accident injuries, aircraft mishaps, drownings, major burns, assaults, and suicides—alcohol has led to impairment of the injured in from 25 percent to nearly 75 percent of the cases. An OHS should be equipped to determine the blood alcohol concentration in injured employees and, as Maull suggests further, should be able to measure the serum r-glutanyl transpeptidase (r-gT) level, for elevations are strongly suggestive of chronic alcoholic intoxication. Appropriate rehabilitative efforts can follow.

MISCELLANEOUS ELEMENTS IN CARE

As there are variations in social thought, so there are differences in the delivery of occupational health care. One large corporation opened a pharmacy in a midwestern city to serve approximately 30,000 employees and dependents. The objective was to lower the prescription costs of a single year amounting to $1.1 million. A cost-containment of 65 percent resulted from the use of corporate space, professional employees, and the stocking of generic drugs [29].

In a Nevada company, Polaroid photographs are taken of the injuries presented by employees, which are then dated, signed by the treating physician, and placed in the worker's clinical record [30].

A petroleum company in Puerto Rico maintains two ambulances, which can be used to transport not only ill or injured workers but also employees' relatives for nonemergency disorders, provided a request has been submitted 12 hours in advance and bears the corporate medical director's approval. By local law, the sick or injured patient must be accompanied by a physician, nurse, or certified paramedic [31].

MEDICATIONS

Because of variation in state laws or regulations concerning the dispensing of medications by professional personnel other than physicians, it is helpful to stock prepackaged preparations of commonly used drugs, which can be given directly to an employee-patient. Most often the so-called industrial or occupational health packs will provide two tablets in a sealed labeled packet, supplied in boxes of 50, 100, 250, or 500 packets.

Currently, dispensing systems are available wherein an OHS can order a wide variety of medications that are provided in a cabinet and can be restocked as needed. One such cabinet has 10 columns each containing about 40 packs,* allowing for slide-out dispensing. These prelabeled plastic containers hold more than a two-tablet or two-capsule dose and provide for a longer period of treatment. In keeping with many state laws, the individual package must bear the following information:

Trade or generic name of the drug
Name of the manufacturer
Complete directions for use
Warnings where necessary
Patient's name
Date prescribed
Name and address of prescriber
Strength of drug
Quantity prescribed
Expiration date

Because of the ready access to most OHS offices or examining rooms, special care should be taken with blank prescription forms. Certain guidelines have been offered in safeguarding these forms and ensuring their proper use [32]:

- Store all unused prescription pads in a safe place where they cannot be easily stolen.
- Minimize the number of pads in use at one time.
- Have prescription blanks numbered consecutively when printed so that one can tell if sheets are missing.
- Never sign prescription blanks in advance.
- Write prescriptions in ink or indelible pencil to prevent changes.
- Write out the actual amount of medication prescribed in addition to using an arabic or roman numeral to discourage alterations.
- Do not use prescription blanks for writing notes or memos, which can be erased for reuse.
- Do not leave prescription pads in unattended examining rooms, office areas, or the physician's bag or car, where they can be easily taken.

*Available from MDS-Medical Dispensing Systems, 2720 Monterey Street, #403, Torrance, CA, 90503, (213) 328-8732.

STAR OF LIFE AMBULANCE

On September 23, 1973, a distinctive emergency care symbol was adapted by the National Highway Traffic Safety Administration of the U.S. Department of Transportation, so as not to be in conflict with emblems used by the American National Red Cross and as authorized by Congress [33]. The symbol bears the staff of Aesculapius, the Greek god of medicine, in white on a primary blue, six-barred cross. The bars, numbered clockwise from the 12 o'clock position, represent the functions of the emergency medical service: (1) detection, (2) reporting, (3) response, (4) on-scene care, (5) care in transit, and (6) transfer to definitive care. The registration mark R appears between the third and fourth bars and represents the registration with the Commission of Patents and Trademarks for an initial 20 years.

The symbol is used as a certification mark on emergency medical care vehicles, indicating that such vehicles have met U.S. Department of Transportation standards, as provided by *Federal Specification Ambulance—Emergency Medical Care Surface Vehicle,* KKK-A-1822A, Apr. 1, 1980. In addition, it may be used as identifying insignia by emergency medical care personnel, certifying that they have been trained to meet the standards. Further, the symbol is authorized for use on road maps and highway signs to indicate the location of or access to qualified emergency medical care services. Such uses take the form of decals, uniform patches, printed materials, plaques, pins, buckles, name plates, and the like [33].

The primary point being made is that an ambulance owned and used by a company should meet the specifications of the standard, which cover not only the structure, mechanics, and performance of the vehicle, but the lighting systems, cots or litters, stowage accommodations, extrication equipment, oxygen units, and medical equipment. It is the duty of the manufacturer to provide the purchaser with an authenticated certification document and label for all ambulances certified as "Star of Life" ambulances. Symbols can be purchased locally, and they must meet the standards as to dimensions and placement on the vehicle [33]. The specifications given by the standard carry the endorsement of the Ambulance Division of the Truck Body and Equipment Association [34].

PHYSICIAN'S EMERGENCY BAG

Whether the OHS possesses a fully equipped ambulance or other emergency vehicle, there should be one or more emergency bags available for transport to the site of injury. The contents of such a bag should be determined by the medical director or consultant, and medications kept in such bags should be checked periodically against their dates of expiration.

ADJUVANT SERVICES

One of the activities of a Chicago bank conducted through its employee health service, targeted toward cost-containment, is a set of guidelines provided employees who seek or are about to obtain outside treatment. One such list is a compilation of surgical procedures that should be carried out as outpatient services, for example, arthroscopy, fracture with closed reduction, laryngoscopy, and so on.

A companion list given employees, when appropriate, comprises various surgical procedures for which the employee-patient should seek a second opinion, for example, spinal fusion, cholecystectomy, cardiac surgery, and the like.

Patients requiring inpatient care are given a checklist to record services received while in the hospital, so that bills may be compared with actual experience.

Finally, the patient to be hospitalized is provided with a blank request form so that an itemized hospital bill can be obtained. Such documents are not always given the patient on discharge.

SPECIAL REPORT FORMS

It might be helpful to refer to some special forms relating to emergency medical care. A blank developed for use at the Continental Illinois Corporation [35] serves as the occupational injury/illness investigation report. The form requires completion by the employee health services and further entries by the division to which the employee-patient belongs. Copies are forwarded to the company's safety committee. In addition to identifying information, it includes diagnosis, time of reporting of injury, lost time, action taken, disposition, body part affected, site of occurrence, and preventive measures to be taken. All entries are coded so that the data are ready for computerization.

A second form resolves the difficulty encountered so frequently in industry of having the treating physician return the injured employee to "light duty," a status usually without meaning to a first-line supervisor. The blank, titled "Light Duty Work Activity Level," developed by the medical facility of Teledyne in Albany, Oregon [36], requires the physician to indicate the amount of activity, by category of physical requirement, to be undertaken by the employee being returned to less than full duty. By use of exact limits, the supervisor is guided in the assignment of tasks to the individual. Such a form is advised for use in any work area where postinjury employees can resume a portion of their previous job.

DEATH ON THE PREMISES

Because of the multiplicity of circumstances at the work scene—aging employees, physical hazards, power equipment, hostile environments, flouting of safety regulations, mechanical failure, overextension of human energy, emotionally disturbed personnel, and delayed preventive maintenance, among others—a death may take place on the premises of the organization. Occupational physicians and nurses long identified with practice in industry will, in a lifetime, probably experience the loss of a worker during a regularly scheduled shift.

While the facts of the event might challenge credibility, it nevertheless has been the experience of seasoned OHS professionals to have been faced with fatalities from naturally occurring disasters and accidents, sudden vascular occlusion, suicide, and murder. As these events are always unscheduled, an immediate state of acute anxiety is created, at first among workers close to the scene and eventually throughout the total workforce. Since most of the plant personnel are inadequately equipped emotionally or by training to provide leadership in such an emergent situation, it becomes the task of the medical director or a designated representative to initiate the appropriate actions.

It would be wise, if the death is not accidental, to have the body brought to the OHS and away from fellow workers, in whom some psychogenic illness readily could appear. However, if it is believed that the death is a "coroner's case," then the body should not be moved without permission of that office.

NOTIFICATION OF PLANT PERSONNEL

The order of notification is not necessarily that as given, for local circumstances will dictate a judicious approach befitting the plant population, location, geography, security classification of the work performed, and so on. The following personnel or offices should be notified: chief executive officer (CEO), clergyman, security director, coroner/medical examiner, safety director, workers' compensation unit, insurance unit, personnel department, private physician, and the family.

THE FAMILY

This step in the complex system of notification is usually the most difficult, for it involves direct confrontation with the surviving spouse, parent, adult progeny, or young children. Such a task should not be relegated to unfeeling or emotionally incompetent supervisors or even friends of the deceased. If the task has not already been cared for by a workmate friend of the deceased, then the medical director and an occupational health nurse should visit the employee's home immediately to apprise the family of the event.* Such action is difficult and should be undertaken by persons accustomed to the relaying of unexpected, distressing news.

Not every such scene follows the neatness of a television script, for the exact response can never be anticipated. The author recalls, as a house officer assigned this task, of having to notify a highly emotionally labile family that their father had expired during a gastric procedure carried out by an eminent surgeon. The women members of the family turned and, almost in concert, literally beat their heads against the tiled walls of the corridor.

Obviously, the news is relayed with the gentlest of feelings, with emphasis on the absence of suffering or pain, and with the offer of all assistance from both the medical personnel and departments on behalf of the employer. No counsel at this point will cover all situations, for, as indicated, one cannot know or even guess what the response might be to the message. It could even be welcome news, for after decades of involvement in occupational health, one has learned that anything can happen with people and that, soon or late, it does and is not surprising.

THE PRESS

If there is an accidental death—particularly if there are multiple losses—there will be calls from the media. Early on, the director of public relations (information), if there is such a position, should be given the details so that there will be a consistent release of information from a single source. The CEO might prefer to provide the print and broadcast media with

*A stinging comment is made by two nonphysician writers—a Ph.D. of an unidentified discipline and a nurse—who state [37]: "Survivors interviewed indicated they would rather be informed by a nurse who seemed to care that their loved one had died and who seemed to understand that the deceased was someone important to the survivor than to be told by a physician who was knowledgeable as to why the individual had died but who seemed not to care that the death occurred."

the details, and if so, such information will already have been given to that office.

OTHER EMPLOYEES

A group frequently forgotten during the upsetting event of a death is the other workers stationed near the deceased or who were closely and jointly involved in the business of the company. They become upset and apprehensive and, irrespective of the cause of death, can be helped if the physician were to meet with them. Questions can be answered, the group can be given whatever support seems needed, and if there are certain members known to the OHS as unstable or labile persons, they might be asked to come in for additional comfort.

Such a meeting, held early, can prevent the spread of false information and will effect a more rapid return to assigned duties. Most troublesome to these work-related employees is not being given answers or being informed by someone not considered in an authority position. One respected authority is a representative of the union, preferably an officer, particularly if the deceased was affiliated with one of the locals at the plant. Ill rumors can be rectified, and a wise person will aid in controlling the spread of conceptions or perceptions not founded on fact.

Particular emphasis is given this element of the notification protocol if fellow workers are foreign born and have a language barrier or have religious beliefs or folklore credos that could lead to truly upsetting behavior. In this situation it would be best to have one of the group's own, preferably an opinion-maker who is bilingual, aid in the meeting.

MEDICAL IDENTIFICATION AND PERSONAL RECORDS

IDENTIFICATION DEVICES

In our contemporary society, the need has emerged for individuals to make known their medical disorders for fear of therapeutic mishandling. From this need has grown a moderately wide choice of identification devices that can provide pertinent information helpful in the treatment of the ill or injured person. Also, as our body of knowledge concerning the health effects of work contacts with hazardous substances enlarges, there should be at hand a continuing history of a person's work—maintained by the worker—for a quicker diagnosis when an etiologic search is undergone at the time of a possible, or alleged, occupationally related illness. Lastly, there should be available, as a referent, a regular annotated health history when medical care is being sought. An OHS can be helpful either in initiating the development of such documents or in actually supplying them if the usual constraints of budget and personnel permit.

When emergencies arise, particularly if a person is away from home and out of contact with family members or colleagues from the place of employment, it is important that specific medical information be available relating either to certain clinical disease states or known disorders subject to acute emergent change. Persons in certain occupations would benefit by such identification, such as law enforcement and firefighting personnel, construction workers, oil-field workers, truck drivers, and salespersons who use the freeway considerably. Benefitted also would be travelers. Various devices have been created, either to be worn or to be carried, that convey medical information or provide a telephonic source of further health intelligence.

CONDITIONS WARRANTING USE

Several types of identification devices have been developed, some by nonprofit organizations, others as commercial products. Common to them all would be the diagnostic rationale for carrying such items. The conditions warranting the immediate availability of medical information are multiple and include not only a wide spectrum of disease states but also medications being taken and other needs such as hearing loss, non-English-speaking person, contact-lens wearer, and the like. Appropriate to all indications would be such adjunctive information as that relating to the recency of pertinent immunizations and physician's name, address, and telephone number. In nearly all instances, an information blank is provided by the organization or vendor for completion by the employee, patient, or applicant.

The devices are available in several modes, including wallet-size cards, wallet-size sealed plastic data containers, plastic bracelets, and metal devices (chains or bracelets). The items can be obtained commercially or from foundations established for the purpose of having such data on record and available.

PERSONAL HEALTH RECORDS

Many agencies have, as a public service, issued small brochures that provide indicated spaces for the entry of health information. Such a document, if maintained accurately and currently, will serve as a reference when consulting a physician, when hospitalized, or when completing certain applications requiring health information. One advantage to the maintenance of a record of this type is the avoidance of repetitive test procedures or excessive exposure to diagnostic ionizing radiation.

A company, again within fiscal constraints, could provide a small printed brochure not exceeding eight pages overall but would provide spaces for the following entries:

Name and additional identifying information
Physician's name, address, telephone number
Dentist's name, address, telephone number
Life insurance—carrier, policy numbers
Health insurance—carrier, group and coverage designations, effective date
Blood donations made
Immunization record
Medication allergies
Other allergies (foods, insect bites, pollens)
Medications currently taken
History of communicable diseases
Accidents
Hospital admissions
Family history—by known relative, disease, and cause of death
Travel outside United States—by country visited, date, and duration
Special laboratory tests
X-ray examinations
Special problems—for example, transfusion reactions, bleeding tendency

Employees should be encouraged to initiate and maintain such a record on each family member, and medical episodes known to the OHS should undergo entry into the personal health record.

WORK HISTORY

Although the details of an occupational history will be presented later, a brief discussion is included in this review of personal medical records. Before the mid-twentieth-century upsurge in public and professional concern with job-associated disease, and prior to the wider application of the epidemiologic method to the study of the health effects on handlers of certain work contactants, there was little need for an accurate recall of previous employments. With the broadened knowledge of delayed tissue changes and the role of chemicals in serious work-generated illness, it is important that all individuals—particularly persons subject to frequent blue-collar job moves—maintain an ongoing record of their various employments.

When efforts are made to develop such histories with workers who have moved about the country or the world, one learns that rarely are there sharp memories of employers, worksites, or production materials. To those manual workers so involved, names, places, and dates do not imbed themselves so deeply as they do with individuals for whom written language is a strong element of a job assignment. Frequently, wives will have more detailed recollection of the sources of pay if they carried the responsibility of family bookkeeping.

Personnel of an OHS should encourage the origination of individual work histories of all employees when they make professional contact. Such documents will be of help not only to the patients themselves but also to the OHS whenever a question of an occupational disease arises, whether symptomatic or evidenced only by laboratory test or radiographic examination findings. Blank forms with some ruled columns and headings would be helpful to employees in organizing their thinking regarding a 20-, 30-, or 40-year work history. Such a form should provide for entries under these headings:

Name
Date of birth
Social security number
Home address, telephone number
Next of kin, address, telephone number
For each period of employment or job, beginning with the first:
  Name of employer, name of plant
  Location of worksite, state, county, city, street address
  Inclusive dates of employment
  Job title
  Materials worked with
  Physical hazards (noise, vibration, and so on)
  Protective devices worn or used
  Physical examinations by company

The employee should be motivated to keep the record current and store it with other important personal or family files.

DISASTER PREPAREDNESS

While the noisy expostulations and destruction occasioned by the rebellious youths of the 1960s have moved into history with the maturing of the involved

TABLE 9-1. *Disasters Affecting Industry*

Man-made disasters	*Natural disasters*
Aircraft collisions and crashes	Avalanches
Bombings, fire bombings, terrorism	Cyclones
Bridge collapses	Droughts
Building collapses	Earthquakes
Civil uprisings	Frosts, freezes, and snowstorms
Construction cave-ins	Heat waves
Dam collapses	Hurricanes
Derailments and overshootings of rail terminus	Landslides
Drownings	Lightning
Explosions	Rain, floods, and subsequent mudslides
Fires, arson	Storms, global and local
Hazardous material emissions from truck or train or from fixed installations	Tornadoes
Industrial accidents	Tsunamis (tidal waves, seismic waves)
Marine disasters—collisions, sinkings, shipwrecks	Volcanic eruptions
Mine disasters	
Nuclear reactor accidents	
Oil spills	
Riots	
Sabotage	
Satellites crashing to earth	
Terrorist attacks, other	
Traffic accidents	
War with conventional weapons	
War with thermonuclear weapons	

generation, other acts against humankind—natural or man-made—continue to kill and disable. Industry was the target of many bombings, representing as it did "the establishment." While the planting of destructive devices has diminished in the United States, terrorist activity abroad continues to harm Americans, and manufacturing installations in this country are still subject to and ravaged by the hazards of the so-called acts of God.

Early in the same decade of youthful chaos there came the emphasis on civil defense, but following this period of preparation, there came a lull with the anxieties of the oil embargo and the recession of the 1970s and '80s. However, a resurgence of concern has appeared with the arms race and depictions by the broadcast media of the devastation secondary to nuclear war. While such a massive destruction has not taken place, fortunately, there have been a number of disasters that directly or indirectly have affected employed groups. That there must be a preparedness plan in which a plant's medical arm participates is one of industry's givens.

VARIETIES OF DISASTER

Between 1941 and 1980, there were nearly 5,000 catastrophic accidents causing almost 50,000 deaths [38]. The types of disasters that can affect or have involved workers or their sites of employment are shown in Table 9-1.

While some events may not produce mass casualties, the potential is present for injuries and possible involvement of OHS personnel. Even in strike situations medical personnel have been allowed through picket lines to provide care as needed. While a heat wave may not affect most of a workforce, certain individuals beyond average retirement age or with cardiovascular disease may succumb. Bomb threats, although not necessarily productive of injury, are disruptive and unpredictable as to their effect on emotionally vulnerable persons.

During the 1970s, security was increased in manufacturing plants and in the metropolitan headquarters of many large companies, obviously adding considerably to the cost of doing business. Similarly, the injuries sustained by persons at work altered the workers' compensation experience and cast new views of the insurance risk. Even when workers are injured or killed in catastrophic accidents away from the place of employment, the company is involved by virtue of hospitalization coverage, indirect costs to production, disability benefits or disability retirement or both, life insurance, and death benefits, in addition to the effect on the morale of coworkers.

DISASTER DATA

Included in the disasters cited were several events affecting people at the worksite, such as nightclub fire, explosion of ammunition ships, circus fire, gas tank explosion, mid-air collisions of planes, dam collapse, hotel fire, coal mine explosion, and earthquake. These catastrophes were in addition to the hurricanes, floods, tornadoes, and snowstorms, which affected both employed persons and nonworkers.

While railroads are diminishing as prime passenger carriers, the fatalities resulting from accidents persist in their occurrence. In the period 1969 to 1978, 1,428 employees on duty and 77 employees not on duty were killed [39].

Employees undertake recreational activities, and while aquatic deaths and injuries do not relate to disaster preparedness, companies engaged in ship repair, underwater salvage operations, and oil (or other marine mineral) exploration should plan for emergency care. In 1980, there were 7,000 drownings, and sadly 47 percent of adults who drown give evidence of alcohol in their bloodstreams [40].

An aberration among the causes of lethality was the eruption of Mount St. Helens in 1980. Following a Richter scale measure of 5.0, the mountain exploded, blasting 600 feet of rock off its summit and generating a mushroom cloud of volcanic ash that was to drift across the continental United States [41]. By July 4, nearly 7 weeks after the May 18, 1980 eruption, there were 25 volcano-associated fatalities, and 40 other persons were listed as missing. In 17, death was due to inhalation of ash [42]. The types of personnel exposed included clean-up crews (equipment operators), rubbish workers, forest and agricultural workers, and law enforcement personnel [43].

Although high in the 1970s, actual and attempted bombings have diminished greatly in number. During 1984, 853 explosive and 206 incendiary incidents were reported, with 10 deaths, 126 injuries, and property damage of $39,970,000. While the deaths and injuries were fewer than were reported the year before, the property damage increased nearly fivefold. Of the total incidents cited, 208 had commercial operations or office buildings as their targets [44]. Different motives for the bombings have included revenge, mischief, personal animosity, extortion, political extremism, labor unrest or disputes, insurance fraud, harassment, attention getting, vandalism, reprisal, malicious destruction, protest, employment disputes, crimes, and disgruntlement, among others. Fortunately, many of the devices emplaced were dismantled or detonated in a safe area.

It is advisable, if the fear of a bomb threat pervades a work group, to have a checklist imprinted on the inside of the front cover of the company telephone directory, providing for such information as time and date of call; recipient of call; exact language used; time, place, kind, reason or identity of bombing caller; type of voice (accent, sex, age, and so on); and background noise. The number of the emergency coordinator should be given.

While 72 percent of fire deaths occur in residential occupancies [45], there are fires in industrial installations. In an early study (published in 1973), the experience for 1970 to 1971 was detailed, and of an average annual number of building fires of 994,300, 4.9 percent or 48,750 were in industrial structures and 7.3 percent of 72,750 were classified as "mercantile and office." Of the nearly 1 million fires, 70,650 or 7.1 percent were caused by other flames and sparks (welding and cutting torches, sparks from machinery, friction, thawing of pipes, and miscellaneous open flames and sparks) [46].

Of immediate pertinence here is the need for an evacuation plan from the OHS. The placement of a medical facility will range from a metropolitan high-rise structure to a freestanding building near the epicenter of a plant's acreage, a lone aid station in a desert terrain, or an enclosed suite in the middle of a manufacturing activity. Irrespective of the typology or the locale, it is essential that fire drills be held with regularity.

Most exercises of this type, be they in industry, on board a cruise ship, or in an office building, rarely are taken seriously. Employees amble out leisurely, offering gallows-humorous or deprecatory remarks while en route, and there is little realization of the seriousness of the trial run. It is advised that such drills be held on a quarterly basis, for an OHS has the additional tasks of assisting patients who may not be fully clothed—individuals receiving physical therapy or undergoing examination—or providing care as required by the disaster preparedness plan.

A fire warden should be appointed whose task is to search the facility and assure the director that all persons have left the premises for a safe area. A further responsibility would be the sounding of the drill signal, the closure of the practice session, the timing of the exodus, and preparation of a critique of the group's effort, which would be impartial and objective.

OHS ROLE IN DISASTER PREPAREDNESS

It was concluded some years ago after a community disaster exercise [47] that the three major factors contributing to death and permanent disability of persons following catastrophes were poor rescue, including improper handling and related problems in the transportation of victims, inadequate first aid at the scene, and inadequate or improper medical care at the hospital. It is possible, with planning, to obviate most of these operational deficits and save lives and minimize residual disablement.

THE GENERAL PLAN

In preparation for a catastrophic event, the OHS participates in the general plan developed by the security personnel of the company. This plan should fit the needs of the organization in light of (1) its location (urban, rural, isolated); (2) its adjacency to sources of definitive medical care; (3) the structural configuration of the plant (high rise, loft, centralized one- to three-story freestanding factory buildings, wide dispersion of structures, fixed complexes such as an oil refinery); (4) nature of raw materials, intermediates, finished products (toxic substances, sources of radiant energy, explosives, laboratory reagents, nonhazardous materials); (5) communications capability; (6) adjacency to civil defense authority; and (7) vulnerability (highly industrialized area, coastal or inland waterway location, development near seismic fault, hurricane/tornado locale, adjacency to potentially riotous populations).

Healy [48] has listed the procedures to be considered in the development of a disaster preparedness plan, and those items germane to the OHS follow:

Select corporate and plant civil defense advisory committees.
Issue corporate policy directives establishing the civil defense program.
Train civil defense coordinators and committees at office of Civil Defense (OCD) schools.
Establish a control center and communications system.
Provide fallout shelter for employees and the public.
Plan for mass movement of employees to shelter.
Organize employees into special groups for self-help.
Enroll these groups into departments of local government as auxiliaries.
Train for shelter management, radiologic monitoring, first aid and medical self-help, decontamination, rescue, and firefighting.
Join with neighboring plants in organizing industrial mutual aid associations.
Plan for continuity of each important company function.
Assign emergency duties to department heads and appropriate employees.
Plan for emergency repair and restoration.
Develop plans for quickly training employees following attack.
Prepare a manual of company and plant civil defense plans.
Tell employees about the company civil defense plan.
Test the disaster control plan with drills and exercises.
Inform and educate employees in methods of personal and home survival.
Publish stories about civil defense in company and employee publications.
Urge discussion of civil defense at employee meetings.

In addition, cooperative arrangements should be made with adjacent plants for both establishment of casualty stations and use of health care personnel.

The specific functions of an OHS are to (1) assist with the rescue of the injured, (2) give emergency medical care at the scene or at a designated aid station (first aid), (3) carry out triage, (4) dispatch the most seriously injured to a hospital, (5) provide definitive care for the injured if hospital facilities not available, and (6) care for the emotionally distraught or bereaved ("psychological first aid"). The considerations that follow are applicable to non-nuclear disasters. Comments regarding the ultimate in international warfare will be offered later.

NEEDED INFORMATION

There must be established leadership in the OHS, along with known task assignments, if a disaster should befall the company installation. It is advisable that all persons responsible for activities during an emergency have their names posted, with both residence and office telephone numbers, in the OHS, with copies also for posting in the office or building that will serve as a command post and in the security headquarters, in addition to copies for each person named in the listings.

It is important that the location of specific hazards be known so that special precautions can be taken in rescue operations in the event of process disruptions.

The completed building-by-building list should be posted in the OHS and in the disaster command center.

Information regarding available facilities for the collection of casualties either in numbers beyond the capability of the OHS or if the medical unit has been destroyed should be part of the publicized plan. Buildings such as warehouses or storage areas, cafeterias, gymnasia, large offices at ground level with movable equipment, garages, or conference rooms without fixed seating can be designated as disaster collecting points or stations.

For purposes of transport of the injured who are in need of definitive care, there must be knowledge not only of local hospitals and their capacity but also of installations at considerable distance. Adjacent facilities can fill rapidly, and transport by helicopter or airplane may be needed to a moderately distant site. As an example, at the time of the 1947 Texas City disaster (570 deaths, 3000 injured, 2,500 left homeless, $50 million in property damage) [48], injured persons were hospitalized not only in that city but also in Galveston and Houston and possibly elsewhere. In a similar vein, information must be at hand regarding ambulance availability, including fire stations with paramedics, and their special capability if other than the standard equipment.

PERSONNEL ASSIGNMENTS

Members of the OHS staff will serve in both a supervisory and working capacity, as determined by the scope of the destruction or threat. The medical director should function as the director of emergency care, and other professional personnel should be charged with transportation, hospital liaison, records, and emergency surgery (the latter when more than field first aid is needed). As additional persons are needed, employees trained in first aid should be called into service as part of the OHS staff. In addition, there should be designated in each work unit certain individuals as litter bearers who will know the location of litters, their preparation for use, and their mode of handling. Also, in each work area to be used as a collecting or casualty station, there must be designated at least two disaster wardens whose task it would be to clear the area of desks, tables, and the like, so that the injured can be brought to the building.

It should be the responsibility of medical records personnel to log the injured and their disposition either home or to the hospital. At the Texas City explosion the disposition of employees was not known, and individual hospitals had to be checked regarding admissions [49]. Of vital importance is the use of an emergency medical tag,* which, in addition to identifying information, indicates the type of injury and first aid treatment, its diagnosis and treatment at the second echelon of care, and the classification of care required. The tags are completed in duplicate—one accompanies the patient, and one remains at the plant, being collected by the person responsible for records. It is essential that the tag show all medications given, to avoid duplication or overdosage.

SUPPLIES

It is necessary that a cache of emergency medical supplies be maintained in each casualty or collecting station in addition to comparable sets of materials that are in a central point and can be transported to certain locations for use—either sites of maximum injury or as substitutes for stations that may have been destroyed. An inventory must be maintained of the location and items comprising the supplies and equipment. A monthly check must be made by professional personnel—preferably occupational health nurses—to determine that expiration dates of medications have not been exceeded and that there has been no loss due to theft, water damage, deterioration, mold, or extreme heat. Replacements must be made of nonusable dated materials, and the date of inspection is to be recorded in both a master inventory and on the container. At an installation where the author served, a large wooden chest, approximately 74 in. (181 cm) in length, 30 in. (73 cm) in height, and 24 in. (59 cm) in depth, was devised for such use. Attached carrying handles extended from either end to facilitate transport, and the lid was so hinged and constructed that its top could be used as worktable, holding opened supplies. Two trays supported on inside ledges could be removed, permitting access to the larger items kept below [50].

In addition to the chest, there were at each location a box for 12 blankets, a box for four folding litters, a 10-gallon cask of drinking water, and a pair of folding supports for the placement of a litter, for use as an examination or treatment table. The supports were merely a variety of a carpenter's folding horse, hinged at the top, notched to hold the rounded ends of the littler poles, and kept upright by a single connecting rope between the two lower crossbars. The containers were painted white, carried the designation "Medical Supplies," "Stretchers," or "Blankets" and bore the legend in red lettering, "Emergency Equipment for Use by Health Division Only." The

*Tags are available from METAG *(Journal of Civil Defense)*, Starlee, FL 32091; local or area Office of Civil Defense; and Precision Dynamics Corporation, 3031 Thornton Avenue, Burbank, CA 91504.

number of such assemblies is determined, of course, by the plant area, the explosion potential of certain operations, the availability of medical care, and the transportation capability of the plant. The contents of such an emergency supply station should be determined locally. As it is not possible to forecast with any exactitude the amount of equipment or number of supplies needed, it is better to overestimate generously what might be required.

TRIAGE

Triage is the sorting out and classification of casualties to determine priority of need and proper place of treatment. One patient classification scheme has been described by Cowan [51] as follows:

Code I Minor injuries and/or illnesses with delayed treatment.

Code II Major injuries and/or illnesses where treatment can be delayed for life-threatening injuries, such as lacerations, simple fractures.

Code III Critical injuries and/or illnesses in persons who must be treated immediately, such as severe burns, open abdominal wounds, cardiac arrest, airway difficulties.

Code IV Deceased persons, or persons in whom death is imminent.

Colored emergency medical tags will aid in identification and avoid retriaging. After emergency care is rendered, Code III patients are transported first, followed by Code II patients. Code I patients may be transported or may be asked to use a taxi or private car to an emergency service or to their own physician. As pointed out by Cowan [51], triage involving trauma is complex, for one patient may be covered with blood, in need of intravenous fluid and a pressure dressing. Another patient may need a Military Anti-Shock Trousers (MAST) suit, intravenous fluid, and surgical repair of a severe internal injury, yet no sign of injury appears on the surface of the patient. Blunt trauma, he states, is one of the most overlooked killers by persons performing triage. It must be emphasized that the disposition of patients described here is the *civilian* mode of triage, and not the military where patients are treated sequentially by code classification in order to return as many men as possible to combat.

EXERCISE OF THE PLAN

Most important in any plan is repeated drills or exercises to familiarize personnel with their expected duties and to evaluate their performances. For example, in the Hartford, Connecticut exercise alluded to previously [47], several deficits became apparent. Agencies with shortwave radios operated on different wavelengths and could not communicate with one another. As there was no medical authority at the disaster scene, evaluations revealed great need for someone to make decisions about the order of treating and transporting patients, administering analgesics, reducing shock, and determining the extensiveness of wounds for notification of the hospitals. There was no recognized leader for purposes of integration of effort. Patients were lifted and transported with little regard to the type or site of injury and were handled unnecessarily, which could produce additional injuries. Some victims were carried out and placed on wet ground, picked up later and placed on a tarpaulin, and then handled a third time when placed in an ambulance. Other persons brought out by litter were removed from the litters, placed on the ground, and subjected to further handling because of the shortage of litters. Some of the injured lay uncovered for 20 to 30 minutes.

Further, ambulance litters were not interchangeable between ambulances, which required patient removal from an ambulance litter at the hospital before the ambulance could return to the disaster site. Also, most modern ambulances cannot accommodate the standard field stretcher because of its length. Some of the injured brought out of a building were placed in positions that blocked traffic or were so close to the disaster site that a building collapse would increase the injuries or kill the victims. No one stayed with a specific victim to give comfort or reassurance, and triage by first-aid personnel was puzzling and inadequate.

Ambulance drivers from out of the city did not know hospital locations, and the ambulance coordinator lost control of half of the vehicles, as they did not follow instructions to return to the rendezvous site. Each ambulance company had its own shortwave frequency, and once an ambulance left the site, communication was nullified. Finally, it was observed that there was inadequate number of state highway and city street signs providing direction to the four general hospitals.

These defects in a scheme can be detected only through trial runs that are repeated on several occasions and are thoroughly evaluated.

MENTAL HEALTH ASPECTS OF DISASTER

Numerous psychiatrists and some others have observed the behavior of persons experiencing a catastrophic event, the emotional state and accompanying difficulties being described as "disaster fatigue," "psychological effects of disaster," "psychiatric aspects of civilian defense," "post-disaster morbidity of the bereaved," "patterns of panic," "mass disruptive reactions," "psychiatric air-raid casualties," and as given in *DSM III* [52], "post-traumatic stress syndrome." Psychiatric observations have been made of major disasters apart from descriptions relating to the Vietnam war [53].

STAGES OF RESPONSE

Singer [67] has reviewed many of the pertinent writings and has summarized the stages of response. In spite of beliefs to the contrary, most victims do not panic, become immobilized, or display psychotic symptoms. Often, organizing behavior is evoked, and the victims' behavior is adaptive, directed toward protection and care of families, friends, and themselves. Reactions to disaster do differ, and they have been linked by various observers to such factors as constitutional predisposition, previous life influences, the nature of the catastrophe, and the culture, folklore, and type of community in which the disaster was experienced. Among persons showing some signs of emotional disturbance as an immediate reaction, the responses are staged, that is, the period of impact, its period of recall, and the post-traumatic period. These stages were originally articulated by Tyhurst [68] over 30 years ago and have held with time.

"PSYCHOLOGICAL FIRST AID"

In view of the responses manifest during mass emergency situations, which may in some instances prove enduring, recommendations have been proposed for care at the scene. First, certain characteristics of coping behavior have been noted, upon which emotional support can be built. Henderson and Bostock [60] in their study of a group of shipwreck survivors felt that a coping capability had these qualities: (1) It consists of anticipating relief from distress either through one's own action or intervention by others; (2) within a group, hope is likely to be more powerful if it is verbalized, since this action enhances its potency through suggestion and confirmation; (3) a leader may express hope to sustain morale while not necessarily believing in what he or she says; (4) the principal function of hope is to control mood, which in turn determines what other behaviors a survivor will undertake to increase his chances of rescue.

The treatment that is offered in disaster settings, as Wilkinson [66] has observed, is based on the assumption that those individuals seeking help were predominantly healthy persons whose psyches had been overwhelmed by a traumatic event for which there could not have been a previous referent. The stress resulting from the event overloaded or exceeded the stimulus barrier, leaving the victim in a state of constant or recurrent stress that would remain until the facts of the experience and the accompanying excitation could be processed.

Certain basic principles must be understood for one to be of maximum service to an emotionally disturbed person, particularly one who has become distraught in a community catastrophe: (1) Accept every person's right to have his/her own feelings; (2) accept a casualty's limitations as real; (3) size up a casualty's potentialities as accurately and as quickly as possible; and (4) accept one's own limitations in a relief role [69].

While these principles are almost trite to the knowledgeable counselor, there will be emergency personnel new to the functions of emotional support who suddenly face a mass of people and who may be unaware of the basics needed in this kind of "first aid." In keeping with the first precept, no one is to be blamed or ridiculed for feeling as one does. In rendering assistance, the task is to help in coping with feelings and not to tell people how they *should* feel. It is not possible to tell *why* individuals feel as they do, but one can determine *how* they feel at a particular moment. Having victims know that one wants to understand *how* they feel can be the first step toward helping them. "It's the collapse of *his* world that distresses him. He will not trust you very far if you deny his world by telling him he has no need to feel the way he *knows* he feels" [69].

As to the second principle of accepting the casualty's limitations as real, there is no place for the scolding, goading type of "reassurance" of "It's all in your head," "Snap out of it," or "Pull yourself together." These ceaseless admonitions went out with the early sophistication of medicine. An emotional wound hurts. Accept it.

Principle three involves identification of victims' potential. Find out quickly something of their pasts, their occupations, and treat them as valued members of the disaster team by assigning tasks befitting their experience—messages or records for the clerk, straightening up of the area by a manual worker.

Last is acceptance of one's own limitations in the relief setting. In the midst of the pressures of a disaster, one's own personality deficits may trip one up so as to have resentments, prejudices, skewed judgments, deep sensitivities, or impulsivity preclude one's carrying out the role of support agent. One must look to one's own defenses, so that "If you understand yourself reasonably well, you may justifiably hope to endure and control your own anxieties in the midst of a community-wide disaster" [69].

Caldwell and his coworkers [55] have summarized well the treatment of true psychiatric casualties. There must be planning to reinforce constructive group and social mechanisms, and emphasis should be placed on (1) preserving the individual's identification with his/her community, job, and family; (2) minimizing the secondary gain of neurotic illness; and (3) avoiding suggestions of illness and disability. For the attainment of these objectives, there must be controlled screening, treatment, and evacuation of psychiatric patients. Hospitalization should be afforded as close to the scene of disaster as possible and should be short. All attitudes of support personnel should promote the expectation of rapid recovery.

Penultimately, in planning for disasters, there must be greater participation of psychiatrists; more frequent participation of psychiatrists during actual rescue operations; wide distribution of some kind of "psychological first-aid manual," possibly using the American Psychiatric Association publication cited previously [69]; and a more intensive training in "psychological first aid" of all emergency workers, particularly the staff of an OHS.

COOPERATION WITH COMMUNITY AGENCIES

In a review of the Buffalo Creek, West Virginia mining disaster of February 26, 1972,* Koplin [70] concluded that occupational and community health were inseparable and that a person's working environment is not of significance to him alone but is inextricably tied to his family's opportunity and his community's health. This concept leads to the consideration of the plant as a disaster site in relation to a plethora of agencies bearing close connection to the workers.

At the time of rescue, the assistance of many organizations is needed. Even though a plan of preparedness has undergone repeated drill, success in the saving of lives and in the minimizing of morbidity rests in the assistance of outside public and private groups. The agencies that can be called on for aid and the roles or functions that they can exercise are the following:

Agency	*Role or Function*
Ambulance companies	Transportation of injured
American National Red Cross	Emergency clothing, feeding, shelter, cleaning supplies, welfare inquiries, comfort kits, supplementary medical care
Civil air patrol	Patrol
Civil defense	Disaster control, evacuation and warning systems
Clergy	Counseling, administration of last rites
Coast Guard	Rescue by water
Fire department	Fire suppression, rescue, paramedic care, care of fallen live wires, clean-up of chemical spills
Hospitals	Medical care
Industrial hygienists	Surveillance of hazardous chemical release
Law enforcement agencies (police, sheriff)	Security, traffic control, supervision of evacuation
Medical examiner/coroner	Recovery, identification
Mental health authority and agencies	Psychological triage and "first aid"
National Guard	Security, prevention of looting
National Weather Service	Weather advisories
Print and broadcast media	Reporting of disaster rescue progress and needs, public relations
Public bus lines	Transportation of personnel
Public health authority	Safety of drinking water, surveillance for possible epidemics of communicable disease, immunization
Public utilities	Shutting off gas lines, maintenance of electrical service
Public works department	Clearance of debris
Radiologic health personnel	Surveillance of radioactive sources, contamination
Roads and streets departments	Clearance of transport and evacuation routes, directional signing
Social Security Administration	Claims, payment for injuries, fatalities
State highway patrol	Traffic control
Workers' compensation underwriter	Claims payment for industrial injuries, fatalities

*Following a rupture of a dam, 117 lives were lost, 500 persons were injured, and 31 were still missing some 16 days after the flood.

The agency concerned at a national level is the Federal Emergency Management Agency (FEMA), which "was created to provide a single point of accountability for all Federal emergency preparedness, mitigation, and response activities" [71]. The agency has been chartered to enhance emergency preparedness and response resources at all levels of government—federal, state, and local—in the meeting of the full range of emergencies, whether natural, manmade, or nuclear, and to integrate into a comprehensive framework all activities concerned with hazard mitigation, preparedness planning, relief operations, and recovery assistance. FEMA provides training and education for governmental personnel in the functions cited through a resident program at a central campus facility, the National Emergency Training Center in Emmitsburg, Maryland. Through an outreach program, courses are available at state and local levels.

In addition to administering the National Flood Insurance program through the Federal Insurance Administration (FIA), FEMA provides a federal reinsurance program against property insurance losses sustained through riots and other civil disturbances. The National Preparedness Programs Directorate is another agency program office, and it administers also the President's Disaster Relief Program.

Regional offices of FEMA are located in the 10 standard federal regions in these cities: Boston, New York, Philadelphia, Atlanta, Chicago, Denton (TX), Kansas City (MO), Denver, San Francisco, and Bothell (WA).

To be sure, not all of the listed agencies will be needed participants in a rescue operation, but selected personnel or unique functions may be required, and assistance should be sought through the disaster command post.

MANUAL

A special disaster preparedness manual should be prepared by, and for use in, the OHS and should cover in detail (1) the general plan, (2) functions of the OHS in a disaster, (3) personal assignments by function, (4) maintenance of postal rosters, (5) maintenance of emergency medical supplies, (6) training, (7) plan review, (8) distribution of manual, (9) emergency care protocols, and (10) map of transportation network.

SURVIVAL IN NUCLEAR WAR

In the Peace Memorial Museum in Hiroshima there is a diorama-like exhibit replicating in chilling reality some severely injured persons fleeing from the scene of the first nuclear bomb burst. The ragged, bleeding, escaping figures challenge the coping capacity of many of the visitors to the museum, for the depictive detail tells in visual precis the horrors of such warfare. Artifacts display the physical damage to structures from the blast and heat, but their impact does not imbed itself in the viewer's mind with the same searing intensity that do the lifelike doomed victims of that August 1945 strike. Just before the second red air-raid alarm was about to be sounded, the explosion took place. The announcement was to contain this message: "Chugoku District Army Information at 8:13 A.M.: three enemy Superfortresses proceeding westward over Saijo area. *Strict precautions should be taken*" [72] (emphasis added).

Precautions cannot be taken. In a masterful writing, Abrams and Von Kaenel [73] provide a sequential review of the medical problems confronting the survivors of nuclear war. The picture is described of the effects of radiation sickness, superimposed as it would be in over one-third of the millions already suffering from trauma and burns. Malnutrition and starvation, dehydration, exposure and hardship, the compromise of sanitation, the uncontrolled breeding of flies, and the presence of corpses all lay the groundwork for death from communicable disease among 20 to 25 percent of the survivors. General disorganization will follow the lengthy residence in shelters, depleted stocks of antibiotics, and the destruction of laboratories. The authors conclude that although no data exist to prove that catastrophic epidemics would ensue, the matter is one of overwhelming importance and uncertainty. They continue, "What is certain is that infection will pose a substantial threat to health and recovery for all those injured by blast, heat, and radiation, and that the resources to grapple with this threat will be inadequate" [73].

In criticism of a Pentagon plan to provide care for future large-scale war overseas, even exclusive of mention of nuclear weapon usage, the Executive Committee of the Physicians for Social Responsibility [74] present it flatly—to think of any plan that could cope with this unprecedented devastation is the height of folly. There is no preparedness plan for this form of human insanity.

The Hiroshima event of 1945, as described by an eyewitness, gives the picture [75]:

> I climbed Hijiyama and looked down. I saw that Hiroshima had disappeared . . . was shocked by the sight . . . what I felt then and still feel now I just can't explain with words . . . I could see Koi [a suburb at the opposite end of the city] and a few buildings standing . . . But Hiroshima didn't exist—that was mainly what I saw—Hiroshima just didn't exist.

Treatment of so massive a catastrophe is beyond the scope of this writing, but efforts toward total prevention are within the capabilities of every living being, including elected or designated leaders.

REFERENCES

1. *The Why and How of First Aid.* Los Angeles: American National Red Cross, Los Angeles Chapter. [n.d.]. P. 1.

2. Occupational Safety and Health Standards. Subpart K—Medical and First Aid § 1910.151 Medical Services and first aid, derived from 41 CFP 50-204.6; Subpart D—Occupational Health and Environmental Controls. §1518.50 Medical services and first aid, and §1926.50 of the Construction Standards.
3. Federal Mine Safety and Health Act of 1977, Public Law 91-173, as amended by Public Law 95-164, §115 Mandatory Health and Safety Training.
4. Byers, L. H., and Hutchison, M. *First Aid.* Safety Manual No. 3. Washington, DC: U.S. Department of the Interior, Mine Enforcement and Safety Administration, 1979.
5. *First Aid.* NMHSA-CE-006, Vol. 1, Work Book and Vol. 2, Answer Book. Washington, DC: U.S. Department of the Interior, MESA, 1976.
6. *Education and Training Programs and Materials.* Washington, DC: U.S. Department of Labor, MSHA, NMHSA, 1982 (for First Aid Instruction Course—73 Overhead Transparencies, and for First Aid Instruction Course—73 35-mm Slides).
7. *Training Films.* Washington, DC: U.S. Department of Labor, MSHA, Education and Training Directorate, Division of Audio Visual Services, 1981–1982 (for series of eight films on first aid).
8. *First Aid Book.* Washington, DC: U.S. Department of Labor, Mine Safety and Health Administration, 1980.
9. *Standard First Aid and Personal Safety* (2nd ed.). Garden City, NY: Doubleday, 1979.
10. *American Red Cross Multimedia Standard First Aid—Workbook.* Washington, DC, American Red Cross, 1987.
11. *Guide for First Aid in Industry.* Jackson, MS: Mississippi State Board of Health, 1972. P. 2.
12. *Scope, Objectives, and Functions of Occupational Health Programs* (rev.). Chicago: American Medical Association, 1971.
13. *Company Medical Policies for Occupational Health Programs* (rev.). Chicago: American Medical Association, 1973. P. 4.
14. *The role of medicine within a business organization JAMA* 210:1446, 1969.
15. Scope of occupational health programs and occupational medical practice. *J Occup Med* 21:497, 1979.
16. Schwab, J. R., cited in Visual acuity exam important in eye trauma. *Intern Med News* 13:30, June 1 1980.
17. Cohen, R. C. Responding to toxic exposure emergencies. *Occup Health Saf* 49:35, 1980.
18. Patterson, R., and Valentine, M. Anaphylaxis and related allergic emergencies including reactions due to insect stings. *JAMA* 248:2632, 1982.
19. Squibb Corporation Medical Department Policy, Apr 8, 1985, courtesy of Allan E. Garb, M. D., Vice President and Corporate Medical Director, Squibb Corporation, New York, NY.
20. Cain, H. D. *Flint's Emergency Treatment and Management* (6th ed.). Philadelphia: Saunders, 1980. P. 103.
21. Brand, D. A., Frazier, W. H., Kohlhepp, et al. A protocol for selecting patients with injured extremities who need x-rays. *N Engl J Med* 306:333, 1982.
22. Pitt, M. J., and Speer, D. P. Radiologic reporting of orthopedic trauma. *Med Radiogr Photogr* 58:14, 1982.
23. Martin, B. H. Communication with the radiologist. *JAMA* 242:1361, 1979.
24. Albert, R. K., and Condie, F. Hand-washing patterns in medical intensive-care units. *N Engl J Med* 304:1465, 1981.
25. Maki, D. G., cited in Hand washing curbs nosocomial infections. *Intern Med News* 18:2, Aug 15–31, 1985.
26. Foster, J. D. and Lauria, D. B. Waiting times and public satisfaction with medical care. *N Engl J Med* 301:1349, 1979.
27. Wasson, J. H., Sauvigne, A. E., Mogielnicki, P., et al. Continuity of outpatient medical care in elderly men: A randomized trial. *JAMA* 252:2413, 1984.
28. Maull, K. I. Alcohol abuse: Its implications in trauma care. *South Med J* 75:794, 1982.
29. Pringle, R. W. Personal communication, March 9, 1981.
30. Kreister, L. Personal communication, Feb 20, 1981.
31. Bravo, A. A. Personal communication, Feb 8, 1985.
32. Medd, B. H. *The Well-Protected Prescription—Guidelines.* From an advertisement of Roche Laboratories, Nutley, NJ 07110.
33. *"Star of Life" Emergency Medical Care Symbol: Background, Specifications, and Criteria.* Washington, DC: U.S. Department of Transportation, National Highway Safety Administration, Office of Driver and Pedestrian Programs, 1979.
34. Schwartz, L. R. Personal communication, July 20, 1983.
35. King, J. C. Personal communication, May 13, 1986.
36. Martin, R. A. Personal communication, 1980.
37. Jones, W. H., and Buttery, M. Sudden death: Survivors' perceptions of their emergency department experience. *J Emerg Nurs* 7:14, 1981.
38. Catastrophic accidents: A 40-Year Review. *Stat Bull Metropol Life Insur Co* 63:3, Apr-June 1982.
39. Railroad accident fatalities. *Stat Bull Metropol Life Insur Co* 62:4, July-Sept 1981.
40. Aquatic deaths and injuries—United States. *MMWR* 31:417, 1982.
41. Lewis, R. MD's, hospitals feel effects of volcano. *Am Med News* 23:2, May 30, 1980.
42. Follow-up on Mount St. Helens. *MMWR* 29:312, 1980.
43. Follow-up on Mount St. Helens. *MMWR* 29:334, 1980.
44. FBI Bomb Data Center. *Incident Summary for the Month of December 1984.* Washington, DC: U.S. Department of Justice, Federal Bureau of Investigation, 1985. P. 1.
45. Fristrom, G. *Fire Deaths in the United States: Review of Data Sources and Range of Estimates.* Washington, DC: National Fire Data Center, National Fire Prevention and Control Administration, U.S. Department of Commerce, 1977. P. ii.

46. Mortality from fires and conflagrations. *Stat Bull Metropol Life Insur Co* 54:6, Dec 1973.
47. Menczer, L. F. A community disaster exercise in Hartford, Conn. *Public Health Rep* 83:288, 1968.
48. Healy, R. J. *Emergency and Disaster Planning.* New York: Wiley, 1969. Copyright © 1969 by John Wiley and Sons, Inc.
49. Felton, J. S. The Texas City Disaster: Early Impressions. *Ind Med* 16:304, 1947.
50. Felton, J. S. Prepare for the worst. *Occup Haz* 12:16, July 1950.
51. Cowan, W. Triage: What it is and how it works. *Emerg Product News,* vol. 8, Apr 1976.
52. *Diagnostic and Statistical Manual of Mental Disorders* (3rd ed.). Washington, DC: American Psychiatric Association, 1980. Pp. 236–238.
53. After disaster: What about survivors? *Mod Med* 43:63, Dec. 1 1975.
54. Brown, F. Civilian psychiatric air-raid casualties. *Lancet* 1:686, 1941.
55. Caldwell, J. M., Ranson, S. W., and Sacks, J. G. Group panic and other mass disruptive reactions. *US Armed Forces Med J* 2:541, 1951.
56. Cohen, R. E., and Ahearn, F. L. *Handbook for Mental Health Care of Disaster Victims.* Baltimore, MD: Johns Hopkins University Press, 1980.
57. Friedman, P., and Linn, L. Some psychiatric notes on the *Andrea Doria* disaster. *Am J Psychiatry* 114:426, 1957.
58. Gleser, G. C., Green, B. L., and Winget, C. *Prolonged Psychosocial Effects of Disaster: A Study of Buffalo Creek.* New York: Academic, 1981.
59. Greenson, R. R., and Mintz, T. California earthquake 1971: Some psychoanalytic observations [among analysands]. *Int J Psychoanal Psychother* 1:7, 1972.
60. Henderson, S., and Bostock, T. Coping behavior after shipwreck. *Br J Psychiatry* 131:15, 1977.
61. Lowenberg, R. D. Psychological reactions in an emergency [Earthquake]. *Am J Psychiatry* 109:384, 1952.
62. Lucas, R. A. *Men in Crisis: A Study of a Mine Disaster.* New York: Basic Books, 1969.
63. Sims, J. H., and Baumann, D. D. The tornado threat: Coping styles of the North and South. *Science* 176:1386, 1972.
64. Trichopoulus, D., Katsouyanni, K., Zavitsanos, X., et al. Psychological stress and fatal heart attack: The Athens (1981) earthquake natural experiment. *Lancet* 1:144, 1983.
65. Weil, R. J., and Dunsworth, F. A. Psychiatric aspects of disaster: A case history. Some experiences during the Springhill, N.S. mining disaster. *Can Psychiatric Assoc J* 3:11, 1958.
66. Wilkinson, C. B. Aftermath of a disaster: The collapse of the Hyatt Regency Hotel skywalks. *Am J Psychiatry* 140:1134, 1983.
67. Singer, T. J. An introduction to disaster: Some considerations of a psychological nature. *Aviat Space Environ Med* 53:245, 1982.
68. Tyhurst, J. S. Individual reactions to community disaster: The natural history of psychiatric phenomena. *Am J Psychiatry* 107:764, 1951.
69. American Psychiatric Association Committee on Civil Defense. *Psychological First-Aid in Community Disasters.* Washington, DC: The Association, 1954. Pp. 9–15. Appeared also in *JAMA* 156:36, 1954.
70. Koplin, A. N. Dam burst shows occupational, community health linked. *Nation's Health,* Apr 1972. P. 2.
71. *U.S. Government Manual 1986/87.* Washington, DC: Office of the Federal Register, National Archives and Records Administration, 1986. Pp. 517–520.
72. *The Outline of Atomic Bomb Damage in Hiroshima.* Hiroshima: Hiroshima Peace Memorial Museum, 1978. P. 3.
73. Abrams, H. L., and Von Kaenel, W. E. Medical problems of survivors of nuclear war. *N Engl J Med* 305:1226, 1981.
74. Executive Committee, Physicians for Social Responsibility Medical Care in Modern Warfare. A look at the Pentagon plan for the civilian sector. *N Engl J Med* 306:741, 1982.
75. [Professor of history] cited in Lifton, R. J. Hiroshima and ourselves. *JAMA* 254:631, 1985.

10. WORKERS' COMPENSATION

Someone said, "What do you say concerning the principle that injury should be recompensed with kindness?"

The Master said, "With what then will you recompense kindness?"

"Recompense injury with justice, and recompense kindness with kindness."

Confucius

The contemporary system of workers' compensation (WC) has been functioning in the United States for three-quarters of a century. Yet, in spite of maturation and growth of the system, medical practitioners experience considerable discomfort in fitting their concepts of medical practice into the legalistic structure that the early considerations of worker welfare produced. While it is expected that physicians in industry will be experienced with the requirements of the compensation mechanism, they frequently face differences in definition as understood by law and medicine, they find that certain practitioners are thoroughly biased in their medical judgments as determined by their claimant or defendant affiliation, and they encounter workers who are inclined to "use" the system to a point of greater personal gain. Frequently, there may be issues of fraud that will require difficult resolution.

Because of these influencing factors and others of an administrative nature, many physicians will not see patients whose medical care is provided through WC, thus depriving certain occupational health services (OHSs) of needed, highly qualified consultative assistance. The physician in industry cannot be similarly selective, for the primary segment of his or her professional activity may involve constant interaction with the administrative or adjudicatory needs of the insurance plan. In essence, it is a way of life that cannot be disregarded but must be learned, understood, and accepted.

The need for a workable method of compensating the work-injured employee will persist, even with our current efforts in accident and disease prevention. As Somers and Somers [1] have expressed it, "Modern technology makes use of stupendous forces—steam, electricity, chemical agents, and the most powerful of all forces thus far discovered, ionizing radiation—that multiply human power and effectiveness a thousandfold when under control but are equally destructive when out of control. Even when controlled, they may cause serious injury through gradual and undramatic erosion of vitality or body damage." It is this last insidious harm to the worker that is causing the greatest consternation to the many agencies concerned with WC.

ADMINISTRATION

The placement of the personnel responsible for the administration of the WC program may vary from company to company, but usually it is a function of the director of industrial relations, assigned in the larger organizations to the director of personnel, who in turn may have the activity exercised in an insurance section, an employee's benefits section, or a separate unit dedicated exclusively to WC. Often the office having that responsibility is located in juxtaposition to the OHS, so that the injured worker will not have an undue amount of travel for the completion of necessary records. In one installation with which the author was connected, clerks from the WC unit were located in the medical facility, which greatly expedited the administrative processing of reports and claims.

Some companies allocate both the safety and WC functions to a single component of the industrial relations department, a placement that normally allows an immediate investigation of an injury-producing accident. Whatever the organization style, the objective is the immediate processing of claims and transmittal of reports to the insurance carrier. Whether medical care is provided in-house or by an outside treating physician, every effort should be made to avoid delay in the forwarding of disability pay to the injured worker. In the seriously traumatized employee, there is sufficient anxiety and disruption of normal relationships in the home to cause emotional and physical hardship without adding the concern of a weakened fiscal base.

The system utilized in the underwriting of WC, whether through a state fund, a commercial carrier, self-insurance, or by being permissibly uninsured, does not change the basic method of submitting initial, periodic, and final reports. To be avoided, particularly in cases of temporary disability, is a lag time between the date of injury and the first payment. As an example of on-time performance in one state (California), it was reported [2] that the average delay in payment during the period of January to June 1982 was 27.3 days, 8 days longer than in a comparable 1981 period. While these particular values represented changes in programming rather than in performance, the effects on the workers, many of whom are paid on a regular weekly basis, can be severe.

PREPARATION OF REPORTS

Physicians' reports make up the basic foundation on which a successful WC system is built. It makes little difference as to the role of the physician who is writing the report, for he or she may be the treating specialist, the independent medical examiner (IME), the agreed medical examiner (AME), or the consultant who reviews the total case history, with or without examination of the patient concerned. Report preparation is discussed in some detail, for the in-plant health care personnel should know what is expected in WC reports.

In light of the above, requests for examinations, reviews, or reports may come from WC underwriters, the state WC authority, attorneys, other physicians (in practice or in industry), or the WC personnel of a company that may or may not have medical personnel. Irrespective of the source of referral, or even if it is necessary to summarize the history of an employee receiving care from the OHS, the same care should be exercised in preparing the communication. Physicians are identified after awhile as those practitioners whose reports are considered good and those whose summaries are skimpy, poorly prepared, inadequate, or failing to provide answers to submitted questions. All reports are valuable and can determine the amounts of money committed or paid in awards, litigation costs, and disability payments, in addition to exerting an effect on the employability of the involved patient.

All reports are legal documents in addition to being medical records and should be prepared with the knowledge that they may be introduced as evidence during a hearing, the taking of a deposition, or a trial, if a third-party suit is undertaken in the future. When such a report is read in toto or in part into the record, the person who has written the report will have his or her professional skills judged by the content, the attention to detail, and the accuracy, clarity, and conciseness of the statements entered in the document. A poorly prepared report from a physician may prove confusing to the issue, may result in injustice, and may be harmful to the reputation of the individual practitioner and of the profession in general [3].

FIRST REPORT OF OCCUPATIONAL INJURY OR ILLNESS

The first report submitted by the physician often is prepared in a thoroughly inadequate manner and, as expressed by one WC authority, is frequently of no worth, is not accurate, is incomplete, and is filled out hastily by the physician or sometimes a clerk [4]. Accuracy at this point in a patient's course through an injury or illness serves the best interests of all persons involved—the patient, the treating physician, the patient's employer, the WC authority of the state, and at a later date if litigation follows, the concerned attorneys and judges. Failure to submit such a report, in some jurisdictions, within 5 days is a misdemeanor.

The physician's first report usually calls for the following information:

Insurer.
Employer.
Address of employer.
Nature of business. (It is conceivable that some patients may not know the kind of business the employer is engaged in, and a call to the company will be necessary.)
Patient's name, sex, date of birth.
Patient's address, telephone number, occupation or job title, and social security number. (Again, the worker may be vague about his or her job title and report a generic designation such as laborer, which conveys little knowledge regarding exposures, job demands, and the like.)
Place of injury (full address of place where injury was sustained).
Date and hour of injury or onset of illness.
Date and hour of first examination or treatment.
Date when last worked.
Previously treated (by reporting physician)?
History (in patient's words, including exposures if chemicals or contactant compounds involved).

Medical findings, including subjective complaints, objective findings, and radiographic and laboratory findings.

Diagnosis. (This statement must be accurate, if it can be given with assurance. The terms *aggravation* or *recurrence* can be used to clarify any relationship of the injury to preexisting conditions. If an exposure to a toxic agent is alleged, but no immediate verification of such contact is possible, the designation can be used of "suspected exposure." If the etiology of the illness is known, it should be stated. No diagnosis should be included that cannot be substantiated. If an injury, give exact type, location, and severity. Never state, "Diagnosis deferred.")

Question: Are findings and diagnosis consistent with the history of the injury or onset of illness? (If discrepancies appear, they should be noted with the first report. The allegiance is to the truth, not necessarily to the patient.)

Question: Is there any current condition that might impede or delay recovery? (This question might present a problem because it involves the disclosure of the presence of a disorder, such as diabetes mellitus, representing information that is privileged. Such divulgence should be carried out only with the patient's signed authorization. While information relating to the occupationally incurred condition is essentially "in the public domain,"—privilege is waived when the patient seeks damages for personal injury or seeks compensation—any other medical data are personal. If a preexisting condition is residual from a previous injury and the new injury might represent an aggravation, it should be so stated.)

Treatment: office, hospital outpatient department, hospital inpatient. (Indicate all surgical procedures, number of sutures or length of laceration, splints, casts, immunizing injections, medications, and particularly instructions regarding follow-up care.)

Question: Further treatment required? Physical therapy? (Overestimation is preferred to underestimation.)

If inpatient—hospital, location, date admitted, expected stay.

Work status: Return to usual work? If not, estimated date of return to work (RTW): Regular work? Modified work?

Physician's name, degree, address.

Physician's signature. (The report must be signed by the physician himself. The responsibilities to the patient, the employer, and the physician him- or herself are too great to delegate this signatory function to anyone else.)

Telephone number.

Date of report.

Internal Revenue Service employer identification (if incorporated).

Social security number (if not incorporated).

Some report forms may require additional information [3]:

Precise statement of disability. (Both subjective and objective factors should be included, with accurate measurements of function, when subject to mensuration. The physician's own evaluation of the validity of the apparent disability factors should be stated when indicated.)

Estimated duration of disability (or disfigurement), total or partial. (Overly optimistic prognoses are to be avoided, for they cause unnecessary and costly reappraisals and are discouraging to the patient, the employer, and the carrier. If some permanent disability is expected, it should be stated on the first and each subsequent report and estimated as accurately as possible.)

Care should be given the completion of the report, for it provides significant information to several concerned agencies engaged in estimating replacements, RTW, disability pay, amount of reserves to be allocated, and scope and cost of rehabilitation, among other cost-producing effects of the injury or illness. Also, as Clark [4] has pointed out, attorneys and judges consider the first report in some ways the most valuable, as the history given is more likely to be accurate because it is fresh in the mind of the worker and was related before any possible alteration could be affected by contact with counsel.

GENERAL GUIDELINES IN REPORT PREPARATION

Anyone who has had to testify in a WC case learns immediately that words are what the attorney uses to practice the profession of law. Although the medical lexicon is structured—irrespective of its multiple etymologies—to provide exactitude and specificity in meaning, and it is perfectly clear among physicians, it is frequently dissected by attorneys in their effort to have it fit legal definitions, or it is misunderstood or not understood. Loose, interchangeable usage in medical records of the terms *impression*, and *diagnosis* can lead to 30 minutes of exasperating questions and answers in the providing of testimony. A radiologist's interpretation of a radiograph of a pneumoconiosis that is worded, "consistent with the inhalation of . . ." can be argued about ceaselessly whether that phrase is equivalent to "a diagnosis of. . . ."

Further, while most attorneys who practice WC law are well primed in the particular body of trauma or pathophysiology involved in the case under discussion, there may be lacunae of ignorance that will require clarification. One should not introduce the results of a sophisticated new test or an old but rarely used test without explaining the objective of the test, precisely what it is supposed to measure, and the relationship of the findings to the case at hand. Whatever it is that is referred to must be clear, as though all readers were laypersons.

As one is instructed at the beginning of any testimony, one must not guess, so in reports one must never say that one is "guessing, or speculating, or surmising, or conjecturing" [4]. One writes, instead, "Based on my experience, my opinion is. . . ."

SPECIFIC GUIDELINES IN REPORT PREPARATION

One cannot assume that because a worker has stated his or her job title that one knows precisely what the person does on the job. A physician's understanding of a craft or an occupation might be minimal, outdated, or totally in error. Many occupational designations have roots deep in history, but now, several centuries later, the job elements are thoroughly modern although subsumed under traditional labels. The term *teamster* comes to mind, as does *mule-spinner*. One must ask precisely what the job functions entail so that the recommendations regarding the time off work, or the RTW, will make good sense, as will an estimate of permanent disability. A partial disability in one worker may totally preclude a return to the job on which the injury was incurred, while a comparable level of disablement will have no bearing on a second patient's fulfilling the requirements of a job. One cannot assume total knowledge of the demands of a job without inquiring fully into the details of the work performed.

It would be helpful to visit the worksite where the patient sustained the injury to ascertain that the work process is precisely the same as when the employee was engaged in his or her regular craft or occupation. Again, as Clark [4] has indicated, the workplace might have been changed greatly between the date of injury and the time of the treating physician's visit; a thorough cleaning of the work area might have removed the agents causative of either the trauma or the chemical-substance intoxication.

Many individuals occupying blue-collar jobs in industry carry out comparable craft activities either at home or in second, "moonlighting" jobs. With the same demands for energy expenditure, such persons are just as subject to injury in these after-hours locations as they are in their regular work. One must ascertain as carefully as possible the true location where the injury was sustained, for certain individuals will seek medical care for conditions arising outside the jurisdiction of their regular employer. If the trauma is severe, or if an attempt is made at litigation, the case can present many unwanted medical or legal complications.

To be avoided in any report is criticism or sarcastic comments regarding previous physicians who had seen the patient prior to his or her being referred currently. Derogatory statements have no place in a report, any more than do gratuities, snide remarks, or "cutesy" commentaries regarding the patient. The inclusion of such rhetoric tells more of the person preparing the report than it does of the patient and does a disservice to both physicians. The report is supposed to be the result of an objective, scientific study and not an intemperate diatribe against other practitioners.

Certain words have behavioral or emotional connotations and are best omitted. For example, one need not say that the patient "alleges," "claims," or "denies," because implicit in such words are disbelief or doubt on the part of the physician. An uncharged statement that indicates no bias is simply, "The patient says, [or states] that. . . ." Clark [4] offers another good example of the fine line between words when he points up the choice in the descriptions of "He moves reluctantly" or "He moves slowly." Much more is inferred from reading the former, and one should be sure of the action before phrasing the retelling in that manner.

Finally, the issue of truth comes up once again. If one believes that the patient is not telling the truth, one should say so, but give a reason for making such a statement. There need be no malice in one's comment, but there should be a sound basis for the observation. In a similar vein, if it is felt that the patient is not cooperating, one can say that in one's opinion the patient did not make his or her best effort.

PERIODIC REPORTS

If a patient is undergoing treatment over a prolonged period or a consultant has been asked to conduct an evaluation of a patient who had an untoward exposure to a known or unidentified substance, a progress report is indicated. The terms used may vary, from "supplemental report," to "progress report," "monthly report," or "reexamination report." Such a report may be needed to establish eligibility for further benefits, and written information is needed to document the status of a patient's care [5]. Changes in diagnosis, prognosis, or expected permanent residual should be indicated. Important statements to be made are the date of full recovery and the expected date of RTW.

The detailed progress report may be required when the patient is discharged from care or when the condition in question has reached maximum improvement or, in the words of WC administration, has become "permanent and stationary." A full description is expected of any residual impairment, including measurements of the range of motion in affected joints. If the injury has ipsilateral involvement only, measurements should be made and reported also of motion on the sound, contralateral side. One should determine which system of impairment measurement is used in the state jurisdiction to which one submits reports—the system provided by Packard Thurber [6], that of the American Medical Association (AMA) [7], or even those of other rating bodies. The labor code of the state will indicate the acceptable method of measuring impairment. Most jurisdictions and physicians are utilizing the AMA's guidelines [7].

A final report is submitted when treatment is terminated and the patient is discharged. Such a report must carry the physician's opinion of the patient's condition at the time of discharge.

REPORT OF CONSULTANT OR INDEPENDENT MEDICAL EXAMINER

A report is prepared after evaluation of a patient by a consultant or independent medical examiner. The details of report preparation are reviewed here because, as indicated earlier, the medical director of a company should know what to expect in such a document, as copies will come to him after certain actions. For example, after an involved employee has been examined by a specialist selected by the medical director, the company's WC personnel, or the company's counsel or selected representative and the claimant's attorney by joint agreement during litigation, the medical director may be asked to interpret portions of the report or even to explain the findings and opinion to the employee. The medical director may have to testify and, therefore, should be familiar with all medical documentation. The medical director may use such a report to guide the attorney who is defending the company.

The report should contain the following information:

Name of patient.
Patient's address, telephone number.
Patient's social security number.
Patient's date of birth.
Employer's name, address, telephone number.
Source of referral (carrier, medical director, state WC authority) with address and telephone number of contact person.
Date and place of examination or consultation.
Reason(s) for referral, consultation, or examination. (There may be included here the questions for which specific answers are wanted through the consultative process.)
Patient's complaint(s).
History of injury or illness.
Past medical history.
Occupational history (of particular importance if patient presents with possible occupational illness; indicate all previous employments, duration, exposures, etc.).
Physical examination.
Laboratory test results.
Radiography results.
Review of previous medical care (chronologic summary of previous examinations and conclusions). (It is desirable to list at this point all documents reviewed, for example, medical history furnished by John J. Jones, M.D., hospital record furnished by Smith Community Hospital, and so on. It is helpful in the review to indicate the name, address, and telephone number of the physician whose record is summarized so that, if necessary, contact can be made conveniently with that source of care.)
Discussion (with rationale, of cause-and-effect relationship, differences in opinion, and reasons, from conclusions reached by previous examiners; opinions at variance; and answers in response to specific questions asked under reasons for referral).
Summary.
Conclusions (to include diagnoses, degrees of severity, impairment, anatomic and functional, total or partial, and permanent or temporary status of disability).
Recommendations (in regard to treatment, specialty referral, rehabilitation, or RTW, regular or modified, and the like).
Signature of physician, with a statement to the effect that the report was prepared by the signatory.

With the addition of nurse practitioners or physician's assistants to the staffs of certain sources of health care, some of the history taking and conduct of the physical examination might have been delegated to such "physician extenders." It must be pointed out that, in some jurisdictions, an additional rule has appeared regarding reports. In essence, it states that if any person other than the physician who has signed the report has participated in the examination of the injured worker or in the preparation of the report, the name of such person(s) and the role performed shall be stated, including the name of the person(s) who took the history, performed the physical examination, or drafted, composed, or edited the report in whole or in part.

It is apparent that in some instances the only role of the physician was to sign the report, while others completed their variously assigned parts. The WC judges are concerned with the quality of the evidence and wish to be able better to evaluate the reliability of the evidence by knowing who the participants were in the examination and evaluation of the patient.

As many of the concepts in WC regarding level or status of disability or need for treatment or rehabilitation have other factors at play—social and economic—and may have different definitions in different jurisdictions, one should know how these various concepts are defined so that the WC judge is better able to compare one medical report with another, for all employ the same understandings. It must be remembered that disability is usually defined in the WC system as an inability to compete in the open labor market. Not only must one indicate what functions in the occupation the patient was performing at the time of injury he or she is now unable to carry out, but there must be indicated also any residuals from the injury that would preclude performing other types of activities, even though the worker would not be called on to carry them out in the particular occupation shown. This point gives emphasis to the definition of disability as inability to compete in the open labor market in any occupation [8].

The disability can comprise both subjective and objective factors or be based exclusively on one set of factors alone. In classifying disability, as indicated previously, the term is divided into *temporary disability* and *permanent disability* and further into *temporary total, temporary partial, permanent total,* and *permanent partial* disability. Additional definition might be helpful. A partial disability is generally an inability to perform some occupations or certain functions of the occupation in which the injury occurred. Total disability implies a complete inability to perform any occupation.

Temporary disability usually has no exact statutory definition but is considered as disability that has not yet reached a chronic or stationary stage. Healing is continuing, but during the process, it is wholly or partially labor-disabling. If the patient is declared temporarily disabled, the physician must give the best estimate or best reasonable medical probability as to how long that will continue into the future and how long it had existed in the past, if already terminated [8].

Consideration must be given subjective disability, for its recognition affects significantly decisions in some jurisdictions. In California, for example, subjective disability is identified by [9]

A description of the activity that produces the disability.
The duration of the disability.
The activities that are precluded and those that can be performed with the disability.
The means necessary for relief.

The gradations in pain are given the following meanings [8]:

Formal	*Informal* [8]
A *severe* pain would preclude the activity precipitating the pain.	Precluded
A *moderate* pain could be tolerated but would cause marked handicap in the performance of the activity precipitating the pain.	Marked
A *slight* pain could be tolerated but would cause some handicap in the performance of the activity precipitating the pain.	Some
A *minimal* (mild) pain would constitute an annoyance, but causing no handicap in the performance of the particular activity. Would be considered as nonratable permanent disability.	Nuisance

Additional information needed in a report involving subjective disability, in order to reduce the level of pain into a percentage and in turn into dollars, includes a statement regarding frequency of the pain. Descriptors that meet this requirement are

Occasional	=	25% of the time
Intermittent	=	50% of the time
Frequent	=	75% of the time
Constant	=	100% of the time

Gradations between any two levels can be used. The importance in pinpointing the intensity and frequency of the pain can be readily seen when given dollar values. It is further advised [8] that one use the standard newspaper reporter's questions of "who," "what," "when," "where," and "why," to give greater description of the symptom. What kind of activity produces it? Where does it occur? When does it occur? How often does it occur? What brings relief to the symptoms? How long do the symptoms last?

Tying in with the preparation of a cogent report is the wording used relative to guidelines for work capacity which apply to pulmonary and heart disease, abdominal weakness, spinal disabilities, and disabilities of the lower extremities (guidelines 7 and 8, below). Again, in California, the levels of work allowed have been delineated as follows [10]:

1. *Disability Precluding Very Heavy Lifting.* Contemplates the individual has lost approximately ¼ of his* pre-injury capacity for lifting. (A statement, "Inability to lift 50 pounds," is not meaningful. The total lifting effort, including weight, distance, endurance, frequency, body position, and similar factors should be considered with reference to the particular individual.)
2. *Disability Precluding Very Heavy Work.* Contemplates the individual has lost approximately ¼ of his pre-injury capacity for performing such activities as bending, stooping, lifting, pushing, pulling, and climbing, or other activities involving comparable physical effort.
3. *Disability Precluding Heavy Lifting.* Contemplates the individual has lost approximately ½ of his pre-injury capacity. (Statement under #1 above is applicable.)
4. *Disability Precluding Heavy Lifting, Repeated Bending and Stooping.* Contemplates the individual has lost ½ of his pre-injury capacity for lifting, bending, and stooping.
5. *Disability Precluding Heavy Work.* Contemplates the individual has lost approximately ½ of his pre-injury capacity for performing such activities as bending, stooping, lifting, pushing, pulling, and climbing, or other activities involving comparable physical effort.
6. *Disability Resulting in Limitation to Light Work.* Contemplates the individual can do work in a standing or walking position, with a minimum of demands for physical effort.
7. *Disability Resulting in Limitation to Semi-Sedentary Work.* Contemplates the individual can do work approximately ½ the time in a sitting position, and approximately ½ the time in a standing or walking position, with a minimum of demands for physical effort whether standing, walking or sitting.
8. *Disability Resulting in Limitation to Sedentary Work.* Contemplates the individual can do work predominantly in a sitting position at a bench, desk, or table with a minimum of demands for physical effort, and with some degree of walking and standing being permitted.

In substance, the report must provide fairly definitive guidelines to those persons responsible for converting some loss of work capacity into a monetary value. Every element needs a statement in keeping with the rating scales shown. Persons engaged in WC activities should seek comparable guidelines in the jurisdiction in which they practice.

Clark [11] has offered some guidance in the preparation of WC reports that are to the point of accurate response to a request for evaluation. His sage counsel follows:

"Injury" includes "aggravation," "acceleration," and/or "precipitation" of symptoms of disability from previous disease.

Obtain a formal job description of the patient's work if it will assist in formulating a sound conclusion.

Histories obtained by others should be reviewed but should not be repeated or summarized. If differences are detected between the history obtained currently and those elicited previously, they should be explained.

Verbatim quotation of complaints and symptoms without comment may serve in place of a paraphrased retelling.

Report joint function as a fraction, injured/uninjured.

If patient is not trying his best in the determination of grip strength, say so, but give an estimate of what is the true grip strength.

Specific questions that should be answered in the report, with Clark's comments, follow:

What is the relation between the condition(s) found and the claimed occupational injury or exposure? Give reasons for the conclusion, avoiding "possibly" and "maybe." "Probably" represents 51 percent or better chance that something is so. If the disorder being considered had several causes acting conjointly, and the occupational injury or exposure was one, the occupational event will be considered as causal. Do not state, "Disability is due to an industrial injury," for that is a legal determination. Say that, "Disability is the result of the injury described that occurred on January 20, 19XX."

In your opinion, during what periods of time was the worker, as a result of the medical conditions, you found, unable to work?

Is the condition(s) permanent and stationary, and on what date did it become so? If not yet, when will it be so? If treatment will improve the condition, what is it and what are the expected benefits? (Give separate information for separate but coexisting injuries.)

Is there permanent disability now?

Summarize factors of disability, subjective and objective, as indicated earlier. Obtain a list of psychiatric disabilities and standard ratings from the state rating authority. In describing factors of disability, mention need for appliances such as canes, crutches, braces, elastic stockings, and so on, as they may interfere with the patient's ability to compete in the open labor market.

*Equally applicable to women.

Apportion, if appropriate, in permanent disabilities, the present disability to the claimed injury and any preexisting conditions.
Avoid any discussion in the "Summary" and "Conclusions," and offer no differential diagnoses.

The AMA in its publication *The Physician and Workers' Compensation* [12] has provided, in outline form, its view of the kinds of information that should be found in each report. The medical evaluation consists of the following:

A narrative history of the medical conditions with specific reference to onset and course of the condition, findings on previous examinations, treatment and responses to treatment.
The results of the most recent clinical evaluation including any of the following which were obtained:
physical examination findings
laboratory test results
electrocardiogram [interpretation]
x-rays [interpretation]
rehabilitation evaluation [findings]
other specific tests or diagnostic procedures and, in the case of psychiatric disease, the results of mental status examination and psychologic tests.
Assessment of the current clinical status and plans for future treatment, rehabilitation, and re-evaluation.
Diagnoses and clinical impressions.
Estimate of the expected date of full or partial recovery.

An analysis of the findings consists of [12]:

Explanation of the impact of the medical condition(s) on life activities.
Narrative explanation of the medical basis for any conclusion that the medical condition has, or has not, become static or well stabilized.
Narrative explanation of the medical basis for any conclusion that the individual is, or is not, likely to suffer sudden or subtle incapacitation as a result of the medical condition.
Narrative explanation of the medical basis for any conclusion that the individual is, or is not, likely to suffer injury or harm or further medical impairment by engaging in activities of daily living or any other activity necessary to meet personal, social, occupational or legal demands.
Narrative explanation of any conclusion that restrictions or accommodations are, or are not, warranted with respect to activities of daily living or any other activities required to meet personal, social, occupational or legal demands, and if they are, an explanation of the therapeutic or risk avoiding value of the restrictions or accommodations.

If the examiner elects to use the AMA's *Guides to the Evaluation of Permanent Impairment* [7], then the following (a comparison of the results of analysis with the impairment criteria) should also be included in the report:

Description of specific clinical findings related to each impairment with reference to the relevance of the finding to the criteria of the chapter. Reference to the *absence* of, or inability to obtain, particular findings is essential.
Comparison of the clinical findings with the criteria for the particular body system contained in the *Guides.*
Explanation of the basis for each quantitative impairment rating with reference to the criteria.
Summary list of all impairments with ratings.
Combined "whole person" rating when more than one impairment is present.

THE PSYCHIATRIC REPORT IN WORKERS' COMPENSATION

While the report concerning a claimant's psychiatric evaluation is not greatly different in format, it does involve certain history details not entering into the reviews of patients with physical injury. Whipple [13] has discussed the needed input for a psychiatric report, highlighting pertinent past events that may be significant in the understanding of both the claim and behavioral factors that may have influenced its filing.

Whipple [13] places emphasis on the childhood education, military, marriage, and employment histories, "not merely to form the basis for a diagnosis, but to determine what problems, handicaps, impairments or disability the individual might have encountered early in life." Data that can prove useful are such elements as family relationships, including both family upheavals and past mental illness, school performance with peer and authority figure conflicts, academic performance, extracurricular involvement, courses taken, dates completed and degrees or units obtained, and last scholastic undertaking and performance. Whipple [13] indicates that if the individual is claiming disability for the recent past and yet the applicant was performing academically, there may be implications concerning impairment in the education or cognitive realm.

In exploring the military history, one should determine the inclusive dates of service, the branch of service, the rank attained, any disciplinary action taken, combat experience, and any service-connected disabilities that were incurred. From the information "one might discover pre-existing authority conflict, impulse control problems, or even awarded disabilities on a percentage basis" [13].

From the marital history, there should be documented the dates of marriage(s) and dissolution(s), in addition to the ages of all children, whether natural, adopted, or step, their current whereabouts and health, and the health of the current spouse. Of importance is the outside employment of the spouse—the location and employer, length of service, and attitude toward that position. Is the present relationship smooth, or have there been discussions of, or actual, separation or divorce?

Whipple [13] comments that inquiry should be made concerning work attitudes, reasons for job change(s), number and kinds of promotions, demotions, discharges, and disciplinary actions. Was the job left for economic, geographic, health, or other reasons? This segment of the total is of worth in illustrating levels of functioning in various capacities and possible preexisting symptoms or even disability.

The examiner should seek information concerning serious or repetitive trauma, arrest records, relationships with coworkers and supervisors, and performance evaluations. In documenting symptoms, Whipple [13] investigates each one as to onset, duration, frequency, intensity, precipitating factors, and any changes over time. Further, the claimant should be asked about his or her view of returning to work, the future, retirement, impairment, disability, and even causation. Also to be included is a query as to what might be wanted out of the present litigation. The response might be money, revenge, retirement, nothing, or even, "I don't know."

In formulating the diagnosis, it should be taken from *DSM III* [14] with a discussion of how the applicant fulfills the guidelines and criteria for a *DSM III* diagnosis. There can be no psychiatric disability without a psychiatric disorder.

To fit these discussion points into the format of the report, it would be helpful to see Whipple's outline for the document [13]:

Introduction
Referring source
Format (including the various histories)
Present illness or industrial injury or description of the cumulative situation
Collateral contact (validation or repudiation of information by spouse)
Mental status examination
Review of records
Psychological testing
Diagnosis
Disability
Causation
Apportionment
Future medical care
Rehabilitation
Paramedical (indication of coworkers in developing the history, performing the examination, or preparing the report)
Conclusion
References

While it will not be the task of in-plant physicians to prepare such reports, similar documents will come to their attention, and with this kind of expectation of quality they will be able better to judge the quality or completeness of the reviews of referred employees.

REHABILITATION OF THE INJURED

In some jurisdictions, rehabilitation has been mandated by the state workers' compensation act. In 1974, for example, California became the first state to enact, as an integral part of the law, a mandatory vocational rehabilitation benefit. Unique to the WC philosophy, in contradistinction to other programs of social insurance, is the goal of returning beneficiaries to the world of work [15].

In a 5-year period, nearly 22,000 severely injured workers had their employability restored through vocational rehabilitation services provided under the law. In most instances, the services are offered to those persons who will benefit, that is, workers whose injury has prevented their returning to their usual occupation or whose injury, when combined with other factors, may preclude "any meaningful attachment to the workforce" [15]. Even with certain physical limitations, nearly half of all the workers undergoing rehabilitation returned to work with earnings greater than those received prior to injury.

While rehabilitative measures in the past have been introduced for the more seriously injured worker—spinal cord injury with resultant paraplegia, for example—now workers with lesser injuries, but possibly more challenging to the restorative team, are undergoing the service. Although the costs have been high, WC has finally offered something beyond medical care and disability payments. It has been the author's experience that often rehabilitation of currently working persons will bring about their vocational elevation to better paying and more prestigious positions.

With this new legislation, rehabilitation counselors, formerly found almost exclusively in state agencies, have entered private practice and have been both diligent and successful in their evaluation of clients, the supervision of the rehabilitative process, the preparation for return to work, and final placement. Casualty underwriters have added rehabilitation nurses to work in parallel with the counselors to return the injured worker to gainful employment.

A problem faced by all the members of the rehabilitation team has been the "worker's disability syndrome" [16], wherein an individual's psychological reaction to injury and the effects of the secondary gains can disable as much as the original trauma. The injury has solved many preexisting life problems, and the removal of symptoms and regaining of health through rehabilitation can spell a return of the former difficulties, both fiscal and psychosocial. The reason for including discussion of rehabilitation at this point is based on the support that can be given the rehabilitative process by the OHS staff. By virtue of previous contacts with employees who have sought health care, the counsel of a physician, nurse, or psychologist can be extremely helpful in underscoring the objective of an early return to work. As Denehy [17] expressed it, when learning that the average period between injury and referral for rehabilitation was 27 months—a length of time that bespeaks poor results—"Rehabilitation commences on the day of the accident," an aphorism that is still true, meaning early motivation for treatment and return to work. "Unfortunately, legal advice has often been 'Don't have rehabilitation, we will get a larger payout,'" he observed.

The concerned OHS member can initiate RTW goals before trade union friends or attorneys can exert influence toward maintenance of a soul-destroying chronic, disabling state. Symptoms must be maintained as convincing evidence in the seeking of an award, and little does the patient/claimant realize the hazards of perpetuating disability. A dedicated occupational health group will provide support and motivation from the beginning and will continue the nurturing during the healing process and the rehabilitation program. The instilling of positive attitudes early represents some of the most insightful and rewarding practice of true occupational health. A person who has been productive throughout a lifetime most often finds a retirement because of disability a blow to self-esteem, often demasculating, and dissatisfying because few manual workers are prepared for the inactivity and the retention of an artificial role.

TESTIMONY, DEPOSITION, AND CROSS-EXAMINATION

Attorneys were queried as to why physicians might be subpoenaed for cross-examination. Some of the reasons given follow [11]:

The history given was incomplete, inaccurate, or conflicted with other reports, and the areas in conflict were not explained.

The examination was incomplete or inaccurate or conflicted with other reports, and the conflicts were not clarified.

The report had internal inconsistencies and contradictions.

The reasons for the physician's conclusions either were not given or were unclear.

The physician "waffled" in his discussion, suggesting that he might not be certain of his conclusions.

The physician's ideas on apportionment did not follow the law or were not supported by the evidence.

In light of this explanation, sooner or later, any physician or other occupational health professional who is engaged in an aspect of WC health care will be called on to give testimony, either in the form of a deposition or before a hearing officer, referee, judge, or possibly a jury. Physicians with great frequency will avoid such confrontations because the attorney-witness relationship, while commonplace to the lawyer, can be extremely emotiogenic to the physician. As implied previously, many physicians refuse to accept patients in the WC system because of the constant threat of participation in the litigation process. The belief is, and often substantiated, that the interrogating attorney is intent on embarrassing, discrediting, confusing, abusing, unsettling, and humiliating the physician, who is on unfamiliar turf and frequently is intentionally angered, creating further upset in this unaccustomed role.

Yet, there are some physicians who look forward to the interchange as an intellectual exercise and who enjoy jousting with opposing counsel. Whatever the attitude of the witness-to-be, there are some fundamental principles that, when followed, can release the situation of some of the anxiety and tension that are frequent concomitants of the inquirer-respondent relationship. Even experienced medical witnesses find testifying a drain, as expressed by psychiatrist Terr [18], long familiar with the courtroom setting: "Testifying is about five times as hard, takes about five times as much emotional energy as my patients. I may not move a muscle when I'm on the stand, but I've expended lifeblood there. Afterward I have to watch a Western movie on tv or get a stiff drink because I'm shot."

Even though an excellent report might be submitted by a physician, there still will be a call for cross-examination. It was observed by a WC official [19] that on occasion attorneys just wish to test the physician, and sometimes they just want to prove to their client—the applicant or the insurance underwriter—that "they are really trying hard, even though they aren't going to get anywhere trying to break down your testimony." Another reason might motivate the action. There may be a feeling that they can induce the physician to change his opinion.

Calvert [19] has commented that if, in a cross-examination, an attorney tries to discredit the physician, the more likely result, if the witness knows what he is doing, is that the lawyer will be more discredited by the end of the inquiry, for he is talking about medical matters, which is the arena familiar to the physician. Occasionally, an attorney will bring the physician in for examination because he wishes to present new facts of which the practitioner was not aware, in an effort to see if the opinion will be changed, as based on those facts. This situation can be avoided by a listing in the report of all the documents that have been reviewed. A cross-examination may be called when there is a problem in the physician's report, if it is incomplete or contains ambiguities or inconsistencies that leave the attorney with "reasonable and legitimate bewilderment as to what the true opinion of the doctor is" [19].

The question arises in certain cases as to whether, in testimony, the physician-witness should offer opinions outside of his specialty. Ordinarily, a response to the effect that one is not qualified in the other specialty will stop a line of questioning that might lead to difficult extrication. It has been suggested though [19] that if the physician believes the claimant is grossly exaggerating symptoms or disability and states that, when asked, an opinion would lie outside his customary specialty, then both sides proceed to seek psychiatric reviews, and long delays will ensue. A better response, which might preclude such action, is, "Yes, it is possible that these complaints are on an emotional or psychiatric basis, but I really don't think so, and I really don't see any need to go to a psychiatrist in this case." Another expression that could lead to psychiatric examinations and is better omitted is "functional overlay," which is not exactly within current nomenclature anyway.

It is advised by WC authorities that one should avoid the use of the term *possible* and distinguish carefully between *possibility* and *probability*. The standard in some jurisdictions is "reasonable medical probability," not "reasonable medical certainty." As anything is possible, saying so adds nothing and is telling nothing. The question usually placed is, "Is this probable; is it more likely than not?" The use of the term *possible* often leads to cross-examination, and such a time-consuming activity can be avoided if the correct standard is offered and if the question cited above is addressed.

Another bit of counsel offered [19] is that a physician should not become identified consistently with one side or the other, so that the appearance of neutrality and objectivity can be maintained. It is wise, when an opinion of a specialist is being sought by an attorney, to inform the lawyer that the case will be reviewed and that there is no guarantee that the resultant opinion will be in his client's favor, for the honest physician will "call it exactly as he sees it." Most attorneys will accept this stance gladly, for they want sound guidance. Their response usually is that if the opinion is not favorable, they will change the physician's role from expert witness to consultant so that the opinion will not have to be introduced as evidence.

On being asked—or subpoenaed—to give a deposition, it is wise to make oneself available at reasonable and convenient times, and thus cross-examination may be avoided. In preparing for testimony, one must be knowledgeable about the issues. All medical files should be reviewed in advance, and particularly one should be familiar with the records of other physicians, especially if one does not agree with them. As it has been pointed out, frequently one rejects certain theories in favor of others that one has adopted, and one is likely to "put them out of mind." Occasionally one will be asked to explain why the ideas of others are not acceptable.

It was indicated previously that one should never guess; looking up a fact in a medical record while on the stand is perfectly acceptable. One must be sure of one's statements before making them, and one should not try to defend a position that is shown to be founded on incomplete or inaccurate facts. One can be receptive to new facts or assumptions not previously available, and "The ability or willingness to change your mind and to do it publicly in the course of the cross-examination when new facts are submitted to you is a sign of integrity and believability and is generally so regarded" [19]. Finally, there are several precautions to be followed by a witness:

Make sure the question is understood and is clear. One can ask to have it repeated or clarified.
Respond as briefly as possible.
Do not talk too fast.
Avoid medical jargon. Explain medical terms, if used.
If the answer to a question is in one's report, refer to it rather than repeating it. Make sure the question is accurate if opposing counsel is citing from your report or record.
Allow the attorney to complete the question, even though the question and the response might be obvious. Do not "jump on his lines." Further, it gives the other attorney time to object.
Do not be emotional.

Do not fight with opposing counsel; stay cool under pressure.
Do not be defensive.
Be serious, avoid jocose remarks, dress appropriately conservatively,* avoid undue familiarity, and do not patronize.
Do not be an advocate.
When on the stand, look at the jury, if there is one, or at "the trier of fact," the judge or hearing officer.
Avoid new theories or unusual points of view.
Ask counsel to define loose terms like "heart attack."
Avoid "unfounded optimism on the patient's progress" [20].
Remember—one is paid for one's time and not for one's testimony.
In spite of legend, one can respond to the demand for a yes-or-no answer by turning to the court and saying, "If the court please, that question cannot honestly be answered by either yes or no." Generally the court will instruct the witness to answer in his or her own way and qualify the answer.
Do not bring notes to the stand that have not been introduced as an exhibit.
Do not volunteer.
Be modest.
As a witness, do not ask to "go off the record."

A practice not usually discussed is one encountered with a claimant's attorney who has his clients complete a form titled, "Instructions Concerning Medical Examination by Defendant's Doctor." The directive asks that the client be cooperative, tell the truth, and "be careful in telling about other doctors." Under the section headed, "Client's Report of Medical Examination," the patient responds to the following:

Client's name
Date of examination
Examining doctor
What time did you get to the doctor's office?
How much time was spent in the waiting room?
How long were you actually with the doctor?
How much of this time was spent answering questions?
How much of this time was for physical examination?
What time did you leave the doctor's office?
Were you questioned by a nurse before seeing the doctor?
How much time did that take?
Were x-rays taken? If so, how many?
Please give any questions you remember the doctor asking you and what your answers were.
Please give any comments the doctor made to you about your case, your injuries, or his opinion.
Other comments or information about the doctor or examination.

Needless to say, irresponsible, unprofessional, discourteous, or other untoward behavior may return to haunt if the physician were asked to give testimony.

FINALE

As every writing in medicine should concern itself, at least in part, with prevention, the following aphorisms of Gerson [21], a clinical psychologist concerned with WC evaluations, are offered as near guarantees of producing a WC claim:

Prior to an actual injury or psychological breakdown, ignore complaints coming out of a department or increased absenteeism from that area.
If an employee's performance slips noticeably or is injured in minor ways repeatedly, assume it is nothing to do with work; rather, he/she is careless or is having problems at home that are spilling over into the work setting.
Once there is an injury or emotional breakdown, minimize it and shirk all responsibility.
Once the person is out with a disability, make sure nothing goes right for him/her and that no one cares.
When all else fails, fire him/her.
If and when the employee returns to work, put him/her back at full capacity right away and/or make him/her feel guilty for the time out.

Lastly, in substance, a knowledge of the WC system is mandatory in occupational medicine, and every physician engaged in the specialty must be familiar with its philosophy, pitfalls, and administrative problems. With this familiarity, there still must

*In an excellent review of the manner of speech in the courtroom (Conley, J. M., O'Barr, W. M., and Lind, E. A. The power of language: Presentational style in the courtroom. *Duke Laws* 6:1375, 1978), the writers make comment regarding the areas of the lawyer, and the point is equally applicable to the physician witness: "Resort by counsel to stylistic extremes creates a particularly serious danger that the jury will be diverted from its theoretical role of evaluation of the facts and induced to engage in speculation and emotional reaction."

be compassion for the worker who has suffered the indignity of being injured or made ill while pursuing a livelihood.

REFERENCES

1. Somers, H. M., and Somers, A. R. *Workmen's Compensation*. New York: Wiley, 1954. P. 7. Copyright © 1954 by John Wiley and Sons, Inc.
2. *California Workers' Compensation Institute Bulletin*. No. 83-2, March 2, 1983. P. 1.
3. Committee on Occupational Health, California Medical Association. The industrial "blank check." *Calif Med* 97:122, 1962.
4. Clark, W. L. Writing the History and Physical Examination. In *Proceedings of the Workers' Compensation Seminar for Physicians, May 19, 1979, Los Angeles*. San Francisco: California Department of Industrial Relations, Division of Industrial Accidents, 1979. Pp. 58–65.
5. Whiting, W. B. *The Physician and Workers' Compensation*. San Francisco: State Compensation Insurance Fund, (Sept) 1977.
6. Thurber, P. *Evaluation of Industrial Disability*. Oxford: Oxford University Press, 1960.
7. *Guides to the Evaluation of Permanent Impairment* (3rd ed.). Chicago: American Medical Association, 1988.
8. Walsh, E. Writing the Report-Framing Conclusions. In *Proceedings of the Worker's Compensation Seminar for Physicians, May 19, 1979, Los Angeles*. San Francisco: California Department of Industrial Relations, Division of Industrial Accidents, 1979. Pp. 65–73.
9. Description of Disabilities. *California Labor Code*. Title 8. Division of Industrial Accidents: Administrative Director—Administrative Rules. Subchap. 1, Article 2, §9729. Subjective Disability (Register 66, No. 20-7-2-66).
10. *Guidelines for Work Capacity: Schedule for Rating Permanent Disabilities*. San Francisco: Division of Industrial Accidents, Permanent Disability Rating Bureau, 1973. P. 1-A.
11. Clark, W. L. *Guidelines for Medical Examination and Report* (rev.). San Francisco: California State Department of Industrial Relations, Division of Industrial Accidents—Workers' Compensation Appeals Board, (Apr) 1985.
12. *The Physician and Workers' Compensation*. Chicago: American Medical Association, Environmental and Occupational Health Program, 1983. Pp. 5–6. Copyright 1983, American Medical Association.
13. Whipple, F. L. The workers' compensation psychiatric report. Typescript and *Audio-Digest-Psychiatry*. Workers' Compensation Psychiatric Evaluations. Vol. 12, No. 7, April 11, 1983, Side B.
14. *Diagnostic and Statistical Manual of Mental Disorders* (3rd ed.). Washington, DC: American Psychiatric Association, 1980.
15. *Vocational Rehabilitation: A Report to the Industry*. San Francisco: California Workers' Compensation Institute, 1983.
16. Hanson-Mayer, T. P. The worker's disability syndrome. *J Rehabil* 50:50, 1984.
17. Denehy, W. H. [Untitled letter to the editor.] *J Soc Occup Med* 33:100, 1983.
18. Cited in Footlick, J. K., Sendza, R., Foote, D., et al. Trials of the medical expert. *Newsweek* 99:58, Feb 8, 1982.
19. Calvert, R., Walsh, E., Laws, R., et al. Panel on Cross-Examination. In *Proceedings of the Worker's Compensation Seminar for Physicians, May 19, 1979, Los Angeles*. San Francisco: California Department of Industrial Relations, Division of Industrial Accidents, 1979. Pp. 73–81.
20. Medical experts should strive to be honest, specific, complete. *Intern Med News* 15:2, March 1–14, 1982.
21. Gerson, A. Increasing the chances for a compensation claim. *Occup Health Saf* 49:39 (May), 1980.

549405

11. EMPLOYEE COUNSELING

If our leg or arm offend us, we covet by all means possible to redress it; and if we labor of a bodily disease, we send for a physician; but, for disease of the mind, we take no notice of them.

Robert Burton

Medicine never has been followed wholly in the scientific spirit. Science serving mankind needs and has had another expression that can be called humanism. It implies an understanding of the mental state of the patient and a sympathy for him as a purposeful being. It is this that distinguishes the physician from the barber-leech.

Frederick A. Coller, M.D.

The gathering of large groups of disparate peoples at work involves the introduction into the site of employment a broad variety of personal and cultural characteristics that somehow must be fused into a compatible productive force. The United States, in addition to being the amalgam that it is, is undergoing even further change through the daily infusion of immigrants and students from Southeast Asia, the South Pacific, the Orient, Mexico, Puerto Rico, and the Middle East.

Resulting from these population drifts is a cultural mix that bespeaks different attainments in experience and education, dissimilar mores and religious credos, divergent personality patterns, antithetic political backgrounds, diverse socioeconomic levels, varying views of gender roles, and frequently, antipodal concepts of the work ethic. Somehow, it is expected that this strange matrix of a work body will fit the constraints of a long-established business enterprise, with each employee fulfilling smoothly and well every task delineated in the formal job description.

Unfortunately, as every supervisor knows, few are the days spent in any commercial, manufacturing, research, or academic arena that are totally free from the effects of human mismatchings, the friction of supervisor-worker interaction, the slowdown of poorly motivated employees, and infrequently, the breakdown of a production process. From this melange of people, supplies, equipment, and regulations emerge human problems in desperate need of resolution so that not only will the mission of the organization be fulfilled, but also, it is hoped, the workers will accrue some sense of satisfaction and worth from their labors.

Not all the sources of conflict are internal to the company, for persisting extramural stressors have their effect on the enterprise: a shaky, wandering economy; the conversion of a society from an industrial state to one replete in information/service organizations utilizing computers and robots wherever possible; closure or downsizing of the industries that characterized American productivity, with the mergers, the reductions in force, bankruptcies, and moves to foreign fabrication sites that follow; and, lastly, as voiced by one industrialist, the overall uncommon period of unpredictability [1]. These pressures are felt soon or late by individual employees who, with their own domestic or fiscal imbalance, begin to manifest some impairment of their job performance.

DETECTION OF HUMAN SLIPPAGE

In most human undertakings that have involved a screening—acceptance at school, admission to advanced training, granting of employment, making a team—applicants usually have met all the prerequisites essential for success in the program such as scholastic level, experience, training, capability of learning, and the like. Yet, in spite of these near guarantees, there will be failures. When reviewed, it may be discovered that an emotional problem has arisen that has served as a deterrent to completion of a program or achievement in a job.

Because of this fact and the clinical findings from several studies showing the great amount of psychogenic illness among patients presenting with presumably frank physical disorders, it is essential that people be provided with a support structure that might aid in reversing some of their emotional disruptions. Disputes on the job, withdrawal from work, and impaired performance are costly and totally counterproductive. A knowledgeable occupational health service (OHS) staff will identify those workers who are manifesting telltale behavioral signs of an adjustment disorder or, with lesser frequency, a frank psychotic state.

The signs that will lead one to consider an employee as currently troubled may be subsumed under the heading of symptomatic behavior (Table 11-1).

Any of the behaviorisms indicated in Table 11-1 can be detected by a member of the OHS staff, managers, first-line supervisors, or even coworkers. Unfortunately, apart from most immediate supervisors, employees are reluctant to involve themselves no matter how extraordinary the behavior or how destructive it might be to the organization. The networks being as tightly knit as they are in industry,

TABLE 11-1. *Symptomatic Behavior Indicative of Emotional Impairment*

WITHDRAWAL FROM WORK	
Chronic absenteeism	Wandering from assigned jobsite
Chronic tardiness	Crying spells
Prolonged "breaks"	Job abandonment
Injury repetition	Delayed return from vacation or business travel without adequate rationale
Sleeping at work	
IMPAIRED TECHNICAL PERFORMANCE	
Increased number of errors	Repeated inability to complete task or meet deadline
Increased amount of scrap	Decreased concentration among executives and "think-tank" personnel
Destruction of tools/equipment	
IMPAIRED INTERPERSONAL RELATIONSHIPS	
Inability to motivate supervised work group	Increased criticism of superordinates
Alienation of both superordinates and subordinates	Disparity or inequity in making job assignments—"favoritism"
Inability to function effectively with peers	Undersocialization
Refusal to follow orders or regulations	Failure to communicate needed work information
Excessive reliance on supervision	"Closed-door" policy
Insensitivity to needs of subordinates	Manifest ambition with "destruction" of fellow-workers
Lack of recognition of subordinates' or peers' contributions	
Refusal to grant reasonable requests of subordinates for needed time off	
PHYSICAL RESPONSE TO STRESSORS	
Sudden change to slovenly, unkempt appearance	Inordinate postoperative convalescence
Evidence of poor personal hygiene	Chemical-substance abuse
Recrudescence of stress disorders	Beverage-alcohol dependence
Arthritis	Street-drug abuse
Atopy—dermatologic, pulmonary	Excessive use of prescription medication
Peptic ulceration	Increased tobacco dependence
Headache uncontrolled by appropriate medication	Break in weight-reduction program, smoking cessation, alcohol abstinence, or control of compulsive gambling
Sudden untoward weight gain	Fear of business travel
Sudden unexplained weight loss	Attempted self-destruction
Increase in off-the-job accidents and accident-related injuries	
In youths, exacerbated acne	
In adults, failure of dermatologic disorders to heal	
MISCELLANEOUS	
Adult antisocial behavior	Repeated wage garnishments
Theft (community or company property)	Passing of "bad" checks
Kleptomania	Problem behavior of employee's children
Excessive number of traffic violations and outstanding warrants	Felonious behavior
Extensive records at social welfare agencies	Unresolved bereavement

workers fear retributive action and prefer to remain silent. However, rumor spreads quickly in a plant, and word of an aberration soon will reach the OHS, where action can be initiated. While employees may not share feelings with fellow workers, they frequently will apprise trusted medical, nursing, or technology personnel of an OHS, for it is known that the source will not be revealed.

The OHS is the logical locus for recognition of the troubled employee, as many such persons develop physical symptoms, and such symptoms are taken for resolution to a source of medical care. It is at that point that the shrewd observer will begin to ferret out significant events to distinguish between the organic illness and the manifestation of an upset worker. The concerned professional will not resort to tranquilization but will take the first steps toward preparation of the patient for wiser and more productive exploration.

PREPARATION OF THE EMPLOYEE-PATIENT

Without question, the most important step in the sequence of Recognition, Reassurance, and Referral—as "R'ed" by Dr. Harry Levinson—is reassurance of the employee. Much of the success in the interaction between the professional person and the patient is a reflection of the personality of the physician or occupational health nurse, the comfort felt and displayed in reviewing the problem with the patient, and the confidence placed in the counseling or psychotherapeutic process. Obviously, anyone who feels that psychological or psychiatric care is a silly waste of time is not going to effect a serious, well-intentioned, or visibly concerned interview or referral.

Probably the reason for physicians or nurses abdicating from the role of counselor in the past and either delegating the function to others or allowing this form of care to go by default to paraprofessionals has been the discomfiture felt on discussing close, personal issues with employees. While the physician or nurse is not necessarily trained to serve as counselor, he or she must accept the role of referring agent so that the benefits can accrue to the person in need.

INTERVIEWING

Much can be done to make troubled employees feel at sufficient ease to verbalize their difficulties, if known. Frequently, the worker is referred to the medical director by an imperious foreman who is without the wit or training to face an employee whose job performance is on the decline. The worker, in essence, is ordered to "go see the Doc," often with no explanation, as good communication often is not one of the skills of the first-line supervisor. When such individuals reach the OHS, they are angry and puzzled and have become completely hostile to the maneuver. The first task is to defuse the highly charged situation, and the best opener is, "You certainly seem to be angry. Would you like to tell me why?"

Recalled from years past was a young woman, a clinical laboratory technologist, who was ordered to the employee health service of a medical center to have a physical examination. The nurse apprised the physician in advance of the obvious anger displayed by the person, in spite of her having said nothing. The examination was conducted in absolute silence, and she was asked to come back to the office when dressed. She came in, took the proferred chair, determined to remain mute. The opener indicated above was used, and that released a flood of tears. Spread for review was the tale of months of interpersonal difficulties with the laboratory chief, against whom the unexpressed anger was developed. When given the opportunity for release, the story emerged, and the reason for the displacement of feeling became obvious. Through counseling of both the worker and the supervisor, talent and productivity were preserved.

In much the same way—that there must be preparation for any personnel action involving the deep concerns of an individual—the OHS professional can open up an acceptable referral path to a mental health professional for the employee having problems. Interviewing skills can come with practice, but a few general objectives of the process should be borne in mind, as expressed by Dr. Stewart Wolf [2] many years ago:

To make the patient feel comfortable and secure.
To enable the patient to trust the doctor's skill and judgment, his respect for confidential material, and his personal motivations.
To make it easy for the patient to talk freely and frankly.
To direct the discussion along the most pertinent and profitable lines for diagnosis and treatment [or referral].

Some basic principles to be followed are suggested.

Preparation for the Interview

Review records in advance to permit familiarity with the problem and to obviate scanning a folder while the patient waits anxiously, not knowing exactly what is going to take place. If the patient has been referred by a supervisor, obtain additional information regarding events having taken place between the initial call and the appointment.

Clear one's desk of the usual stacks of papers and journals, to demonstrate a concentration on the problem at hand.

If the office, by chance, faces the outside at ground level—or if higher and close to an adjacent building—draw the blinds or curtains so that the patient will feel the privacy of the setting.*

Have a chair available for the employee near the chair of the physician or nurse, preferably behind or alongside the desk, and not in front of the desk, which then becomes a barricade, physically and emotionally.

Arrange to have telephone calls and staff visits held so as not to disrupt the flow of the interview.

The Interview

When the patient enters or is escorted in, arise and greet him or her, shake hands warmly, not limply, close the door, and usher the employee to the chair indicated above, taking the coat, hat, hard hat, tool, or whatever accompanies the worker, and placing it conveniently.

If the patient feels that the clinical record contains material that is being withheld from him or her, the record can be placed in full view so that a perusal, if needed, can be conducted openly and jointly, sharing whatever entries have been made that are germane.†

Do not "play" with anything on the desk, such as pens, paper clips, or rulers, as the action is distracting and indicates a lack of attentiveness on the part of the interviewer.

Look at the employee, and maintain eye contact. Do not look at the desk, the wall, the floor, or the ceiling. Avoid looking distracted or fatigued. Nonverbal messages are inhibiting.

Do not check the time periodically, particularly avoiding scrutiny of one's wristwatch. If necessary, keep a clock behind the patient or in an unapparent line of sight.

Avoid the usual opening pleasantries or preamble about the weekend fishing or the most recent big-league game, for it is difficult at best to get to the subject without derailing the conversation even momentarily. Get on with it! Do not apologize for the interview.

Look, listen intently, give the appearance of concerned listening, and learn.

Avoid generalities, and talk about specific, pertinent things.

Talk about the patient, not yourself.*

Avoid emotional involvement even though the employee angers you, is defensive, or slanders you or "the system." Avoid being resentful or defending yourself, and do not try to put the employee down. Explore the basis of the feelings shown.

Observe the employee's hands, eyes, skin, posture, and anything that will reveal feelings or attitudes. Nonverbal communication frequently tells more than conversational content.

Let pauses remain as pauses without rushing in to fill the gap. If there is no inclination to continue after a long stop, rephrase as a question what was said last, or repeat as a question the patient's terminal clause. Patient: "That was when he came over to my bench." Pause . . . Counselor: "He came over to your bench?"

Responses should be neutral: "I see," "Uh-huh," "I see what you mean," or "I understand."

Save the employee's "face."

Emphasize what the individual can do, rather than what he or she cannot do.

Avoid questions readily answered "Yes" or "No." Use more of the why, who, when, where, what, and how queries.

If one is asked questions, turn them back with, "What do *you* think?" or "What do you *mean*?"

Do not argue, interrupt, give advice, take sides, scold, or be authoritative.

If you say, at one point, "I'll look into that," be sure to follow up.

Always have a box of tissues at hand.

Be yourself.

Summarize the interview, and arrange for a return.

Some decades ago Cook [3] classified interviewers as follows:

*Although such a point in preparation is not possible when an OHS installation is complete, there can be a correction made in the planning stage. An arrangement to be avoided in the layout of the physical plant—and this error has been seen—is to place the interviewer's office next to a restroom. As material is being discussed of a highly personal or confidential nature, the trend of thought and speech is punctuated by intermittent fixture-flushings next door. In a comparable vein, an office has been seen where a call bell had been placed just outside the physician's office to direct field personnel to a telephone, in a situation without radio or beeper communication. Again, a continuous interview could not be held with staccato interruptions.

†As no observational impressions of *character* should be entered in the file, there need be no hesitation in sharing the document.

*The author had a staff physician once who was supposedly interviewing his patient. As the office door was open, one could not avoid hearing the conversation. The professional was unburdening himself endlessly of all of *his* problems so that the patient had no opportunity to talk; he reached for his hard hat and left.

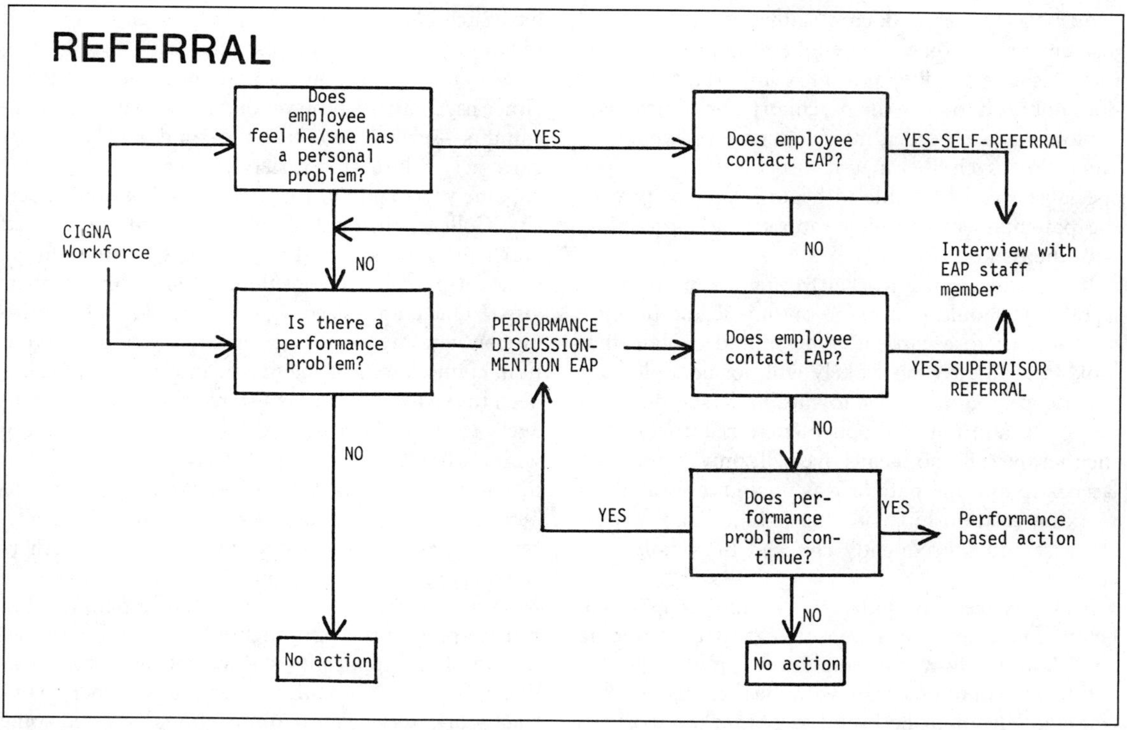

FIGURE 11-1. *Mechanism of referral to employee assistance program, as developed in one organization. (Courtesy of Brady C. Hartman, M.D., Corporate Medical Director, Rohr Industries, Inc., Chula Vista, California.)*

Poker-face interviewer: challenges the employee-client to make him or her smile. "I dare you to move me to any show of emotion."

Smart-aleck interviewer: sacrifices anything for a wise crack.

Interviewer with a power drive: considers people as objects; never admits being wrong; uses the words "definitely" and "absolutely."

Oh-so-charming interviewer: attempts to win everyone; overuses a smile; agrees with last person spoken with; sets one person against another.

Mr. Milquetoast: lacks poise, putting burden of interview on interviewee; filled with fear and self-depreciation; facial expression and gestures say, "Please, like me."

Good interviewer: measures ability as an interviewer by drawing people out, getting them to talk, and helping them to gain self-confidence.

It is obvious that the first five types of interviewers will accomplish little in their efforts to assist workers in trouble.

PREPARATION FOR REFERRAL

If the employee is in need of counseling and such a service is available within the OHS, if there is an employee assistance program (EAP) in the company, or if there is need for outside referral to a psychologist, psychiatrist, or other mental health specialist, the patient must be prepared for such a suggested change in health care. One must be certain that all efforts at identifying a physical cause for the behavioral problem have been carried out and that no evidence of organic disease has been encountered. Such a move is particularly important because, in industry, most companies have a policy whereby a supervisor can request a determination of physical fitness of an employee when there is evidence of a downslope in job performance.

When the worker is declared physically fit, yet the problem remains, it is the task of the OHS professional to familiarize the employee with some of the entities, in general, that make for emotional difficulties. Such a presentation should be made in a compassionate, empathic manner, with the focus at all times on the benefits to accrue to the patient—better health, job retention or improvement, better relationships at home, and the like.

The mechanism of referral at one organization is shown in Figure 11-1.

The counselor must be honest when he is suggesting referral to a mental health specialist, and such a professional must be identified by discipline—a psychiatrist, a psychologist, a family or marriage counselor, a psychiatric social worker—and not erroneously as a nerve doctor, someone with special instruments, or some other euphemism that skirts the issue dishonestly. Preparation is important, for one does not wish to have the psychiatrist or clinical psychologist waste needed interview time in explaining what the psychotherapeutic process involves. The specialist should be able to begin immediately with the patient in establishing rapport and proceeding with the issue.

In introducing the worker to the possibility of referral, one should not be too optimistic and promise a variety of rose gardens. One should explain that looking at oneself most likely will not be a pleasant experience, that the move toward understanding will be uphill, and that the patient may not always like the therapist. By no means oversell, only to find at a later date that the patient was unable to establish a working relationship with the psychologist or psychiatrist and subsequently chucked the whole concept.

The physician in industry or the occupational health nurse must be supportive and encouraging and should follow the employee's progress by remaining in communication with the therapist *and* the employee. It might be useful to obtain the worker's permission to tell his or her supervisor that special care is being obtained in the hope of resolving the behavioral problem at work. If there are difficult periods, the supervisor will be more understanding and tolerant.

ROLE OF THE MENTAL HEALTH SPECIALIST AS CONSULTANT TO INDUSTRY

Many companies have used the services of specialists in mental health both in the OHS and as consultants to the management group. Such assistance is sought usually when the medical director is comfortable with the behavioral aspects of illness and is not a pure somaticist. Even though it has long been understood that most illnesses are multifactorial in etiology and that there are both physical and psychological factors at causative play with disease—and injury—many long-seasoned physicians are still reluctant to explore some of the less obvious reasons for a person's becoming ill.

A consultant may be added also when the chief executive officer is comfortable with such a specialist and is free from such disorders as alcoholism, which might be detected readily with a knowing person in the plant. The presence of mental illness in the family of the medical director occasionally has embittered him toward psychiatry and negated any effort to have such in-plant help at hand. A last consideration, of course, is budgetary constraint.

Several of the nation's largest companies have had either psychiatrists or psychologists as part-time consultants—several were full-time—and they have been extremely helpful in a variety of areas.

Some years ago Dr. Roger Tredgold of the University College Hospital, London, visited the United States [4] and discerned readily the operating differences of psychiatric consultants "according to their gifts." One emphasized morale, selection, and training, and another was concerned with crisis intervention, counseling, and diagnostic interviews. So it has been that some consultants were asked to train managers to have them upgrade their skills in working with and motivating people or, as Longaker [5] put it, to improve their managerial interpersonal competence and provide them some capability in identifying behavioral breaks in their workers. Others were asked to serve in a more clinical sense—to see worker-patients who had emotional difficulties that were impairing their productivity or to aid in the selection of job applicants who were headed for sensitive positions (law enforcement, government contract work, service abroad) or who manifested some obvious behavioral aberration that might contraindicate the anticipated placement. In addition to the diagnostic and short-term counseling functions, they could also conduct training of OHS staff personnel to increase their sensitivity to symptomatic behavior, to become somewhat more self-reflective, and to develop a supportive tolerance for the worker beset by an emotional or personality disorder.

Workers, by virtue of the mission of an organization, are placed in a social institution—business or manufacturing—or, better yet, in a social matrix, and "treatment, to be most effective should occur with a minimum of dislocation of the individual from his usual social matrix" [6]. Serving the employee at the customary worksite makes for an easier rapport where the operations, the language, and the relationships are known bilaterally by the patient-client and counselor.*

One of the most valued contributions of the psychiatric or psychological consultant is the review

*A long-employed shop foreman became well-known to a medical director, for he was an overweight person with diabetes headed eventually for complications. As he visited the OHS in his customarily creased work clothing, comfortable on familiar turf, he confided his life's joys and sadnesses. But in a private medical office downtown, he would be attired in a slightly ill-fitting, rarely worn but pressed dark suit, bereft of his cap of authority, and reticent in sharing his 60 years. Is this the same man? Or readily accepting of counsel as before?

of patients with the physician or nurse who has attended the particular workers. This cooperative one-to-one effort provides a strong educational opportunity that far exceeds the knowledge fallout from seminars, conferences, or workshops. Not only does this kind of teaching allow a better treatment of the emotionally disturbed person, but also better care for all patients, irrespective of the problem presented. If necessary, the consultant can meet briefly with the patient to provide greater substance to the case review process.

Who is the consultant to be called? The choice may be difficult, but Coodley [7] has viewed the contemporary scene and opines in this way:

> In Southern California, we certainly have a potpourri of so-called therapists, ranging from out-and-out slobs to con artists and quacks to melodramatic show-business characters and eventually to the legitimate therapists. One crucial source for choosing a psychotherapist originates from advice of other patients, at least those in a stage of positive transference to the therapist. Essentially, if the therapist combines teaching experience with board certification, publications, and public and professional participation—coupled with doing a good job with one's current patients receiving psychotherapy—chances of continuing and maintaining a healthy patient load are automatically enhanced. The likelihood that such a therapist will benefit his patients is definitely on the high side.

Such a person can be attracted to industry, for the work setting provides an exciting new theater of operations, a living laboratory for research, and an opportunity to share in the emerging segment of psychotoxicology or behavioral toxicology. But stepping into this new locale cannot be accomplished without a learning period. The consultant must become familiar with the company, its organization, its informal structure, its physical plant, and most particularly, the patois and jargon of the shops. Until these informational nuggets can enter discourse appropriately, the consultant will still be viewed as an outlander, an outsider. The psychiatrist must understand "the employee's environment with its stresses and supports, his rational and irrational reactions to it, and the probable circumstances of his job situation and when he can return to it" [8], for acceptance is the needed element in successful treatment [9]. The point is given further emphasis by Tanay [10], in a discussion of the use of consultants by the occupational physician, when he comments, ". . . many consultants utilized by the major corporations are the outstanding men in the field; they are the blue ribbon experts who are more familiar with blue blood clientele than blue collar workers. They are frequently unable to communicate with factory workers and are uninformed about the work setting." This point must be remembered in soliciting consultative assistance.

Irrespective of the medical or behavioral science discipline of the consultants, specialists can be of immeasurable professional assistance, provided they understand the ethos of the plant and the company of which it is part and become known to the working personnel, irrespective of the color of the collar.

STRESS AND TODAY'S WORK CULTURE

Practitioners of occupational health in decades past have been fully aware of the negative reception given anything smacking of psychology or psychiatry. Trade union leaders fought the introduction of counseling into companies because they feared that their membership would be "brainwashed," being converted through that procedure to the viewpoint of management and no longer obedient followers of the labor movement. The author had an indelible experience in 1949 when appearing on a panel in Detroit, along with representatives of the nation's largest unions. The counseling program that had been introduced at the Oak Ridge National Laboratory was described in some detail, as part of the larger occupational health effort. A fellow panelist who followed called me an absolute liar because, in his eyes, no company would ever have anything that advantageous.

It would take some years before one of the country's outstanding labor leaders—president of the Oil, Chemical and Atomic Workers' International Union [11]—would deliver an address that contained these statements: "We must insure that our proposed standards produce no mental, as well as no physical, harm. The criteria for setting standards should include the comfort and mental ease of the worker. Not only should the work environment be free of toxic chemical and physical hazards, it should also be free of psychological stresses." He concluded by saying that the basic philosophy of his union was "to measure well-being not by increases in productivity, or by increases in gross national product, but by the health and mental well-being of the people who work in industry and live in the community."

Old fears die slowly. But in the mid-1970s one word was decanted off Hans Selye's lifelong research to become a buzzword in all circles—"stress." All of the words plucked from previous lexicons, such as psychological problems, emotional distress, nervousness, emotionally upset, even counselor, and the like, which had been used for years and had been feared and shunned by employees in need of care for their behavioral disruptions, now had a successor. The introduction and popularization of the word (and the concept of) stress might possibly be attributed to the fact that the deficit within the worker can now be laid on external circumstances—the job, the spouse, the foreman, the anonymous "they" or "them," the times we live in—and thus the worker is freed of any blame, any guilt, any error, any deficiency. It is now the fault of the external force that is causing the worker to react—to develop a stress response to all those terrible stressors pressing in on him or her.

With this kind of new perception, plus the consolidation by industry of all of its counseling functions into an activity called an employee assistance program (EAP), the stigma has been removed of one's having to be referred to a psychologist or psychiatrist. After all, does not everyone, at one time or another, have need of "assistance"?

Another feature of this move must be brought to light. For years, even decades, most OHS personnel have avoided involvement with workers in need of counseling or referral for psychotherapy, as mentioned earlier. Whatever the reason might have been, efforts to help such employees have not been forthcoming from the health arm of the organization. Certain efforts at departmental aggrandizement combined with the lethargy displayed in this area by many occupational health professionals led to the development of EAPs by other units in a company, most often under the aegis of the industrial relations department or the personnel division.

The creation of these programs allowed the subsumption of all counseling activities under a single designation, bringing alcoholism rehabilitation counseling, counseling for other chemical substance abuse, counseling for emotional or behavioral problems, and even guidance in certain other areas, such as budgeting and family relationships, together into one unit.

Not all EAPs are to be found within industry, for labor unions have established assistance programs, most of which focus primarily on alcoholism. A national organization has brought together many counselors from occupational alcoholism programs under the heading of ALMACA, the Association of Labor-Management Administrators and Consultants on Alcoholism.* Other offshoots of the programmatic movement are seen in academe, where efforts are made to reach the impaired or troubled academician, and in the medical profession, where considerable recent attention has been directed toward the impaired physician [12,13]. On one university campus, a memorandum was distributed directly from the chancellor in which the new Employee Assistance Services (EAS) was announced and full support of the program was encouraged [14]. The EAS would "provide confidential assessment and referral services, free of charge, to employees and their families who experience problems on the job or in their personal lives. Such problems may include marital, family, emotional, financial, legal or those related to alcohol or drug abuse." The chancellor continued, "It is recognized that problems such as these, though not directly associated with a person's job, can have an effect on job performance. Frequently, people are able to overcome such problems on their own; however, sometimes professional help may be necessary."

Such openness on a university campus is a far cry from the days when faculty members objected to voluntary physical examinations offered by a medical center's employee health service because they felt them to be an infringement on academic freedom—a freedom to die from preventable disease or to spread an identifiable infectious process to others.

The personnel who staff EAPs may be psychologists at the doctoral level, social case workers at the master's or doctoral level, or as indicated previously, consultant psychiatrists. The unit designation may be other than simply EAP. Variations course from worker health program to employee health advisory program, to members assistance program, to a variety of direct or euphemistic titles used in the private sector.

EMOTIONAL STRESS AT WORK

The literature on stress has enlarged beyond belief in recent years [15–18], partially because there has been increased interest in what is now an "acceptable" concept among workers and managers, because of heightened concern among occupational health professionals who were more recently trained, and unfortunately, because stress reduction, mediation, or management has become a highly marketable service, and in almost every jurisdiction one finds endless numbers of seminars, symposia, or conferences being offered at great tuition cost.

A few simple ideas regarding stress should be recalled that are of value in familiarizing or attuning workers to human needs. The way people or managers respond to stressors varies; no one works well with a total absence of stress, and no one works well with extreme, prolonged stress. Each person has a

*Located at 1800 North Kent Street, #907, Arlington, VA 22209.

middling level of stress that is optimal for him or her, a level at which that individual's productivity and feeling of satisfaction are greatest, people peak at different levels, for what is optimal stress for one person may be excessive for another, and boring for a third.

Another complication that muddies a discussion is that what is a stressor to one employee is a source of satisfaction to another. Common, readily recognized sources of stress may be *work environmental* or *human interactional* in origin. The first includes many of the physical aspects of the work setting such as heat, illumination, vibration, noise, or the demands on one's physical strength. While there are considerable individual differences in response to these environmental entities, nearly everyone does react to them as stressors.

In the category of the human interactional sources of stress, reactions are more diverse. Some workers thrive on frequent contacts with the public, for example, while other employees shrink from such tasks, preferring to work, and usually most efficiently, when isolated from such demands. Because of these wide personal variations, the most that a supervisor can do in a practical sense is to analyze carefully the demands of a job and to explore with employees their subjective characteristics in relation to the range of potential job situations. An analysis of stressors arising from interactional sources should consider the following measures:

Isolation–interaction: To what extent does the job entail working with others? What is the level of interaction with the public? With supervisory personnel? With peers and subordinates?

Autonomy–direction: How much independent action does the job require? Is there continual direction from supervisors? Are the decisions to be made spelled out in a usable book of directives, or is there a great demand for "playing it by ear"?

Originality–precedence: To what extent do things have to be done for the first time? Are the actions of the employee well laid out by tradition and past experience, or are a number of new, unique, creative responses needed?

Negative contacts–positive contacts: How many of the interpersonal contacts on the job are inherently negative? Does the employee have to handle primarily complaints or give people bad news? How much opportunity is there in the contacts with people to grant them their wishes?

External support–demand for self-sufficiency: How much help, encouragement, and support will be available on the job? Will the employee have "to go it alone" most of the time?

The categories given above do not cover all work situations, but they do represent some of the basic desiderata to be considered in job placement. Discussion with the job applicant, and later with the incumbent, will aid in determining the elements that are employed and the ones that are repellent, so that a more intelligent placement will result, with less opportunity for the job to be productive of stress [18a].

OBJECTIVES OF A COUNSELING PROGRAM

Whether the counseling function is OHS-based or is conducted by qualified staff of an EAP, certain goals should be stated and made known to supervisory personnel. The objectives follow.

PRIMARY OBJECTIVE

The primary objective is reduction of emotional ill health through early recognition of behavioral problems that impair job performance and the provision of counseling or treatment for those workers desirous of undertaking such care.

SECONDARY OBJECTIVES

To offer responsive, easily accessible, and readily obtained short-term counseling for the employees of the company, including crisis intervention for emergent states.

To offer counseling, education, referral, and follow-up support to employees experiencing problems related to alcohol and other chemical-substance usage.

To offer counseling, education, referral, and follow-up support to employees experiencing problems in living that affect their emotional health, behavior, or attitudes.

To provide an alternative to discipline for the supervisors of employees experiencing problems in job performance, attendance, or work attitudes.

To offer referral to community mental health resources for employees whose problems extend beyond the scope of short-term counseling.

To conduct educational and training sessions for supervisors, union representatives, and employees in substance use and abuse.

To conduct training sessions in communication for supervisors and managers.

To work closely with supervisors to assist them in confronting and motivating an employee toward recognition of a behavioral problem and acceptance of appropriate treatment.

To work with pertinent community organizations in the presentation of special programs, such as women's health, behavioral aspects of accidents, alcoholics anonymous, and gamblers anonymous.

SPECIFIC PROBLEMS

ALCOHOLISM

Although alcoholism is recognized as a problem requiring inclusion in any counseling program, the only way a rehabilitation effort will succeed is to have strong managerial support. Such assist, in turn, is obtained solely by having a written policy that spells out exactly the understanding of the organization regarding this particular illness and the mechanisms that are available for providing help to the problem drinker.

The document that is developed should include discussion of such topics as program objectives, the conceptual base (responsibility, recognition, referral, evaluation, counseling, and referral to outside resources), and personnel action (applicants for employment, employees, community agencies, and reports).

Such a written policy covers nearly every issue that may be presented by a problem drinker, with the appropriate personnel action to be taken. The written policy and "Procedure on Alcoholism" of a company with many decades of experience in support of a rehabilitation program (since 1947) offer several points worthy of iteration [19]. First, the procedure provides for

Early recognition of the employee with a drinking program—departmental responsibility.
Rehabilitation of the employee if feasible—medical department responsibility.
Establishment of a basis for termination of employment whenever rehabilitative efforts are rejected or prove fruitless—disability panel action.

The definition that is provided makes a good, working statement [19]: "Alcoholism is a chronic and relapsing but treatable illness, characterized by preoccupation with alcohol and loss of control over its consumption, which results in progressive emotional, physical and social impairment and deterioration in job performance and abnormal behavior."

The cost of alcoholism, beyond the health of the involved individual and family are given as follows [19]:

Lost production
Reduced efficiency
Absenteeism
Lost time on the job
Lateness
Overtime pay
Faulty decision-making
On-and-off-the-job accidents
Theft
Impaired morale of fellow workers
Friction among workers
Impaired consumer and public relations
Early retirement
Premature disability and death
Personnel turnover
Loss of skilled and valued employees
Cost of insurance programs, including life, health, and disability and property-damage insurances

The cost to industry of an alcoholic employee is estimated to reach as much as 25 percent of the individual's salary per year. Placement of the employee on the alcoholism procedure is the responsibility of the worker's department and not that of the medical department. If the condition reaches a stage that requires work restrictions, the employee's department will be notified by a medical department memorandum that the limitations are due to the "chronic sequelae of an avoidable illness." A comment addressed to supervisors is pointed [19]: "Supervisors who are indecisive about placing these employees on procedure for reasons of loyalty and concern, follow a tragically misguided and self-defeating practice. Initiating full cooperation in the rehabilitation process sooner, before the most serious symptoms develop, is a more constructive expression of concern, kinder to their families and far more beneficial to each employee and the department."

For the use of the supervisor, the procedure lists the signs and symptoms of alcoholism that are observable on the job and that should create a high index of suspicion that the individual's problem is related to alcoholism. Care must be exercised in determining that none of the observed symptoms or signs might be caused by a coexisting disease process, unrelated to the overusage of beverage alcohol.

As a further note of emphasis, it has been fairly common experience that in localities where highly specialized team-staffed alcoholism clinics do not exist—they usually are found in large metropolitan areas—the most effective referral is to Alcoholics Anonymous (AA). The person "who has been there" is much more cognizant of all the diversionary tricks used by the problem drinker and of the lies that, to the knowledgeable person, are so patently transparent. The changes seen in the job performance of a person who has "gone on the program (AA)" and has had a successful recovery are striking and thoroughly rewarding.*

Frequently personnel in an OHS would like to administer a screening questionnaire to employees tentatively believed to be problem drinkers. The first set of questions was developed at Johns Hopkins University Hospital and is shown in Figure 11-2.

Supportive counseling is mandatory for both the recovering and the recovered employee who is a problem drinker; in contradistinction to emergency care for other medical conditions presented by workers, alcoholism is not gone after two or three visits. The disease is perpetual, but the drinking can be controlled through the kind of help offered by a knowledgeable counselor and an understanding employer, provided the worker will accept the challenge.

DRUG ABUSE

In the early 1970s industry was faced with the problem of drug abuse, as addiction to both street drugs and prescribed medications (controlled substances) rose rapidly. Companies accustomed to identifying and referring their alcoholic employees for care were encountering new difficulties with the narcotic user. Problems of screening new employees—who were addicts and who were pushers?—evoked the issue of testing. Thefts and break-ins became commonplace, as costly habits required money. Turnover increased, adding to the overhead charges in industry. One company reported that in 1969 the cost of turnover resulting from the release of addicted employees was $75,000. Absenteeism increased, work performance became poorer, insurance rates were elevated, and security forces were added where none had been needed before. Taxes on business were greater because of the need for augmented police, social, medical, and mental health facilities to treat drug abusers [20]. Further, changes in physical plants were needed to augment security. Other concomitants of drug usage were accidents, property and equipment damage, disability claims, and damage to company images and morale.

At that time, some employees who had been retained were being cared for in methadone clinics, and alcoholism counselors began to see drug abusers as they were assisting the company's problem drinkers. With the growth of the EAPs through the United States, the programs were broadened in scope to include both the soft- and hard-drug abusers. But workers who are addicted are still on payrolls, and company premises are still the sites of dealing. Compounding the picture is the acceptance by younger workers of marijuana use as a way of life. Further, the habituation is not limited to any particular employee group, for blue-collar, white-collar, and professional workers are all involved.

Although the drug abuser is more difficult to detect than the chronic alcoholic, certain telltale signs can become apparent to the supervisor attuned to the problem. Rowan [21] gives these behavioral changes prominence:

Absenteeism and arriving late to work three times as often as fellow employees.
Frequent trips to the washroom.
Falling asleep on the job.
More carelessness, mistakes, and errors in judgment. A drug user is involved in accidents about 3½ times more often than other workers.
Abrupt changes in mood and overreaction to criticism.
Inconsistent work quality and lowered productivity.
Deterioration of personal appearance, along with increased complaints about problems at home.
Constant financial problems.

Referrals of suspected users should be made to the OHS so that appropriate assistance can be provided through the in-plant facility or by secondary referral to community drug-abuse treatment or rehabilitation facilities. While the frank user might be identified, a problem remains in the detection of the occult abuser. Also, as Bensinger [22], former Administrator of the Federal Drug Enforcement Administration, has put it, industry has a problem with the recreational drug user, including, as mentioned, the recreational user of marijuana. "The whole concept of drug use as recreational," he observed, "—even marijuana—flies in the face of medical reality. There is nothing recreational about the use of substances that affect motor coordination, slow brain synapses, im-

*A *National Directory of Alcoholism and Drug Addiction Treatment Program* is published annually by *Alcoholism,* a national magazine, 2100 North 105th Street, Seattle, WA 98133. In addition to treatment facilities, it lists AA central offices and intergroups, state authorities, national organizations, and self-help groups. Comprehensive data are provided for each treatment institution, including capacity, medical model used, detoxification, and the like.

If an employee is on travel status on business and contact with Alcoholics Anonymous is desired, a listing of AA chapters in the United States and in 30 foreign countries can be obtained. There are four directories—Eastern United States, Western United States, Canadian, and International—obtainable from General Service Board of Alcoholics Anonymous, 468 Park Avenue South, New York, NY 10016.

ARE YOU A PROBLEM DRINKER?

- Do you lose time from work due to drinking?
- Is drinking making your home life unhappy?
- Do you drink because you are shy with other people?
- Is drinking affecting your reputation?
- Have you ever felt remorse after drinking?
- Did you get in financial difficulties as a result of drinking?
- Do you turn to lower companions in an inferior environment when drinking?
- Does your drinking make you careless of your family's welfare?
- Has your ambition decreased since drinking?
- Do you crave a drink at a definite time daily?
- Do you want to drink the next morning?
- Does drinking cause you to have difficulty in sleeping?
- Has your efficiency decreased since drinking?
- Is drinking jeopardizing your job or business?
- Do you drink to escape from worries or troubles?
- Do you drink alone?
- Have you ever had a complete loss of memory as a result of drinking?
- Has your physician ever treated you for drinking?
- Do you drink to build up your self-confidence?
- Have you ever been to a hospital or institution on account of drinking?

— If you have answered YES to any 1 of the questions, there is a definitie warning, YOU MAY BE AN ALCOHOLIC.

— If you have answered YES to any 2 of the questions, the chances are YOU ARE AN ALCOHOLIC.

— If you have answered YES to any 3 of the questions, YOU DEFINITELY ARE AN ALCOHOLIC.

Don't confuse the issue by believing you have to be a bum on skid row or a habitual drunkard to be an alcoholic. Those places on skid row are just the future addresses of the alcoholics who are not wise enough to arrest their disease.

FIGURE 11-2. *Screening questionnaire developed at Johns Hopkins University Hospital for potential problem drinkers. (From* Guidance in Handling the Problem of Alcoholism. *Publication 157. Washington, DC: Post Office Department, 1970. Pp. 5–6. Modified version of "The Liquor Test," with 35 questions, as seen originally in R. V. Seliger, in collaboration with V. Cranford, and edited by H. S. Goodwin, Alcoholics are sick people: A guide for the bewildered and perplexed.* J Clin Psychopathol Psychother *6:145, 1944.)*

pair memory and peripheral vision, and slow time perception."

As emphasized with alcoholism rehabilitation programs, the motivating force for referral is impaired job performance, and every supervisor has that basic and supportable reason to request action with a suspected user.

There has been much discussion about urinalysis at the jobsite, conducted for the detection of a single drug or a series of substances present in the urine.* If urine testing is undertaken, certain legal questions may be raised. Was the specimen obtained truly from the individual being checked? There must be no break in the custody of the sample from donation to analyses, and appropriate labeling must identify the specimen at each point. Surveillance during production of the sample by the same individual who follows the specimen through to the end point may be necessary, particularly if there is a possibility that non-drug-containing urine may be substituted for the requested sample.

At one time, the issue of invasion of privacy was raised, but the author has always interpreted this test procedure as no different from any bioassay undertaken on prospective or current employees, be it a standard urinalysis or a blood chemistry battery. With on-site testing, extraordinary care must be used to determine that confidentiality is scrupulously maintained by personnel involved in the test protocol. Findings must be guarded, for erroneous reports are possible, and airing such information can be permanently damaging. Positivity in the test results cannot be used as a basis for discharge but should serve as the reason for referral to a counseling resource.

Counseling by a trained professional is the next step, and as indicated, the referral system is comparable to that for the problem drinker. If the testing proves positive for marijuana, and the employee indicates "recreational" use of the drug the previous weekend, counseling can be used to familiarize the worker with some of the undesirable side effects.

*The urine testing system, the Emit/ST Drug Detection System, is available from Ayva Company (a Syntex Company), P.O. Box 10058, Palo Alto, CA 94303-0847. Assays are available for the testing of amphetamines, barbiturates, benzodiazepines (Valium, Librium), cannabinoids (marijuana, hashish), cocaine metabolite, ethyl alcohol, methadone, methaqualone (Quaalude), opiates, (heroin, morphine, codeine), phencyclidine (PCP, "angel-dust"), and propoxyphene (Darvon). Anyone considering in-plant testing should consult the advisory from the Centers for Disease Control, Public Health Service. See Urine testing for detection of marijuana: An advisory. *MMWR* 32:469, 1983.

Before beginning a system of testing, employees must be informed, and one must have as a rational basis for the decision one of three reasons: (1) the employee holds a position of public trust; (2) the employee is involved in public safety; or (3) it is a business necessity that employees be fit for duty, unimpaired by drugs [23].

In keeping with the comment regarding prudent behavior concerning discharge, there is the strong likelihood that the employer would be accused of releasing a person with a handicap, an action contrary to the dicta of the Rehabilitation Act of 1973. As indicated before, all personnel action must have a sound footing in the demonstration of impaired job performance.

If a company decides to add a subprogram to its alcoholism rehabilitation policy, the contemplated addition should be reviewed with the unions in advance, in the "meet and confer" mode. Failure to obtain their support can prove disastrous. If the new policy is agreed on, it must be given wide publicity—posters, bulletin board notices, articles in house organs, training sessions for supervisors, tailgate conferences, and the like. The message, the declaration of policy, must be repeated periodically to freshen the memories of incumbents and to apprise newly hired workers.

In essence, a program involves

Declaration of a policy.
Training of supervisors.
Adding drug abuse to the EAP.
Establishment of an intramural system of referral.
Establishment of an extramural system of referral when needed.
Development of a system of discipline for workers failing to improve job performance by virtue of continuing chemical-substance abuse and failing to follow the offered rehabilitation program.

SMOKING

Industry is being used as the site for smoking-cessation programs for employed groups. That such disease preventive efforts are justified is given substance in an editorialized summation. Pollin [24] has pointed out that the 350,000 excess deaths per year that are attributable to cigarette smoking constitute more than all other drug- and alcohol-abuse deaths combined, seven times greater than the annual number of automobile-accident fatalities, more than 100-fold the deaths recorded from the acquired immunodeficiency syndrome, and more than all of the American military fatalities resulting from

World Wars I and II and the Vietnam War put together.*

Even though the percentage of adult Americans who smoke diminished from 37 percent in 1980 to 29 percent in 1983, of those persons who do smoke, 29 percent still use over one pack a day [25] and thus put themselves at continuing risk at the workplace, where there is an opportunity for interaction between smoking and their occupational exposure to a variety of physical and chemical agents. Again, even though tobacco use has declined over the years, the number of potentially hazardous jobsite exposures has increased. The modes of interaction are postulated by the National Institute for Occupational Safety and Health (NIOSH) as follows [26]:

Certain toxic agents in tobacco products and/or smoke may also occur in the workplace, thus increasing exposure to the agent.

Workplace chemicals may be transformed into harmful agents by smoking.

Tobacco products may serve as vectors by becoming contaminated with toxic agents found in the workplace, thus facilitating entry of the agent into the body by inhalation, ingestion, or skin absorption.

Smoking may contribute to an effect comparable to that which can result from exposure to toxic agents found in the workplace, thus causing an additive biologic effect.

Smoking may act synergistically with toxic agents found in the workplace to cause a much more profound effect than that anticipated simply from the separate influences of the occupational exposure and smoking.

Smoking may contribute to accidents in the workplace.

Additional interactions that have been hypothesized are between smoking and exposure to cadmium, chloromethyl ether, and beta-naphthylamine and other aromatic amines [26].

With these potential interactions of smoking and work exposures, it behooves the OHS staff to counsel all smokers seen, either for care or a surveillance procedure, in an effort to have them cease the risk habit. Also, the OHS can encourage smoking-cessation group-counseling courses or conferences, to be facilitated by a physician, a nurse, or a representative from a community agency (American Cancer Society, American Heart Association, or American Lung Association) skilled in this kind of group leadership. The fees are usually low when an outsider comes to the plant. The advantage of the group method is that, like all support-group efforts, the participants can share problems, successes, and encouragement [27]. Whether the worker selects to go it alone or attempt cessation with a group, the OHS should provide supportive counseling while the smoker is attempting to control the injurious addiction.

While the matter of declaring a company policy of no smoking at the workplace is a sensitive issue currently, it seems that with the increase in municipal mandates, in the near future employers may have to follow the wishes of nonsmokers and local ordinances. Although this kind of control or total proscription is a matter for both the legislative and judicial branches of government to decide [28], the OHS can support efforts to eliminate smoking from the workplace.

OVEREATING

In some individuals, environmental stressors may lead to weight gain of some proportion. The modality of self-help groups has been applied in an effort to have the members lose weight through a support system comparable to that used in smoking cessation, gamblers anonymous, and the like.

The group method was used by the author with first-year nursing students at a university medical center, where it was found that the stressors present in the beginning of professional training both exacerbated latent acne and led to nearly a universal weight gain. The same technique may be used in industry, with leadership provided by an interested OHS staff member with the assistance of a nutritionist.

A variation of the usual group format was reported by Brownell and coworkers [29], in which weight-loss efforts at the workplace were enhanced by establishing competitive efforts (1) among three banks and (2) between employee teams selected at random or between divisions of a single company. The result was successful, for both employees and managerial personnel reported positive changes in morale and employee-management relations, and the competition was considered important to the success of the program. The cost-effectiveness ratio ($2.93

*Other estimates of the costs of smoking are the following: cigarette smoking will results in approximately $65 billion in lost productivity and health care costs, roughly amounting to $2.17 per package purchased according to the Congressional Office of Technology Assessment (OTA says smoking costs $65 billion per year. *Nation's Health* 15:3, Oct–Nov, 1985); and the number of deaths caused or accelerated by smoking cigarettes is roughly equivalent to the number of fatalities that would be associated with the crash each day of three fully loaded 747 jumbo jets (Dinman, B. D., in review of Urquhart, J., and Heilmann, K. *Risk Watch: The Odds of Life*. New York: Facts on File, 1984. *JAMA* 254:1378, 1985).

per 1-percent reduction in percentage overweight) was considered by the investigators as "the best yet reported."

As with the other substance abuses, a creative OHS will initiate or nurture efforts of this type in the company setting. The self-help group is Overeaters Anonymous,* and it utilizes the same principles in goal attainment as Alcoholics or Gamblers Anonymous.

COMPULSIVE GAMBLING

Another behavioral disorder that will impair job performance and will require attention of an OHS is compulsive gambling. The definitions that are most descriptive of this addictive problem come from Gamblers Anonymous (GA), a fellowship that is closely patterned after AA, and are offered in the question-answer format [30]:

What definition of gambling is generally accepted by the members of Gamblers Anonymous?

Gambling is defined as follows: For the compulsive gambler, any betting or wagering whether for money or not, no matter how slight or insignificant (where the outcome is uncertain or depends upon chance or skill), constitutes gambling.

What is compulsive gambling?

. . . compulsive gambling is an emotional illness, progressive in its nature, which can never be cured, but which can be arrested.

The compulsive gambler is a person who is dominated by an irresistible urge to gamble. Coupled with this is the obsessive idea that a way will be found not only to control the gambling but to "make it pay" and enjoy it besides. We compulsive gamblers often express a desire to quit forever, but inevitably we find ourselves back in action. For most of us there are days, weeks, or even months when we are certain that we have gained control. These intervals invariably are followed by long periods of all-out, uncontrolled gambling during which a process of deterioration in almost every department of our lives becomes evident. This deterioration is most acute in the relationships with our wives and husbands, friends, relatives and employers.

The structure of the GA recovery program, as indicated, is similar to the twelve-step program and the twelve traditions of AA, and referral can be made to a representative, listed in the local telephone directory under "Gamblers Anonymous." As it is estimated that there are about 6 million compulsive gamblers in the United States, it is likely that at some time either an employee or an employee's relative will be brought to the attention of the OHS.

ABSENTEEISM

A vexatious problem to all industrial managers is that of repetitive absenteeism from work of certain employees. As the cause of such episodes is alleged to be illness, the OHS becomes involves, although the problem of so-called illness-absence rarely involves the true acquisition of disease. Over a decade ago, Teeling-Smith [31], then Director of the British Office of Health Economics, said, "The real cause for concern is the impression that the pattern of sickness absence seems increasingly to reflect a pattern of job dissatisfaction, frustration and anxiety." He added that the process of becoming ill is more and more "the consequence of a social decision rather than the result of specific medical events."

For those practitioners in industry who have been the recipients of everything from simple raillery to caustic comments from their anguished managers, it has been difficult to explain that it is not possible to prevent the so-called illness-absence when it really has little to do with illness, but represents deficits in work attitude. Again, to refer to the British observers, this statement seems to state the case with clarity [32]: "Because of the personal, social, economic and other factors involved, 'absence from work *attributed to sickness*' [emphasis added] is a more accurate description of the phenomenon commonly called 'sickness absence': 'sickness absence' implies that absence is due to and caused by illness alone."

How much absenteeism is there? We seem to accept a range of 2 to 4 percent as inevitable and immutable, and industry carries an additional payroll burden to compensate for those workers who decide not to report in during a particular period. It is estimated, therefore, that there is an excess of 20 to 40 workers needed for every 1,000 on the payroll.* What is known from research that has been conducted? Before responding, a few definitions might be useful [33]:

Absence	The failure of an employee to report during the hours normally scheduled for work.

*The World Service Office of Overeaters Anonymous is located at 2190 West 190th Street, Torrance, California 90504, and local groups are listed in telephone directories.

*Plummer and Hinkle in a classic study of absenteeism (Plummer, N., and Hinkle, L. E., Jr. Sickness absenteeism. *AMA Arch Ind Health* 11:218, 1955) reported that of the total labor force of 75,000 New York Telephone Company employees, there is an average of 3,000 absentees. Counting all direct costs, this absence carried a price tag of $10 million per year, in 1955 dollars. See also, by the same authors, Medical significance of sickness and absence in an industrial population. *Ann Intern Med* 39:103, 1953.

Tardiness	The occurrence when an employee is not on the job at the time work is normally scheduled to begin.
Excused absence	Occurs when an employee notifies the immediate supervisor of an upcoming absence for an acceptable reason such as illness, personal or family emergency, or the like. The supervisor must give the employee permission to be absent—and note such permission in writing—for the absence to be considered "excused." Rare exceptions are permitted in cases where employee notification is lacking.
Unexcused absence	Occurs when an employee fails to notify the immediate supervisor of absence prior to the normally scheduled work time, or when an employee decides to be absent when supervisory permission was not granted when requested in advance.

The concept of "illness-absence" is one of administrators, economists, sociologists, psychologists, and statisticians who are not necessarily close to medical bases of operation, as pointed out by Adelstein [34]. The problem is multifactorial in causation, with elements of social, economic, and cultural concern and of morale.

In any review, one looks at absenteeism as unplanned lost work time, including tardiness and wandering. Some of the conclusions are the following:

There is less absence among the handicapped. Thousands of workers with severe, impairing physical or functional residua lose no time at all.

A concerned, dedicated worker does not want to be absent. Offered by Darrow [35] as a hypothesis for research is the following: Overachievers (those persons with income superior to education) are too busy to get sick and thus deny illness, but underachievers (those persons with education superior to income) use the secondary gains of frequent illnesses to excuse their shortcomings.

Absences are fewer in December and higher in January: Do workers wish to attend in-plant parties? Do they want all available earnings for Christmas?

More absences are seen among persons manifesting stress responses, such as peptic ulceration, atopic states, essential hypertension, and the like, than among workers with less fragile personalities who are able to cope with the stressors of the work and home environments.

Employees under age 30, while the healthiest, have the greatest amount of absenteeism [36]. Have they yet to establish a work ethic, or do they believe that these early jobs are merely stepping stones where performance does not matter?

Those workers engaged in a greater amount of overtime have much less absenteeism.

Absenteeism seems to be related more to perceived health problems—those disorders tied to social or emotional health—than to objective health problems involving pain or limitations in physical mobility.

Cultural factors dictate work practices, as seen among certain employees who receive a paycheck, absent themselves until the money runs out, and then return to work for another paycheck. In the days when the utilization of the hard-core unemployed was of governmental concern, a few young members of certain ethnic communities would be punished for leaving gang membership to go to the outside world for work.

The greater the level of employment, the greater the absenteeism; the larger the work group, the higher number of absences; and employees reporting to women supervisors have 30 percent more absenteeism [36].

Work no longer is of a central value in society, for other activities offer greater creative outlets. There is insufficient responsibility in most jobs, and many workers lose their initial level of motivation.* Further, absenteeism can be contagious in an individual work unit where leadership is lax.

"Patients" manipulate their physicians to grant them certificates justifying their absence; in some cases, the workers were never seen by their practitioners, the notes† being issued by clerical or nursing personnel. In most instances, these statements from the physician are meaningless.

There are great inconsistencies in the periods of convalescence as perceived by the treating physician. Frequently the patient will be asked, "When do you want to return to work?" A post-hemorrhoidectomy period of recovery may range from 2 to 8 weeks, and the time elapsing after repair of an inguinal hernia could vary from 51 to 70 days before a return to work [37]. Low-status workers expect, in advance, greater exemption from work when ill,

*As John Ruskin put it, "Labor without joy is base." (Ruskin, J. *Time and Tide*. London: George Allen & Unwin, 1867. P. 29.)

†Called the $1-letter during World War II.

or as termed by one observer, they demonstrate "anticipatory incapacity."*

Keeping in mind that there is a continuum here, in that "high absenteeism (lateness and absence) appears to be an earlier sign, and turnover (quitting *and* being fired) the dying stage of a long and lively process of leaving" [38], what can be done to break the pattern?

There is absence legitimately caused by illness and attendant medical or surgical care. As just indicated, the periods of convalescence vary considerably, and few organizations have attempted to establish standards. The Cleveland Clinic Foundation of Cleveland, Ohio has attempted a listing of normal convalescence periods (disability) following certain medical disorders and surgical procedures in its "Disability Guide." Through the courtesy of Jody Moss, Ombudsman for the Foundation, a few examples follow:

Ureterostomy, unilateral	4–6 weeks
Shaft of humerus fracture, hanging cast	12–16 weeks
Knee arthroplasty	16–20 weeks
Removal of foreign body from surface of cornea	3 days
Hepatitis, acute	2–4 weeks
Postgastrectomy syndrome	1–3 weeks
Toe amputation	1 month
Dermabrasion	3 weeks
Hemorrhoidectomy	14 days
Cholecystectomy	6 weeks

With such a guide, which is conservative, judgments can be reached regarding excessive amounts of time taken following substantial illness.

Reporting and Recording

There must be accuracy in the data regarding withdrawal from work. In a previous communication [39], an effort was made to dissect out the fallacies inherent in the collection of absence information.

*The issue of unnecessarily prolonged periods of recuperation is given further testimony by Brandaleone who wrote that an employee who had a circumcision done was given 4 weeks off postoperatively, and another man was considered disabled for 4 months by his physician "because of some mild angina." When the electrocardiogram was requested for review, the company's medical director was told that it showed little change from normal. When the practitioner was asked why the employee did not return to his sedentary job, he replied, "If he had to go back to his own business, he would have been back three months ago, but since this is not his own business, he is taking his time off." (Brandaleone, H. Personal communication to the author, March 11, 1981.)

Most categorizations of absence attributed to illness list respiratory disease and gastrointestinal illness as the lead and secondary nosologic causes of the nonappearance at work. It is believed that the popularization of "a cold" or "flu" allows a socially acceptable reason for not coming to work. How many workers tell their foremen, "I was out yesterday because of gonorrheal urethritis," or "My herpes was bad." "Flu" and "stomach flu" usually cause no further questioning.

There is faulty communication. The reporting of an absence may be mandated as a call to the supervisor, the medical service, the department head, or the insurance section. The message may be telephoned by the ailing worker's spouse, child, or neighbor, each giving a personalized slant to the true condition. Further, when received, there can be additional interpretation or modification, depending on the recipient's understanding of the message.

Even with certification by a physician, the true diagnosis may be simulated, for example, "gastrointestinal upset" for acute alcoholism and detoxification. The certificate may offer only a statement that "Mr. Jones has been under my care from ______ to ______," or "Mr. Jones is fit to return to work." These notes maintain the confidentiality of the care situation but lend no substance to the absence recording. On some occasions when certified reasons for absence have read "anemia," or "low blood pressure," OHS personnel have been unable to confirm such findings. Frequently employees visit therapists other than physicians, and statements made by the less scrupulous of these "healers" furnish nothing knowledgeable regarding the worker's absence.

The orientation of physicians to stressor-induced illness varies, and one practitioner may pin a physical diagnosis label on the disorder while another, more acutely sensitized to the patient's illness patterns, will identify a psychogenic condition, and so the data are skewed.

Company sick-leave policies often do not cover preventive medicine procedures such as periodic examinations, diagnostic tests, or even immunizations, so the treating physician will provide an illness designation that will allow the worker to have sick leave or sick pay coverage. Obviously, there was no illness-absence, as such.

Sick-leave policy is riddled with whimsical discrepancies so that an hourly worker's illness might be investigated at some length, while a high-level manager's unsubstantiated statement will be accepted without question.

Even in those companies where clearance through the OHS is mandatory after an illness, the professional personnel are seeing the worker after the fact, and no tell-tale residual may be present as evidence of recent disease. The resulting statistic may be strictly a surmise, gathered from a late inspection and the patient's history.

Another factor that confounds the recording is the job to which an individual is returning. A clerk will be able to return to the job within a few days after a certain illness or injury, while with the same disorder, an underground miner would have to defer reporting for work until several days later. Yet, the condition causing the absence was identical in the two employees.

As indicated previously, one surgeon, overly cautious, will keep a postoperative patient in a convalescent state for 6 weeks, while another will allow a patient to return to work in half the time. Again, the classification of the causative disorder is the same.

Many companies make no provision for a worker to carry out urgent personal business—to see an attorney, to have a conference with her child's teacher, to visit a bank. The result is that the time is taken and the loss is attributed to a fabricated illness.

Lastly, there should be a standardized method of recording absences. Any period of absence alleged to be illness in origin should be reported and recorded, whether it is of a half-day's duration or 8 days. Some organizations do not record 1 to 3 days absence, believing that they are inconsequential for it is only the severe illnesses that are costly. It is essential that these brief absences be made a matter of record, for it is among these short withdrawals from work that one finds the repeaters, the employees in greatest need of counseling.

A Solution for Alleged Illness-Absence

Several steps can be taken in which the OHS can be helpful, but reversal of the problem rests with managerial rectification and control. The OHS should not be made the scapegoat for deficits in company administration or individual supervision that end as apparent medically related causes for failure to come to work.

1. There must be some sense of worth put into a job that is credible, that can be conveyed to the worker in full sincerity. Such action may require joint consultation, job enrichment, praise, or a general concern with and genuine elevation of morale.
2. Get at the cause of the absence so that one determines the true reason for withdrawal rather than the proffered, rarely questioned illness rationale. Such action requires confrontation, a difficult undertaking for many supervisors. This face-to-face review includes query of the Monday absentees immediately on their return to work. As Gerson and Skipper [40] expressed it interestingly, "Absenteeism 'on the line' [in the automobile industry] is so high on Mondays and Fridays that informed people sometimes refuse to buy a new car coming off the assembly line on those days of the week due to the higher number of imperfections in production."
3. Counsel employees whose lifestyle causes temporary departures from scheduled work time, to include direct discussion with and referral of workers whose problem drinking or smoking patterns cause an excessive number of absences. While only 28 percent of nonsmokers experience respiratory disease absence, 40 percent of smokers are away from comparable illnesses. Further, smoking magnifies the effects of occupational exposures to inhalable particulates. This type of counseling includes discussion with abusers of other chemical substances.
4. Encourage supervisors to review absence recidivists with the medical director early, while there is a possibility of reversing the behavioral pattern. Physical fitness determinations can be requested by supervisors in cases of excessive absenteeism, and usually no *medical* reason for the recurrences will be identified. The examination situation provides an opportunity to initiate discussions—with the employee *and* the supervisor—regarding the faulty attendance habit. If the supervisor receives certificates from the treating physician, these notes should be shared with the OHS.
5. Periodically at staff meetings, orient supervisors to the nature of the problem of absenteeism, and present disguised case examples so they become aware of the sociopsychologic reasons for repetitive absences.
6. Identify special problems to determine if solutions are possible, such as that of certain working women with a demanding role at home in addition to their full-time jobs or workers who wish to change jobs, but their accrued benefits preclude their leaving.
7. Endeavor to shorten prolonged periods of convalescence by temporarily allowing return to work in less physically demanding jobs.
8. Work closely with union representatives in connection with employees known both to them and to the company as poor attenders at work.
9. Redo the orientation programs for new employees so that the emphasis is less on all of the wonderful benefits the company grants a worker, and more on the expectations regarding workload,

attendance, promptness, job performance, and the like. The medical director should attend and participate in the presentations [41,42].
10. Develop detailed medical and absence histories so that there might be some prediction of absence recidivists by virtue of the determination of trends.*
11. Prior to elective surgery, have the treating physician inform the patient and medical director of anticipated period of convalescence prior to return to work.
12. Correct, insofar as possible, errors in the reporting system so that accurate information can be used as a basis for epidemiologic studies of absenteeism.
13. Make contact with the treating physician whenever suspect certifications of illness-absence are received relating to either questionable periods of professional care or the use of euphemistic diagnoses. Particularly to be verified are certificates from other "healers."
14. Formalize the personnel procedure of having any employee who is ill or injured report to the OHS before going home. Obviously, workers experiencing true trauma emergencies will not be detained in the same manner.
15. Train supervisors in identifying behavioral causes of impaired performance in a way similar to that outlined for chronic alcoholism.
16. Interview and counsel in the OHS or refer any worker who is absent allegedly owing to illness two or more times in a single month.
17. Apprise managers each month of the absenteeism in their departments and of the amount of time lost, by various characteristics, such as sex, age, marital status, shift, job title, diagnostic category, number of absences, days lost, by number and day of week, size of work group, gender of group supervisor, and rates derived from the above (frequency and severity).

The rates (in 17, above) to be developed are the following:

Frequency rate (FR) reveals the absences per employee per unit of time. The number of absences (also referred to as episodes or spells) often is multiplied by 1,000 or 1,000,000 in the maintenance of statistics.

$$FR = \frac{\text{number of absences}}{\text{average number of employees}} \text{ per unit of time}$$

Severity rate (SR) reveals the time lost per absence.

$$SR = \frac{\text{number of days of absence}}{\text{number of absences}}$$

Disability rate (DR) indicates the units of time lost per employee per unit of time.

$$DR = \frac{\text{days of absence}}{\text{number of employees}} \text{ per unit of time}$$

Proportion (or percent) of absence (P) indicates the amount of time lost per amount of time scheduled. Absence is multiplied by 100, as a percentage is sought. A rate of 3 percent or less is "generally considered excellent, and it has been calculated that 70 percent of this, or 2.1 percent, usually is sick absence" [43].

$$P = \frac{\text{number of days of absence} \times 100}{\text{number of days scheduled}}$$

The procedures given above represent the participation of the OHS in an absence control program. Omitted are the disciplinary steps that may be taken, which are personnel actions to be exercised by the worker's department. Primarily, having people come to work regularly and on time is the task of top managers. When they formulate and support a strong program of control, absenteeism drops. Whey they relax, the absence rates creep slowly back. The matter of absenteeism as an issue of behavior is closed on the gloomy note of Browning [44], who wrote, "We should not expect to make jobs into situations for self-expression or self-fulfillment: jobs should be recognized and accepted as primarily opportunities to earn a living. If they also afford many people a way to express and fulfill themselves constructively, so much the better, but let's keep the realities in clear sight."

MASS PSYCHOGENIC ILLNESS

The occurrence of mass hysteria has been reported in the last several years in both school [45–47] and industrial populations. As pointed out by Levine [48], the group disorder is one in which affected individ-

*For a record form for the notation of incidental sickness absence, see Bews [36]. Also, Froggatt, cited in Absence from work (editorial), *Br Med J* 2:383, 1970, suggests that (1) short-term absences may simply be the overt expression of a desire to work discontinuously, and (2) the pattern of 1-day and 2-day absences in individuals is immutable, and that this is probably true when it has been established for many years.

uals identify with a model of hysterical behavior by exaggerating the significance of similar feelings within themselves. Characteristic of such manifestations, he continues, has been the preponderance of affected women, hyperventilation, emesis, abdominal cramps, paralysis, tremors, convulsions, abnormal movements, chorea, analgesia, pain, paresthesias, contractures, echolalia, echopraxia, globus, laryngismus, cough, laughing, crying, running, dancing, rash, and pruritus.

In the industrial setting, several outbreaks of mass psychogenic illness have been encountered [49–52], and two episodes have been reported from abroad, one in Singapore [53] and the other in Israel [54]. While in one writing an effort was made to direct attention to the possibility of low-level industrial intoxication [51], the essence of most of the reports is that there should be a complete investigation of the psychosocial, ergonomic, and organizational stressors at the worksite where the mass illness has occurred.

While these group affections are not to be belabored, they are mentioned because they require empathic inquiry and understanding of the etiologic factors. The author had experience with at least four such episodes wherein groups of workers—in all instances women—reported illness, primarily pruritus. The first episode dates to World War II when the blue pigment used in an early document-duplicating method allegedly "poisoned" the workers, who offered the skin stain as evidence of the untoward effect. Much investigative effort went into the study to disprove the presence of any environmental toxicants. The working conditions in that unit were those of hastily converted offices on a pier on the San Francisco waterfront, devoted exclusively to the shipment of materiel to the Pacific theater.

The next two events were encountered about 1970 when a group complained of the presence of "paper mites," allegedly encountered in the supply area of a large office operation. Again, studies revealed nothing positive to explain the pruritus of the arms, on which there were no visible lesions. An area spray with an insecticide eliminated the complaints. Within a year, the complaints recurred, and on this occasion a placebo spray was used and the symptoms subsided. The office was one of a municipal government where individual personalities mattered little, and first-line management was unfeeling.

About 1976, a variation of the theme was played, only this time the site of complaint was a women's restroom with the women, some 12 of them, stating that they had acquired either pudendal or vaginal irritation or infection from the toilets. Investigation by knowledgeable sanitarians disclosed no incriminating agents, although they did comment that the facilities were old and esthetically unappealing. All the workers were invited to come to the OHS for examination by a woman physician. The physical evaluation disclosed no lesions, no signs of inflammatory response, no evidence of infection or infestation. A repainting of the entire restroom put the problem to rest.

Emphasis is given this mass response to stressors, for these episodes require sympathetic and compassionate handling, with no derogation of the complaints. Somewhere, the etiologic factors will be found, usually in insensitive supervisors, most commonly male. As in the Israeli "mysterious illness" [54], there might be a triggering odor, not toxic, but suggestive of toxicity, and it would be wise to eliminate such a source early if it can be identified. Immediate concerned action is warranted, particularly in highly litigious jurisdictions.

EMOTIONAL ILLNESS AND WORKERS' COMPENSATION

Since the theory of cumulative injury began to attain reality in workers' compensation claims, the concept of "stress" as a job-generated injury has become popular.* In the California Labor Code, for example, such an injury is defined as "repetitive mentally or physically traumatic activities extending over a period of time, the combined effect of which causes any disability or need for medical treatment." The maximum of tension was described by E. Grey Dimond, M.D., in an essay directed to eminent physician members of the coronary club [55]:

> Endless commitments to speak, to serve on committees, to be on planes after a full day's work in an effort to make the next commitment. Days, weeks, years, and finally complete careers of attempting to handle editorships, manuscripts, research protocols, patient appointments, lecture dates, ward rounds, the press, transcontinental and intercontinental travel, presiding on panels, attempting wit and wisdom at the grand banquet at the end of a long, long day, doubling the tempo when one actually has a free day in an effort to catch up on the correspondence, accepting an unnecessary dinner date because you can't always say no and because sometimes you have to admit you have a wife and family, leaving one meeting late to get to another across town and feeling tension build up as you get slowed by traffic, consciously telling yourself to ease up, take a deep breath, relax, be careful . . . a bona fide sense of oppression as your desk accumulates unan-

*The so-called "stress injuries" rose in California from 1,282 in 1980, 0.3 percent of the total, to 4,236 in 1984, or 1.1 percent of the total (California Workers' Compensation Institute, *Bulletin,* No. 85-7, Sept 4, 1985).

swered problems, your briefcase bulges, a second briefcase bulges, your study at home bulges. No time to even write checks and balance your books, an uneasy awareness that you are not really making much money doing all this and that you really do need to think about the family and about your own future . . . but right now there is today, there goes the phone—I'm behind on my appointments—I'm speaking at Grand Rounds—I'm due in Washington tonight and haven't even packed—don't worry, I'll take care of those other things such as family and self later when I have more time. Right now I'm healthy, I'm obligate, I don't have time, my commitments won't let me slow down.

But the lifestyle described was that of many contributing professionals. How comparable are the stress, the tension, the fatigue felt by workers in dull, dreary blue- or white-collar jobs? In *McDonald* v. *International Paper Co.* [56], the Supreme Court of Louisiana held that, "It is well established that an unexpected and catastrophic effect upon an employee, such as death by heart attack, produced by extraordinary mental or emotional work-related stress, is compensable." The applicant, in this case, for several weeks before his death, had been subjected to "extraordinary emotional and mental stress" associated with the impending closure of his mill, the possible termination of his job, and the increased difficulty of doing his job because of shorthanded, dilatory work crews and poorly maintained equipment. The myocardial infarction was deemed employment-related.

In an earlier case [57] the Missouri Court of Appeals held that workers' compensation benefits were due a claimant injured on the job. Although the original claim covered orthopedic injuries, there was a later amendment that alleged that, as a result of the fall, the applicant had suffered a "depressive reaction." The court indicated that a depressive reaction was a condition involving the mind, that "mind" and "psyche" were synonymous, and that the evidence clearly supported the conclusion that the claimant had suffered a depressive reaction.

In a case where physical and verbal harassment was experienced by a woman worker at the hands of her supervisor, and which occurred concurrently with marital difficulties at home, the applicant had benefits reinstated by the West Virginia Supreme Court of Appeals for the claimed "depressive neurosis." The court held that the claim was compensable, as it met three coexisting elements: it was a personal injury; the injury was received in the course of employment; and the injury resulted from that employment. The court added that "one does not have to be struck by a truck or deluged by a slate fall to receive a compensable injury within the contemplation of our compensation law" [58].

That stress can be experienced at all levels was given evidence in 1975 when Stanley K. Hathaway, who had been sworn in as Secretary of the Interior 6 weeks before, was hospitalized for "moderate depression brought about by physical exhaustion and fatigue," after suffering "an emotional collapse" from the strain of the fight to win Senate confirmation of his nomination and from the pressures of the Cabinet post [59].

Finally, even a suicide led to an award of death benefits by the Michigan Court of Appeals [60], when it determined that the claimant's employment, following demotion from a high-level supervisory position to a simple desk job, aggravated, accelerated, or combined with his state of mind ultimately to result in his suicide.

These cases are cited because they point up the increasing leniency of the workers' compensation judges and referees—and the jurists, on appeal—in granting awards to workers developing emotional disturbances. The need here is for early recognition of stress responses and either to alleviate the source of stress inherent in the job situation or to attempt stress reduction in the employee. Certain recommendations have been offered either to lower the effect of stressors at work or to eliminate them from the job setting [61]:

Match the person's capabilities to the job requirements. By matching, boredom and frustration, both stress producers, can be avoided.

Provide worker participation, as much as possible, in determining how a job should be performed.

Set up machine-paced jobs so that the operator is not altogether a captive of the machine. If such a move is infeasible, arrange the process so that the operator is not cut off from social interaction with fellow workers.

Avoid rotating shifts, to lower the number of injuries and illnesses sustained by workers on such shifts.

Provide workers with clear-cut responsibilities, thus avoiding the stressor of role ambiguity.

Although the above recommendations are the indicated actions for management, the attention of operating heads can be directed to these potential changes when such process deficits have led to symptoms presented to OHS personnel. The steps indicated in the care of workers manifesting a stress response are, as noted previously, recognition of the situational reaction, reassurance, and either counseling or referral for counseling. If there is capability in the EAP to work with such stressed individuals, it is incumbent on those counselors to apprise managers of the effects of the current operations and the workers' compensation claim and litigation potential.

THE "WORKAHOLIC" AND "BURNOUT"

This new word "workaholic" was added to the pseudobehavioral vocabulary to describe individuals who work more intensively and longer than they must but, on occasion, may exceed their ability to recover when symptoms develop.*

The characteristics of such a worker, as expressed by Mow [62], follow:

You work more than the average person, sometimes putting in 50 to 60 hours a week. You're at work early, leave late, and when you leave, it's often to go to dinner with business associates, and you usually bring work home to do in the evening.
As your hours tend to be irregular and you are often traveling on business, you seldom have a chance to see your family and never seem to have the time for family activities or vacations.
You seldom take more than one week's vacation a year—if that much—because you get "antsy" with nothing to do.
What few vacations you do take are typically active like your job—backpacking, tennis, sailing, sightseeing.
You tend to travel a great deal and may have been all over the world, but most of your trips are short and business-oriented.
You have few hobbies and, although you probably read a great deal, your reading is usually related to your work.
You can't imagine being retired. Since you have no strong outside interests, you may feel you will be literally bored sick with no work to do.
You are probably well educated, in a professional or managerial job, and you have a strong sense of responsibility to your work and to your family in your role as provider.
Because you are probably in a financially comfortable and socially prominent position, you no longer need to work for money or recognition, but continue to work just as hard or harder than you used to because you enjoy your work and get the greatest satisfaction out of a job well done.
You are intellectually curious and would probably enjoy a chance to "clear your brain" and explore other interests or do more reflective work, but your job seems to monopolize your time and energy even when you would like to get away from it for a while.

Such persons, usually on the managerial ladder, should be seen periodically by the OHS, and if there are indications for intervention—impending impairment of health, physical or emotional—counseling or referral should be initiated.

Similarly entered into the professional lexicon has been "burnout," a medical syndrome . . . characterized by exhaustion on all levels—physical, emotional, and attitudinal" [63]. When this state is reached, one may encounter impaired performance, fatigue, insomnia, depression, increased susceptibility to somatic illness, alcoholism, chemical-substance addiction, and even suicide. It has been most commonly associated with the professions—health care personnel, administrators and managers, judges, attorneys, rehabilitationists, educators, and social workers [64–77].

Some generalizations have been offered in coping with the stressfulness of striving. Moss [77] has suggested the following as personal controls:

Maintaining personal fitness.
Increasing respect for leisure time.
Reducing workload.
Not taking on too much work or behaving as if one had unlimited capacity to cope with stressors.
Cognitive coping—analyzing stress-producing situations to decide what is worth worrying about and what is not.
Delegating workload.
Establishing daily goals and setting priorities to reach most important objectives.

More must be done, external to the individual, for like the workaholic, the individual headed for burnout will not alter his lifestyle. Kind, pursuasive intervention by perceptive occupational health personnel may shed some light on the person headed for physical or emotional destruction.

BEREAVEMENT

Parkes has written extensively on the stress response resulting from the loss of a spouse or close relative [77–79]. As noted in the frequently cited Holmes and Rahe scale of social readjustment [81], death of spouse ranks number 1 and death of a close family member number 5 among 43 life events that demand some adaptive or coping behavior. Parkes and coworkers [78] demonstrated that the death of a spouse is frequently followed extremely soon by the demise of the surviving mate. In some studies, intervening counseling was brought to play to counteract or prevent both the resulting morbidity and mortality following a loss.

While with the County of Los Angeles, the author, in association with Joe Yamamoto, M.D., trained the

*The term "workaholic" was coined by Oates, a minister and psychologist, in *Confessions of a Workaholic,* New York: World Publishing, 1971.

nursing members of the OHS in bereavement counseling of employees. Although the data are unpublished, it was the consensus that much of the usual grief-period morbidity was lessened. The surviving spouse had an opportunity to share or express the grief or, in rare cases, to explode with expressions of joy that he or she had finally been freed from an intolerable situation.

It is suggested that this kind of counseling can be undertaken by the OHS, particularly by those physicians or nurses who are most interested in the human condition and who can confront or comfort grieving workers at their greatest time of need—immediately.

REPRISE

If, by now, it is still felt that emotional difficulties do not arise in one's organization, note two situations with which the author had personal contact. In the first, a large institution, the following stress responses were encountered among executive personnel in different departments within a 2-week period:

An administrative department
- Executive A—cerebrovascular accident
- Executive B—memory loss and lack of ability to concentrate
- Executive C—testy, short-tempered, "no longer any fun on the job"
- Executive D—conversion reaction, twice, simulating cerebrovascular accident with hemiparesis
- Executive E—excessive weight gain
- Executive F—irreversible "acute" hypertension

A law-enforcement department
- Executive G—extreme anxiety and fear of impending myocardial infarction

A technical department
- Executive H—recurrent anxiety, preparation for retirement

A service department
- Executive I—"pressure," unrelenting

A legal department
- Executive J—constant anxiety
- Executive K—anxiety, tension, cardiac surgery, retirement

In the second organization, with a completely different work orientation, the head of a large department, upon which nearly all of the mission of the total installation depended, reported to the medical director one day that he could not sleep and listed his current concerns:

A $2.5 million lawsuit filed against him by a grieving employee.
Murder of one of his employees by a hitchhiker.
Suicide of a third employee.
Surgery undergone by a valued supervisor for a protruded intervertebral disk.
Cardiac valve replacement in another supervisor.
Applications submitted for disability retirement by three good, but burned-out, supervisors.
Two grievances filed against him for alleged unfair labor practices.
Two discrimination complaints filed against him with the equal opportunity authority.
One employee recovering from street-drug overdosage.
His own old back injury "acting up."
Personnel action being initiated to release an employee manifesting near-psychotic behavior.

He was given some medication to allow sleep at night. The remaining problems he thought he could handle. He was known as a concerned, dedicated executive, fair in his administration and his decisions. What would the box score be were he uncaring, impersonal, and ruthless?

By way of closure, one recalls the highly germane comment of Reiser in a review of a book of essays for George Rosen, the late, distinguished medical historian [82]. He closes his critique in this way:

> We maintain an uneasy relation with our current knowledge of the social causes of illness. We usually give them lip service while placing most of our therapeutic apples in the biologic basket. Ultimately, we hope that complete biologic solutions to the problems of illness will eliminate the need to confront personal habit, work, custom, government, and the rest of the tangled skein representing the social aspects of life in disease.
>
> Thus we are far from achieving the integration of social and biologic factors that George Rosen wrote of and hoped for. His work stands as an eloquent reminder of our failure and our potential.

REFERENCES

1. Douce, W. C., cited in Goodbye, Henry Ford, hello. . . . *Shield* [Phillips Petroleum Co.] 8:16, 1983.
2. Wolf, S. Talking with the patient. *Current Med Digest* 19:21, 1952.
3. Cook, A. R. Face to face: What of the interview? *Ind Med* 14:635, 1945.
4. Tredgold, R. Current activities in occupational mental health in the United States. *Occup Ment Health Notes,* Feb. 1968. P. 3.

5. Longaker, W. D. Occupational psychiatrist: A job description. *Occup Ment Health Notes*, June 1970. P. 1.
6. Longaker, W. D. The full-time psychiatrist in industry. *J Occup Med* 14:216, 1972.
7. Coodley, A. Choosing a psychotherapist. *JAMA* 243:329, 1980. Copyright 1980, American Medical Association.
8. Modlin, H. C. The occupational physician and the psychiatrist. *JAMA* 226:50, 1973.
9. Modlin, H. C. Put the psychiatrist on the team. *Occup Health Saf* 45:34, Jan/Feb 1976.
10. Tanay, E. Psychiatric aspects of the role of industrial physicians. *J Occup Med* 14:207, 1972.
11. Grospiron, A. F. What has to be done to protect the worker. Address delivered in Los Angeles, 1972. Typescript, pp. 18, 31.
12. Shore, H. J. The impaired physician: Four years after probation. *JAMA* 248:3127, 1982.
13. Gualtieri, A. C., Cosentino, J. P., and Becker, S. S. The California experience with a diversion program for impaired physicians. *JAMA* 249:226, 1983.
14. Aldrich, D. G., Jr. Employee Assistance Services. Irvine, University of California, unpublished memorandum, Feb 1, 1982.
15. Kieffer, S. N., Yolles, S. F., Carone, P. A., et al. *Mental Health and Industry: Planning for the 1980's*. New York: Human Sciences Press, 1980.
16. Egdahl, R. H., Walsh, D. C., and Goldbeck, W. B. *Mental Wellness Programs for Employees*. New York: Springer-Verlag, 1980.
17. Warshaw, L. J. *Managing Stress*. Reading, MA: Addison-Wesley, 1979.
18. Moss, L. *Management Stress*. Reading, MA: Addison-Wesley, 1981.
18a. Montgomery, H. Emotional Stress in Work, unpublished memorandum, [n.d.].
19. *Con Edison Personnel Practices and Procedures, Subject: Procedure on Alcoholism*. New York: Con Edison, Apr 15, 1977. Pp. 1–14.
20. *Drug Abuse as a Business Problem*. New York: New York Chamber of Commerce, 1971. P. 7.
21. Rowan, C. T. Drugs at work. *The Almacan* 14:12, June 1984.
22. Bensinger, P., cited in *Drugs in the Workplace: Solutions for Business and Industry*. Employee Relations and Human Resources Bulletin. Report No. 1540, Section III, Special Report. Waterford, CT: Bureau of Business Practice, 1983. P. 14.
23. Angarola, R., cited in *Drugs in the Workplace: Solutions for Business and Industry*. Employee Relations and Human Resources Bulletin. Report No. 1540, Section III, Special Report. Waterford, CT: Bureau of Business Practice, 1983. P. 18.
24. Pollin, W. The role of the addictive process as a key step in causation of all tobacco-related diseases. *JAMA* 252:2874, 1984.
25. Percentage of adults who smoke down over past 3 years. *Intern Med News* 17:40, June 1–14, 1984.
26. *Adverse Health Effects of Smoking and the Occupational Environment*. Current Intelligence Bulletin 31. Cincinnati: U.S. Department of Health, Education, and Welfare, Public Health Service, Center for Disease Control, National Institute for Occupational Safety and Health, 1979. Pp. 2–5.
27. *Searching for a Way Out: Smoking Cessation Techniques*. New York: American Council on Science and Health, 1984.
28. Goerth, C. R. Clearing the smoke through law, courts. *Occup Health Saf* 52:54, Sept 1983.
29. Brownell, K. D., Cohen, R. Y., Stunkard, A. J., et al. Weight loss competitions at the work site: Impact on weight, morale and cost-effectiveness. *Am J Public Health* 24:1283, 1984.
30. *Gamblers Anonymous* (3rd ed.). Los Angeles: GA Publishing Inc., [n.d.]. Pp. 18–19.
31. Teeling-Smith, G., cited in Sickness and discontent. *Occup Health* 24:153, 1972.
32. "Absence from work attributed to sickness." *Occup Health* 21:39, 1969.
33. Employee Attendance. In *BBP Personnel Policy Manual*. Waterford, CT: Bureau of Business Practice, 1981. Sec. 32.000. Pp. 173–181.
34. Adelstein, A. M. Absence from work attributed to sickness. *Br. J Ind Med* 26:169, 1969.
35. Darrow, W. W. Sick role, status, and acute respiratory illness. *JAMA* 229:266, 1974.
36. Bews, D. C. A medical program to assist management in the control of absenteeism. *J Occup Med* 8:243, 1966.
37. Semmence, A., and Kynch, J. Hernia repair and time off work in Oxford. *J R Coll Gen Pract* 30:90, 1980.
38. Melbin, M., cited in Lyons, T. F. Turnover and absenteeism: A review of relationships and shared correlates. *Personal Psychol* 25:271, 1972.
39. Felton, J. S. Illness-absence recording: Accurate or inaccurate? *Arch Environ Health* 5:495, 1962.
40. Gerson, L. W., and Skipper, J. K., Jr. Job status and expectations of exemptions from work due to illness. *J Occup Med* 15:633, 1973.
41. Felton, J. S. Orienting the new employee in the services of the health department. *Ind Med* 16:519, 1947.
42. Felton, J. S. Orientation of the new employee by the health division of an atomic energy research laboratory: A four-year review. *Ind Med Surg* 21:107, 1952.
43. The physician and sickness absence. *JAMA* 199:413, 1967.
44. Browning, G. G. Sickness absence certification. *J Occup Med* 18:219, 1976.
45. Levine, R. J. Epidemic faintness and syncope in a school marching band. *JAMA* 238:2373, 1977.
46. Small, G. W., and Nicholi, A. M., Jr. Mass hysteria among schoolchildren. *Arch Gen Psychiatry* 39:721, 1982.
47. Small, G. W., and Borus, J. F. Outbreak of illness in a school chorus: Toxic poisoning or mass hysteria? *N Engl J Med* 308:632, 1983.
48. Levine, R. J. Is the presence of low-level environmental contamination a sufficient excuse for not diagnosing mass hysteria? *J Occup Med* 23:597, 1981.

49. Colligan, M. J., and Smith, M. J. A methodological approach for evaluating outbreaks of mass psychogenic illness in industry. *J Occup Med* 20:401, 1978.
50. Murphy, L. R., and Colligan, M. J. Mass psychogenic illness in a shoe factory. *Int Arch Occup Environ Health* 44:133, 1979.
51. Faust, H. S., and Brilliant, L. B. Is the diagnosis of "mass hysteria" an excuse for incomplete investigation of low-level environmental contamination? *J Occup Med* 23:22, 1981.
52. Colligan, M. J. Mass psychogenic illness: Some clarification and perspectives. *J Occup Med* 23:635, 1981.
53. Chan, M., and Kee, W. C. Epidemic hysteria: A study of high risk factors. *Occup Health Saf* 52:55, March 1983.
54. Kempster, N. U.S. team says hysteria caused West Bank illness. *Los Angeles Times* I:1, Apr 26, 1983.
55. Dimond, E. G. What price glory? *Multimedia J* 4:1, Nov 1972.
56. *McDonald* v. *International Paper Co.*, 406 So 2d 582 (1981).
57. *Gunnerson* v. *Kansas City Structural Steel Co.*, 535 S.W. 2d 585, (Missouri) Missouri Court of Appeals, Kansas City District, March 29, 1976. Cited in *Ment Health Court Digest* 20:3, Nov 1976.
58. *Brenda C. Breeden* v. *Workers' Compensation Commissioner et al.* [West Virginia Supreme Court of Appeals]. Cited in Work-related neurosis nets benefits. *Occup Hazards* 44:113, Apr 1982.
59. Shaw, G. Interior Secretary Suffers "an Emotional Collapse." *Los Angeles Times* I:1 (July 23) 1975.
60. Irene Lopucki v. Ford Motor Company [Michigan Court of Appeals], cited in Did Suicide Bar Death Benefits? *Occup Hazards* 44:63, May 1982.
61. Coping with Stress. *Occup Hazards* 43:75, Apr 1981.
62. Mow, A., cited in Zimmerman, D. Are you a workaholic? *Mainliner* 19:35, Nov 1975.
63. Medd, B. H. The "burnout" syndrome. *JAMA* 249:1433, 1983.
64. Chermiss, G. *Professional Burnout in Human Service Organizations.* New York: Praeger, 1980.
65. Edelwich, J., and Brodsky, A. *Burn-Out: Stages of Disillusionment in the Helping Professions.* New York: Human Sciences Press, 1980.
66. Kiev, A. Burnout among physicians. *Med Trib* 24:42, Apr 27, 1983.
67. Communication held key to reduce stress in intensive care. *Intern Med News* 14:40, Sept 1, 1981.
68. Freudenberger, H. J. *The Staff Burn-out Syndrome.* Washington, DC: Drug Abuse Council, Inc., 1975.
69. Paulson, R. Fatigue in medical personnel. *JAMA* 246:124, 1981.
70. Vash, C. L. *The Burnt-Out Administrator.* New York: Springer, 1979.
71. Neville, S. H. Job stress and burnout: Occupational hazards for services staff. *College Res Libraries* 42:242, 1981.
72. Heddesheimer, J. Multiple motivations for mid-career changes. *Pers Guidance J* 55:109, 1976.
73. Judges found to be prone to "burnout." *Los Angeles Times* I-C:8, Oct 29, 1981.
74. Maslach, C. Burned-out. *Hum Behav* 5:16, Sept 1976.
75. Emener, W. G., Jr. Professional burnout: Rehabilitation's hidden handicap. *J Rehabil* 45:55, Jan/Feb/March 1979.
76. Tabor, M. Job burnout rates higher for social service professions. *Occup Health Saf* 53:51, Mar 1984.
77. Moss, L. The Burnout Syndrome. In *Management Stress.* Reading, MA, Addison-Wesley, 1981. Pp. 66–68.
78. Parkes, C. M., Benjamin, B., and Fitzgerald, R. G. Broken heart: A statistical study of increased mortality among widowers. *Br Med J* 1:740, 1969.
79. Parkes, C. M. *Bereavement: Studies of Grief in Adult Life.* New York: International Universities Press, 1972.
80. Glick, I. O., Weiss, R. S., and Parkes, C. M. *The First Year of Bereavement.* New York: Wiley, 1974.
81. Holmes, T. H., and Rahe, R. H. The social readjustment rating scale. *J Psychosom Res* 11:213, 1967.
82. Reiser, S. J. In review of *Healing and History: Essays for George Rosen.* New York: Neale Watson Academic Publications, 1979. *N Engl J Med* 302:698, 1980.

APPENDIX 11-1 GUIDE FOR SUPERVISORS

Supervisors in either office or craft functions are usually not prepared adequately to assist their employees who have work performance problems. The EAP of the County of Los Angeles has made available some guidelines to air in the confrontation with and the referral of workers in need of counseling. The following is provided through the courtesy of Homa Mamoudi, Ph.D., former director of the EAP.

DO'S AND DON'TS FOR SUPERVISORS

DO apply steady, firm pressure by insisting that the employee discharge satisfactorily all job performance requirements.

DO document job performance.

DO point out that help is possible and available at no cost to the individual through the Occupational Health Service Counseling Section.

DO make it clear that we are concerned only with job performance. Unless performance improves, the employee's job may be in jeopardy.

DO explain that the employee must decide for him-self/herself whether to accept assistance.

DO emphasize that all aspects of the Employee Assistance Program are completely confidential.

DON'T try to diagnose the problem.

DON'T discuss drinking unless it occurs on the job.

DON'T discuss personal problems unless they manifest themselves on the job.

DON'T moralize.

DON'T be misled by sympathy-evoking tactics, at which the alcoholic becomes an expert.

DON'T pin a label (alcoholic, neurotic, addict) on anyone who has not first labeled himself/herself.

DON'T cover-up for a friend. Misguided kindness can lead to a serious delay in real help reaching him/her.

JUST REMEMBER THAT . . .

the sooner the problem is identified and dealt with, the more likely is a satisfactory solution, and this will be of benefit to you as a supervisor, the employee, and the County.

549406

12. MEDICAL RECORDS AND DOCUMENTATION

Faithfulness to the truth of history involves far more than a research, however patient and scrupulous, into special facts. Such facts may be detailed with the most minute exactness, and yet the narrative, taken as a whole, may be unmeaning or untrue. The narrator must seek to imbue himself with the life and spirit of the time. He must study events in their bearings near and remote; in the character, habits, and manners of those who took part in them. He must himself be, as it were, a sharer of a spector of the action he describes.

Francis Parkman

RECORDS AND FORMS

In the continuity of the relationship between the occupational health service (OHS) and an employee, the medical record—or the health record, as the purists would have it—is the sustaining nurture. The record should reflect the chronology of the worker's career at the enterprise, encompassing much more than a detailed recording of examination findings or laboratory test results. A good record tells one something about the individual as a person and how that particular employee lives the many lives of worker, husband or wife, father or mother, son or daughter, hobbyist, community citizen, churchgoer, moonlighter, student, or homemaker. A cold series of clinical notes without annotation as to the person's concerns and worries, progress on the employment ladder, honors or other recognitions, or extramural job assignments reveals little of personality, character, or development.

It will be argued by the hassled clinician that time precludes the inclusion of lengthy biographic material, and besides, what do such notes have to do with the worker's health? They have much to do with health, for a careful perusal of an entered series of events may predict and forestall a psychiatric break, may reveal areas of impending behavioral change, or may be indicative of inadequate, oppressive, or erroneous supervision. Further, if the OHS can serve as a warm and welcoming representative of the employer or institution, personal items will allow the member of the OHS team to individualize the visits the worker makes to the health facility, which, it is believed sincerely, will lead to better mental health and even some growth. Most physicians and nurses at work daily in an OHS tend to minimize their roles as change agents. A well-documented record will allow the occupational health professional to be much more effective in the support that is provided the employee who seeks counsel.*

The move toward computerization of medical records will make for a better study of the cause-and-effect relationship between exposure and the appearance of symptoms or findings both in the individual and the group, but will not facilitate the preservation of observations made by an astute occupational health practitioner. If behavioral toxicology will one day mature, the recorded impressions of the sensitive health care practitioner may aid materially in pinpointing subtle changes undetected by conventional methods.

*Feinstein (*Intern Med News* 13:2, Jan 15, 1980) has deplored the medical profession's nearly sacred regard for "hard" data, which has led to the omission of "soft" data of equal worth in medical records, and subsequently, a loss to research. His plea is for the inclusion of the humanistic aspects of treatment and decision-making which have been considered erroneously as invalid additions. As examples, when it is noted that the patient is not working, the reason for the lack of gainful activity should be included; was he cautioned by his physician to cease work or were symptoms aggravated by working? Why was medical attention sought at this particular time, even though chest pain had been noticed for 6 months? Was the visit occasioned by the death from coronary artery disease of a brother just the week before? Feinstein asks that *all* related information be included, along with the hard data, so that research can produce a comprehensive and compassionate improvement in patient care. In substance, a record should reflect the patient not just diseases.

OBJECTIVES

As with any system that is instituted for frequent application and use, there must be certain declared objectives or goals, against which progress can be matched and which can serve as guidelines for continuing operation. In the maintenance of a clinical-record system, the following can serve as such a declaration of purpose.

A well-maintained health record will

Provide a chronologic register of health events in the life of the employee.

Serve as a memory of examination results or other findings pertinent to the continuity of medical care.

Be a repository of any information germane to the life of the employee that relates in any way to present or future health patterns.

Aid in the provision of care when, on a repeat visit, the attending professional is a different one from the therapist who initiated the treatment plan.

Serve as the source of data for statistical compilations of employees seen and services provided.

Authenticate the claimed visits made to the OHS by an employee but whose expenditure of time is questioned by a supervisor.

Allow comparisons of clinical measurements over time so that trends of change in health status, visible through juxtaposed entries of findings, can be detected readily.

Indicate compliance with appointments made for mandated surveillance procedures.

Serve as the evidence that an employee was informed of the need for a clinical procedure, of the effects of a work toxicant, of the precautions to be taken in the form of work practices, and of the schedule required for completion of mandated tests and examinations.

Document all counsel given a worker regarding continuing treatment at the OHS, procedures to be followed at home, medications to be taken (dosage, frequency, and duration), and any modification, temporary or permanent, of job activity.

Note the actual time spent by an employee in need of care at the OHS.

Be the basic document for the placement of data needed in epidemiologic study.

Supply the essential health data needed in occupational health research other than that involved in epidemiology.

Serve as a repository of health queries asked by the employee of OHS personnel, both intramurally at the health unit and extramurally, and of the responses given.

Function, under the unit record system, as a file for all communications concerning the health of the individual received from a personal physician, referred specialist, hospital, or health or welfare agency.

Be the place of retention of all fiscal records of medical care if the OHS is involved in the payment process concerning care authorized by the OHS from outside sources.

Provide needed documentation of findings and services in the event of litigation and the introduction as evidence of segments of the record in the form of claimant's or defendant's exhibits.

Act as a repository of all environmental measurements relating to employee's alleged or real exposures to work substances and of actions taken regarding new or continuing corrective or control measures.

Note all details concerning referrals of the employee-patient to outside sources of care, such as name, address, and telephone number of physician or hospital, day and time of appointment, and patient's or employer's responsibility for payment.

Be a source of information for the inclusion of data in the various forms of personal clinical identification such as wallet cards, identification bracelets, and the like.

Provide assistive data for job placement.

Contribute information for program evaluation and improvement.

FILE CABINETRY

As records cannot be allowed to accumulate on desk or table tops, there must be provision made for the orderly retention of the records that will allow both reasonably rapid filing and retrieval of the documents. The type of file device will, in great part, be determined by the record prototype used (for example, standard manila folder, 5 × 8 inch card). Also, space constraints will dictate the format to be adopted. Some of the determining factors of the system to be used, and thus the file cabinetry, are the following:

Number of employees.

Population served—employees only, or employees and dependents.

Company mission—involving hazardous exposures or white-collar office procedures.

Composition of OHS staff—physicians, nurses, emergency medical technicians (EMTs), or some of each discipline.

Type of potential occupational health hazard.

Location—isolated or urban.
Research potential.
Extent of mandated medical surveillance.
Available space.
Need for retention of inactive records.
Load-bearing potential of supportive flooring.
Frequency of retrieval of records.
Available support funding.

No fixed criteria can be provided for the selection of file retention facilities, for added to the determinants given above is the frequently unassailable factor of personal preference, which, difficult though it might be to believe, is often based on personality needs formed early in life.* Many types are commercially available.

STANDARD FILE CABINETS

Standard file cabinets have tiers of two to five pull-out drawers, accepting 9 ⅜ × 11 ¾ inch folders or equipped to store hanging folders of the same dimension, if desired as carriers only. These cabinets require permanent bolting to a support wall to avoid tipping when one or more upper drawers might be pulled open for use. Inexpensive models are difficult to open when the drawers are full and are short-lived. Better models with good side-slides may be operated by both unimpaired and impaired personnel. Flush fronts with recessed fingergrip pulls are available and make a pleasing appearance in multiples. There may be a safety factor present in that the pull handles may obviate immediate release of the user's fingers.

HORIZONTAL OR LATERAL FILES

Horizontal or lateral files accept the same size of folder. The distinct advantage of these files is space conservation. Even in the open position, less floor space is required than with the standard file cabinets, and banks of files can be placed opposite each other with a minimal need for access space. These cabinets must be fixed to the backing wall. Certain makes have a locking device that precludes opening more than one drawer at a time. For compliance with security precautions, lockable drop-shelf fronts are desirable. The preferred form of lateral file is that with the roll-out drawers, which bring the files to a position in front of the cabinet.

While in most lateral file cabinets with pull-out shelves and fixed or receding doors, records are placed at right angles to the cabinet, the folders can be placed parallel to the shelving, with the tabs facing forward, allowing three rows of records to be read directly, front to back, without having to read the tabs from the side of the opened shelf. Suspension files can be used with either positioning.

Another feature to be considered is the type of door. Covers for the shelves can be added so that they can be either locked individually or gang-locked, ensuring security. Also doors are obtainable that can be opened to a horizontal position and retained for use as a reference or writing shelf, but still can be completely retractable.

To be mentioned is the alternative use of suspension rods to accommodate hanging file folders. While the file is convenient for the extraction and replacement of folders, the suspension hooks, it is believed, are inconvenient as folders are bunched or stacked in use or placed in receptacles awaiting use with patients yet to be seen. In all such cabinets, compressors can be obtained to keep files upright on a partially filled shelf.

MULTI-TIERED ROTARY FILES

Another space-saving file that will accept the standard clinical folder is the multi-tiered rotary file. In this configuration, in place of a vertical or horizontal file line, the cabinet consists of two to six open shelves that rotate independently, allowing access to one or more persons seeking records, from either a seated or standing position. Color-coding of the file ends (or tabs) facilitates placement and retrieval.

In another type of rotary file, a double bank (back-to-back) of seven or eight adjustable shelves is held in a fixed frame that rotates—as does a lazy-susan tier of kitchen shelves—within an exterior cabinet, so that access can be had to one side or the other, or both, if the cabinet is freestanding in an open office area. When the unit is turned 45 degrees, the sides will then present as closed panels that permit locking, thus ensuring full security.

SMALL FILE DRAWERS

Small file drawers, holding envelopes containing 5 × 8 inch record forms, are available as individual or multiple units and can be placed on a desk top for use in a small plant or can be supported by a multiple drawer stand. The disadvantage of these small storage containers is that they demand small records, and such cards tend to deter more than the most abbreviated of clinical entries. Their use might be legitimized in a small plant where a single nurse provides services and over-the-counter medications are used primarily. The unit would not allow the usual complete recording of pertinent information and would

*Although one cannot supply a supportive research base, a study of blank forms, as designed by occupational health users, frequently will reveal differences of extreme crowding, free open spaces, compulsive linear demarcations, and the like.

not prove of worth in most occupational health installations.

OPEN-SHELF CABINETS
With open-shelf cabinets, file folders require end coding or identification. Open shelving holds great numbers of records and can be obtained to fit the full floor-to-ceiling height, which then demands stepstools or ladders, portable or fixed for horizontal rolling on a high rail. As the shelves do not pull out for great access or label identification, their use may be slightly difficult.

A variation in filing systems may be used with cabinetry that gives the impression of shelving, but actually long rods are substituted for the supporting shelves. The rods or rails, in pairs, course the full length of a single cabinet, usually 36 inches (91.4 cm) wide, and by means of hooks, hold suspended folders into which medical records can be placed. Folders of different thicknesses can be held in orderly position with such a suspended system. Identification or indexing is accomplished by means of end labels in angled holders.

VERTICAL AUTOMATED MOVABLE FILE SYSTEMS
In a system described by the author nearly four decades ago [1] and subsequently commercialized into highly utilizable and popular record storage and retrieval devices, folders can be obtained without the operator's having to move from a single, fixed position.

While costly, these systems permit the storage of vast numbers of records, which rest on carrier trays. The tray, when called for by pressing the wanted number on a key pad, presents itself at an aperture on the front of the device, and the record can be removed by the operator while at a seated work station. There is versatility, in that the folders may be filed as in a horizontal file or placed in a series of adjacent drawers that accommodate the folders as in a vertical file. The individual trays may be pulled out like drawers or removed completely for work elsewhere. Such equipment should be considered only for an OHS serving many employees—perhaps 20,000 or more. If a built-in safety device becomes inactive, indicator lights point to the corrective action needed. Computerized displays can provide the same information as the employee's file number.

SPACE-SAVING MOVABLE FILE CABINETS
In this system, records are stored in ceiling-height, open-shelved cabinets that are mobile, moving on tracks so that aisles can be opened or closed between lines of cabinets. These high-density storage and filing systems allow the opening of an aisle where needed, either manually or electrically.

A system such as this one is utilized best where space conservation is of prime importance and where the number of filed records is in multiples of thousands or where inactive files must be maintained with those folders in use. The space saved is 50 percent over that needed for open-shelf files and 75 percent over that required by vertical file cabinets. These cabinets may serve also for the storage of radiology files.

HORIZONTAL AUTOMATED MOVABLE FILE SYSTEMS
In another configuration, ceiling-height open shelving revolves horizontally around a continuous oval track. The method allows access from a seated desk position at the end of the loop, and an automatic file selector will allow movement of the appropriate set of shelves. The presence of aisle space allows multiple, simultaneous access.

Again, such a mode for filing should be reserved for installations with tens of thousands of employees, and today such companies have become rare.

In nearly every system of shelving, dividers or supports are available so that groups of records may be kept in the vertical position. Ordinarily, slotting is available so that dividers can be placed at different intervals.

FILE FOLDERS

There are cabinets to meet all needs, but the plea is made that, irrespective of the size of the occupational health facility or the number of employees served, standard-size file folders holding 8½ × 11 inch sheets should be used. Small cards tend to defeat detailed notations, and with the rapid increase in epidemiologic studies in industry, one should be able to supply all needed data. A card will not accomplish this task. Such entries as "Cold treatment given. F.X.C." should never be encountered on audit in today's level of occupational health culture. Such notes bespeak ignorance, laziness, archaism, and most importantly, vulnerability.

Folders of the size indicated are available in a variety of configurations, all subject to the methods of retention just described, either vertical or horizontal filing, and with top- or end-identification markers. They may come equipped with metal fasteners or left as is, or they may be doubly or triply so equipped so that, in fact, one has a triptych. The choice of record folder depends on several factors, such as

The accidental injury rates, necessitating a capacity sufficient to hold notes of continuing OHS visits.
The number of visits made for nonoccupational illness, particularly if there are many women employees or service is provided also to dependents.
The volume of workers' compensation report forms and correspondence.
The volume of correspondence received from outside health and welfare agencies.
The overall diligence with which surveillance procedure results and environmental measurements are transcribed into or posted in the record.

It has been the author's choice over the years to use standard-size manila folders with color-coded pages and to trust to a page-numbering system to avoid the confusion of reassembly on those rare occasions when a loose record is dropped and contents veer to all compass points. Metal fasteners require (1) time for punching of new pages; (2) lowering of valuable lines at the top of a form; (3) printing of all pages in flipstyle, otherwise reading of a record is difficult; and (4) the use of several folders, for a thick record is impossible to use, as the greater the number of added pages, the less visible are the individual sheets that make up the record. There are many persons in occupational health and in medical records administration to whom the use of metal fasteners becomes a life-and-death issue.* A slightly time-consuming compromise for smaller records is the use of gummed tabs liftable from a parent gummed strip placed next to the inside of the folder crease, which will hold individual sheets in place, but this method is not feasible in thick folders.

Many OHSs use a double, heavy stock folder, with a metal fastener at the top of the left-hand side of the open folder and second clip at the bottom of the right hand inside cover. The two sides separate occupational from nonoccupational disorders and care, and the placement of the metal precludes one-ended bulking of the contents. In other institutions, usually not engaged in occupational health, the triptych folder is used, particularly when there is considerable correspondence to be filed concerning claims. Such folders, ordinarily of a firm, colored fiberboard or pressboard stock, are costly and are rarely needed in an OHS, particularly if the use of the facility is not excessive.

*For those persons who wish to multiply their use of fasteners, there are the so-called Siamese fasteners, which will bind two groups of paper back-to-back, without taking more space than a single regular fastener.

RECORD IDENTIFICATION

Numerous systems have been developed that will permit ready location of a medical record. Most services prepare and issue to each employee a plastic registration card approximately the size of a credit card, 2 ⅛ × 3 ⅜ inches (53 × 8.5 cm), which provides the name, social security number, and employee number or medical file number, in addition to other information if needed. The use of imprinting devices in all departments of an OHS will permit identification of every page newly added to the record and will avoid misfiling. In smaller systems, a vertical file of a 3 × 5 inch (7.6 × 12.8 cm) card index will be maintained that will provide the patient's file number. A visible cardex system, with the inserted overlapping card displaying the bottom edge and the filing title maintained in pull-out trays or on a one- or two-tier rotating columnar file, will serve the same purpose.

Health records can be filed utilizing any of these alphabetic or numeric methods:

By last name, alphabetized
By social security number
By terminal-digit filing
By numeric sequence, using the year as a prefix
By employee number
By OHS number
By a combined name and alphabetic-numeric sequence

STRAIGHT ALPHABETIC NAME FILE

Such a system can be used in a small facility with a limited number of employees, but it does not function well with a large worker population. Common surnames appear in great number, such as Johnson and Williams, and there are many instances of duplicate names. Silver [2] points out also the problem with alphabetic filing or sorting out the McPherson/MacPhersons and the Gray/Greys.* He advocates the use of a 3 × 5 inch index card, bearing a file number, for the need of this additional step still takes less time than attempts at retrieving misfiled records. Further, the pulling of such a card allows the opportunity for

*The Soundex System has been used in surveys to obviate this kind of confusion in similarities in spelling and name and also can be used as guide cards in a filing system that allows clumping of names that sound alike but are spelled differently, for example, Burk, Burke, Birque, Bourque, Borque, Berke, Berc, Berck, Bork, Birke, Bourk, Burque, Birck, Birk, Bourke, Buark, Berk, Bourk, Borck, and Buerck. The system is of historical interest but is no longer available. It was originally made by Remington Rand.

updating, for example, "Is your address still 123 Elm Street and your telephone still (207) 918-6115?" Other identifying information can be carried on the card. In short, alphabetic filing is not recommended except for use with small groups of employees. Silver, a practice management consultant, states emphatically, "I do not believe it [alphabetic filing] is ever preferable in medical records."

If an alphabetic system is employed because of a personal preference or other rationale, the filing is aided by the use of expandable alphabetic divisions, which may increase the number of letter guides from 25 to as high as 3,000, or even more. Such alphabetic dividers may have straight tabs continuous with the guide itself, or they may be angled to increase their visibility. One simple rule to follow in determining need is to count the number of records starting with the letter *B* or *S* and multiply by 10, as each represents 10 percent of the alphabetic names. About 10 records should be allowed for each guide. If the actual number exceeds the guide cards on hand, consideration should be given an expanded set of divisions.

An aid to filing in this mode is commercially available* in what is termed "around-the-vowel" color-coded filing. Folders are provided in five different colors, coded around the second letter in the patient's list name. In this system there are 130 divisions, expandable to 650 divisions by coding to the third letter. This method obviates the need for a name-number cross index, for names are found readily and misfiling is quickly rectified.

FILING BY SOCIAL SECURITY NUMBER

Certain difficulties are encountered when efforts are made to file records by the social security number. Many computerized record systems continue to use this number, the belief being that it really is the only universal personal identification for all Americans. Some persons will not supply the number on request, feeling that such a solicitation is an invasion of privacy, even though the number is needed and used by nearly every employer in the payments to or withholding for the social security system.

The American Hospital Association some years back [3] presented reasons in support of its position against the use of the social security number. First, the Social Security Administration will not validate or confirm a specific number at the request of another person or organization using the number for data-bank or identification purposes. The number given is really not verifiable. An estimate indicated that at least 4 million persons have two or more social security numbers, since there was no law prohibiting multiple issue before 1972. Also, because of these multiple numbers and erroneous information, the Social Security Administration makes 2.5 to 3 million corrections in social security numbers yearly.

Also, it is believed that a great number of persons are using the same number, having adopted the number indicated as the sample social security card supplied with new wallets. Hospitals indicate that upward of 45 percent of patients being admitted either have no social security number or are unable to remember or find it. As it takes 3 weeks to obtain a social security number, hospitals find that they are forced into a dual identification numbering system. Lastly, the social security number is felt to be too long at nine digits to guarantee error-free use [4].

The rationale for the use of social security numbers for filing would have to be cogent and strong to legitimize their use for this purpose.

TERMINAL DIGIT FILING

While not a new method of numbering, terminal digit filing (TDF) is an improved method of filing sequentially issued numbers [5]. The system allows an even distribution of records as they are added to the file. In contradistinction to conventional numbering systems, the assigned numbers are used in reverse order. If one uses, as an example, the number 158,642, which has been issued in the usual sequence, one knows that ordinarily it is read from the left to right. In TDF, it is read from right to left in two-digit groups. The last two or terminal digits, 42, become the primary digits; the middle two, 86, become the secondary digits; and the two remaining, 15 become the tertiary digits.

The file is divided into 100 sections, from 00 to 99, on the basis of the last (terminal) digits on the right. All records ending in 00 are filed together, all records ending in 01 are filed together, and so on, thus allowing equally sized spaces for records and almost ensuring that a record is in the right section (Fig. 12-1).

Within each section, the records are arranged in numeric order on the basis of the digits to the left of the two terminal digits, thus allowing an infinite number of records to be added. The first sort of the file folders with the example given would be by the first number of the terminal (primary) digit, or 4; the second sort would be by the second number of the terminal digits, or 2; the third sort would be by the first number of the secondary digits, or 8. The tertiary 15 is filed in numeric order.

As there are only 100 possible combinations of any

*Biffers Systems, Inc., 1300 N. McDowell Boulevard, Petaluma, CA 94952.

Tertiary	Secondary		Terminal or Primary	
15	8	6	4	2
Straight Numeric Order	Third sort 0.1% of filing area	Fourth sort 0.01% of filing area	First sort 10% of filing area	Second sort 1% of filing area

FIGURE 12-1. *Distribution of records when using terminal digit filing.*

two-number group, 00 to 99, each sort of the file leads to a further breakdown of the previous sort. The exemplary file number given, 15-86-42, would be placed between 14-86-42 and 16-86-42.

TDF lends itself to both retention of records because of mandates regarding the maintenance of files of workers with specified exposures and to periodic purging because of terminations or retirements. The system is aided by color-coding the ends of the record folders with color bars, so that by utilizing 10 distinct colors to represent the digits 0 through 9, single or in any combination, a single color will represent each group of terminal digits. As an example, in a vertical banding of three colors, folders with terminal digits 20 to 29 would have a blue band in the middle position. The same 10 colors would be repeated in the lower position and would correspond to the last number of the terminal digits. Again, as an example, terminal digit 20 would be blue in the middle position but red in the lower position, and terminal digit 21 would show blue in the middle position but gray in the lower position. The same 10 colors would be used in the top position, corresponding to the first number of the middle digits.

The system of color coding eliminates filing errors in the sorting, refiling, and locating of lost records. Folders that are prenumbered and precolor printed are commercially available, as are radiograph envelopes or jackets utilizing the same TDF and color-coded systems. For small operations, pressure-sensitive labels in 10 colors are available in dispensers for local application on TDF folders.

FILING BY ANNUAL NUMERIC SEQUENCE

A method utilized successfully in both small and large facilities and also by many pathology departments consists of assigning numbers to employees as they report in for their preplacement examinations. For example, the first new employee to be seen in 1988 would be given the number 88-1, the second would be 88-2, and so on until the arrival of 1989, when the first new employee receives the number 89-1.

The advantage of this system is that it precludes the use of lengthy numbers, and for whatever statistical purpose it might serve, one always knows instantly the number of new employee-patients added in a year or in any part of a year. The use of this method requires, of course, a file of names and numbers for record identification at the time of need for a folder.

FILING BY EMPLOYEE NUMBER

A filing method using the employee number or badge number as the significant identification can be considered only if employee numbers are not reissued. If numbers are reassigned after a worker leaves an organization, such a system is nullified. (It is to be noted that old-time employees take considerable pride in having and displaying their "low" numbers, and reissue works against a simple method of increasing morale.)

FILING BY ASSIGNED OHS NUMBER

Implicit in this method is the assignment of a special series of numbers that usually become known locally as one's "medical number." While there may be unique indications for this extra set of identifying digits, the system only adds another to-be-remembered depersonalizing number to the social security number, the employee number, the locker number, driver's license number, and so on.

FILING BY ALPHANUMERIC SEQUENCE

Although usually not seen in an OHS records system, folders can be filed under an alphabetic sequence, with arabic cardinal numbers further dividing the letter file. It is mentioned only for completeness.

USE OF RECORD COVERS

The actual folder in which the record contents are maintained may serve different purposes. As indicated earlier, it might be made from a cream-colored or off-white (manila) stock of different weights, or the folder might be fabricated from colored stock or even from pressboard in a variety of colors. The cut of a folder, or tab for identification or labeling, may be of single or double thickness and may be full-cut (full length or straight-cut), double-cut (half-cut or in right and left positions), third-cut, or one-fifth or two-fifths cut. Tabs smaller than one-third of the width of the folder may be too small for ease in identification. The tab may be on the top or side of the folder. If records contain a great number of documents assembled over the years, expansion pressboard folders might prove more efficient than overexpanded standard manila folders. Fasteners, if used, can be placed in any one or more of eight positions, in parallel with each edge of the front and back covers, and can even be placed on flaps that allow flip-flop turning of the entire record within the folder.

The folders need not serve solely as a blank document that holds an assemblage of various reports. The cover can be used for a variety of purposes, provided it is of stock other than heavy pressboard.

FRONT COVER

Imprinting of Identifying Information

Identifying information such as addresses, names, and telephone numbers can be imprinted on the front cover. As these change, multiple blocks should be provided for the insertion of new data.

Record of Physical Examination

Some OHSs have used the front cover as the record of physical examination findings. Continued use of a record—handling, retrieval, delivery, updating, transferring information, refiling—may abrade the ink-recorded notes so that the record would not be legible within a few years. In one instance, the front cover was imprinted for the recording of the results of five periodic or reexaminations, while the preplacement examination results were given space on the inside back cover.

If the OHS is such that an employee rarely seeks counsel except at times of annual examinations or is stationed at a considerable distance from the medical facility, then the cover will not be subject to the handling and wear that are inevitable with dispensary visit recidivists or in operations where accidental injuries are frequent.

The front cover is the ideal site for a warning concerning specific allergies or atopic states.

INSIDE FRONT COVER

Several different uses for the inside front cover are feasible and have been seen in practice.

Pocket to Hold Plastic "Charge-Card" Identification

A transparent envelope slightly larger than the card itself and with an end opening can be offered so that it is both visible and readily accessible for imprinting new pages or reports to be added to the record.

Identification Photograph

As nearly every organization takes, in multiples, and issues color photographs of employees for inclusion in clear-plastic sealed identification badges, it is possible to obtain one of these photographs for the OHS. The picture is affixed to the inside front cover, and appropriately sized rectangles can be printed to accommodate the photos. As new ones are taken, a second or third updated likeness can be added to the folder.

These photographs have been invaluable in the immediate recognition of employees who communicate by telephone and allow the OHS respondent to be more knowledgeable when answering, after obtaining the record. Further, when records are pulled in preparation for scheduled examinations or surveillance procedures, a sense of warmth is conveyed when an individual is asked directly to accompany a staff member because he or she is identified, rather than having a name bellowed out impersonally, fully remindful, to use the Hollywood casting term, of a "cattle call."

Another use of the photograph, particularly when a secular sequence is obtained, is to note certain clinical changes that are apparent: weight gain, undue evidence of aging, weight loss, increased pigmentation, and the like.

Lastly, the photograph does, in fact, identify the individual seeking care and precludes the substitution, as indicated in the discussion of the preplacement examination, of a more medically acceptable candidate for one less physically fit.

Record of Physical Examination

The inside of the front cover may be imprinted for the recording of findings elicited at the time of the preplacement medical examination. This use is satisfactory, but it precludes the entry of future examination results, important in the visible matching of findings obtained serially. The initial examination, while important at the time of hire, becomes dated because of aging, the adverse effects of work exposures (illness or injury), or the changes resulting from significant intercurrent nonoccupational disease.

Diagnostic Index

The inside front cover can provide immediate access to a list of various diagnoses made of an employee. A ruled imprint allows, in a four-column format, the recording of the date, code number, the diagnosis, and the signature of the physician or attending nurse. If such a listing is used, the diagnosis entered should be in conformity with *ICD·9·*^{CM}, The International Classification of Diseases, 9th Revision, Clinical Modification, so that the information can be computerized. The "up-front" entries obviate the need of

	500	1000	1500	2000	3000	4000	6000	8000	Screen
R									
L									

Audiometrist Date

FIGURE 12-2. *Form for recording the results of an audiometric examination. The printing of several such forms on a page allows comparison of findings over time.*

search throughout the record for diagnostic information needed in statistical summaries or epidemiologic studies.

Problem List

When the problem-oriented record is used in an OHS, rather than a source-oriented record, the inside front cover can carry an imprinted set of columns for entry of the following:

Column 1:	Problem number
Column 2:	Problem
Column 3:	Date noted
	Date resolved
Column 4:	Inactive problems

The formulation of the problem list is accomplished by a physician acting on information derived from the data base or from subsequently obtained data, in keeping with the framework of the "SOAP" flow: *S*—subjective data; *O*—objective data; *A*—assessment; and *P*—plan (diagnostic, therapeutic, educational). As indicated by Schall [6], the entries are statements of the objective level of diagnosis of a particular problem, not a guess or an assumption. The problem may be a symptom (headache); it might be a laboratory test result (blood glucose 134); it might be a physical finding (enlarged thyroid); the problem could be a physiologic diagnosis (congestive heart failure) or an etiologic diagnosis (arteriosclerotic cardiovascular disease—atrial fibrillation—angina pectoris class III-C).

Immunization Record

The inside front cover of the folder has been used to record skin test results and the immunizing injections given.

Laboratory Test Results

Various laboratory procedures may be listed on the inside of the front cover and the findings on periodic testing recorded, allowing future comparison.

INSIDE BACK COVER

Again, as with the second side of the record folder, use is made of the inside back cover.

Past Medical History

In some applications, the third side is used as a questionnaire for the job applicant, including a check-off set of various clinical disorders. Often this history form carries a statement to be signed by the applicant to the effect that the information provided was true and complete and that falsification may be considered sufficient cause for termination.

Record of Physical Examination

The record of physical examination may be located on the inside back cover instead of side one of the file folder.

Record of Periodic Examinations

As previously described, space is provided for columnar recording of findings for sequential comparison over time.

Record of Audiometry and Vision Testing

While space does not allow, even with reduction, many complete audiogram blanks to be reprinted, the curve can be entered, thus allowing temporal comparison. To be preferred, however, if this form of entry is needed or desired, is the transfer of data from the audiograms to a simplified version (Fig. 12-2).

Questions can be added, at least for the initial examination, covering history of hearing, noise exposure, hobbies, and so on.

A reduced version of the record card used with the several vision-screening devices can be reprinted on side three of the file folder.

BACK COVER

The back cover has been employed primarily for the recording of examination and test results, but its use is discouraged because of the wear potential of this side of the folder, particularly in cases of extensive usage of the medical facility by certain workers. Any part of a record is subject to copying for introduction as an exhibit in litigation, and a worn surface will not have the desired clarity, particularly in the second-generation format. In general, it is suggested that the back cover be left blank.

Straight-Cut Tab
In relatively small operations, "follow-up" file folders with a full-cut tab can be obtained bearing an imprinted line of the names of the months and days of the month (1–31) in addition to a blank space, protected by a clear plastic strip stapled into position. The edge of the folder acts as a slide for the insertion and placement of colored plastic signals, which can be moved into position for recall purposes. The signal would be positioned over a month and day or, if no longer needed, placed in the blank area or removed entirely. This system would be too cumbersome in a large facility, where a regularly issued computer printout would serve the purpose of apprising the OHS of employees needing recall for examination, surveillance, and so on.

CONTENTS OF MEDICAL RECORD

The purpose of the folder—or envelope jacket—is to serve as housing for all documents relating to the health of the worker while employed by the company. Copies of all pertinent forms relating to health care, surveillance, or administrative actions necessitated by changes in health status should be retained, actually with no exception, for one can never tell which document might provide the pivotal evidence in a litigious action.*

Before discussing the forms that can make up a full record, it might be advantageous to identify some precautionary measures in connection with the maintenance of clinical records.

Use standard, letterhead-size pages, except for clinical laboratory report forms, for small slips are difficult to file and to find, and they may be lost. Any form less than standard size should be ticked in, in overlapping fashion. Even with what is an obvious partially covered display, as with laboratory reports, copying agencies for attorneys have photocopied entire pages of such reports, resulting in the most recently filed document being the only one that is visible, the remainder comfortably hidden underneath, not having been subjected to individual duplication.

Always use full signatures of attending staff members, for initials are puzzling, particularly in years to come.

Identify each page with the employee-patient's name and number.

Strive for legibility. Markovits [7] put it pithily when he wrote that "the doctor's illegible scrawl is a cliché in practice as obsolete as leeches" and that, in these days of extensive communication—backed up in the military for a guarantee of comprehension by the verbal phonetic alphabet—illegible handwriting is symptomatic of affectation, egocentricity, or irresponsibility, none of which should have any place in medicine. It is particularly important that signatures be clear and reproducible by contemporary photocopy devices, which implies the use of a dark ink.

Number each "continuation" page in sequence.*

Place a newly used page or form in the folder in which it belongs. Mix-ups have been encountered where important clinical information was placed in the wrong folder—one of a stack awaiting refiling.

Although this caveat goes beyond the individual folder to the total system of record usage, it is strongly advised that every record be returned at day's end to the records section for accountability, centralization, and security.

The use of "out" cards facilitates refiling. Outguides are available in colored plastic, making possible a distribution system indicative of either (1) the day of the week the record was signed out or referred or (2) the section using the record. The use of colors will allow a more rapid retrieval. A clear plastic envelope over the colored backing permits the holding of material to be filed on return of the record. A smaller, superimposed clear plastic holder on the outguide permits insertion of a 3 × 5 inch (7.7 × 12.8 cm) card that records the destination of the folder.

Copies of prescriptions, return-to-work forms, signed authorizations to leave work because of illness, and signed receipts for loan of crutches, splints, bed boards, and the like must be maintained in the record folder. There have been many occasions when it would have resolved certain difficulties if the stamped times of reporting to and departing from the OHS would have been made part of the permanent record, rather than on a "medical pass."

Whenever possible, combine an examination or test request and report on a single form.

*At the height of the initial filing of claims for asbestotic disease, the author's appointment book for one full year was photocopied for distribution to a great number of involved defense attorneys.

*The blank ruled pages used for continuation of the clinical entries are given different headings such as Chronological Record of Medical Care; Progress Notes; or History, Diagnosis, and Treatment Record.

RECORD FORMS

Certain forms make the daily function of an OHS possible.*

Examination Forms

Airman medical certificate
Audiogram
Authorization for medical examination (issued by personnel department)
Clinical laboratory test request and report forms
Electrocardiogram mount and report form
History questionnaire
Management health examination record
Motor vehicle operator examination record
Periodic medical examination
Preplacement examination
Radiography report
Range of motion, lower extremities
Range of motion, upper extremities
Record of medical examination
Record of pulmonary function test
Record of special histories and examinations (dental, podiatric, psychological, optometric)
Record of vision screening
Report of physical fitness determination
Sobriety examination report
Special medical surveillance examination report (exposure to lead, manganese, carcinogen, and so on)
Visual fields examination

Laboratory Reports

Blood chemistry
Blood grouping
Erythrocyte sedimentation
Feces
Hematology
Microbiology
Miscellaneous
Parasitology
Serology
Tissue Report
Urinalysis

Treatment Forms

Completed prescriptions forms
Continuation record form for nonoccupational injury or illness
Continuation record form for occupational injury or illness
Immunization record
Record of physical therapy
Regional anatomic diagrams (total body, eye, hand, face, and so on, available as printed charts, rubber stamps for imprinting, or diagram-transfers)
Workers' compensation report form (physician's first report of injury)
Workers' compensation report form—supplemental

Administrative Forms Relating to Patients

Authorization of release of information from OHS
Authorization of release of information to OHS
Authorization of company transportation
Blood type card
Classification of health status (for use after preplacement or periodic examination)
Consent form for clinical photography
Consent form for surgical care
Form for receipt of treatment equipment on loan
Identification card for record imprinting
Instructions to patients in preparation for blood chemistry test procedures, 24-hour urine collection, and so on
Issue of hearing protective devices
Medical identification cards
Order forms for safety eyewear
Parental consent for examination/treatment of minor
Pregnancy statement by private physician
Prescription blanks
Record of recreational injuries*
Referral to outside treatment source
Refusal of medical care
Report of animal bite
Report of communicable disease
Request for clinical photography
Request for other photography
Return appointment forms
Return-to-work authorization, with restrictions (as needed)
Sick-leave authorization

Administrative Forms for OHS Use

Absenteeism records
Ambulance travel record
Calibration record for audiometers
Daily log of patients seen

*For samples of many of these forms, see a 1984 publication of the American Medical Association's (AMA) Environmental and Occupational Health Program, *Guide to the Development of an Occupational Medical Record System,* available from the AMA, 535 North Dearborn Street, Chicago, IL 60610.

*Persons who are interested in a detailed system of recording sports injuries sustained in company-sponsored recreation programs should consult J. F. Kraus and F. D. Burg. Injury reporting and recording: Some essentials in the collection and retrieval of sports-injury information. *JAMA* 213:438, 1970.

Daily log of services provided*
Equipment inventory
Individual section record of services rendered (number of radiographs taken, biochemical procedures, patients seen in counseling, and so on) for statistical summary of case load
Narcotic inventory and record forms
"Out" cards for use in record files
Personnel time cards
Purchase order
Radiology filing envelopes
Request for approval of new form (forms control)
Requisition for supplies
Supply inventory

FORMS INDEX

Because of the multiplicity of record forms needed in an OHS, it is helpful if an index of the forms is prepared, and annotated when necessary, which can become a separate chapter in the OHS manual of policies and procedures. A listing would provide such information as the form number, the source, the title of the form, the user, and the quantity to be stocked.

As forms are used that originate outside the OHS, such as the Motor Vehicle Operator Examination Record (available from a state agency) or Requisition for Supplies (a company-wide form), it is helpful if separate indexes are prepared as follows:

1. OHS-numbered forms index
2. Non-OHS-numbered forms index
3. Unnumbered forms index
4. Index of forms used by OHS section

A description of each form and its use should be included in the OHS manual chapter devoted to forms (see Chap. 13) and should provide the following information: title of form, purpose, sample of form, size (possibly reduced in size), source (origin), section of use or user originator, quantity to maintain in supply, quantity to order, method of use, number of copies, distribution of copies, retention period, classification or access, and periodicity of review of need.

*In the daily log form, space should be provided to indicate first visits and repeat visits. The reason for this coding is that the resulting data will be used to demonstrate that the OHS truly is providing emergency medical care—particularly in connection with the evaluation and treatment of patients presenting nonoccupational conditions—and is not seeing patients who rightfully should be receiving care from their own physicians. In most tabulations, "first visits" usually outnumber by far the "repeat visits."

NEW FORMS

There are frequent requests by staff members for new forms to be prepared, and to avoid the excessive generation of additional documents, it would be wise to ask the questions indicated by Soukhanov and Haverty [8]:

What purpose will this form serve? Do we really need such a form? Why?
Does the form contain all necessary information and no unnecessary information?
Is there wasted space on the form? Could this form be combined with another one?
Will the form save time for the data recorder and retriever?
Is the content logically organized? Are terms and symbols clear and unambiguous?
Is the format appropriate? Are the data arranged so as to permit continuous recording from left to right and from top to bottom?
Is related information grouped together? If more than one person is responsible for entering data on the form, are the blocks for these data arranged in sequence?
Is the form identified with an appropriate title, briefly but clearly indicating the function and purpose of the form?
Has the data-entry method (that is, handwriting versus typing) been considered in determining the appropriate size of the spaces for entering the information?

From a review of many OHS forms seen in various organizations, a few generalizations might be offered:

Identify every form with the designation of the OHS, using the same name, not Occupational Health Service on one, and Medical Department on another.
Include the name of the organization.
If the OHS has a logo, use it on the forms, for it ties all activities (medical care, health education, community services, and so on) into a single unit.
Develop a sequential series of OHS form numbers, and place them in the same area on all forms, for example, in the lower left-hand corner.
Color-code the forms for ease of identification.
Make every effort to have the forms in the same configuration, either vertical or horizontal, to avoid unnecessary rotation of record during use.
Encourage the inclusion of the union "bug" if printing is accomplished extramurally.
Any form that has an outside distribution should include a return address.

SPECIAL FORMS

Laboratory Reports

By now, it has become fairly commonplace to file individual laboratory report forms, if one-half sheet or smaller, in order of receipt on a master report form, beginning at the bottom of the page. Master forms are commercially available that will hold 12 overlapping reports that require no gluing. A pair of tabs is removed for each report in need of filing, and two pressure-sensitive, adhesive areas remain to which the report form will adhere firmly.

Also available from commercial printers are forms that present several discrete areas for recording of laboratory test results and that also provide a sufficient number of blocks for four to six different sets of test results. Such a display allows a ready scan of previous findings for comparison with the most recent values, but transfer of the data is required, which is both time-consuming and subject to error. The juxtaposition of past and current levels is mandatory for the ease of reference to results that might determine a change in job assignment.

If the laboratory results are returned on computerized printout forms, they usually will be of the same size as other sheets in the folder and can be retained in their appropriate order.

Referral Form

A situation often leading to misunderstanding between the OHS and the employee, between the OHS and an outside treating physician, or among the patient, the OHS, and the practitioner is the responsibility for the professional fee. A form was developed by the author and was used successfully when the patient was referred to a specialist for care. The employee was asked to confirm that the conditions expressed were understood. It was then hand-carried to the treating specialist. The form is seen in Figure 12-3.

Report of Sobriety Test

Because the determination of sobriety is an important step in the evaluation of a worker's ability to function in an assigned job, a standardized procedure is necessary for equal application to all persons suspected of having consumed beverage alcohol just prior to coming to work or while on duty. The form shown in Figure 12-4 was developed to meet such a need. The same form, with changes, or a similar form can be used in the assay of an individual suspected of being under the influence of drugs.

Narcotic Records

Two types of records are essential in the use of controlled substances. The first relates to the inventory of the medications, and the general format of the record for each preparation should show the date of action, voucher number (shipping list, receipt, numbered prescription for a specific patient, or number from the Narcotic Register described below), quantity issued, balance, and signature of responsible staff member.

A second form, the Narcotic Register, is used as a record of the individual dispensing of a controlled medication and includes the following information: number, date, patient's name, patient's address, and narcotic dispensed or administered, quantity or dosage, diagnosis, person authorizing use, and person dispensing or administering narcotic.

Authorization for Preplacement Examination

As indicated earlier in the discussion of the placement examination, there must be an authorization for the conducting of the examination before final employment. One reason is to avoid examining persons who do not plan to apply for work and merely wish a medical review at no cost, and the second is to be assured that—as mentioned in the discussion of the identification photographs—the right applicant is being examined and not a substitute. The authorization can be a simple request for examination, bearing the signature of a representative of the personnel department. The response from the OHS comprises a classification of the applicant and, if job modifications or limitations are indicated, a listing of the restrictions, such as in Figure 12-5. This list may be expanded, as needed, in light of specific work exposures.

Patient Routing Slip

A form that has been found helpful is a small card for temporary use that is affixed to the front cover of the employee's record folder. The form lists all of the examinations and test procedures to be undergone either as a new employee or as an incumbent who is being given a multitest battery or a surveillance protocol. Various boxes or parentheses allow clerical or other personnel the opportunity to indicate which are required procedures and which have been completed. As the order of tests is not fixed, an equitable distribution of examinees throughout the OHS is thus obtained. If the radiology section is busy, the employee might be seen in the clinical laboratory, and so on. The form is not retained when the examination protocol is complete.

Blood Grouping Record

Frequently, certain blood donors are needed as determined by a critical patient's condition, content of surgical procedure, or inventory of the local blood

ABC BRASS FOUNDRY
123 ELM STREET
EAST NUTMEG, PT 98765

TO: ______________________________ DATE ____________

______________________________ TELEPHONE ____________

Our employee M______________________________ OHS No. ____________

has (been advised)(chosen) to consult you because of

( ) Personal Illness. The ABC Brass Foundry assumes no liability in connection with the consultation and any expenses incurred will be on his/her personal account or that of the insurance company carrying his/her health insurance. It would be appreciated if these forms could be completed and returned to the undersigned. One may be retained for your files.

( ) Occupational Injury. Customary reports and statements for services rendered should be mailed immediately to the DEF Casualty Insurance Company, 456 Pine Street, East Nutmeg, PT 98765, telephone (909) 432-1100. Copies of all reports forwarded would be appreciated, mailed to the undersigned.

( ) Determination of Occupational Origin of Injury or Illness. For evaluation of the patient's condition in order to assist in determining liability under workers' compensation laws. Please send reports and bills to the DEF Casualty Insurance Company, and copies of the reports, in addition to these forms, to the undersigned.

History and Impression ______________________________

____

____

A

FIGURE 12-3. *A. Patient referral form, obverse. B. Patient referral form, reverse.*

bank. Depending on the size of the organization, the blood groupings of employees can be kept either in a 3 × 5 inch (7.7 × 12.8 cm) card file or entered into the data bank. If an employee or a dependent is in need of blood, plant personnel of the appropriate group can be sought by searching the file and their contributive assistance solicited. A simple card will meet the need by recording the following: name, department, OHS number, badge number, blood group, type and Rh factor, office telephone, and dates of donation.

Authorization of Care for a Minor

Young persons are employed during vacation or as part of a work-study program, which means that underage personnel may be hired at any time throughout the year. As they are minors, parental consent must be secured for both the initial examination for placement and for subsequent emergency care, if indicated.* While it is advisable to review the issue with company counsel, in view of possible different local requirements, it is suggested that a form be prepared in which the parent or legal guardian gives

*State law must be consulted regarding the concept of the emancipated minor, one who although below the chronologic age of majority has assumed the lifestyle and responsibility of an adult (see A. J. Rosoff, *Informed Consent.* Rockville, MD: Aspen, 1981. Pp. 190–191). Emancipation may be accomplished by marriage or the cessation of one's being dependent on parents for support, or both. In some jurisdictions, the minor's becoming a parent automatically confers emancipation.

If occupational injury, date ______________________________

Remarks ______________________________

Should, for any reason, prompt communication with the undersigned be desired, please telephone (909) 543-2200.

______________________________ M.D.

Report of Consultation

History, Examination, Diagnosis and Treatment:

Disposition:

( ) Hospitalized at ______________________ Hospital

( ) Modified work; details ______________________________

( ) Regular work ( ) Sent home

Further treatment to be secured at:

( ) OHS, Brass Foundry ( ) Office ( ) Hospital

Estimate of disability:

( ) Partial ______________________________

( ) Temporary __________ Days

( ) Permanent ______________________________

______________________________ M.D.

B

FIGURE 12-3 *(continued)*

consent to the furnishing of health services to the minor. Certain procedures, such as taking a blood specimen, may be noted specifically. The signature should be witnessed by a person other than a parent or guardian.

Confirmation of Visit to the OHS

Because of the infrequent need of proof of an employee's visit to the OHS, a form providing confirmation might be used. It should indicate the times of arrival and departure of the worker either seeking care or undergoing medical surveillance. A time stamp can be used appropriately here.

Multipurpose Form

A method introduced by the author some years ago to facilitate the recording of a patient's visits, without necessitating a multiplicity of forms, involved the design of a multipurpose record that utilized a lateral

ABC BRASS FOUNDRY
Occupational Health Service

________________ 19___

SUBJECT: Report of Sobriety Test
TO:

____
Name Badge No. Department and Foreman

Was examined at ______ _.m. _____________ 19__, for evidence of alcoholic intoxication. The procedures composing the test and the results obtained are noted below.

A. To determine if alcoholic beverages were consumed:

1. Odor of alcohol on breath:		None	( )	Slight	( )	Marked	( )
2. Suffusion of conjunctivae:		None	( )	Slight	( )	Marked	( )
3. Flushing of face:		None	( )	Slight	( )	Marked	( )
4. Drying and furring of tongue:		None	( )	Slight	( )	Marked	( )
5. Salivation:		Normal	( )	Excessive	( )		
6. Admission of having taken alcohol:		Admitted	( )	Denied	( )		
7. Tremors:		None	( )	Present	( )		
8. Tachycardia:		Pulse ( )					
9. Condition of pupils:	Right:	Dilated	( )	Contracted	( )		
		Reacts to normal light: Yes			( )	No	( )
		Reacts to bright light: Yes			( )	No	( )
	Left:	Dilated	( )	Contracted	( )		
		Reacts to normal light: Yes			( )	No	( )
		Reacts to bright light: Yes			( )	No	( )

B. To determine if consumption of alcoholic beverages has affected normal behavior:

1. Loss or confusion of memory:		None	( )	Confused	( )		
		Complete amnesia	( )				
	Oriented as to time:			Yes	( )	No	( )
	Oriented as to date:			Yes	( )	No	( )
	Oriented as to place:			Yes	( )	No	( )
2. Impairment of speech	Unimpaired		( )	Sluggish	( )	Slurred	( )
	Boisterous		( )	Profane	( )	Obscene	( )
3. Errors of coordination:							
Finger-to-nose test:		Normal	( )	Fair	( )	Inaccurate	( )
Finger-to-finger test:		Normal	( )	Fair	( )	Inaccurate	( )
Picking up object from floor:		Normal	( )	Fair	( )	Inaccurate	( )
Sitting down:		Normal	( )	Fair	( )	Inaccurate	( )
Ability to walk a straight line:		Normal	( )	Wavering	( )	Unable to	( )
Romberg test:		Positive	( )	Negative	( )		
4. State of consciousness		Conscious	( )	Semi-	( )	Comatose	( )
5. Cooperation		Normal	( )	Fair	( )	Uncooper.	( )

A

FIGURE 12-4. *A. Report of sobriety test, obverse. B. Report of sobriety test, reverse.*

pinfeed document in sextuplicate that served these record needs:

1. Visit for occupational disability
   Visit for illness
   Visit for injury
   Visit following absence because of illness
2. Visit for nonoccupational disability

Additional determinations:

Blood pressure: Systolic ( ) Diastolic ( )
Temperature: ________ degrees C ( ) F ( )
Signs of injury: ( ) None ( ) Signs observed were:

Signs of recent or concurrent illness: None ( )
Signs observed were:

Following clinical survey of the above patient, the IMPRESSION is that:
He/she is drunk ( )
He/she is not drunk ( )

A blood alcohol test was taken with the results as follows: _____ %
From this blood examination, it has been determined that:
He has consumed alcohol recently ( )
He has not consumed alcohol recently ( )

With due consideration being given the clinical survey and the blood alcohol report, it is CONCLUDED that:
He/she is drunk* ( )
He/she is not drunk ( )

The following treatment was given to the patient:

Disposition of the patient was as follows:

________________________ M.D.

* The term "drunk is defined as follows: The person concerned was so much under the influence of alcohol as to have lost control of his/her faculties to such an extent as to render him/her unable to do safely the occupation he/she may be called upon to perform by virtue of his/her employment at the Foundry.

B

FIGURE 12-4 *(continued)*

Visit for illness
Visit for injury
Visit following absence because of illness
Visit following absence because of injury

3. Report of disposition of patient (regular or restricted work, to hospital, to private physician, retained in OHS)
4. Report of injury
5. Discharge (from injury) note

The form is reproduced in its entirety in Figure 12-6. The placement at the top of "Non-Occupational Disability Diagnosis," with limited carbon-paper interleaving, preserves confidentiality, for the entry appears only on the copy retained in the OHS. The distribution was as follows:

Original—employee's medical record
Copy 1 (blue)—insurance section on initial report of injury

LIMITATIONS: Not to be assigned to any job requiring:

[ ] 1. Anything other than seated work.
[ ] 2. Any pushing, pulling or lifting over ___ pounds.
[ ] 3. Repeated bending or cramped positions.
[ ] 4. Prolonged kneeling or squatting.
[ ] 5. Any kneeling or squatting.
[ ] 6. Continuous walking.
[ ] 7. Walking up any steps.
[ ] 8. Walking up steps other than to work level.
[ ] 9. Continuous standing.
[ ] 10. Work on ladders or overhead.
[ ] 11. Arms above shoulder level.
[ ] 12. Exposure to dust including buffing of metals or plastics.
[ ] 13. Exposure to chemical fumes.
[ ] 14. Accurate far vision.
[ ] 15. Accurate near vision.
[ ] 16. True color perception.
[ ] 17. True depth perception.
[ ] 18. Squeezing of hand tools.
[ ] 19. Good hearing.
[ ] 20. Exposure to excessive noise.
[ ] 21. Work around moving machinery.
[ ] 22. Operation of moving machinery.
[ ] 23. Operation of motor vehicle.
[ ] 24. Use of vibratory tools.
[ ] 25. Finger dexterity.
[ ] 26. Exposure to solvents, greases, thinners or sealers.
[ ] 27. Exposure to oils, resins, or fiberglass.
[ ] 28. Bicycle riding.
[ ] 29. Mental tension or responsibility.
[ ] 30. Any industrial type of physical activity.
[ ] 31. Altitude over ______ ft.
[ ] 32. Other ______________

THIS PERSON MUST WEAR:

[ ] Properly Fitted Glasses
[ ] Properly Fitted Safety Eyewear
[ ] Contact Lenses ______ Approved ______Not Approved

FIGURE 12-5. *Listing of job restrictions on a preplacement examination form.*

Copy 2 (pink)—safety department on initial report of injury

Copy 3 (yellow)—supervisor on initial report of injury

Copy 4 (green)—insurance section with discharge note completed at time of discharge from care of injury

Copy 5 (goldenrod)—safety department with discharge note completed at time of discharge from care of injury

The register carrying the continuous two-folded forms was made of lightweight metal and proved to be no burden as it was carried from patient to patient. As a number of registers were maintained, a partially completed report could be retained in the register until final disposition of the patient was determined or the treatment was complete.

Dental Examination

The health status of the teeth is of importance in certain workers who are exposed to heavy metals or acid vapor, and notations should be made of the dentition as examined periodically. As most OHS personnel are not too familiar with the content of such a review, the following represent the items to be checked and noted on the record:

Identifying information

Pictorial schematic display of teeth, numbered as follows:

Upper	1	2	3	4	5	6	7	8	9	10	11	12	13	14	15	16
Lower	32	31	30	29	28	27	26	25	24	23	22	21	20	19	18	17

The diagram for an individual tooth may be shown and comments concerning these elements should be made, when appropriate: texture of teeth, caries, roots, fillings, position of teeth, mastication or occlusion, attrition, gums, anchorage of teeth, radiographic findings, dental calculus (tartar), oral hygiene, remarks regarding occupation, general remarks, and other.

If there is a dental section in the OHS, then a form for survey purposes can be designed professionally.

Radiology Records

The maintenance of a file of radiographs requires a filing system comparable to the one used for medical records. The same alphabetic or numeric system should be paralleled in the radiology section, for the visible edge of a filing envelope can carry the same color-coding and application of letters and numbers as the tops or ends of the clinical folders.

Every envelope, on its face, should bear the name of the employee and the identification number that is used elsewhere in the OHS. There should not be two systems of designation in use. In some services, on the face of the envelope, there are printed blocks or lines to allow entry of the date and type of examination.

In some sections, the exposure data are entered into a logbook and cross reference is made by entering the book and page numbers in line with the date and type of examination on the face of the file envelope. As radiographs frequently are put on loan to private physicians or other sources of care, the original file folder should be retained and identified with an "OUT" marker. Needless to say, all radiographs, as part of the imaging system, should show the name

MEDICAL REPORT

NON-OCCUPATIONAL DISABILITY DIAGNOSIS

LAST NAME	FIRST NAME	INITIAL	BADGE NO.	PAYROLL NO.	AGE	SEX	RACE	MARITAL ST.

OCCUPATION DEPARTMENT FOREMAN OR SUPERVISOR HOME ADDRESS

OCCUPATIONAL DISABILITY		NON-OCCUPATIONAL DISABILITY	
DISPENSARY VISIT FOR ILLNESS ☐	DISPENSARY VISIT FOR INJURY ☐	DISPENSARY VISIT FOR ILLNESS ☐	DISPENSARY VISIT FOR INJURY ☐
ABSENTEEISM EXAM. BECAUSE OF ILLNESS ☐	ABSENTEEISM EXAM. BECAUSE OF INJURY ☐	ABSENTEEISM EXAM. BECAUSE OF ILLNESS ☐	ABSENTEEISM EXAM. BECAUSE OF INJURY ☐

PERIOD OF ABSENCE NUMBER OF DAYS ABSENT

FROM TO

DISPOSITION - PHYSICALLY FIT TO RETURN TO:

REGULAR WORK ☐ RESTRICTED WORK ☐ FOR DAYS UNTIL

DETAILS

GENERAL HOSPITAL ☐ OTHER HOSPITAL ☐ PHYSICIAN'S OFFICE ☐ REST WARD ☐

REPORT OF INJURY

DATE & HOUR OF INJURY	EXACT LOCATION OF THE PLACE IN WHICH INJURY OCCURRED	DATE & HOUR OF FIRST VISIT

CAUSE OF INJURY, EMPLOYEE'S OWN OPINION:

HISTORY TAKEN BY

WITNESSES TO INJURY:

PHYSICAL EXAMINATION:

DIAGNOSIS, FIRST VISIT:

X-RAY DIAGNOSIS:

IS ACCIDENT ABOVE REFERRED TO THE ONLY CAUSE OF PATIENT'S CONDITION? IF NOT, STATE CONTRIBUTING CAUSES:

INITIAL TREATMENT:

PROBABLE DURATION AND EXTENT OF DISABILITY:

WILL THE INJURY RESULT IN A PERMANENT DEFECT? IF SO, WHAT?

DATE TO RETURN:

DISCHARGE NOTE

IN	OUT

DATE OF DISCHARGE DISCHARGE BY

FINAL DIAGNOSIS

CONDITION ON DISCHARGE

M.D. R.N.

FIGURE 12-6. *Multi-purpose OHS visit record form.*

of the patient, date of examination, identifying number, and designation of the organization and the OHS.

The radiology departments of hospitals and large medical centers include much more information on the envelope face, but this detail—anatomic field, loan record, diagnosis, date of birth, ACR (American College of Radiology) index number, and so on—is not believed necessary in the usual OHS. Some files contain a second smaller envelope on the front to hold reports. If a "Pathology/Teaching File" is needed or would be of worth, such a separate collection can be maintained, even if duplicate copies of original films are made to meet this need. An elaborate system of maintenance is not indicated.

Radiograph file envelopes measure 14 ½ to 14 ¾ inches in height by 18 ¼ inches in width (36.7–37.4 cm × 46.2 cm) and can be obtained in a variety of colors, other than kraft, if there is aesthetic or filing need.

In some installations, where occupational exposure to ionizing radiation is of significance, a detailed record of diagnostic x-ray exposure is maintained on the face of the filing envelope in addition to the usual alphanumeric identifying information. Many radiologists do not believe that such a record is valid because of the great differences among various pieces of diagnostic radiologic equipment, gross variations in technique, and the lack of standardization in delivered dosages. With greater engineering controls in worksites involving radiant energy and with the lowered exposure levels and numbers of radiographs taken on employees, such records may not be indicated.

A combined radiography request and report form can be used, conserving time and labor.

OSHA REQUIREMENTS

Certain records need to be maintained for report purposes for forwarding either to the Federal Occupational Safety and Health Administration (OSHA) or the equivalent state agency. This material will be discussed under Reports in Chapter 13.

RETENTION AND STORAGE OF INACTIVE RECORDS

The files of individuals who are no longer employed ordinarily would be placed in inactive storage and possibly later be destroyed, in parallel with company policy, with the exception of the records that are mandated for retention by OSHA Regulation No. 1910.20 [10]. The OSHA standard requires that each employee's medical record be preserved and maintained for at least the duration of employment plus 30 years. An employee medical record, as defined in the standard [10],

> . . . means a record concerning the health status of an employee which is made or maintained by a physician, nurse, or other health care personnel, or technician, including medical and employment questionnaires or histories (including job description and occupational exposures), the results of medical examinations (pre-employment, pre-assignment, periodic, or episodic) and laboratory tests (including x-ray examinations and all biological monitoring), medical opinions, diagnoses, progress notes, and recommendations, descriptions of treatments and prescriptions, and employee medical complaints.

Excluded from the record for retention purposes are physical specimens, such as blood and urine samples; records concerning health insurance claims if maintained separately and not accessible to or identifiable by the employer; and records concerning employee assistance programs (EAPs) if maintained separately from the medical program and its records.

Record is defined further as "any item, collection, or grouping of information regardless of the form or process by which it is maintained (e.g., paper document, microfiche, microfilm, X-ray film, or automated data processing)" [10].

The standard does not dictate the mode of preservation of the record so long as the information is retrievable, with the exception of radiographs, which must be preserved in their original state. In substance, x-ray films will not meet the federal requirement if reduced to microfilm. Under consideration at present is a modification of the rule regarding retention of exposed film as originally obtained, so that microfilm storage under certain approved circumstances would meet the requirement [11].

Innumerable commercially available containers and methods of storing records can be used for the retention of records.

When records are removed to storage, locator file cards should be maintained so that ready access can be had to inactive records. A few guidelines for record retention are in order [12]:

Inventory records being stored.
Schedule retention periods. (As employees terminate at different times, the 30-year retention mandate will represent staggered time periods.)
Store records conveniently.
Make maximum use of floor space.
Select files that are easy to reference.
Select a system that meets the needs. (In light of the continuing need for records in cases of asbestos-related disease undergoing litigation, the files should not be stored in old salt mines, reactivated

for such purposes, miles from the site of the originator.)

Select files that are structurally sound. (Shelving may be needed to preclude the collapse of heavy cartons that are self-stacked.)

Most companies dispose of over-age records in landfill projects, at the least cost. If security is an issue, records can be incinerated (where pollution contracts permit) or shredded. Records may be sold for recycling if metal-free and if other methods of destruction have not been developed three decades hence.

Records no longer needed or not mandated for retention can be microfilmed or reduced to a microfiche format, but a cost-benefit study should be conducted to determine the advantages of such handling. More importantly, the storage in a computer data bank should be considered if retention in that mode is feasible or even possible. Medical records are living documents as long as a worker is subject to a repeated and somewhat stochastic frequency of use. To have to resynthesize a record with each visit, to search a microfilm or microfiche, or even to supply each physician with a terminal to bring up the record of the last visit or previous medical needs seems highly impractical. For other forms of documentation, computerized records are mandatory, and this issue will be addressed shortly.

RUBBER STAMP IMPRINTING

Repetitive entries in clinical records can be made by means of rubber stamps, and a collection of the imprints of stamps in current use should be included in the section on medical records in the OHS manual, to be discussed under Manuals in Chapter 13.

Rubber stamps may be used in the following instances:

Instructions on envelopes containing dispensed medication.

Entry note regarding immunizing injections, showing name of antigen, dose, and route of administration.

Stamp for near-universal use reading "Confidential."

Entry of date of visit or service.

Entry of time of arrival or departure of patient, using a time-stamp.

Name in block letters for imprinting below signature of physician, nurse, or other occupational health personnel rendering a service that is recorded in the patient's file and signed.

Identification of library holdings.

For recurrent dispatch or transport of documents, the name and address of recipient.

Designation of OHS section visited or type of service provided.

Signature stamps when originals are not required legally.

ORDER OF RECORD CONTENTS

Another issue in record maintenance that has caused considerable variation of opinion is the order in which record elements are maintained in the folder. This subject has led to great embitterment between the personnel responsible for the stewardship of the records and users of the folders in the OHS.

Custom has had it that records of examinations are given a position of primacy, followed by the chronologic notation of various usages of the OHS made by the employee, with laboratory and radiography reports in the penultimate position, and correspondence the final documents in the folder. This order of march seems to have been satisfactory and is altered only by certain firmly entrenched position-takers who feel that an OHS will collapse unless entries relating to occupational disorders or surveillance procedures are left totally apart from notes covering non-work-related information.

The author has favored no particular change in the pattern mentioned but has preferred color-coding of the progress notes or continuation sheets, the ruled "Record of Nonoccupational Injuries and Illness" being printed on one color of heavy stock, and the "Record of Occupational Injuries and Illness" being given another color. The simple separation of just the two areas of cause and care has allowed a more expedient review of the lesion currently being treated. At one time consideration was given the insertion of laboratory reports within the record following notation of the reason for the test or examination, rather than the usual time-sequential gathering of the slips toward the back of the folder; the practice seemed to work well and matched immediately diagnostic test results with physical examination findings. The system is worth a trial.

CONFIDENTIALITY AND RECORD ACCESS

That the medical record is a confidential document, except in cases of work-generated injury or illness, is challenged by no one in health care, but many in managerial ranks believe that they should be made privy to its contents when there is interest in an individual employee. Reference must be made to Standard No. 7 of the American Occupational Medical Association (AOMA) Code of Ethical Conduct (adopted July 23, 1976), which reads:

> Treat as confidential whatever is learned about individuals served, releasing information only when required by law or by overriding public health considerations or to other physicians at the request of the individual according to traditional medical ethical practice, and recognize that employees are entitled to counsel about the medical fitness of an individual in relation to work but are not entitled to diagnoses or details of a specific nature.

Emphasis is given to the point made previously that diagnostic information is *not* needed for placement or for a change in character of work assignment because of altered health status. The role of the physician, as pointed out by Bews [13], is that of interpreter of medical facts and findings, converting a knowledge of health states into guidelines for work placement. Stating that an individual is physically and emotionally fit for all work or that an employee should not be given an assignment working at heights (ladders, roofs, staging) meets the needs of company administration and in no way alters the privilege of the medical information in the possession of the OHS.

This exact point was expressed well by May [14], who stated:

> Following illness or accident, in association with advancing age, or on change of job or promotion, the employer is entitled to know . . .
>
> 1. Ability to continue with present employment or carry out proposed duties;
> 2. Suitability or need for alternative work;
> 3. Limitation on activities (temporary or permanent);
> 4. Existing disability (temporary or permanent);
> 5. Future prospects (long- or short-term); and
> 6. Expectation of life (if appropriate).

May concludes that the above six items can be known "without the disclosure of actual details of health."

The separation of the "occupational" and "nonoccupational" record notations, indicated in the discussion Order of Record Contents, is of assistance when third parties need copies of the record, insofar as portions relate to a litigated claim of work-related injury. Personal medical history having no connection with the job-generated injury is readily set aside at time of photocopy, and privilege is preserved.

A point must be made that relates to personal experience of the author and is supported by Bundy [15]. Try though one might in an active OHS to exercise every means of retaining confidentiality, including closed offices during consultation, private examination rooms, and even cryptic or euphemistic entries in the clinical record, word seems to spread regarding an employee-patient, and often the OHS is blamed for releasing information. Not only have employees been overheard freely discussing their conditions while waiting in a reception area, but the same workers whose medical intelligence was being guarded carefully will relate their disorders and treatment to other personnel in the organization, with no regard for the confidentiality of the information. Patients must be instructed that they, as well as the OHS, must retain the privilege of the relationship.

No discussion of confidentiality is complete without reference to the OSHA standard regarding access to employee exposure and medical records. No recent issue in occupational health and safety has created the opposition, the discussion, the testimony, and the heat that did the proposal for this invasion of privacy. The issue compounded one that has been brewing much longer, and that is the potential loss of confidentiality through computerization of medical information in the development of data banks.

Fiscina [16] clarifies understanding when he indicates that before a physician-patient privilege is legally recognized, the existence of a "confidential communication" must be demonstrated. Such a communication involves *information* acquired through the physician-patient relationship needed to treat the patient professionally. The statutes regarding privileged communications are designed to protect persons who consult physicians from a disclosure of secrets imparted in such consultation and "to prevent physicians from disclosing information that might result in humiliation, embarrassment, or disgrace to the patient." Not only are these untoward feelings to be avoided by imprudent disclosure, but also possible action undertaken by the employee-patient because of the generation of such feelings.

The matter of confidentiality has been adumbrated by the growth of several different sources of concern. Records will be needed on an extremely long-term basis because of linkages between dangerous substances and reproductive dysfunctions, which, as Westin [17] observes, are the kinds of things that are most sensitive in terms of people's feelings about privacy. Next, records become part of large automated data systems, which are inviting targets for governmental regulatory agencies, courts, law enforcement officials, and endless others who "view such easily retrieved and extensive data as a resource for their own self interests." Westin points out the other players in this arena: The individual worker is concerned because of the possibility that leakage of such information will affect his or her mobility and transferability. The personal physician and the community health facility* may not be able to execute their responsibilities properly if not possessed of certain exposure information never previously divulged. The union has its interest because of the hazards to which its membership is exposed, and the employer, of course, is "caught in a dilemma and whipsawed between two forces." On one hand, pressure is placed on employers to conduct studies that might detect adverse health effects from exposure to their processes, and on the other they are "subject to tort liability under which the courts and juries decide at what point in time an employer received due notice of a dangerous situation."

Other concerned parties are the health and safety agencies, the health insurers who have actuarial interest, and the public-interest groups.

So, it comes down to the medical director or the physician who is guardian of the OHS records. The primary point of contention has been the release of information to the exposed worker. Much of the difficulty has arisen because there have been exposures to hazardous substances that have resulted, or can result, in impaired health, and employers have not wished potentially litigious situations to be aired. Yet, the basic premise of occupational medicine (or occupational health or industrial hygiene) is to control a hazardous situation so that harm will not accrue to the exposed employee.

The matter of loyalty arises, and the physician faces a choice—to provide information or to keep data from the employee. The OSHA standard [10] states as its purpose to provide employees and their designated representatives a right of access to relevant exposure and medical records and to provide the Assistant Secretary of the U.S. Department of Labor (DOL) the right of access "to yield both direct and indirect improvements in the detection, treatment, and prevention of occupational disease." Being a matter of law, the standard mandates observance, and the issue is no longer one of choice.

It has been the personal philosophy of the author that employees have the right to know their health status as determined by the present methods of environmental and medical measurement. Clinical records have been shared, for it has been the belief that, if there is free disclosure, the employee will not suspect the medical facility of retaining information that, in the opinion of the physician as representative of the employer, the worker should not have.* It has been found that efforts at preventive medicine will be more successful if there is a shared relationship in health care.

While this participation of individuals in their own health planning is encouraged and eagerly sought, the content of the record is scrupulously guarded so that it becomes known to no person unauthorized by the patient. Any violation of the principle that becomes known to plant personnel will soon lead to a break with the OHS, and the warm relationship that existed between the workers and the health personnel will disappear. Complaints will arise from shop stewards, there will be increased noncompliance with surveillance appointments, and destructive rumors will be circulated regarding the medical unit.

Counseling records present a problem, for there might be information concerning psychiatric states that could readily be misunderstood by a disturbed worker or one who is emotionally distressed. An eminent psychiatrist once fielded the question regarding the sanctity of records when he stated that "the record is whatever we say it is," and "my notes are not my records." In a university hospital, the records on psychiatric patients were considered "part of the educational process" and were not to be considered as medical records as such. In most situations in the author's personal experience, health care personnel conducting counseling were requested to enter into the worker's record a note, reading only the date of the visit and "Counseling session held." Whatever back-up notes might have existed were unknown to the director of the OHS.

Before leaving the issue of confidentiality and access to medical records, the essence of the OSHA standard might be recapitulated by stating that as of August 21, 1980, OSHA† and each worker or his or her representatives who have received written consent would be permitted to examine and copy an employer's records of exposure to toxic materials, per-

*Simmons [18] worded it well when he commented, "The interlocking domains of privacy, confidentiality, and informational requirements are receiving both extensive and intensive scrutiny. . . . The central and most pervasive principle governing wise resolution is this: Appropriate *balance* must be sought between a person's fundamental right to a degree of privacy and society's acquisition of information about itself in order to guide its activities, and, indeed, to assure its freedom."

*For a parallel thought, "Open knowledge of the record removes the patient's fantasies about treatment—fantasies that can lead to paranoid thinking and even to litigation." (See J. J. Brophy, Patients should be responsible for their own medical records. *N Engl J Med* 307:1530, 1982.)

†It must be noted that it has been ruled in several federal court cases that the National Institute for Safety and Health (NIOSH) has the right to subpoena employee medical records for occupational health investigations [19].

sonal medical records, and analysis based on those records. Access was to be provided no later than 15 days after a request. The standard applied to all general industry, construction, and maritime employers subject to OSHA 1970.

Lest it be forgotten, from the *Oath of Hippocrates,*

> Whatever, in connection with my professional practice, or not in connection with it, I may see or hear in the lives of men which ought not be spoken abroad I will not divulge, as reckoning that all such should be kept secret.

INFORMED CONSENT

The need for informing employee-patients in keeping with the concept of informed consent is probably less in an OHS than in a health care source where extensive diagnostic procedures—many of them invasive—are carried out and where major elective and emergency surgery is conducted. The principle does apply in certain aspects, however; if a test is advised as part of medical surveillance, and the employee refuses the procedure, the patient must be told of the consequences of omitting a recommended test. A note must be made in the patient's record indicating that a certain injunction was given. If there are alternatives to either a particular screening procedure or examination, the patient should be informed of the choice, and the entry note should reflect the discussion.

The doctrine enters into the administration of immunizing injections, the use of mydriatics and miotics in an occupational eyewear program if given by an ophthalmologist, the application of plaster jackets, and the prescribing of medications, among other activities. Every instruction or warning given a patient should be recorded in the folder and appropriately dated and signed. These annotations, if regularly recurring and standardized, can be imprinted by a rubber stamp.

It has become particularly significant in litigation that the date an employee was informed of a diagnosis be determined with exactitude, for the importance lies in its relationship to the statute of limitations. The application of this need is given special attention in cases of occupational disease where, in contradistinction to the sudden occurrence of an accidental injury, the disease will have an insidious onset.

It was the author's experience to convey to employees the results of a chest radiographic survey where the concern was one of asbestos-related disease. Because it was not possible to meet with the individual workers—there were 8,000 who were studied [20]—group sessions of about 100 workers were held weekly, and a notation concerning attendance and content of the meeting was made in each attendee's clinical record with a rubber stamp imprint. The note has passed scrutiny in depositions, being referred to without question by attorneys for both the claimants and the defendants.

In essence, whatever is given the employee in the way of instruction, interpretation, explanation, diagnosis, numerical or qualitative result, examination finding, or precautions regarding prescription medication side effects must be entered in the record. Further, when the information given may be negative—for example, an aberrant blood level of a substance, radiographic evidence of a disease process, or an important electrocardiogram (ECG) interpretation—the patient's acceptance, response, or emotional reaction must be noted. This reaction noted in reports has been brought to light for discussion during the giving of testimony. No interchange between OHS personnel and patient should remain unrecorded. It is time-consuming to be sure, but protective of all: the employee, the employer, and the occupational health physician or nurse. It has been suggested that the instructions given to the patient be signed, in the record, by *both* the physician and the patient, to avoid litigation. This procedure will often minimize or eliminate a patient's claim that he "was not told" or did not understand specific instructions [21].

CORRECTION OR CHANGE OF RECORD NOTATIONS

Entries in clinical records can be changed if an error is discovered in the original notation or if certain wording should be added. In the case of change, the words to be corrected should be lined out, leaving the original words legible, and the date and the signature of the person making the change entered just above the alteration, or in the margin or other clear space. Placing the word "Error" above the changes or in the margin will add to the clarification. Initials can be used only if the signator name appears close by, perhaps 2 or 3 inches below. If words are to be added, the same principle holds: Indicate the position of insertion with a caret (^), add the material, date, and sign. In California, any practitioner who alters a record with fraudulent intent is guilty of a misdemeanor [22], and one physician's insurance exchange will place a 50-percent surcharge on the professional liability policy of a physician if a medical record has been tampered with, for it makes a case virtually indefensible.

Under no circumstances should an entry be erased,

be covered with opaquing fluid, or have paper pasted over it. On one occasion a staff physician performed a preplacement medical examination and noted that the applicant presented a unilateral inguinal hernia. For some reason the attention of the medical director was brought to the new employee, possibly for verification of the finding, and after extensive reexamination with positional change, strain, and cough, no hernia was found, and the original physician was so informed. Rather than having an additional entry reflect the change of finding or difference in opinion, he clumsily erased the inked entry on the colored stock of the record form and noted the normality of the area, with blurring of the new inking. Another entry had to be made to clarify and explain the glitch if the record might ever be brought into court.

OTHER PRECAUTIONS

Ever since the push in medical school days to record lecture notes, physicians have developed their own shorthand systems in addition to the abbreviations commonly employed throughout the health care system. In clinical record maintenance, however, the use of abbreviations is to be discouraged, except for the ones that present no possibility of ambiguity in their interpretation.

There have been court cases with adverse decisions where the records were either inadequate or the initials used as abbreviations could be interpreted differently. Irrespective of the publication of several monographs listing medical and related abbreviations, a word or phrase should be spelled out completely if there is a chance of misreading.*

The selection of words appearing on printed forms can convey feelings and meanings. One OHS that uses a report form for the recording of data regarding an injury shows, in a space occupying one-quarter of the page, an outline diagram of the body, anterior and posterior views, to indicate the site of injury. Above the two illustrations appears the word "Alleges," which indicates immediately a lack of belief in the patient's history, implying that all injuries are alleged and never genuine.

In another installation that was being visited with students, it was noticed that the medical records bore colored tabs. On questioning, it was learned that the colors indicated various chronic disease states such as diabetes, epilepsy, hypertension, and so on. When asked what the black tab represented, we were given the code, and we read opposite that indicator, "medical nuisance"; with that bit of intelligence, the entire point of view of that particular service was given away. Presumably, there was no effort made to keep that information from the patients involved.

Nothing judgmental should be included in the record, and there should be no emotional interjections. An example of such an entry was cited by Parker [23] in a review of defective records: "How can I continue to treat this person in this hospital when lab studies I order never show up back on the chart? I don't know whether this patient has LE and I can't possibly know." Parker [23] comments, "The patient may or may not have had lupus, but if there were any suspicion of an injury and that chart goes to court, the credibility of the doctor, the conscientiousness of care and the organization of the hospital will be open to very high criticism. These notes have nothing to do with the care or treatment primarily; this is one doctor getting mad at the system."

Not to be included are remarks regarding previous treating physicians. It is customary for medical students and some house staff members to view all outside practitioners, dubbed L.M.D. (local medical doctor), as less than bright or knowledgeable. On occasion, deprecatory comments will appear in the record indicating that Dr. X "should have picked up this diagnosis." A record of this order cannot be defended, again, as far as credibility or conscientiousness of care might be concerned.

The expressions commonly employed in medical histories of "Patient denies such-and-such," or "disclaims X," or even "admits such-and-such" should not be used. They smack of accusations or challenges. The wording of "Patient states that he has not had herpes" frees the narrative of the near-adversary relationship.

Not too much has been said concerning the actual style used in medical records. While they need not reflect publishable material or the quality of articles in peer-reviewed journals, the content will possibly surface in a workers' compensation hearing, a third-party suit, or an action alleging malpractice. The document must make sense and must be useful. Warshaw [24] described the problem accurately when he wrote:

> History taking is an art in which many health professionals are not accomplished and recollection is often faulty. Records are often incomplete, handwriting illegible and entries made anonymously or signed by initials now not recognized. Individuals tend to get labeled on the basis of complaints rather than a considered diagnosis. Records

*For example, *NP* can mean "new patient" or "neuropsychiatric"; *PM* can stand for "afternoon," or "evening," or "prostatic massage"; *AA* is either "arteries" or "Alcoholics Anonymous"; and O might be "zero," or "normal," or "or." (These meanings are real and are taken from Office procedures: Write your standards for back-office work. *Patient Care* 8:168, 1974.)

are notoriously lacking in follow-up information. Decisional information that explains why physicians begin, stop or alter treatment, or why patients sometimes reject diagnostic or therapeutic proposals is frequently absent. Another frequent omission is some note of the communication between the patient and the doctor that might illuminate the perceptions of both with respect to the information they share.

Jargon, while understandable to fellow practitioners—members of the primary health care institutions—should be avoided because of the possible use of the record by members of other professions, employees' representatives, unions, or whatever person or organization to whom the patient has authorized the document's transmittal. As Bromage [25] indicated, functional communication assumes as its obligation the transfer of information and thought with brevity and exactitude. She observes, "It is not the conscious display of in-group phraseology that is the usual problem as much as the instinctive, taken-for-granted use by the hurried, unthinking, engrossed writer." The notes on which the record is built must be comprehensible and make sense irrespective of where they are being read.

A federal judge, Jack Weinstein [26], was irked with the continued use of bewildering verbiage when he ordered the government to rewrite the letter in which Medicare recipients are given the reason for reduction or rejection of their claims. He said, "The language used is bureaucratic gobbledygook, jargon, double talk, a form of officialese, federalese, insurancese, and double speak. It does not qualify as English." The same principle of clarity he sought is applicable to the preparation and maintenance of medical record contents.

Wish [27] emphasized the need for uncorrupted English and clear documentation when he wrote:

> Since the medical record is a legal document we owe it to ourselves not to hold the medical profession up to ridicule should such a record require deciphering in a public forum. We are witnessing increasing public pressure that financial, insurance and other legal documents be written in plain English, and the advent of "medical consumerism" with increased public access to patient records will no doubt lead to similar pressure on the medical profession. Only after we succeed . . . in being able to talk to one another will we be able to respond to the pressure from an increasingly sophisticated and demanding public.

COMMENT

A few of the standards regarding medical record services promulgated by the Joint Commission on Accreditation of Hospitals [28] are applicable to the OHS and summarize much of what has been said:

Standard I—An adequate medical record shall be maintained for every individual who is evaluated or treated.

Standard II—The record shall contain sufficient information to identify the patient, to support the diagnosis, to justify the treatment, and to document the results accurately.

Standard III—Medical records shall be confidential, secure, current, authenticated, legible, and complete.

HISTORICAL NOTE

Finally, through courtesy of a forgotten British writer, some lines of Shakespeare are cited, indicating that the need for written records is not a new concept [29]:

> Lady Macbeth: Yet here's a spot.
> Doctor of Physic: Hark! she speaks: I
> will set down what comes from
> her, to satisfy my remembrance
> the more strongly.

COMPUTERIZATION OF OCCUPATIONAL HEALTH INFORMATION

For a broad variety of reasons, it is necessary that industry be able to review expeditiously the data that have accumulated, and are currently being gathered, concerning the findings of the clinical and environmental examinations of multiple workers and workplaces. Regulatory agencies at the federal and state levels have mandated the collection of data involving both the workforce and the worksite. More occupational health data are being generated now than ever in the past, and they are being used not only to assess the present-day relationship of exposure to morbidity or mortality, but also to provide an information base (1) to aid in the control of untoward health effects, (2) to assist in future epidemiologic studies, (3) to serve certain current and possible future legal needs, and (4) to determine the health status of the labor force. The awareness of health hazards in contemporary and industrial processes has increased, and the public, most likely through both the print and broadcast media, have been acutely sensitized to the potential of chronic health changes secondary to long-term exposures to the stressors encountered at work—chemical, physical, biologic, and psychological. As public opinion in a democracy leads to legislative response—with openly declared policy and fiscally supported enactments for control—occupational health programs have multiplied in the clinical and environmental arenas.

From the operation of these efforts in preventive medicine have emerged vast bodies of data that defy handling and analysis by any system but electronic processing, with its various modes of access functions, software, and entry and output features.

There are other difficulties present with current data collection, and McDonagh, Smith, and Gutierrez [30] have epitomized these well:

Medical records, useful in managing the health aspects of individuals, are inadequate for population studies and for the evaluation of the safety of a process or a product.
Incomplete toxicologic data and a lack of awareness of all potential hazards can lead to the accumulation of inappropriate information.
Incomplete work histories preclude the establishment of associations between work exposures and health status.
Industrial hygiene exposure data may be inadequate.
Occupational health records in the paper mode do not lend themselves to extensive study.
Handwritten records often are indecipherable.
Data are not recorded in a standard manner within one site or from site to site.
Industrial hygiene monitoring data are not collected in a consistent manner.
Medical records are "diagnosis-oriented" rather than "symptom-oriented," thus compromising the ability to use medical information as an early indicator of disease.
There is insufficient detail in the recording of lifestyle histories and away-from-work exposures, potential contributors to occupational or nonoccupational illness [or potentiators of subclinical illness].

These 10 points make a familiar statement. OHS records are almost useless in population studies and frequently of little value in individual cases. Work histories are often totally neglected, and lifestyle detail is handled in a perfunctory manner that reveals little.

For the OHS director who desires to convert hand or mechanical operations to a computerized system, the picture has not been made any easier by the rush to the marketplace of multiple methods of building data bases and of techniques for extracting wanted answers or reports.

There are, however, certain basic questions to be raised and acknowledged when exploring this vast array of commercially available information systems. Further complicating the matter of simple choice is the presence already in most organizations of a complete data-processing facility, so the matter of program interface for automatic exchange of data with other systems or devices arises for review.

It might be of worth, before discussing methods, to define a data base, the essence of a computer information system. Wiederhold [31] views it simply as a collection of related data that are organized so that useful information can be extracted. A data base comprises certain components such as (1) file storage systems ("software to allocate and manage space for data kept on large computer storage devices, such as disks or tapes"); (2) file access methods ("software to rapidly access and update data stored on those devices"); (3) data description languages ("means to describe data so that users and machines can refer to data elements and aggregations of similar data elements conveniently and unambiguously"); and (4) data manipulation languages ("programs to allow the user to retrieve and process data conveniently") [31].

In an effort to introduce the subject, the director of one of the current occupational health systems has been asked to adapt a previously published paper for inclusion here, which should prove helpful to the neophyte who is beginning to explore the pertinent issues.

OCCUPATIONAL HEALTH DATA PROCESSING SYSTEMS*

Wanda Rappaport, Ph.D., Director, Occupational Health Systems, Flow General Inc., McLean, Virginia

Where does one start in defining requirements for an occupational health system? What functions and characteristics are needed? How will needs change in the future? Should one build or buy a system? How do commercially available systems really differ? These queries are just a few of the questions that companies ask as they decide on an occupational health data processing system (OHDPS).

In developing and marketing one of the major commercial OHDPSs, it has become clear that a group of critical functions and features are universally required in OHDPSs, irrespective of the industry and corporate variations.

OVERVIEW OF A SYSTEM

Occupational health data are automated in large companies as a matter of necessity. When more than a few hundred employees in a company are exposed to potentially hazardous agents, it is impossible to conduct a thorough health-surveillance program manually. The storage, retrieval, and analysis of data become too complex to ensure worker health, and thus the financial stability of the company. Automated systems are essential, and that is why the companies develop, buy, or timeshare OHDPSs.

These systems, such as the one diagrammed in Figure 12-7 support two primary groups of functions: monitoring employee health and workplace conditions. To perform these functions properly, many different types of data are required. Medical and industrial hygiene examination records obviously are needed. Also required is information about personal and workplace protective devices, such as the devices being used, their location, their inspection dates, and so on. What frequently is not realized is the requirement for extensive personnel and inventory data as well. Job and inventory shifts cause changes in employee exposures and are therefore critical to record in a data base. Figure 12-7 shows the relationships among the essential types of data in an occupational health system, and Figure 12-8 shows a typical data-base structure and the types of changes required to maintain up-to-date records within the data base.

The data-base linkages shown in Figure 12-8 testify to the dependence of an OHDPS on other corporate data bases if there is to be an efficient use of resources within the organization. A capability to interface between corporate personnel systems and the new or potential OHDPS is, therefore, an important consideration when systems are being evaluated.

DATA-BASE REQUIREMENTS

No two companies want to store exactly the same data in exactly the same manner. In fact, there often are differences among divisions and plants within a single company, so a system must allow for different data-base structures among users.

Despite the need for data-base variations, the same categories of data frequently emerge when discussing comprehensive requirements with medical staff members, industrial hygiene and safety specialists, epidemiologists, and toxicologists. Across companies and industries, these professionals must know about the health of employees, where they work, and to what environmental agents they are being exposed, at what levels, and for what length of time. Only with these data can the proper analyses be performed now, and in the future, to determine whether illnesses are occupationally related and if appropriate precautions are in effect.

Figure 12-9 shows the major categories of data that should be available in an OHDPS. It is not necessary to organize data into the same three major files, but it is essential that any item of data in any of the three major categories be capable of relating to any other element or elements in the other categories. Moreover, if specific items of data are not included in a system's data base, the capability must be available to incorporate them easily should the need arise among users of the system.

No OHS or industrial hygiene activity should be completely dependent on a vendor or a data-processing department to make such modifications to system records. A successful OHDPS be-

*Adapted from W. Rappaport. Rx for occupational health systems. *Ind Hyg News* 6:42, March 1983.

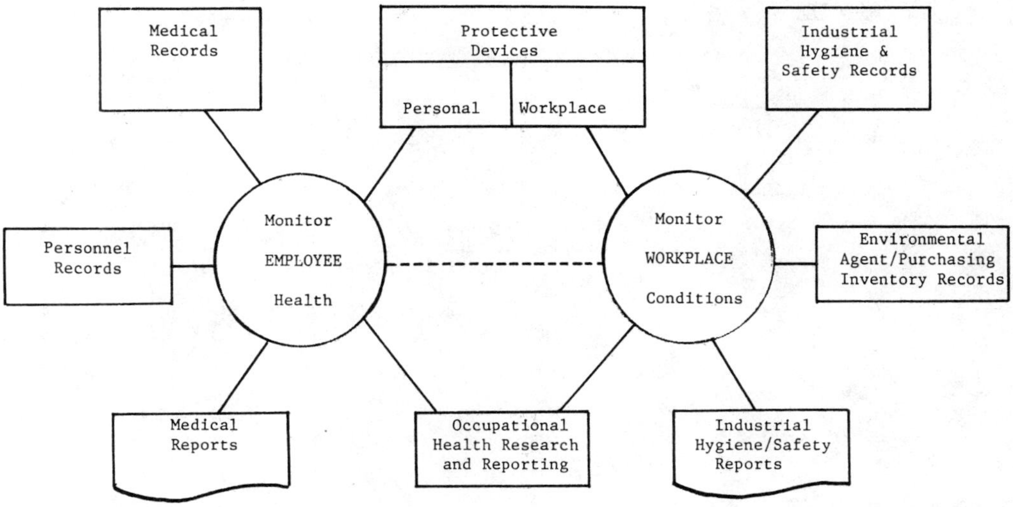

FIGURE 12-7. *Overview of an occupational health information system (OHIS). (Courtesy of Wanda Rappaport, Ph.D., Director, Health and Environmental Systems, Flow General, Inc., McLean, Virginia.)*

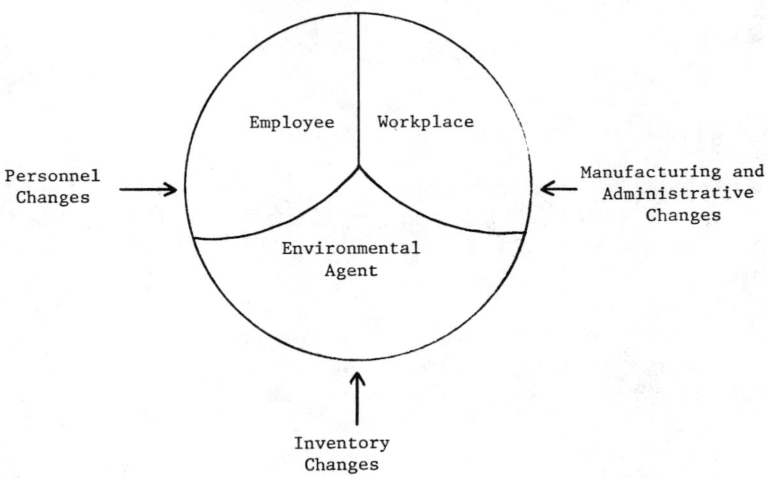

FIGURE 12-8. *Occupational health data base linkages,* Internal OHIS Data. *(Courtesy of Wanda Rappaport, Ph.D., Director, Health and Environmental Systems, Flow General, Inc., McLean, Virginia.)*

comes a part of the professional's performance. Flexibility and user independence in enhancing and modifying the system are key characteristics.

Several other features must be considered in evaluating or designing a comprehensive OHDPS. While standard coding schemes, such as CAS* or RTECS*, may not be required by all companies, the ability to accommodate standard codes, as well as individual company variations and synonyms, is necessary for companies that wish to compare their populations with industry norms and published studies.

*CAS = Chemical Abstracts Service [Registry Number].

*RTECS = *Registry of Toxic Effects of Chemical Substances*. Rockville, MD: U.S. Department of Health, Education, and Welfare (annotated periodically).

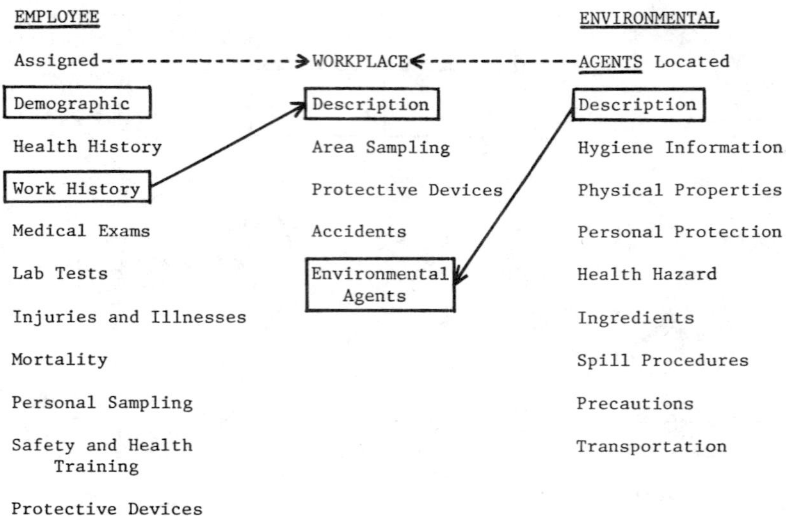

FIGURE 12-9. *Essential categories of data and relationships in an OHIS. (Courtesy of Wanda Rappaport, Ph.D., Director, Health and Environmental Systems, Flow General, Inc., McLean, Virginia.)*

ACCURACY AND CONFIDENTIALITY

Data accuracy, confidentiality, and security are paramount concerns within a medical environment. Data must be carefully edited before they become a permanent part of the data base. An OHDPS should automatically create an audit trail indicating when and by whom all data were entered. The system should ensure that each item is edited for length, character validity, and acceptable range. For some data items, such as date, data should be mandatory, and there should be a provision for key verification of critical items and sight verification of all others.

Confidentiality and security are best achieved by limiting access to system functions and the actual data stored in the system on a need-to-know basis. For example, the authority to change the data-base structure, or even the contents, should be controlled. There is no reason for clerical staff members in other departments to have access to industrial hygiene data. In some cases, it may be necessary to restrict access to specific individuals for selected records, as would be the case with highly confidential psychological or counseling data in an employee's record. In a multi-plant or multi-division environment, users in one location are unlikely to need access to the records of another location. However, corporate staff members charged with aggregating data for the entire company must have access to the data from all locations. All of these options should be regularly available.

RETRIEVAL, ANALYSIS, AND REPORTING REQUIREMENTS

One must be able to retrieve and analyze one's data without restriction. This capability, along with user independence in modifying the data base, is often the key to differentiating one system from another. There is no point in storing data if they cannot be retrieved, analyzed, and used effectively to protect workers and the company. Four major requirements are: (1) a capability for users to modify standard reports, (2) a capability for users to develop new reports, (3) an on-line query function, and (4) a complete statistical capability.

Most systems provide standard reports, but what happens when users do not want reports as they were designed by the system's developer? Some parts may be irrelevant, others may be missing, the users may not like the format, and reference ranges may change. Nothing is static in the occupational health field. In evaluating systems, one must learn how standard reports can be changed and how new ones can be developed. If one must depend on the vendor or one's own data-processing department, it can be extremely costly in terms of both money and time. Does one have to know a programming language to change or develop reports? What happens if federal or state regulations change and a new report is required in 3 months? The vendor may charge thousands of dollars to develop it, and there could be a 6-month backlog in one's own data-processing department, not an unusual situation. Make sure that one can, as a user, be independent of the vendor for changing and writing reports. Ideally, someone in the OHS should be able to perform these functions.

Authorized users of the system should be capable of utilizing a terminal to find out what data are stored for any environmental agent, workplace, or employee and to retrieve all the information about specific groups of workers and work locations, as based on an unlimited set of selection criteria. For example, one might wish to retrieve the complete medical and exposure history of all men and women who worked with a given group of chemicals for a specified period of time and have below-normal pulmonary function. This capability requires a so-called query language—an English language–like set of commands for the retrieval of data based on criteria specified by a nontechnical system user.

Analyzing the data retrieved through the query language requires a statistical capability. A comprehensive OHDPS should include a full range of statistical programs, preferably one of the three most widely used commercial packages.

How are these capabilities evaluated? Time must be spent becoming sufficiently familiar with any system that is being seriously considered to determine the extent to which it meets established requirements. Discover how the system handles routine tasks. It is essential to observe the system in operation and, ideally, to see how it can be tailored to meet one's needs. If a system falls short of requirements, one should note why and what it would take in terms of time and money to overcome the limitations. Also, one should not fail to consider the cost of future changes if there must be reliance upon the vendor.

MAINTENANCE AND OPERATION

Having the right persons to maintain and operate an OHS system is critical to success. One must make sure that an experienced OHDPS vendor, with an excellent track record, is asked for references, which subsequently must be checked. One must have all pertinent details in written form to avoid misunderstandings. Further, one should select and train employees carefully, and vendors must be willing to provide thorough training and immediate help when user problems arise. Experience, service, and people are essential in making a system succeed.

CONCERNS WITH VARIOUS SYSTEMS

The various contemporary occupational health information systems have been analyzed by Adrienne A. Whyte, Ph.D. [32], and as there are frequent enhancements made to the systems, the fact sheets making up the analyses are updated periodically. Whyte, in her review, follows a particular scheme of inquiry, and the features given below should be investigated before final consideration is reached regarding type, cost, interfacing capability, and facility for new programming. The elements entering her comparative analysis include system name, contact person, system components or function, hardware and software environment, type of terminals, language used, type of access, data-entry features, data-output features, codes, security features, software costs, and services included in cost.

One of the issues of concern to most users is that of the confidentiality of data, which in computers means security, or "security features." The following represent the features claimed by various producers or system developers, and one or more of these protective steps may aid in selection:

Client options.
Password access.
Document numbers printed, rather than names or social security numbers.
Back-up tapes held in a protective vault.
Meets federal requirements for security.
User IDs.
Any request that accesses the data base to generate a report requires a second password.
Tied terminal feature.
Restricted access to functions.

Restricted access for programming.
Scrambled social security numbers.
Multiple password-controlled functional access levels defined for each report.
User-defined data access profiles for individual users.
Separate disk drives for data base and transactions (for time-sharing use).
Vault storage of daily transaction tapes (for time-sharing use).
Terminal restrictions under operating system.
Audit trail for segment.
Layered access restrictions.
Patient numbers (unique) needed for access to individual records.
Names of individuals not on master records in the system.
Tied terminals for medical data.
User profile for system activity.
Additional password for access to each module.
Restricted access by module and functions within module.
Available to each user, segregated files and libraries that can be integrated for analyses.
Menu-restricted access.
Access protected at file level.
Managerial specification of each user's input, inquiry, and reporting privileges by system submodule.
Automated time-outs.
Data encryption.
Record restriction, by individual user, based on data item value.

STATE OF THE ART

In light of the increased need and use of computer-based information systems, particularly in companies involved with petrochemicals, to "deal with the individual and collective health experience of employees, with the qualitative and quantitative character of workplace exposures, and with the potential relationship between exposures and health" [33], a group of knowledgeable representatives of such companies was assembled in early 1981 to exchange information on the state of the art. Some salient features extracted from the many papers composing "Supplement on Medical Information Systems" [33], plus some updating, will provide guidelines in the conceptualization, development, and operation of a few exemplary systems.

Finucane and McDonagh [34] indicate the types of information needed for maximum effectiveness in a multidisciplinary occupational health program that comprises occupational medicine, toxicology, industrial hygiene, and epidemiology: (1) detailed worker and job histories and demographic data; (2) an inventory of potential exposures and their possible associated adverse health effects as they relate to specific work locations; (3) worksite exposure data; and (4) employee medical information collected throughout the worker's career, or, optimally, throughout his or her entire life.

A system that is well designed [34] will allow for (1) standardized consistent record-keeping procedures and data collection, thus improving the overall quality of health records; (2) a data base of continuous health and exposure information on employees that will facilitate epidemiologic studies; (3) facilitation and improvement of procedures for the collection and interpretation of workplace exposure monitoring data and the identification of the need for additional environmental controls; (4) efficient handling and analysis of the large amounts of data generated in occupational health programs through electronic data management technology; (5) support of administrative professional activities within the medical department on a daily basis; (6) an effective reporting system that will allow both health professionals and company managers to evaluate potential problems and the effectiveness of programs; and (7) enhancement of the response capabilities of the company to external and internal inquiries and allegations regarding health-related matters.

Sugano [35] approaches the problem of tracking employees, admitting that few employers can provide personal monitoring for every employee, every day, for every possible hazard to which that individual might be exposed, by defining relatively uniform exposure groups. From the identification of these groups, three general types of information can be reconstructed: the type(s) of hazards to which a worker may be exposed, the degree of severity of that exposure, and the time and duration of such exposure.

The employee subsets among which there is a similitude of exposure can be developed through (1) grouping by job description or title, (2) grouping by work location, and (3) grouping by process or activity unit. Sugano [35] points out that most companies attempt to classify worker-exposure groups by combining two of three methods (for example, electrician in Area B, Building 17). Care must be taken in tracking to recognize mobility among workers, where multiple exposures might be experienced, or to sharpen the meaning of duties of such personnel as "mechanics" or "laborers" for the sake of specificity. Generic titles can either cover multiple exposures or allow misassignment of hazardous contacts to workers free of such interactions with toxic substances. The basic qualities that a tracking system should possess, within the local constraints of budget, personnel, and existing data bases, are uniformity within the exposure groups, accuracy in classifying workers into proper exposure groups, adequacy of updating reviews, and cost-effectiveness. The establishment of groups for tracking might best be done conjointly by the industrial hygienist and the epidemiologist.

HEALTH INFORMATION SYSTEMS

OCCIDENTAL CHEMICAL CORPORATION

A system designed as COHESS (Computerized Occupational *H*ealth and *E*nvironmental *S*urveillance *S*ystem) and developed by the Diamond Shamrock Corporation was described initially by Hillman [36–40]. The system, as defined, is a computerized vehicle that codes, stores, and reproduces, according to program data on employee health, the work environment and potential hazards therein, for purposes of surveillance. Basic to the system are the three modules of employees, plant locations, and chemicals or, for ease of reference, *People, Places,* and *Things.*

People-related (employee health) information includes identifying information and all examination findings, personal sampling results (exposure data), and health incidents (clinic visits, laboratory test results, insurance claims information, workers' compensation data, accident episodes, illness-absence information, and death-certificate material). The design allows coding and entry of any useful datum relating to an employee's health. The ANSI 216.2-1962 (R. 1969) Codes (American National Standards Institute Method of Recording Basic Facts Relating to the Nature and Occurrence of Work Injuries) and the H-ICDA Codes (International Classification of Diseases, adapted for use in the United States, 8th revision, Hospital Adaptations) are used or expanded as need dictates.

Places-related information includes worker location, as divided into various geographic areas: corporation, company, division, facility, area, section, structure, and zone (specific place of exposure). In the more finite subdivisions, work activities and potential exposures are similar. An individual may be listed in as many as five zones, for there must be a 100-percent accounting for a worker's time.

In the *Things*-related information module, all information concerning chemicals, agents, and materials is stored, with the appropriately designated grid locations. The CAS (Chemical Abstract Service) numbers are used, and material regarding physical stressors, such as noise, can also be entered. Material Safety Data Sheets (MSDSs) are maintained by means of a Text Management interface.

The system is flexible and versatile, for there can be (1) utilization of existing forms, if desired; (2) change in form at any time without reprogramming; (3) again, without reprogramming, elements deleted or added in parallel with new mandates; and (4) capture of past data at the user's convenience.

A minicomputer in the OHS controls input, and clean data are passed on to the corporate mainframe computer. Scrambled social security numbers maintain confidentiality. As indicated by Hillman [36], the ultimate objective is the surveillance of the health status of employee populations in relation to their work environment, in order to detect the most subtle changes at the earliest possible moment.

COHESS is available through a license or lease agreement, the latter with an option toward purchase.

MONSANTO COMPANY

A system developed at the Monsanto Company of Saint Louis, Missouri, is entitled MEHI (Medical and Environmental Health Information System). As described by Elmer and Coleman and others [41–43], a data storage-and-retrieval capability in occupational health was needed for the usually stated purposes of (1) ongoing health monitoring, (2) tracking and comparing employees' exposures, (3) compliance with current and anticipated regulations, and (4) future epidemiologic studies.

Four of seven independent but integratable systems include (1) the Materials System (all substances in use in corporate inventory, with location, property, process, and health-effects details); (2) the Occupational Exposure System (a combination of personal and worksite monitoring and employee work histories); (3) the Medical System (all derived historical and medical event data); and (4) the Statistical Data Analysis/Epidemiology System (used to identify trends in exposure levels or health deviations). Originally, the Materials System was retained even though a joint agreement was reached to utilize COHESS. More recent system hardware and database modifications have eliminated COHESS programs and have resulted in a sophisticated information retrieval system that integrates data from any of the modules and can be accessed by medical and industrial hygiene functions in all world areas, for inquiry only.

Both CAS and RTECS numbers are used for the ease provided in electronic updating. Mixtures and combinations not possessing registry numbers are entered by a created nine-digit number series. Because of the need for security of company-confidential information—process components, substance locations, volumes, and so forth—a multilevel data-base security system is used. Personal IDs are needed for access by persons with a true "need-to-know."

Care was given the preparation of industrial hygiene measurement information for entry: accurate descriptions of the types of samples taken, including general area or fixed point, source, wipe, personal or breathing zone samples. Other information must define the units used in data collection as well as the type of determination, such as actual or calculated time-weighted average (TWA), ceiling determination, or engineering or job-task determinations. Cognizance must be had of the use of personal protective devices to distinguish between potential and actual exposures. The degree of validation of test methods relating to specific sample data must be noted.

Special forms with a common format for around-the-world use were matched with screens for medical data entry and were designed with checkboxes to reduce entry time. Scrambled social security numbers are employed for confidentiality, and the only resource for unscrambling is contained in the front-end minicomputer. Security is greater than with the traditional hard-copy files.

AMOCO CORPORATION (FORMERLY STANDARD OIL COMPANY [INDIANA])

In another petrochemical company a system was developed earlier than the imitation of many of the record-keeping methods currently in use. At Standard Oil Company (Indiana), Wolkonsky [44] experienced use of the Amoco System approximately since 1975. The sources of data for various inputs in demography, claims information, historical medical and clinical findings, industrial hygiene exposure records, and toxocologic and safety material were essentially the same as for other systems.

In 1982, however, as related by Spies [45], it was apparent that the system was in need of revision and improvement. After 3 years of development, in February 1985, a new computerized record system, the Medical Analysis and Reporting System (MARS), was placed in operation. It is an on-line system developed by Amoco and is tied directly into the company's mainframe computers. As it reacts with the corporate Human Resources information system, there is no need to store demographic data such as name, age, sex, and job title. Some of the system's features include

The ability to store the names and addresses of expatriate employees' dependents.
An on-line code data base that permits the addition of new codes when needed.
Forms designed by the medical department and produced in-house at considerable savings over purchased forms.
Scheduling capabilities for examinations.
Laboratory data tape interface with tapes provided by the testing laboratory.
Sophisticated on-line edits to ensure integrity of the data.
Audit and control reports to identify missing bits of information.
Data audit trails that list all key-entered transactions by users.
Several levels of tight security.

Unauthorized users are "abended" immediately and are listed on a security-violation report, which is produced each day. Monthly activity reports are generated for the medical department, and MARS can tie together all activities of a particular "case." Various clinical summaries are producible, and the system lends itself to statistical analysis and the research required in epidemiologic studies. Further, through the Amoco Audiogram Analysis System, audiometric test tapes produced either by vendors or in-house input can be accepted and analyzed, generating printed reports and employee notification letters. Anticipated in the future is access to industrial hygiene data for the creation of job-exposure profiles.

SMITHKLINE BECKMAN CORPORATION

When the then SmithKline of Philadelphia, a company producing pharmaceuticals, animal health products, consumer goods, medical diagnostics, ultrasonic devices, and eye care products, considered the development of a data processing system, of prime importance in design was the identification of data useful in epidemiologic studies. As reported by Hagstrom and coworkers [46–47], the following criteria were established for key "health effects" components. They must

Be objective and unequivocal.
Be easily measured.
Be reliable or repeatable, or both.
Occur with relatively high frequency.
Be predictive, or indicative, of early changes amenable to preventive measures.
Relate to the company's own unique workplace exposures.
Pose special problems for the pharmaceutical industry.

To be included in a computerized system, a health measure had to possess at least one of the seven characteristics.

Of interest is the job classification that is based on 10-digit codes, reflecting major divisions, departments, groups, and job categories. The objective is to identify workers fairly who have identical or similar jobs at one site, at different sites, or in different departments. As pointed out by Hagstrom and coworkers [46], the job code of a mechanic in pharmaceutical tablet manufacturing would have the same last three digits as those given a mechanic in the packaging department. Comparably, secretaries in those two departments would show the same terminal digits. A problem constantly to be faced is currency in the job codes, for some employees change jobs and others are on rotation.

To develop a methodology for the analysis of periodically occurring laboratory screening results by exposure category, defined by job code, a program utilizing the Statistical Package for the Social Sciences (SPSS), a software package, was written to provide summary measures in tabular form that then could be plotted, using Chart-Master. Each variable is examined in the tables and graphs according to mean, 95-percent ranges, and other values. For example, the varying levels of a standard blood parameter such as serum glutamic-oxaloacetic transaminase can be plotted for workers in different departments. Groups can be compared, and the layout allows readily the detection of group shifts in the distribution of various measures. The original system was designed for installation on a mainframe computer.

Design difficulties that were encountered have included the health professionals' lack of familiarity with computer terminology and the unfamiliarity of the computer staff with the occupational health lexicon. Further, the authors were surprised by the heavy user involvement at all phases of system development, the near impossibility of arriving at accurate cost estimates (no more than ± 50-percent accuracy), and the lack of surety regarding the number of persons needed for maintenance of the system throughout worldwide locations. Fortunately, with the advent of personal computers and fourth-generation computer languages, it was possible to implement the system on personal computers within the department, without further intervention by the systems group.

PHILLIPS PETROLEUM COMPANY

While the Phillips Petroleum Company program at Bartlesville, Oklahoma, Computerized Health and Environmental Surveillance System (CHESS) resembles other systems that have been described, it is of interest to list the types of reports stemming from each of four modules, current or planned, as described by LeBlanc [48].

Medical Module

Programmed reports	*Frequency*
Complete physical examination	On-line and on request
Diagnosis/surgery/cause of death summary	On request
Physical examination summary	Weekly
Temporary restrictions	Monthly
Morbidity forms	Monthly
Morbidity report	Quarterly
Morbidity summary	Quarterly
Morbidity forms list	
Morbidity statistics	Annually
Diagnosis summary	Quarterly
Permanent restrictions	On request
Analysis of physical examinations	Annually
Analysis of diagnosis	Annually
Mortality report	Annually
Mortality summary	Annually
Employee health status	Annually
Other reports by special programming	As needed

Employee Tracking Module (Programmed Reports)

Work history by employee

Work history by plant and by process, listing employees associated with the process, past and present

Correlation of employee-tracking data with data in other CHESS modules

Other reports by special programming, as needed

Toxicology Module (Programmed Reports)

Chemical inventory division, plant, location, employee, and job category

Chemical use rates

Material Safety Data Sheets (MSDS) form replication

Product label information

Industrial Hygiene Module (Programmed Reports)

Plant management, listing all air-sample concentrations

Exposure to principal chemical tested (TWA exposures only)

Greater than or equal to 50-percent Permissible Exposure Limit (PEL) summary

Greater than or equal to 100-percent PEL summary

Greater than or equal to ceiling limit summary

Greater than or equal to Short-Term Exposure Limit (STEL) summary

Location report, results by location and by chemical or contaminant

Employee-notification letters—normal (compliance) or abnormal (noncompliance)

Transmittal letter describing report to plant manager

Follow-up monitoring program status
Other reports developed through special programming, as needed

The system described for use at Phillips Petroleum Company was developed in-house, as it was believed that systems with the scope and flexibility that were needed were not commercially available.

STANDARD OIL COMPANY OF CALIFORNIA

The system developed for use at the Chevron Corporation (formerly the Standard Oil Company of California) [49,50], the Safety and Health Information Management system (SHIMS), resembles many of the methods of data entry and capture indicated previously. A cooking structure interrelates location, job assignment, and chemical-agent data. The SHIMS Control Center staff includes (1) an administrator who is responsible for the SHIMS computer and security, (2) a coordinator who is responsible for the data bases, (3) a user analyst who cares for job assignment and location coding, and (4) data processing assistants who maintain the data bases. The system licenses the Flow Gemini software package from Flow General Corporation and uses also company-developed programs operating on mainframe IBM computers.

SHELL OIL COMPANY

The Shell Oil Company's system, in use at Houston [51,52] was developed for the same surveillance needs as were other programs, but in addition, nonoccupational morbidity and mortality information was to be obtained to address the problems associated with the cost-containment of health care and to permit the conduct of in-house epidemiologic studies. Retrieved data can provide reliably structured responses to (1) employees and unions, (2) customers and the general public, (3) regulatory agencies, and (4) legislative and administrative bodies.

Six modules are linked together to compose an information network; the data bases operate in an Information Management System (IMS) data-base environment in an interactive mode. The six modules include *Personal Attributes* (the demographic data include records not only of current employees but of all pensioners and persons terminated since 1973), *Biometrics* (all medical findings and historical information), *Morbidity* (absence data using ICDA codes), *Mortality, Work Histories* (include a Job Exposure Profile [JEP] and a Work Histories file), and *Exposure Monitoring*.

Certain design considerations have provided for confidentiality, quality assurance, reliability, retrieval flexibility, expandability, and cost competitiveness. The system was developed in-house after an external search failed to disclose a commercially available system that would meet Shell Oil's needs. Within-system security of information is ensured through the use of passwords and data encryption and with the decryption limited to medical terminals. Duplicate copies of medical records are shredded.

The system, as concluded by Joyner and Pack [51], has met user expectations and has operated at less than forecast costs. Maintenance costs will approximate 35 percent of the system life-cycle costs, significantly below the 60-percent range encountered typically in commercial systems.

ALUMINUM COMPANY OF AMERICA

A significant note is sounded [53,54] in the description of the Aluminum Company of America (Alcoa) Health Information System, which is central to computerization efforts: "The System will enable medical and industrial hygiene personnel to divert their manual recordkeeping efforts to increased activities in preventive medical programs and health education." These professionals will have enhanced capability in the monitoring of occupational health in general, and greater staff efficiency and effectiveness were the expected end points.

E. I. DU PONT DE NEMOURS & COMPANY

Epidemiologic studies have characterized the DuPont occupational health program for many years, shedding light on such issues as the work capability of persons with certain chronic illnesses [55–57]. Because of this program strength, remarks concerning the DuPont surveillance program, as reviewed by Bonnet and Pell [58] and Fayerweather [59], will be limited to the use of an information system for purposes of occupational health epidemiology.

The epidemiology program comprises three components: (1) ongoing epidemiologic surveillance to measure morbidity and mortality in the company as a whole and in major manufacturing, laboratory, and office locations; (2) special studies, such as cohort and case-control studies, to investigate suspected hazards; and (3) the evaluation of preventive programs. Four company-wide computerized files serve as data sources, two of them containing the basic morbidity and mortality data collected regularly from all DuPont sites in the United States. One of the files relates to sickness absences that result in disability of 8 or more days, and the second contains information on the deaths among both active and retired employees.

The other two files, derivative of the first two collections, are a cancer registry and a coronary heart disease (CHD) registry. The insurance plan, from which most information is obtained, covers retirees as well as current employees. Morbidity data on the pensioners is important because (1) if there is a latent period between the time of first exposure to a substance and the time a disease caused by such exposure appears, the specific illness may not manifest itself until the period of retirement; (2) employees with a fatal illness who retire early because of disability would not be included in the company's death rates if the mortality data were not inclusive of retirees; and (3) the recent liberalization of pension plans has increased substantially the number of retirees.

The Cancer Registry, including supplemental reports from company physicians, holds such information as work histories both before and after beginning employment with DuPont, smoking histories, methods of diagnosis verification, histologic types of the tumors reported, and histories of exposure to known or suspected carcinogens.

The Coronary-Heart-Disease Registry covers two categories of CHD: acute myocardial infarction supported by ECG evidence and sudden deaths attributed to CHD. Persons with coronary insufficiency, angina, or other forms of ischemic heart disease are not included. Disease registries of the type described surpass clinical medical records as sources of morbidity data for epidemiologic studies because cases are reported by mechanisms ensuring complete or nearly complete case findings, standard diagnostic criteria are used to determine inclusion in the registry, and follow-up procedures are used to obtain missing information or to verify available information.

One additional feature of the DuPont system as it relates to the maintenance of morbidity and mortality files consists of a special computer program that will generate appropriate letters to on-site physicians for further information or for verification or clarification of diagnoses.

EXXON CHEMICAL COMPANY

An issue central to any health information system is the capability of tracking employees. Smith, Gutierrez, and McDonagh [60], in their presentation of the Exxon system, discuss this element of the protocol. The health information system tracks process workers to a post, a specifically designated location within the larger unit (specific grouping of equipment and components related to a specific process, product, or function), for example, chief operator on a chlorobutyl unit. Mechanical workers, in contradistinction, are tracked by area (containing one to three units) and craft (groupings of detailed skills as determined by local custom*), such as metals worker, instrument technician, or rigger. If the mechanical workers are highly mobile, great emphasis is placed on tracking by craft and types of tasks performed. Plant shutdowns for maintenance, possibly thought of as times of lessened exposure, actually are periods of higher exposure risk, and time-keeping codes are used by the system in identifying employees involved in such projects. Not only are employees scheduled for health examinations by the Medical Surveillance Module, as is common to many of the information systems, but they are also computer-scheduled for toxic-hazard training.

INTERNATIONAL BUSINESS MACHINES CORPORATION

ECHOES, IBM's Environmental, Chemical, and Occupational Evaluation System, was designed, as were the previously cited systems, to help collect, store, retrieve, and summarize data related to health and the environment [61,62]. The expressed purposes were to provide a standardized format for the gathering of medical and job-related information, to improve the accuracy of these data, and to facilitate retrieval and comparison with earlier and related information.

While ECHOES as it was conceived originally is not, except for the Chemical Data System, in current use, the concepts inherent in the system are still pertinent to occupational health information systems, so the capabilities will be outlined. The only part of the system other than the Chemical Data System that is presently in use is a revised form of the industrial hygienist's input. There is a good likelihood that with expansion and improvement of ECHOES, many features of the original design will be included.

The Chemical Data System is based on IBM's expanded version of the MSDS, and through a powerful on-line retrieval system, authorized users can access the most recent information. For instance, one could obtain just the medical section data concerning a single substance and have the material displayed on a screen and, if needed, create a hard copy on an adjacent printer. As Hillman [61,62] cites another example, if one wished to scan the entire data base and select only substances used at Plant D that have a boiling point of less than 0° C, that should be avoided by persons with liver disease, that are manufactured by the XYZ Chemical Company, and that are not carcinogenic, mutagenic, or teratogenic, then the user would present those variables to the system.

*As is well-known, certain skills associated with a craft in one area may be assumed by another craft in a different geographic location. Further, craft designations themselves may differ for the same sets of skills.

The entire file would be scanned, and in less than 30 seconds there would be a display (and a printed copy, if desired) of those substances meeting the criteria presented.

An Environmental Summary Form is used to collect information concerning the substances with which a worker is in contact. The employee's manager completes the form, it is machine-read, and the data are entered into the computer. Every substance to which there has been exposure by the worker is entered and retained; a single person may have many unique employee/chemical records, indicative of substances used in the past or to which the worker is presently exposed.

The Environmental Measurement Form, used to record the actual level of environmental exposure, also is machine-processible and is initiated by the industrial hygienist. As indicated, this information, at present, is the only data collected and entered into the system routinely. Machine-readable cards are no longer used, all data entry being accomplished through use of an IBM microcomputer.

Medical department action is determined by a presenting option chosen through medical review. These include *no test required, do usual tests,* or *test regardless.* If testing is required because an exposure level has been exceeded, the system will automatically generate a schedule for the appropriate medical test procedures called for in the Medical Section of the Chemical Data Base. The system will scan the Chemical Data Base for possible synergistic health effects resulting from multiple exposures. If such are found, the medical department is issued a precluding condition report. In addition, a report is generated if the system determines that the employee has a medical condition that should exclude him or her from contact with the substance concerned.

Examinations are scheduled automatically to be conducted in the employee's month of birth. As an individual may be subject to several test procedures, all are clumped to avoid unnecessary examining, to minimize inconvenience to the worker, to eliminate needless time away from the job, and to allow the medical facility to carry out multipurpose reviews. The schedules are provided 1 month in advance.

The IBM system has undergone study after 3 years of operation. Although not readily appreciated, the potential exposures are legion, for as the company moved from the manufacture of time clocks, scales, and tabulating machines to the production of computers and microcircuits, many of the mechanical and electromechanical methods of manufacture were replaced by high-technology chemical processes. Currently over 5,000 chemicals and more than 17,000 formulations are in use, supporting the product line. Timlin, Hillman, and Peterson [63] have discussed the origin of ECHOES, the mode of operation, and some of the functional difficulties.

Many of the products in use represented unknown ingredients' data, which made surveillance scheduling difficult. Manufacturers and formulators were reluctant to disclose various compositions for fear of compromising so-called trade secrets. In place of scheduling an unneeded examination, the system now generates a report indicating a worker's exposure and stating that insufficient health-effects information is available to permit scientifically rationalized examination. Medical judgment is relied upon, and if it is believed that surveillance procedures should be conducted, then an Examination Forecast Card is completed and the system schedules examinations at the indicated frequency.

To allow maximal efficiency of an information system, the personnel data base must be current to reflect employee transfers, shift changes, and even moves to different plants. Without on-line personnel data, ECHOES would schedule workers for examination after a move, post-retirement, or after contact with chemicals had ceased. An on-line, real-time personnel data base is mandatory for medical department currency.

The use of the machine-readable Environmental Summary Form and Environmental Measurement Form allowed entry of contact time and exposure measurement data. These proved to be not so "user-friendly" as desired by involved personnel. The users have "pressed" for local on-line input and output capability in light of the increased availability of personal computers and satellite techniques for improved telecommunication between computers. All medical and industrial hygiene personnel felt that personal computers would be much more serviceable, particularly in day-to-day tasks such as appointment scheduling for physicians and nurses and, in industrial hygiene, in providing assistance in calculations and graphic exposure reports to employees. Another deficit expressed by the users was that ECHOES, because the system used factual, numeric information, failed to accept entry of professional judgment, such as developed by walk-through surveys.

In a special six-plant study, it was found that certain health and safety personnel users were frustrated with ECHOES. Recommended were improved industrial hygiene components, a review for accuracy of all MSDSs, and greater emphasis on statistical and epidemiologic analysis and reporting of data. Subsequently, a special internal team reviewed the system and made several recommendations:

Local and central health and safety information systems were necessary.

A simplified set of MSDSs was needed, with a priority to be established so that greater attention could be given the more hazardous substances.

A statistical analysis and reporting package should be incorporated into the system.

A system should be developed and implemented in a structured and phased manner, with documented objectives, defined tasks, prescribed completion criteria, management decision checkpoints, and realistically estimated time schedules and resource requirements.

An accurate and current personnel system is essential for successful system operation.

A better tracking protocol is needed, to tell "who works with what."

Revision and enhancement are required, better to direct resources toward operations in need of professional health and safety attention.

A health information system is cost-effective through the saving of time, health, and safety of personnel.

This recognition of faults bespeaks an honest analysis of the seminal design and implementation of a large and ambitious system. The authors believe that personal computers will be placed in medical and related facilities, so that terminal entry will replace batch processing of machine-readable documents. End users will be more involved in the information systems, as short-supply programmers become absorbed by large-scale data management applications. The conclusions of the IBM review can serve as guides for those OHSs yet to develop their own systems.

OTHER ORGANIZATIONS

Several other companies have reported on the details of their particular information systems, either in operation or in the planning stages [64–70]. Plucked from some of these reviews are interesting items. A risk code, provided by Stallard [68], offers a gradient in exposure that might prove useful:

Risk Code	*Exposure*
0	None, or negligible exposure
1	Intermittent exposure below an action level
2	Continuous exposure below an action level
3	Intermittent exposure above an action level and below the threshold limit value (TLV) or PEL
4	Continuous exposure above an action level and below the TLV or PEL
5	Intermittent exposure above the TLV or PEL or occasionally above a short-term exposure (STEL)
6	Continuous exposure above the TLV or PEL or frequently above the PEL
7	Past exposure, no current exposure

In the system delineated by Robinson and Wood [65], various chemical modules are given, and some of the data collected are derived from a Health Status Assessment (HSA) form, part of the company's Health Care Management (HCM), defined as the application of business management methods to health care. One of the areas of inquiry is of interest, for the responses are rarely sought in occupational health settings. The form reads, in part:

Patient Attitude Toward:

A.	Life Problems	☐1. Fulfilled
		☐2. Just Coping
		☐3. Overwhelmed
B.	NYT* Medical	☐1. Trust
		☐2. Caution
		☐3. Hostility

In a diagram of health management, a market survey does not seem out of place.

COMMENT

The conference that comprised reports by representatives of 21 companies mentioned previously was summarized by Joiner [71]. Each system proved to be unique, and one could not have served any of the other companies by direct duplication. Even those medical information systems that began with purchase of an off-the-shelf package—COHESS [36–39] or HEMS [44,45]—needed modification before becoming functional in a different setting.

Systems that were successful in meeting local needs were sophisticated interactive programs fully supported by their users, all of whom, irrespective of health or safety or computer science discipline, have been involved in the design. In each system was a compromise between optimum and practical approaches in achieving corporate goals. The successful system was flexible, cost-efficient, and fulfilled current and some future needs of the organization.

Common to all systems was the need for hard work, imagination, and a perception of a void and a mechanism to fill it. Joiner [71] listed the elements of commonality among the surveillance systems as

Flexibility
Interaction

*New York Telephone Company.

User friendliness
Modular design
Valid data base
Economy
Innovation
Key staff
Commitment
Phased approach

Input information must be verified and validated whenever possible, for there is no place for data that are questionable, inaccurate, imprecise, or unreliable. In addition to being applicable, the data must be objective, reliable, replicable, discrete, unequivocal, easily obtained, representative of the workplace from which they were obtained, and quickly and inexpensively collected.

The phases of development of a system, as summarized by Joiner [71], include

1. Feasibility study
2. Planning and identifying of potential users
3. Designing the system and defining components (system development and modification)
4. Implementing
5. Operating
6. Maintaining
7. Upgrading the system

Certain decisions must be made when an organization contemplates development of a health information system. An on-line, interactive system is more costly than the use of batch or off-line transmission; yet, real-time decisions are only feasible with on-line connections—when emergency medical information is needed, for example, for a potentially exposed employee. Usually a compromise position is selected, putting on-line those functions for which there will be immediate need and retaining those activities in an off-line mode when there is no need for urgency.

Time may be the factor in determining if a system should be designed in-house or if a commercial package should be purchased. If time is not constraining, greater efficiency might result from local design.

As in any occupational health–related project, success is ensured only with top-manager commitment and equal dedication by the data-generating and user components of the organization.

In substance, the development of a system is costly, lengthy, demanding of many conjoint efforts, and subject to change on completion, but in the end, the system will result in better health surveillance, improved well-being of the workers, and the greatest opportunity for the practice of true preventive medicine, nursing, industrial hygiene, and safety.

ADJUNCTIVE OR EXTERNAL DATA BASES

As there is a constant need for updated information about the toxicity of certain chemicals, or epidemiologic or clinical findings among exposed worker groups, a variety of computerized data bases can be searched through various libraries on the online network. Charges will vary from none to a modest fee to recover communication costs incurred for staff time and for the time of connection to the National Library of Medicine (NLM) computers.*

The NLM computers can be accessed by computer terminals that are connected to the central computer facility at the NLM. MEDLARS (Medical Literature Analysis and Retrieval System) is available through a network of centers nationwide, located in over 1,000 universities, schools of medicine, hospitals, governmental agencies, and commercial establishments. Information can be reviewed at local terminals, or printouts can be mailed within a day.

Not part of NLM, but still a governmental source, is a reference center developed by NIOSH† (National Institute for Occupational Safety and Health)—with over 120,000 documents in occupational safety and health, the majority post-1973.

Innumerable specialized data bases exist, covering toxicology, oncology, environmental pollution, mental health, and the history of medicine, among others. Referral can be made through contact with a local medical library.

SPECIALIZED APPLICATIONS

While the systems reviewed to this point cover most needs in occupational health, certain types of work exposure may require programming for a single medical surveillance protocol. In hearing conservation activities, on-line audiometers are in use. In the textile industry where the work contactant is cotton dust, considerable attention is given to pulmonary function evaluation, and detailed reports can be generated.

In an application unrelated to the collection of occupational health data concerning workers, clinical findings, exposure levels, and the like is the use of the computer for the establishment and maintenance of an occupational health reference library. While it

*National Library of Medicine, 8600 Rockville Pike, Bethesda, MD 20209.

†NIOSH, Parklawn Building, 5500 Fisher Lane, Rockville, MD 20857, and Division of Technical Services, NIOSH, 4676 Columbia Parkway, Cincinnati, OH 45226.

is convenient to request a literature search through the nearest MEDLARS coordinating center, the information may be needed immediately in hard copy. Further, certain historic pieces will be sought that antedate banking in the mid- to late 1960s, or even in the 1970s.

While a vertical file, maintained in keeping with a detailed index, is of extreme value, items do get misfiled, and cross-indexing is time-consuming and frequently difficult. Mastromatteo [72] has developed a system in which key words are assigned to published articles. Information involving the key word(s), author(s), organization, journal, publication, and so on, is keypunched, and printouts of the various indexes showing accession numbers direct one to the body of literature on file. If the facilities and fiscal support are available, this type of computerized system meets the needs of a specialized reference collection in occupational health. The sequential accession numbers permit great ease in filing, without reference to title, author, or subject matter.

MEDICAL AND OCCUPATIONAL HISTORIES

From the earliest days in medical school one is trained to obtain histories that not only will provide the chronology of the disease entity that one hopes to identify at tunnel's end but in addition will allow one to tease out the many factors that impact themselves on those persons we are privileged to attend. As work is a social activity carried on in an institution, one must learn as much as possible of the worker both as a patient and as a human being, with goals, aspirations, frustrations, anxieties, and hope, who attempts to meet the daily responsibilities in life.

To penetrate the protective wall that many employees erect around themselves requires tact, concern, purposeful intention, empathy, and compassion. With these qualities in evidence, a detailed history is the inevitable goal, fully illuminative of both the individual and the problem presented. Histories in occupational medicine are of two types: (1) the traditional review of past illnesses, the salient health features of the respondent's family, contemporary practices in the use of both prescribed medicinals and habituating substances, and the story of the current difficulty, and (2) the lifetime summation of all work activities with their concomitant exposures to a variety of environmental stressors.

Both history formats are needed in an understanding of the new employee, the incumbent who is seen intermittently, and the worker who presents with a possible job-related illness. An effort will be made to delineate the requirements of productive historical documentation.

MEDICAL HISTORIES

The accustomed gestalt of a medical history is known not only to physicians but also to all who compose the occupational health team. Where the difference lies today in industry is that the history might be obtained by the use of a questionnaire to be completed by the patient or by presentation on the screen of a visual display terminal (VDT).* Rarely, because of numbers, is a medical history obtained through the more time-consuming method of query-response as conducted by the occupational health physician or nurse.

Irrespective of the method of acquiring answers, positive responses are signals for further elaboration, the filling in of missing details, or a need for ancillary information. A "yes" reply that goes by without further expansion might deprive the main body of the history of the significant points needed in the final meaningful assembly of data.

Because so many of today's OHSs employ a printed list of questions—probably eventually to be replaced by a respondent-operated terminal displaying branched queries—a list is offered in Table 12-1 that comprises the main items asked employees, as culled from a large collection of history forms currently in use. The list is offered (1) as suggestions for selected inclusion in a new history layout, if one is being contemplated; (2) for selection and local application, if appropriate to a particular work population or place; and (3) merely as a memory jogger of the areas that can be searched in the structuring of the patient's medical past. Strangely, practice seems to dictate many more questions for executives' health histories than for other personnel.

Printed history forms are available from several commercial sources. These questionnaires are of various styles from single page to brochure, employing carbons or carbonless copy paper, and when completed, some are computer-ready. Each prospective user must determine on a cost and individual basis the best route to follow—local design and production or direct purchase from vendors of available

*An example of an automated self-administered employee medical history is in the Info Med 100 (Besserman "history-taker") available from American Health Sciences Corporation, 6081 North 19th Avenue, Phoenix, AZ 85015.

TABLE 12-1. *Items for Selection and Use in the Development of a Medical History Form**

ALLERGIES	
Allergic to adhesive tape	Allergic to vaccines
Allergic to certain clothing	Asthma
Allergic to cosmetics	Hay fever
Allergic to food	Hives
Allergic to medicines	
BLOOD DISORDERS	
Anemia	Hodgkin's disease
Bad blood	Leukemia
Bleed excessively	Sickle cell disease
Blood condition	Sickle cell trait
Blood disorder	Syphilis
Bruise easily	
CARDIAC DISORDERS AND SYMPTOMS	
Angina	Heart skips beats
Ankle swelling	Heart trouble
Blood pressure high	Leaky heart valves
Blood pressure low	Pain in chest
Feet swelling	Pain in heart
Heart enlarged	Palpitations
Heart goes too fast	Pressure in chest
Heart murmurs	Short of breath
Heart pounds	Sleep on more than one pillow
CHEST AND RESPIRATORY DISORDERS	
Breast trouble	Nose stops up
Breathing blocked on one side	Nosebleeds
Bronchitis	Pleurisy
Clear throat frequently	Pneumonia
Cough	Pus in chest
Cough at night	Raise phlegm
Difficult breathing	Short of breath on a hill
Emphysema	Sinusitis
Fluid in chest	Sneezing
Frequent colds	Spit up anything
Hay fever	Shortness of breath
Heavy chest colds	Sore throats
Hoarseness	Tightness in chest
Lung trouble	Tonsillitis
Nose broken	Tuberculosis
Nose hurts	Tuberculosis contact
Nose runs	Wheezing in chest
ENDOCRINE DISORDERS	
Diabetes—take insulin (sugar diabetes)	Hair coarse
Diabetes—take oral medication	Hair dry
Enlarged glands	Perspire excessively
Goiter	Thyroid overactive
	Thyroid underactive

TABLE 12-1 *(continued)*

GASTROINTESTINAL DISORDERS AND SYMPTOMS	
Abdominal cramps	Hiatus hernia
Abdominal pain	Indigestion
Abnormal thirst	Internal parasites
Appendicitis	Intestinal worms
Appetite good	Jaundice
Appetite poor	Lip sores
Belching	Liver trouble
Bleeding from rectum	Loose bowel movements
Bloody diarrhea	Mouth sores
Bowel trouble	Nausea
Bridges, dental	Pancreas disease
Change in bowel habits	Piles (hemorrhoids)
Cirrhosis	Poor appetite
Coated tongue	Rectal disease
Colitis	Rupture
Constipation	Stomach pain
Diverticulosis	Stomach trouble
Duodenal ulcer	Stomach ulcer
Dysentery	Stools black like tar
False teeth	Swallowing difficulty
Feel bloated after eating	Teeth straightened
Gallbladder disease	Thirst excessive
Gas excessive	Tongue sore
Gas pain	Toothache
Gulp food	Ulcer
Gum infections	Ulcerative colitis
Gums bleeding	Upset stomachs
Gums sore	Yellow jaundice
Heartburn	Vomiting
Hemorrhoids (piles)	Vomiting blood
Hepatitis	Worms
Hernia	
GENERAL DISEASE ENTITIES	
Heatstroke	Sunstroke
GENITOURINARY DISORDERS AND SYMPTOMS	
Abortions	Pap smears
Albumen in the urine	Painful urination
Bedwetting between ages 8 and 14	Pregnancies
Bedwetting now	Pregnancy complications
Bladder trouble	Premature births
Blood in the urine	Prostate trouble
Breast lump	Prostatitis
Bright's disease	Stillbirths
Cesarean sections	Sore on the privates
Change in sexual desire	Stones passed in urine
Clap	Testicle lump
Cystitis	Tubes inflamed
Erection difficulty	Urinate more than before
Frequent urination	Urine changed color

TABLE 12-1 *(continued)*

GENITOURINARY DISORDERS AND SYMPTOMS *(continued)*	
Get up at night to urinate	Urine passed unintentionally
Gonorrhea	Urine smells bad
Kidney stone	Vaginal bleeding
Menstrual cramps	Vaginal discharge
Miscarriages	Vaginal itching
Nephritis	
HABITS	
Beer—glasses/day	Pipes stopped (year)
Whiskey—ounces/day	Snuff/day
Cigars/day	Snuff started (age)
Cigars started (year)	Snuff stopped (age)
Cigars stopped (year)	Chewing tobacco (day)
Cigarettes/day	Medicines taken
Cigarettes inhaled	Exercise taken
Cigarettes started (year)	Sleep/night
Cigarettes stopped (year)	Alcoholism
Pipefuls/day	Drug addiction
Pipes started (year)	
DIET	
Salt/day	Bread/week
Eggs/week	Potatoes/week
Beef/week	Coffee/day
Pork/week	Tea/day
Fish/week	Soft drinks/day
Whole milk/week	Gained weight in last year
Oil/week	Lost weight in last year
Nuts/week	Weight stayed the same in last years
HEARING	
See Chapter 16	
INFECTIONS (BACTERIAL, FUNGAL, VIRAL)	
AIDS	Pleurisy
Amebic dysentery	Pneumonia
Brucellosis	Poliomyelitis
Chickenpox	Rocky Mountain spotted fever
Dengue fever	Rheumatic fever
Diphtheria	Scarlet fever
Epstein-Barr virus infection	Shingles
Encephalitis	Smallpox
German measles	St. Vitus dance (chorea)
Gland trouble	Syphilis
Gonorrhea	Tetanus
Hepatitis	Tonsillitis
Histoplasmosis	Tuberculosis
Infectious mononucleosis (or "mono")	Typhoid fever
Influenza	Typhus fever
Malaria	Undulant fever
Measles	Valley fever
Meningitis	Venereal disease

TABLE 12-1 *(continued)*

INFECTIONS (BACTERIAL, FUNGAL, VIRAL) *(continued)*	
Mumps	Virus infection
Night sweats	Whooping cough
MEDICATIONS	
Aspirin	Laxatives
Appetite depressants	Sedatives
Blood medicine	Sleeping medicine
Diabetes medicines	Steroids
Diuretics (water pills)	Thyroid medicine
Iron	Tranquilizers
Hormones	Vitamins
MENTAL AND EMOTIONAL ILLNESS	
Anxiety	Nervousness
Bored	Neurosis
Cry easily	Not effective
Depression	Migraine headaches
Delusions	People think I drink too much
Feel blue	Relocation is difficult
Feel inferior	Sensitive
Feel lonely	Shyness
Feelings easily hurt	Suicide attempted
Get a raw deal from life	Suicide considered
Hallucinations	Thinking confused
Insanity	Unhappy
Nervous breakdown	Worrisome
MISCELLANEOUS	
Accidents	Military service
Country of birth of parents	Place of birth
Date of birth	Rejected by armed services
Date of last examination by physician	Rejected for employment
Disability pension	Rejected for insurance
Discharged from hospital against medical advice	Results of skin tests
Education	Surgical operations
Hobbies	Surgery recommended, not undergone
Hospitalizations	Travel abroad
Immunizations	X-ray treatments
Lived abroad	Any problem to be talked over with physician
NEOPLASMS	
Cancer	Growth
Lumps	Malignancy
Tumors	
NERVOUS SYSTEM DISORDERS	
Blackouts	Memory loss
Clumsiness	Misunderstood by others
Concussion	Motion sickness
Convulsions	Nervousness
Difficulty in writing	Neuritis
Dizziness	Neuralgia

TABLE 12-1 *(continued)*

NERVOUS SYSTEM DISORDERS *(continued)*	
Epilepsy	Nightmares
Fainting spells	Numbness
Feeling sad or alone	Paralysis
Fits	Parkinsonism
Handwriting changed	Sleepwalker
Hard to concentrate	Speech defect, other
Headaches	Spells of total exhaustion
Head injury	Stammer
Keyed up or jittery	Stutter
Knocked unconscious	Unconscious spells
Lose ability to smell	Wake up tired
Lost "pep"	Weakness
Making up mind difficult	Worry
SKELETAL DISORDERS AND SYMPTOMS	
Amputations	Gout
Ankle injury	Head injury
Arthritis	Knee injury
Back brace worn	Lameness
Back injury	Muscle weakness
Back sprain	Muscular disorder
Back trouble	Neck injury
Backache	Painful joints
Birth defect	Rheumatism
Bone infections	Shoulder injury
Broken bones	Spine trouble
Disc ruptured	Stiff joints
Dislocation of joints	Swollen joints
Feet painful	Trick elbow
Feet weak	Trick knee
Foot injury	Trick shoulder
Fractures	Wear corrective shoes
SKIN DISORDERS OR SYMPTOMS	
Acne now	Nail picking
Acne when young	Numbness of skin
Boils	Persistent sore
Eczema	Pimples
Face flushes	Ringworm
Itching skin	Skin rash
Jock itch	Skin sensitive or tender
Jungle rot	Skin twitching
Moles changing	Sweat in cold weather
Nail biting	Tingling of skin
VASCULAR DISORDERS	
Apoplexy	Phlebitis
Clots in veins	Stroke
Hands and feet cold	Thrombophlebitis
Leg cramp at night	Varicose veins
Leg cramp when walking	

TABLE 12-1 *(continued)*

VISUAL DISTURBANCES	
Artificial eye	Eyesight blacked out
Blind spots	Glasses worn
Blindness	Glasses worn for reading
Cataracts	Glaucoma
Color blindness	Redness of eyes
Contact lenses worn	See spots
Double vision	Trouble seeing at night
Eyes hurt	Vision blurred
Eyes water	Vision changed

*Items can be developed individually, can be mixed by organ system, or can be clustered in response to such questions as "Have you ever had . . . ?", "Have you ever been told you had . . . ?", "Do you now have . . . ?", "Have you ever had or have you now . . . ?", "Please check the appropriate answer (yes, no, don't know).", "Mark an X in the boxes to indicate past or present health problems (past, now).", "Are you bothered with or ever had . . . ?", etc. Questions may use lay equivalents, for example, "nervous breakdown." As pointed up by Vann A. Brewster, M.D. (personal communication, 1980), asking questions in the mode of "Do you have back trouble?" is meaningless and open to misrepresentation. He opts for the more specific, symptom-related, "Have you ever had back pain?" or the action-related "Have you ever seen a physician for back trouble?" or "Have you ever had a back x-ray?" These points should govern history-questionnaire design.

copyrighted forms. Either one will accomplish the goal if adequate instruction is given the respondent. Some of the forms are available in other languages if bilingual need exists. Further, specific history formats are available from some sources, such as questionnaires for cardiac history, respiratory disease review, and the like.

It will be noted in the items shown in Table 12-1 that the same topic for questioning might be phrased in different ways. It is common experience that medical terms are not readily understood by lay persons, particularly manual workers, so that there should be no hesitancy in using words that are in common parlance. It is advisable also that questions be asked in a manner that allows "no" responses to be significant. Often an applicant for a job will go directly down marking every answer "no," believing that positive responses will adversely affect employment. Such a method of reply is, of course, meaningless.

There might be need for phrasing some of the items in the colloquial terminology of the area. For example, in the Southeast people speak of "a rising" (furuncle, cellulitis), a "side ache" (appendicitis), or a "bealed ear" (otitis media). If these cultural variants are commonplace, it would be wise to translate the more correct designations into local folk words.

FAMILY HISTORY

Again, only by way of reminders for form design in the development of history questionnaires, the following are the usual relatives asked about in obtaining a family history: father, mother, brothers, sisters, mother's mother, mother's father, father's mother, father's father, wife or husband (present or former), sons, daughters, and grandchildren.

One covers usually only a certain number of diseases in connection with the family history for two reasons: (1) Rarely is the true cause of death known by surviving relatives, and (2) families are not usually made privy to the correct designations of rare clinical disorders but, instead, are given lay or media equivalents that frequently are not remembered. The diseases that should suffice in this area of history development are the following: arthritis, asthma, bleeding tendency, cancer, diabetes, epilepsy, heart trouble (heart attack), high blood pressure, kidney trouble, miscarriages, nervous breakdown, stroke, ulcer, or intestinal problems.

OCCUPATIONAL HISTORIES

It has become almost a literary cliché to quote Bernardino Ramazzini [73] in this context, but it was he in the early 1700s who verbalized the need to affix another thought to the counsel of Hippocrates when meeting with a patient: "I may venture to add one more question: What occupation does he follow?" In spite of the passage of nearly three centuries since this simple advice was first published, and even with the popularity of Sherlock Holmes's quick identification of a client's occupation from miniscule clues—

via Sir Arthur Conan Doyle, M.D.,* as learned from his mentor, Dr. Joseph Bell of Edinburgh—little attention has been given a person's work by the attending physician. Ramazzini lamented further this lack of inquiry when he wrote, "In medical practice, however, I find that attention is hardly ever paid to this matter, or if the doctor in attendance knows it without asking, he gives little heed to it, though for effective treatment evidence of this sort has the utmost weight."

There have been contemporary comments regarding this lack of search not only for occupational data but also for good historic medical material. Feinstein [75] has complained that history-taking is demonstrated to students less often than almost any other technologic aspect of the medical curriculum. Abrahamson [76] was more incisive in his comment that in practice many histories are inadequate, a proportion useless, and a minority actively harmful. Asked pertinently by Melinkoff [77] was this question: ". . . But is there a seasoned physician who has not seen some patients subjected to the wrong tests, at the wrong times, for the wrong reasons, at great expense and with disastrous results because the original history was taken clumsily or carelessly?"

Mitchell [78], speaking from NIOSH, stated that if he were the "Czar of Medicine," he would decree only one thing in the area of occupational health and that would be to teach all medical students to take a proper occupational medical history. He would try to raise their level of awareness and suspicion about job-related illnesses. Coming from outside the ranks of occupational medicine is a comment from Toewe and Beck [79]: "Since the patient may be unaware of the relationship between job exposure and illness, or may have forgotten about it, the family physician must include occupational causes in the differential diagnosis of almost every adult patient's problem."

Further emphasis is given the need through the retelling of actual case histories, wherein the lack of a complete history, or the unwillingness to pursue the important detail, can be counterproductive diagnostically. Hunt and Young [80] reported plural effusion with pain and fever in a 56-year-old retired army sergeant who was seen in an army hospital. Thoracentesis and pleural biopsy examination did not show the cause of the finding. While being followed subsequently as an outpatient, he developed bilateral pleural thickening compatible with exposure to asbestos. "When initially queried about occupations generally considered pertinent to asbestosis, e.g., asbestos-weaving and steam-pipe lagging, he denied any such occupation. However, when asked to go through his occupational history month-by-month including part-time jobs, he recalled working for nine months at age 16 as a fire-eater in a carnival. This entailed using an asbestos torch, inhaling and exhaling fire from the torch and frequently extinguishing the torch by placing it in his mouth." Were that history obtained initially, the thoracentesis, possibly, and the pleural biopsy, certainly, could have been averted.

Sargent, Jacobson, and Wilkinson [81], on reporting patients with diaphragmatic pleural calcification, commented, "A routine occupational history obtained by the referring physician failed to mention any exposure to asbestos dust." However, detailed questioning by the radiologists who personally made contact with the patient revealed an 11-month exposure as a clean-up laborer, sweeping the decks in the holds of ships after pipefitters had installed asbestos insulation on overhead pipes.

In a second case [81], there was again no mention of asbestos in the admitting physician's history. The radiologist, as before, learned that there was an 8-month exposure when the patient mixed asbestos with cement for an insulation material.

A patient who aspirated a red plastic coffee straw while working in a fast-food restaurant developed "near opacification of the right hemithorax secondary to atelectasis and a large pleural effusion" [82]. As the history was neither volunteered nor elicited, erroneous conclusions were reached when surgical procedures were undertaken, followed by months of repeated courses of antibiotics.

Finally, the frequent derogation of the patient as a "poor historian" belies the inability of the history-taker to derive the tell-tale exposure information. As Coulehan [82] expressed it, "Interview data must be judged by criteria of precision, accuracy, and completeness just like any other medical data. The doctor *is* the instrument of history taking. We must interact with the patient to obtain the most useful, robust data possible. No doubt, there will always be poor historians in medicine, but, if we pay more attention to the clinical art, fewer of them will be the doctors."

*Doyle had a brief experience in occupational medicine, for he made two sea voyages as ship's surgeon. The first was on a whaler to the Arctic, and the second to the West Coast of Africa. He was engaged in the Boer War in South Africa, serving as medical officer to British troops, for which he was knighted in 1902 [74].

OBJECTIVES IN OBTAINING THE OCCUPATIONAL HISTORY

The objectives in this quest for background work data may be summarized as follows.

PRIMARY OBJECTIVES
Improvement of medical care.
Return of worker to gainful employment.

SECONDARY OBJECTIVES
Identification of the correct etiology of the illness.
Determination of anatomic or physiologic (functional) deficits.
Facilitation in formulating the diagnosis.
Institution of appropriate treatment plan.
Correction of hazardous work environment.
- Removal of worker to alternative assignment.
- Removal of offending physical, chemical, or psychological stressors and substitution of nonoffending agents.
- Protection of workers not yet manifesting frank disease.

Establishment of bioassay baselines for use in future comparisons.
Formulation of appropriate recommendations, if indicated, to employer regarding assignment of worker.
Early initiation of rehabilitative measures and prevention of disability.
Documentation of data potentially significant in future epidemiologic study.

WORK DETAILS

To reach these objectives, certain questions must be framed and asked. Of considerable aid, as a first step, is the delineation of the primary elements of the patient's history of employment, beginning with the first job and developing the work experience up to the present time, to include the following:

Company (employer)
- Name; city, county, state (and country, if abroad)
- Type of company; statement of mission or type of product
- Department, division, branch, unit, section, work station, if any one is known

Period of employment—from month and year to month and year
Full-time or part-time work
Job titles or work performed, in detail
Potentially hazardous work exposures:
- Physical
- Chemical
- Biologic
- Psychological
- Sociologic

Personal protective equipment used or devices worn*
Secondary or moonlighting jobs held

Specific areas can be explored then, as determined both by leads obtained from the medical history (present illness) and from the jobs listed.

QUESTIONS TO BE DIRECTED TO THE PATIENT

THE COMPANY
Is there an occupational health program in your company?
Does the company give physical examinations?
What is the industrial hygiene policy or activity?†
Is there a safety program?
Are you informed of the results of examinations or of workroom air samplings?

THE JOB
What exactly were you doing when you became ill?
Were you working your regular shift?
What materials do you work with?
- If they are liquid, do they give off vapors ("fumes"‡) that can be breathed?
- Do they ever spill on your skin?
- Do they ever soak through your clothing?

If you used protective devices, are they maintained by the company?
Do you exchange your respirator when it gets dirty or when you smell the chemical through the mask?
Does the company ever hold information meetings to tell you about the materials you work with?
How do you clean up your workplace at the end of the shift?§
Is any chemical being used near you by other employees?
Do you become ill during the week at work and then get better over the weekend?
Do you get sick when you return to work? After a weekend off? After your vacation?

*Included are protective clothing (impermeable gloves, aprons, shoe guards, disposable uniforms), air-supplied respirators, masks, ear defenders, protective eyewear, safety shoes, face shields, and welders' hoods.
†This question will require reference to technical personnel with instruments, air sampling devices, individual monitoring devices, and the like, for "industrial hygiene" as a professional discipline is not understood by most workers.
‡"Fumes," with thanks to the media, has become a generic term for vapors, gases, mists, dusts, aerosols, particulates, pollutants, and, yes, even fumes.
§The wrong materials may be used as work surface cleaners or topical skin cleansers and prove to be toxic or dermatogenic.

Has any new material been introduced that you work with?
Has the brand of any material been changed?
Has there ever been a spill at your work station?
Has the equipment ever broken down?
Has anything interrupted the usual work process or production line?
Have you ever changed jobs at the company because of your health?
Has there ever been an OSHA inspection of your workplace?
If so, what was found and what action was taken?
Is there ventilation or an exhaust system at your work station?
Does anyone ever take air samples at your work station?

FELLOW WORKERS
Have any of your fellow workers been ill in the same way you are? If so, when?
Have any workers complained of being unable to have children?

HOME, HOBBIES, AND HABITS
What do you work with at home? Glue? Pesticides? Fertilizers? Your car? Furniture refinishers? Paints? Photography chemicals?
Do you smoke? What, where, and how much? What year did you start? If you quit, what year was it?
Do you drink? What, how much, how often?
Do you use firearms?
Do you play rock music? Peak volume? Do you use earphones?
Do you drive heavy farm equipment?
Where do you have your workclothes washed?
Do you have any pets at home?
Do you take any medicines?
Do you live near any manufacturing plants?
Are any of your neighbors ever sick like you?
Does your house paint ever turn color from something in the air?

FEELINGS ABOUT THE JOB
Do you like your job?
Are you still good at your job?
Have you had trouble holding a job?
Do you get frustrated at work?
Do you like shift work when it is assigned?
Is your job more than you can handle?
How do you feel about your supervisor?
Is there much stress in your job?
Do you look forward to retirement?

To be sure, not all of the questions listed are asked, for one is selective in using appropriate leads, as indicated previously. On occasion it is necessary to reword questions, for few workers actually know their role in the overall mission of the organization and not many are familiar with the material or substances with which they work. Most of the liquids carry trade names that convey no meaning, and rare is the employee who ever sees or reads the labels on original containers. An influence that can be adverse is the foreman, pushed for production, who tells his personnel not to worry about potential toxicities—"everything is o.k., go ahead and work!" Or the variation on that theme—"It's all right. You're only going to work with it (or be in there) a short time. Don't worry."

PRECAUTIONS REGARDING JOB TITLES

Certain elements pertaining to the designation of jobs require emphasis. The recorder of the history—physician or nurse—cannot take at first hearing the patient's job title as a full description of what is actually done. It is customary in industry to give certain positions rather generic titles such as mechanic, laborer, clerk, or aircraft assembler. The assignments meted out to incumbents in those jobs are legion and can vary greatly in both the physical and mental demands. The advantage of such a looseness in classification is that the practice permits flexibility and interchangeability in a department. A laborer can be asked to paint a bench, stir up soil, carry ladders, and the like. A helper can be assigned to any of several crafts.

With each task may go different exposures. An assembler may come in contact with a variety of toxic solvents, while another may work exclusively with drawings. The inquiring physician must inquire or else will be led astray by the inexactitude of classifications and will miss identifying the point of contact of worker and hazard.*

*As far back as 1935, Leroy U. Gardner, the eminent Saranac investigator in silicosis made a similar observation: "Ordinary medical histories usually note the present occupation in one or two words with reference neither to previous employment nor to the character of the work involved. The occupation 'laborer' might mean anything but to be of significance it must be qualified by some such phrase as 'in a cement plant, grinding sand' or 'in a pottery, removing china from a kiln,' 'development work, hard rock mine.' Since silicosis may not manifest itself for years after the exposure has ceased it is essential to have a chronological tabulation of all the occupations at which the individual has worked since leaving school." (Pneumonokoniosis. *Int Clin* 45th series 2:16, 1935.) Three

As the parallel of this point, the patient may be tagged with a job title that carries no meaning to the physician. Harrington and Schilling [83] underscored this point in their discussion of the problems of developing accurate histories. The job title, as they use the brewing industry for the example, may go back several centuries, and either a knowledge of the industry or an explanation from the worker is needed to decide truly what is involved in the jobs of masher, wort runner, bottoms presser, racker, titler, stripper, smeller, and trauncer. Or, in comparable vein, how many physicians would recognize at first hearing these job labels—stullman, flumer, yare man, turkish rubber, or grubber, or even ecdysiast? One must seek clarification from the industrial cognoscenti so that hazardous contacts can be identified. Harrington and Schilling [83] point to another trap in the development of an occupational history, and that pertains to the chronology of a product. As they relate it, a physician will know, certainly, what a cooper does—he repairs or makes barrels. But what neither the physician nor the cooper knows is that the barrels undergoing overhaul previously contained white lead. The last job is not necessarily the one causative of disease.

One must be warned in this discussion that there are many myths connected with certain occupations so that some workers believe in work-related health hazards that do not exist. Deeply buried are many time-nurtured untruths regarding dangers in the job. The way to a diagnosis has its pitfalls, for the company representatives, like the foreman cited previously, will tend to depreciate the plant's capacity for causing morbidity, and the employee frequently will exaggerate the hazards attendant upon certain operations.

DETAILED EXPOSURE REVIEW

When it is believed that patients might have knowledge of the substances that are used in their particular job, a questionnaire may be used that lists a broad variety of chemicals—both in elemental form or as compounds. A form can be developed locally, or an "Exposure History Record" is available commercially* that provides checkoff columns for exposures, the specific years of contact, and the total number of years of exposure. A backup page allows for computerization of the patient's notations.

Halen, Hassel, and Ostlund [84] from Stockholm have visualized a person's past occupational enferences in an interesting and succinct manner, as seen in Figure 12-10.

OTHER OCCUPATIONAL HISTORIES

DERMATOLOGY

Adams [85], in a comprehensive and well-reviewed monograph, has provided a form for recording the history and examination findings of a patient with a suspected occupationally incurred dermatosis (Fig. 12-11).

PULMONOLOGY

Because of the increased knowledge of the health effects following exposure to a broad variety of chemical agents and dusts, nearly every OHS is engaged in performing pulmonary function evaluations. Baselines are obtained, and periodic testing is conducted subsequently, at intervals either subject to mandate or as deemed appropriate in light of local work processes and the extent of engineering controls. A detailed respiratory history is needed whether the screening pulmonary function tests are performed in the OHS, the employees are referred to another facility, or after screening, patients are to undergo complete function evaluation by a pulmonary disease specialist. Particularly in the case of referral, considerable time can be saved if the history is obtained in advance.

The format for such a document is not unique, for most of the questionnaires reviewed have been printed with questions on the left and with "yes" and "no" columns on the right. There are specific areas yielding of pertinent information, and from the subjects listed in Table 12-2, a selection can be made and the wording can be matched to fit the intelligence or comprehension levels of the respondents. Once developed, the questionnaire can be translated for use by workers for whom English is a second language. All questionnaires should be devised so as to be computerized.

years later Gardner repeated the plea when he commented on the investigation of dust hazards: "The occupational history of all employees should cover the entire industrial life of every workman. It should include the names of each employer, the kind of job, an estimate of the type and quantity of dust encountered and the approximate dates of each position held." (Etiology of pneumoconiosis. *J Med* 111:1925, 1938.) Nearly half a century later the same tune continues to be played to unhearing ears.

*Published by Miller Communications, Inc., Norwalk, CT 06856.

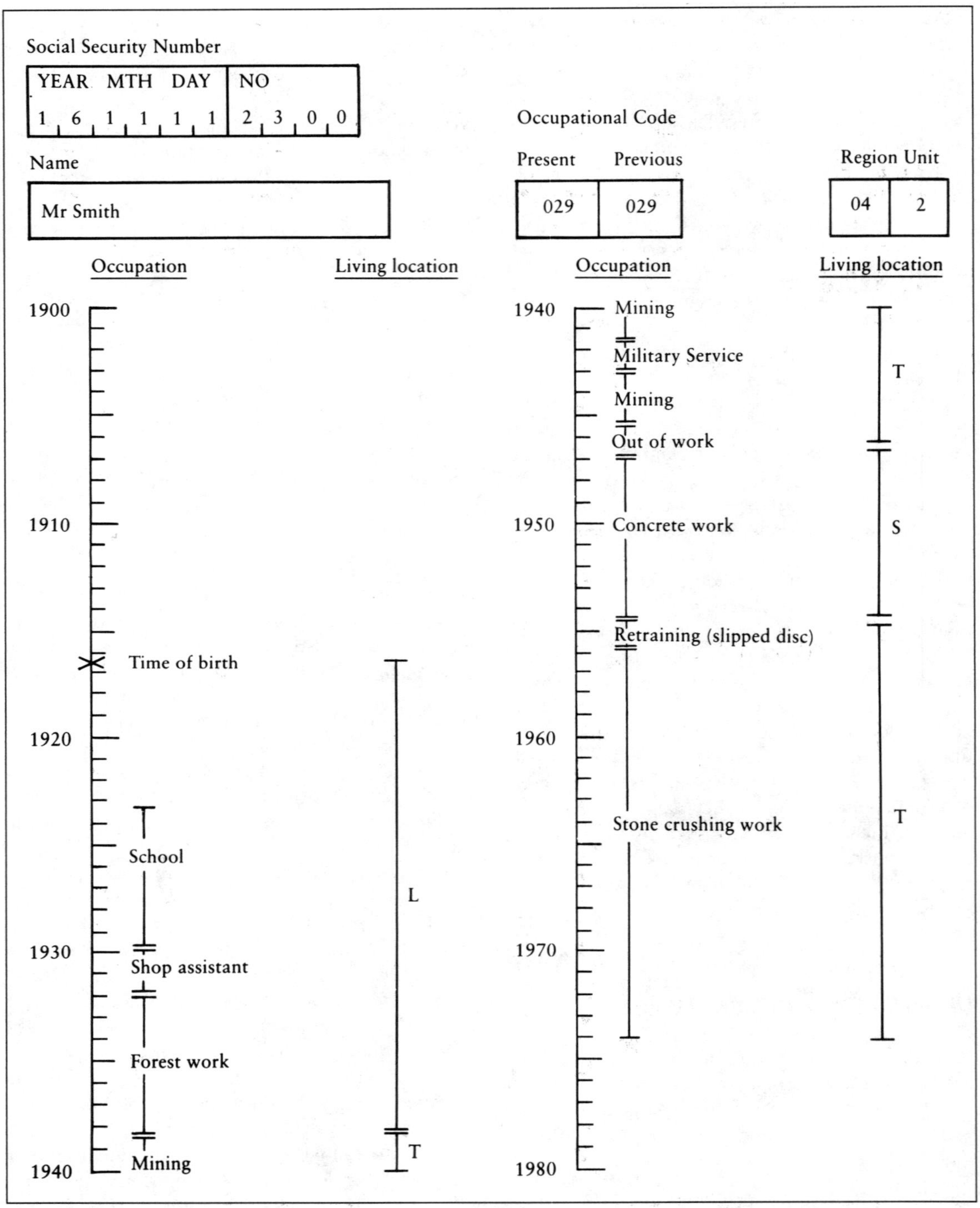

FIGURE 12-10. *Example of total individual occupational/environmental exposure. S = Stockholm; T = Tatort (population center); L = Landsbygd (countryside). (From Halen, M., Hassel, A., and Ostlund, E.* Environment Profiles in the Swedish Construction Industry *[BHF 1976:3] Stockholm: Bygghalsans Forskningsstiflelse, 1976.)*

Name ______________________________ Date ______________
Address ______________________________ Age ________ Sex ________
Home phone ______________ SSN ______________ Referred by ______________
Current employer (name and address) ______________________________
______________________________ Present job title ______________
Employer at onset of injury (name and address) ______________________________
____
Date employed ______________ Date terminated ______________
Job title at onset of injury ______________________________ Date ______________
Insurance carrier (name and address) ______________________________
____

PRESENT ILLNESS

Date of onset ______________ Dates of disability ______________
Location at onset ______________________________
Patient's description ______________________________
____
____
____

Effect of weekends: Improved ________ Unimproved ________ Worse ________
Effect of vacations: Improved ________ Unimproved ________ Worse ________
Duration of vacation ______________________________

PREVIOUS TREATMENT

1. Plant dispensary ______________________________
____
2. Other physician ______________________________
3. Self-treatment ______________________________
____

DESCRIPTION OF WORK

____
____
____
____

FIGURE 12-11. *Form for recording the history and examination findings in patients whose skin disease is suspected of being occupational in origin. (From Adams, R.M.* Occupational Skin Disease. *New York: Grune & Stratton, 1983, pp. 111–113.)*

Materials contacted ____

____

____

Other workers affected? Yes ________ No ________ No. affected ________

How many workers on this job? ________________

Methods of cleaning skin at work (and frequency) ______________________

____

Protective creams (names) ______________________________________

____

Protective clothing ____

PAST HISTORY

Previous compensation claims? Yes ____ No ____ Explain __________________

____

Previous skin diseases ____

Relation to occupation? Yes ____ No ____ Place of birth ________________

Past health ____

Previous compensation claims? Yes ____ No ____ Explain __________________

____

Allergic history: Hay Fever _______ Asthma _______ Eczema _______

Allergic to cosmetics, medications, creams, ointments, jewelry, drugs? (circle which)

Describe ____

Family history of atopy? Yes ____ No ____ Second job ____________________

Hobbies __________________________ Home contactants ________________

PHYSICAL EXAMINATION

General appearance ____

____

Description of disease ____

____

Other skin diseases ____

____

DIAGNOSIS ____

____

Contributing factors ____

SPECIAL TESTS

KOH ______________ Fungal culture ______________ Bacterial culture ______________

Biopsy ____

Patch testing (results) ____

____

____

____ Clinical photographs? Yes ____ No ____

TREATMENT ____

____

DISABILITY Yes ____ No ____ Date may return to work ____________________

REMARKS ____

____

FIGURE 12-11 (continued)

EMOTIONAL STATUS

Ireton has observed that several of the psychological test instruments used to obtain psychosocial information have been either cumbersome or time-consuming in practice or have lacked comprehensiveness [86]. To meet this particular need of providing a brief measure of the patient, current concerns, emotional status, life stresses, and personal functioning, he devised the "Personal Inventory,"* which includes questions pertaining to (1) well-being, (2) life concerns, (3) emotional-mental status, (4) life stress, (5) personality, and (6) life satisfaction/desire for change. The inventory comprises a set of rating scales by which the patients describe themselves and their situations. Completion requires only 10 to 15 minutes, and if the patient has limited reading ability—less than sixth-grade level—the inventory may be used as an interview guide.

Ireton points out that caution should be used in treating the patient's report as literal and valid. In the face of such inquiry, some persons may be defensive, while others may exaggerate their difficulties. With judicious use, however, it should prove helpful in dealing with the psychological aspects of patient care [86].

NEED FOR EMPHASIS

That occupational histories are given short shrift even in medicine's respected institutions was pointed out by Cowles [87], who reviewed 53 case records (from the Massachusetts General Hospital and published in the *New England Journal of Medicine*) from 1971–1972 and a comparable number for the 1981–1982 period. In the early group, occupation was mentioned only in six cases, and in four of the group, job title solely was noted. The later group showed some improvement, with the occupation indicated in 13 cases, but by the job title only in 10. Of interest was the finding that even though several case records concerned childhood cancer, in not a single record was the occupation of either parent given. Further, even when the diagnosis was that of an occupational disease, no complete occupational history was included. As Cowles underscores the point, "Too often the influence of occupation on health and of health on occupation is ignored, despite increased public awareness of the potential adverse effects of work on health."

*Distributed by Behavior Science Systems, Inc., P.O. Box 1108, Minneapolis, MN 55440.

Lastly, in its *Third Annual Report to Congress* [88], the special Task Force on Environmental Cancer and Heart and Lung Disease made this recommendation among others relating to education: "Professional organizations and Federal Agencies interested in environmental and occupational health should work toward the education of medical and nursing students to take a thorough environmental and occupational history."

USE OF INTERPRETERS

In certain areas of high levels of immigration where bilingual relatives or other workers are not available to accompany the patient to the health care facility, it may be necessary to employ an interpreter. Such persons are obtainable for a fee and will remain with the patient during the development of the history and may aid in the delivery of certain instructions during the physical examination.

The use of a third person has not proved entirely satisfactory, for pertinent details do not cross the language barrier. Often one may be given in English the interpreter's understanding of the patient's response, which may not reflect the individual's description of a symptom or the essence of a work exposure. Putsch [89] has explored this issue and has provided guidelines when both the provider in the health care setting and the patient are monolingual.

GENERAL GUIDELINES

Unless one is thoroughly effective and fluent in the target language, always use an interpreter.

Avoid using family members as interpreters.

Learn basic words and sentences in the target language. One must ask interpreters about words or comments that have not been translated to prompt attention to detail.

One should utilize dictionaries of languages used by the patient population, being careful to avoid the brief "definitions" provided by translating dictionaries, for they only serve as labels.

One must become familiar with special terminology used by patients, for specific beliefs, practices, or traditions often are referenced by indirect language, or special terms. Local beliefs and moral tenets may lead to overemphasis on under-reporting of certain symptoms, issues, and events.

One should check the quality of translated health-related materials by having them back-translated.

One should meet with the interpreters on a regular basis, for they will provide both a window and a

TABLE 12-2. *Areas for Inquiry in the Development of a Pulmonary Disease Questionnaire*

History	*Details*
Present condition	Details, date of first symptoms
Cough	When (time of day or night, season, with smoking), duration of single cough, duration in weeks or months, date first noticed, constant or intermittent, other influencing factors
Phlegm (or understandable local term)	When (time of day or night, season, on going out of doors, with smoking), date first noticed, duration during year, increase in recent weeks or months, estimate of amount
Blood	With cough, without cough, blood-streaked phlegm, estimate of amount
Breathlessness	When (hurrying or on level ground, walking uphill, when walking with others at regular pace, when washing or showering or dressing), need to stop when walking, date first noticed, recovery time
Wheezing (whistling noises in chest)	With colds, apart from colds, day or night, date first noticed, associated with breathlessness, corrected by medicine, how brought on, other influencing factors
Hoarseness	Duration, date of onset, influencing factors
Fingernails	Change in color or shape, date of onset
Effect of weather	Any of symptoms affected or brought on by hot weather, cold weather, damp weather, foggy weather, air pollution, associated with breathlessness
Past chest diseases	Any illness that precluded working or going out or that forced bed rest, by duration of illness, with increase of symptoms noted above, medical care obtained, physician's diagnosis
Past specific illnesses	Asthma, bronchitis, collapsed lung, emphysema, hay fever, heart disease, high blood pressure, histoplasmosis, industrial lung disease, pleurisy, pneumonia, sinusitis, tuberculosis, valley fever, whooping cough
Past injuries	Lung injury, fractured ribs
Past surgery	Heart, lungs, chest; bronchoscopy
Skin tests	Type, results, dates
Smoking history	For each item, amount or frequency currently and previously: cigarettes/day; pipe tobacco, ounces/week; chewing tobacco, amount/day; snuff, amount/day; cigars/week, inhale or not Age started; age stopped; if stopped, reason: physician's orders, pressure of spouse, pressure of children, personal concern about health, television messages, ads, other reason Times tried stopping
Drinking history	Glasses of beer, wine, hard liquor/week
Occupational history	As outlined previously
Racial background	Caucasian, black, Asian, Native American, Spanish surname, brown
Parentage	Part of world parents came from
Hobbies	Pets, birds, chickens, cattle, painting, welding, boat-building, jogging, woodworking, other
Allergies	Foods, medicines, pollens, dusts
Birthplace	Where born, where reared, duration and places of residences before working
Chest x-rays	Places, dates, results, last examination

mirror with dealing with another language and another culture.

Personal information often is closely guarded and difficult to obtain. Patients frequently request a specific interpreter or even bring one along.

One must evaluate the interpreter's style and approach to patients. In special cases or problems, the interpreter should be matched to the task.*

One must be patient, for careful interpretation often requires that the interpreter use long explanatory phrases.

GUIDELINES FOR PROVIDER-INTERPRETER-PATIENT INTERACTIONS

One must address the patient directly, avoiding the direction of all comments to and through the interpreter.

One should be certain that the interpreter is thoroughly involved with the patient during the interview.

One should develop alternatives to the taking of histories by means of direct questions. Strangers to direct, western-style inquiry may respond better to conversational modes.

One should invite correction and induce the discussion of alternatives, for example, "Correct me if I'm wrong; I understand it this way . . ." or "Do you see it some other way?"

One should pursue seemingly unconnected issues that the patient raises, for they may lead to crucial information or uncover difficulties with the interpretation.

One should return to an issue if one suspects a problem and gets a negative response. One must be sure that the interpreter knows what is wanted. One can use related questions, change the wording, or come at the issue indirectly.

One should provide instructions in the format of lists, and one should have the patients outline their understanding of the plans.

If alternatives exist, one should spell out each one.

One should emphasize by repetition.

One should clarify one's limitations, for talking about an issue may be misinterpreted as "understanding it" or having the ability to "fix it."

Particularly in closely knit communities, it is important that one assure the patient of confidentiality.

*The writer, nearly totally monolingual, when seeing Spanish-speaking patients and when using "commercial" interpreters has detected a sense of superiority or even arrogance on the part of the interpreter, which will be counterproductive in obtaining a history reflective of the problem.

Unless one devises the correct circumstances, it may be impossible to address certain male/female problems by way of discussion or physical examination.

GUIDELINES FOR LANGUAGE USE IN INTERPRETER-DEPENDENT INTERVIEWS

One should use short questions and comments, avoiding technical terms and such medical jargon as "workup."

When lengthy explanations are necessary, they should be divided and interpreted piece-by-piece in straightforward terms.

One must use language and explanations the interpreter can handle.

One must make allowances for terms that do not exist in the target language (lack of linguistic equivalence).

One must avoid ambiguous statements or questions, abstractions, idiomatic expressions, similes, or metaphors. It is helpful to learn of these usages in the target language.

One should plan one's queries in advance.

One should avoid indefinite phrases that use "would," "could," "if," and "maybe," for they can be mistaken for actual agreements or firm approval of a course of action.

One should have the interpreter comment on the patient's word content and emotions.

REFERENCES

1. Felton, J. S. Modernizing the medical facility in industry. *Ind Med* 16:291, 1947.
2. Silver, M. Alphabetical or numeric filing? *Intern Med News* 9:17, May 15, 1979.
3. Statement against use of social security numbers for hospital medical records. *Hospitals* 48:124, 1974.
4. Curran, W. J. Social security numbers and privacy: New Hospital Policy. *N Engl J Med* 290:556, 1974.
5. *We Can Help You Attain Higher Standards in Record Keeping Efficiency.* Somerville, MA: Ames Color-File, [n.d.].
6. Schall, D. W. Automation of the Problem-Oriented Medical Record. In *Proceedings of the Annual Conference of NASA Clinic Directors, Environmental Health Officials, and Medical Program Advisors, Charleston, SC, Oct. 12–14, 1971.* Washington DC: NASA Headquarters Office of Administration, Division of Occupational Medicine and Environmental Health, 1971. Pp. 135–144.
7. Markovits, A. S. The doctor's scrawl: Affected, egocentric, and irresponsible. *Resident Staff Phys* 17:107, 1971.

8. Soukhanov, A. H., and Haverty, J. R. (Eds.). Patient Records and Case Histories. In *Webster's Medical Office Handbook*. Springfield, MA: Merriam, 1979. Chap. 9.2, p. 149.
9. *Medicolegal Forms with Legal Analysis*. Chicago: American Medical Association, Office of the General Counsel, 1979. P. 93.
10. Access to employee exposure and medical records. *Fed Reg* 45:35212-35303, May 23, 1980.
11. X-ray records. *J Occup Med* 25:11, 1983.
12. *Records Control and Storage Handbook*. Stasca, IL: Bankers Box Records Storage Systems, 1977.
13. Bews, D. C. The occupational physician and privileged communications. *J Occup Med* 8:383, 1966.
14. May, C. R. Confidentiality of medical records. *J Occup Med* 12:51, 1970.
15. Bundy, M. Nurse-personnel-physician symposium: Confidentiality of medical records. The physician's viewpoint. *Arch Environ Health* 19:290, 1969.
16. Fiscina, S. Information about Patients: How Confidential? In C. Wecht (Ed.), *Legal Medicine*. Philadelphia: Saunders, 1980. P. 249.
17. Westin, A. F. Confidentiality of Medical Records. In *Occupational Safety and Health Symposia 1978*. Cincinnati, OH: U.S. Department of Health, Education, and Welfare, Public Health Service, Center for Disease Control, National Institute for Occupational Safety and Health, Division of Technical Services, June 1979. Pp. 9–12.
18. Simmons, W. R. *Issues Regarding Confidentiality of Data in the Cooperative Health Statistics System*. Vital and Health Statistics Documents and Committee Reports Series 4, Number 22. Hyattsville, MD: U.S. Department of Health, Education, and Welfare, Public Health Service, Office of Health Research, Statistics, and Technology, National Center for Health Statistics, April 1980. P. 5.
19. Court affirms NIOSH's right to subpoena medical records. *Occup Health Saf Letter* 10:7, Aug 22, 1980.
20. Felton, J. S. Radiographic search for asbestos-related disease in a naval shipyard. *Ann NY Acad Sci* 330:341, 1979.
21. More M.D.'s sued for bad records than bad practice. *Skin Allergy News* 11:2, 1980.
22. Do's and don'ts of handling late medical record entries. *Calif MA News* 20:5, Feb 14, 1975.
23. Parker, W. A warning on defective, risky hospital charts. *Med Trib* 21:11, Dec 3, 1980.
24. Warshaw, L. J. Confidentiality versus the need to know. *J Occup Med* 18:534, 1976.
25. Bromage, M. C. In Justification of jargon. *Michigan Bus Rev* 20:20, July 1968.
26. Feinstein, J., cited in Newman, E. R. An anniversary. *San Francisco Examiner,* Nov 6, 1984. P. B3.
27. Wish, J. B. Medspeak. *N Engl J Med* 301:507, 1979.
28. *Accreditation Manual for Hospitals, 1981 Edition*. Chicago: Joint Commission on Accreditation of Hospitals, 1981. Pp. 83–92.
29. Shakespeare, W. *The Tragedy of Macbeth*. Act V, Scene I, lines 33–36.
30. McDonagh, T. J., Smith, F. R., and Gutierrez, R. R. Health information systems: A necessary component of modern occupational health programs. *Ann Occup Hyg* 24:303, 1981.
31. Wiederhold, G. *Databases for Health Care*. Berlin: Springerverlog, 1981. P. 1.
32. Whyte, A. A. *A Comparative Analysis of Commercially Available Occupational Health Information Systems* (6th ed.). Falls Church, VA: Bio Technology, Inc., March 1983.
33. Editor's Note, introductory to the Supplement on Medical Information Systems. *J Occup Med* Suppl 24:781, 1982.
34. Finucane, R. D., and McDonagh, T. J. Medical information systems roundtable foreword. *J Occup Med* Suppl 24:781, 1982.
35. Sugano, D. S. Worker tracking: A complex but essential element in health surveillance systems. *J Occup Med* Suppl 24:783, 1982.
36. Hillman, D. W. A computerized occupational health and environmental surveillance system. *J Occup Med* 35:785, 1982.
37. Hillman, D.. W. Personal communication, March 2, 1981.
38. Diamond Shamrock Corporation: Influencing the "need to know." *Occup Health Saf* 49:22, Jan 1980.
39. *COHESS*. Niagara Falls, NY: Occidental Chemical Corporation, 1986.
40. Boutchyard, H., Jr. Personal communication, June 9, 1987.
41. Elmer, C., and Coleman, D. L. Monsanto's Medical and Environmental Health Information (MEHI System). *J Occup Med* Suppl 24:788, 1982.
42. Baxter, R. A., and Henshaw, J. L. Experience with an occupational exposure data recording system. *Ann Occup Hyg* 25:95, 1982.
43. Elmer, C. Personal communication, June 8, 1987.
44. Wolkonsky, P. Computerized recordkeeping in an occupational health system: The Amoco system. *J Occup Med* Suppl 24:791, 1982.
45. Spies, H. W. Personal communication, June 9, 1987.
46. Hagstrom, R. M., Daugherty, W. E., English, N. B., et al. SmithKline Environmental Health Surveillance System. *J Occup Med* Suppl 24:799, 1982.
47. English, N. B. Personal communication, July 7, 1987.
48. LeBlanc, J. V. A Computerized Health and Environmental Surveillance System (CHESS). *J Occup Med* Suppl 24:804, 1982.
49. Judd, S. H. Occupational Health Information System (OHIS). *J Occup Med* Suppl 24:806, 1982.
50. Judd, S. H. Personal communication, June 12, 1987.
51. Joyner, R. E., and Pack, P. H. The Shell Oil Company's computerized health surveillance system. *J Occup Med* Suppl 24:812, 1982.
52. Joyner, R. E. Personal communication, June 4, 1987.
53. Belk, H. D., Sussman, N., and Bonney, T. B. The Alcoa health information system. *J Occup Med* Suppl 24:815, 1982.
54. Belk, H. D. Personal communication, June 8, 1987.
55. Pell, S., O'Berg, M. T., and Karrh, B. W. Cancer epi-

demiologic surveillance in the DuPont company. *J Occup Med* 20:725, 1978.
56. Pell, S. Epidemiologic studies in a large company based on health and personnel records. *Public Health Rep* 83:399, 1968.
57. O'Berg, M. T., Burke, C. A., Chen, J. L., et al. Cancer incidence and mortality in the Du Pont Company: An update. *J Occup Med* 29:245, 1987.
58. Bonnett, J. C., and Pell, S. DuPont's health surveillance systems. *J Occup Med* Suppl 24:819, 1982.
59. Fayerweather, W. E. Personal communication, June 11, 1987.
60. Smith, F. R., Gutierrez, R. R., and McDonagh, T. J. Exxon's health information system. *J Occup Med* Suppl 24:824, 1982.
61. Hillman, G. ECHOES: IBM's Environmental, Chemical and Occupational Evaluation System. *J Occup Med* Suppl 24:827, 1982.
62. Hillman, G. Personal communication, July 23, 1987.
63. Timlin, E. L., Jr., Hillman, G., and Peterson, K. W. IBM's experience with its Environmental, Chemical and Occupational Evaluation System, ECHOES. *Ann Am Conf Gov Ind Hyg* 6:31, 1983.
64. Garrett, R. W. Environmental tracking at Eli Lily and Company. *J Occup Med* 24:836, 1982.
65. Robinson, H., and Wood, L. W. The New York Telephone Company medical information system. *J Occup Med* Suppl 24:840, 1982.
66. Kuritz, S. J. The Ford Motor Company environmental health surveillance system. *J Occup Med* Suppl 24:844, 1982.
67. Walter, D. F. Control Data Corporation's occupational health and safety system. *J Occup Med* Suppl 24:848, 1982.
68. Stallard, C. W., Jr. The SOHIO health information system *J Occup Med* Suppl 24:24:853, 1982.
69. SOHIO's health care monitoring system. *Occup Haz* 44:47, Nov 1982.
70. Rossi, D. A., Cox, J. D., and Seger, M. J. Computerization of medical and exposure records in the semiconductor industry. *J Occup Med* Suppl 24:859, 1982.
71. Joiner, R. L. Occupational health and environmental information systems: Basic considerations. *J Occup Med* Suppl 24:863, 1982.
72. Mastromatteo, E. Personal communication, February 26 and March 22, 1985.
73. Ramazzini, B. *Diseases of Workers*. The Latin text of 1713, revised, with translation and notes by W. C. Wright. Chicago: University of Chicago Press, 1940. Pp. 12–13.
74. Kay, J. D., Shampo, M. A., and Kyle, R. A. Arthur Conan Doyle. *JAMA* 244:2363, 1980.
75. Feinstein, A. R. *Clinical Judgment*. Baltimore: Williams & Wilkins, 1967. P. 299.
76. Abrahamson, D. Procedure reexamined. *Lancet* 1:1153, 1974.
77. Melinkoff, S. M. The physician of tomorrow. *JAMA* 273:1952, 1977.
78. Mitchell, F.L., cited by Snyder, J. How NIOSH can help you spot job-related disease. *Mod Med* 46:57, 1978.
79. Toewe, C. H., II, and Beck, J. D. Occupational Health and Industrial Medicine. In R. B. Taylor (Ed.), *Family Medicine: Principles and Practice* (2nd ed.). New York: Springer-Verlag, 1983. Pp. 1911–1926.
80. Hunt, K. K., and Young, M. B. Fire-eater's asbestosis. *JAMA* 229:23, 1974.
81. Sargent, C. N., Jacobson, G., and Wilkinson, E. E. Diaphragmatic pleural calcification following short occupational exposure to asbestos. *Am J Roentgen Rad Ther Nuclear Med* 115:473, 1972.
82. Kraus, V. B., Fulkerson, W. J., Gowen, M. A., et al. Straw lung. *N Engl J Med* 312:924, 1985.
82. Coulehan, J. L. Who is the poor historian? *JAMA* 252:221, 1984.
83. Harrington, J. M., and Schilling, R. S. F. Work and Health. In R. S. F. Schilling (Ed.), *Occupational Health Practice* (2nd ed.). London: Butterworth, 1983. Chap. 3, pp. 47–53.
84. Halen, M., Hassel, A., and Ostlund, E. *Environment Profiles in the Swedish Construction Industry* (BHF 1976:3). Stockholm: Bygghälsans Forskningsstiftelse, 1976. Figure 1.
85. Adams, R. M. *Occupational Skin Disease*. New York: Grune & Stratton, 1983. Pp. 111–113.
86. Ireton, H. R. A personal inventory. *J Fam Pract* 11:137, 1980.
87. Cowles, S. Inadequate occupational histories in case records. *N Engl J Med* 307:1713, 1982.
88. Task Force on Environmental Cancer and Heart and Lung Disease. *Environmental Cancer and Heart and Lung Disease—Third Annual Report to Congress*. Washington, DC: U.S. Environmental Protection Agency and other Federal Centers and Institutes, Aug 7, 1980. Education Program Recommendations, p. 31.
89. Putsch, R. W., III. Cross-cultural communication: The special case of interpreters in health care. *JAMA* 254:3344, 1985.

APPENDIX 12-1 FUNCTIONS OF AN OCCUPATIONAL HEALTH INFORMATION SYSTEM

In a presentation made in 1984 by Adrienne A. Whyte, Ph.D., of OHIC, Inc., Frederick, Maryland, the functions of an information system were outlined, and the material follows, with permission of Dr. Whyte.

CLINICAL SUPPORT—OPERATIONS

Examination scheduling
Protocol management
  Scheduled examinations

Unscheduled examinations
Examination, diagnosis, and treatment data collection, reporting, and management
Medical history
Multiphasic testing data
Physician's review of systems
Diagnoses
Diagnostic assistance
Treatment data
Follow-up requirements
Analytic tools
Suspense function for incomplete examinations
Data edits
Data validation
Examination reports, including evaluation
Fitness-for-duty notices
Occupational injury and illness reports
Trended profiles
Comprehensive reporting functions
Risk assessment
Records management
Interface between manual and automated systems of records
Management of records requests

ENVIRONMENTAL HEALTH AND SAFETY SUPPORT

Environmental agent management
Chemical, biologic, and physical agents
Agent identification
Agent inventory
MSDS functions
Toxicology information
Emergency management data
Regulatory information
Exposure inventory
Comprehensive reporting functions
Program management
Scheduling of activities
Sampling and inspection data collection, reporting and management
Analytic tools
Incident management
Comprehensive reporting functions

EMPLOYEE TRACKING SUPPORT

Employee demographics
Employee work histories
Employee exposure histories
Mortality data
Prospective measures data
Personal protective equipment
Training

ADMINISTRATIVE SUPPORT

Activity analyses
Log functions
Resource management
Staff
Supplies
Benefits program management

ANALYTIC SUPPORT

Clinical analyses
Environmental analyses
Administrative analyses
Integrated analyses

APPENDIX 12-2
THE ART OF DICTATION

Not directly but tangentially related to medical records is the substitution of dictated notes for the holographic, indecipherable scrawl usually seen in clinical files. McGrath* has listed some guidelines for good dictation:

Identify yourself, the date, the work, and priority. Be as specific as possible. Tell the transcriptionist what the message is (letter, progress notes, insurance form), on what kind of paper you want it (white bond, personal, or practice letterhead), and the number of copies you require.

Make certain all of your notes and reference material are at hand. Consider what you want to say and sequence each thought into a separate paragraph.

Talk loudly enough so the microphone will clearly record your voice. Speak in a normal pitch at your normal speed with your standard inflections. Give your message one phrase or sentence at a time.

Clearly denote plurals, numbers, special capitals, and special punctuation. Spell out the name of the person, the procedure, and unusually difficult street or city names.

*McGrath, B. Dictation: Words are golden. *Skin and Allergy News* 10:22 (Oct), 1979.

Tell your transcriber when there is a new paragraph or special indentation, underlining, or numbering. If dictating a form, indicate that it will be given from left to right and top to bottom. Prescribe whether columns or subparagraphs are desired.

Avoid long pauses, mumbling, smoking, slurring words and endings, and trying to set records for speed talking.

Relax; be as natural as possible, and enjoy the time you are saving.

Periodically audit your dictation. Listen to something you dictated 2 weeks earlier, and make mental notes of what you can do to improve. This is the only way to refine your dictation skills.

No matter how well a physician implements good dictation technique, it is wasted if he or she procrastinates. Medical facts that have accumulated for even several hours tend not to be so complete as those recorded immediately.

When progress notes are dictated immediately and in his or her presence, the patient has the opportunity to hear some of the facts for a second time.

549 407

13. ADMINISTRATION

To succeed, to the full, I believe our plans and programs must include the creative and productive potentialities of trained and skillful workers, of responsible and constructive management and the will to establish and use modern methods, of securing cooperation through responsible labor-management relations.

David E. Lilienthal

PERSONNEL ADMINISTRATION IN THE OCCUPATIONAL HEALTH SERVICE

Long recognized and accepted is the knowledge that the medical director and all of the personnel composing the staff of the occupational health service (OHS) occupy "staff" positions, as opposed to "line" assignments. The incumbents in such positions serve as advisors to the executive person to whom they are subordinate in the hierarchy of the organization. They have no "line" or command function, except as they relate to their own departmental employees and cannot order medical action or other kind of response. Recommendations are submitted to the next level of responsibility, and unless determined differently by local policy, the action that is directed to be taken is done so by the chief executive officer (CEO), the company president, the chancellor, the plant manager, the commanding officer, or whoever has the ultimate designated or vested power to issue orders, develop statements of policy, or devise principles of procedure. As sociologists pointed out, we are an employee society, so that even the chairman of the board occupies that position through election by the directors, and they, in turn, are responsible—mostly in a figurative sense—to the stockholders.

While this structure spells the ladder of control in an organization, the medical director or occupational health nurse (OHN) in charge of other OHS staff, if there is no full-time physician or consultant, does have the assigned authority and responsibility for certain personnel actions in connection with the OHS members. These functions should be understood, and their initiation, execution, and periodic review should not be delegated to a lower level person, who might view the procedures as paperwork movements without feeling for the individuals involved.

Staff members in an OHS are recruited, utilized, nourished, deployed, and severed from service when circumstances dictate. All of these actions, involving people, are to be carried out in concert with the personnel department or the company unit given that responsibility.

ACQUISITION OF PROFESSIONAL PERSONNEL

Staffing of an OHS either from the inception of such a service or at times of growth or needed replacement usually is a joint activity between the personnel department's recruiting arm and the directorate of the OHS. Professional personnel in occupational health are in relatively short supply so that many in-plant physicians know most of the others in the community, state, or nation, and membership of the OHNs in their professional associations allows knowledge of nurses engaged in the same speciality. Further, as frequently there are preceptor programs in both medicine and nursing between the university centers training specialized occupational health personnel and the sites of practice in industry, there is an awareness of the residents or nurses who are about to complete their graduate programs and who will be seeking positions.

This network situation occasionally affects the smooth working arrangement between the health and personnel branches of a company because an agency does not recruit professionals in the same manner as one seeks a number of laborers or clerks. The usual cooperative effort entails completion of a personnel requisition that expresses to the recruiting section the need to fill a vacancy in a certain professional category. If the medical director knows of a physician desirous of making a change, then a first contact between physicians would be the logical seminal exploration, inclusive of meeting the requirements of all existing policies in affirmative action.

If the potential staff member expresses an interest in the position available, a preliminary interview would be in order, for the discussion would clarify both the training and the experience of the candidate and the local occupational health philosophy and principles of operation. If the interest seems intensified from the first interchange, then referral can be made to the personnel department, where both the expectations and the benefits of employment can be delineated and further negotiations can be consummated.

In the recruitment of physicians, many paths seemingly are open, but few lead to desirable end points. While there are many executive search firms, and the number concerned with medical personnel has grown, it has been the author's experience that rarely do staff additions stem from those sources. The recruiters in those organizations usually know of existing vacancies, for they have been asked to find physician replacements. This body of knowledge is broad and firm, but often the candidates they are trying to place may differ in quality from the professionals more recently trained or those persons known to their colleagues as willing to change affiliation. The academicians in university occupational health programs frequently know of both available positions and potential candidates and should be queried regarding recruitment possibilities.

Another source is the placement activity of the American Occupational Medical Association (AOMA), or more recently known as the American College of Occupational Medicine, where a listing is maintained of available physicians and positions, and particularly during the annual meetings the rosters can be searched. Leads can also be obtained from corporate medical directors who may have had to terminate seasoned physicians because of the economic downturn. It is hoped that such professionals will be able to make the move during the period of transition from basic industries to those companies engaged in "high technology."

A final source of personnel would be the advertisements placed in medical journals, although usually there are more notices concerning vacant positions than there are available physicians.

ACQUISITION OF NONPROFESSIONAL PERSONNEL

In connection with nonprofessional staff members, as opposed to the recruitment of professional persons, the personnel authority will take the lead, standard procedures will be followed, and candidates will be referred to the OHS for interview. It is suggested that one be completely familiar with the recruitment requirements relating to affirmative action, the interviewing and testing of applicants, and the character and number of candidate interviews, as established both by regulation and policy. In all instances, any written references should be confirmed by telephone, for former employers or colleagues will speak more freely and will be considerably more direct in their appraisals of performance than when their opinions are solicited in writing. Frequently insightful evaluations are obtained from subordinates as well as peers.*

Rejected applicants should be sent personal letters of appreciation for the opportunity of interview, and any delay in notification should be explained, such as the time taken for additional interviews and the like.

ORIENTATION

Every new employee, irrespective of level, should attend the company's orientation program, if one is held, where it is hoped that the presentations will cover the employer's expectations of the work to be performed in addition to the usual litany of the many benefits that accrue one during a lifetime of service. That there is an *exchange* of salary and benefits for work accomplished, under certain sets of controls, is rarely given the emphasis that is indicated. At this formative period, the idea should be underscored that one is paid for the work accomplished and not for the hours put in while in the organizational setting. The orientation session should give emphasis to the work expectations: Reinforcement can be provided by the new staff member's immediate supervisor in the OHS.

It is the section supervisor's task to orient the new employee to the philosophy underpinning OHS activities, the customary manner of meeting OHS objectives, and the expected quality or level of staff-patient relationships and to provide the training required in procedures that might be unique to the OHS and different from the mode of work in previous medical facilities. In these early days of employment, new staff members should be familiarized with certain personnel actions in which they will be

*In years past when the author was visiting a certain set of national hospitals, it would be the custom to have consultants met at the local hotel and be driven to the hospital. When the driver would be asked about the institution as a place to work, about the director, or about the ambience of the installation, the opinions were found to be solid and close to the target's center point.

involved, either by review of pertinent sections of the company personnel manual or the OHS staff manual, by discussion, or preferably, by both mechanisms.

Copies of pertinent sections of the company manual of policies and procedures or copies of the staff personnel manual, if available, should be given each new employee. If this is not feasible, each staff member should be informed as to which person in the OHS can provide counsel regarding personnel policy. The segments of the personnel manual or employee guide that should be reviewed with, *and* understood by, the new staff member include the following.

EMPLOYMENT AND INTRODUCTION TO JOB

Mission of the organization
Orientation program
Probationary (trial) period
Significance of the preplacement medical examination
Opportunity for improvement
Performance evaluation
Job security
Break in service
Due process—grievance procedure
Union affiliation (if applicable)
Dismissal; retention

WORK SCHEDULE

Hours and days of work
Time cards, attendance records
Excused absence from work for illness
Excused absence from work for urgent personal business
Unexcused absence from work
Lunch periods
Rest periods, coffee breaks
Visits to credit union, OHS, personnel department, cafeteria, snack bars
Time devoted to union activities

PAY INFORMATION

Frequency of pay, days of pay, methods of pay
Overtime pay
Compensatory time off
Step increases
Payroll deductions
Loss of pay

PERSONNEL PROGRAMS

Reclassification
Promotion
Employee development
Shift differential

RULES AND REGULATIONS

Company policies
Departmental policies
Disciplinary measures
Causes for exerting disciplinary measures
Review of cause at termination of discipline
Dual employment
Demotion
Suspension
Layoff
Medical separation

BENEFITS

Insurance
- Health/hospital insurance
- Dental/vision service
- Disability insurance
- Unemployment insurance
- Life insurance
- Workers' compensation, medical care, rehabilitation

Paid holidays, vacation, leave of absence
Retirement—voluntary, compulsory
Athletic programs
Activity programs
Physical fitness programs
Occupational health service
- Examinations
- Surveillance
- Emergency care
- Health education
- Counseling
- Ambulance service

Passes, reduced admissions to telecasts, games, plays, amusement parks, concerts
Credit union
Vacations
Sick leave
Leaves of absence
Cafeterias, snack bars, vending machines
Purchase of company products
Stock options
Parking
Tuition reimbursement
Uniforms
Laundry
Awards
Attendance at conferences
Employee representation

SAFETY PROGRAMS

General safety; specific safety in OHS
Fire prevention

Emergency drills
Housekeeping
Reporting of injuries
Safety rules
Safety committees
Smoking regulations
Safety performance awards

UTILIZATION OF PERSONNEL

Once an individual has been oriented and has an understanding of the requirements of the position, then all the other elements of personnel management should be applied. Errors or deficiencies in performance should be discussed with the employee as soon as detected. It should be determined if additional training is needed and if improvement can be achieved. It might be that different placement or other action will be required for betterment of job performance. If unsatisfactory performance continues, the fact and circumstances must be recorded, and consideration should be given a change of assignment within the OHS or elsewhere in the organization. If efforts prove fruitless, a joint review with the OHS director must be undertaken.

In a parallel sense, a particular task well done, a continued outstanding performance, or a patient contact that resulted in a compliment to the director should be noted immediately, mentioned at a meeting of the staff, or given OHS bulletin board publicity.

If corrective action of a specific type is indicated by company policy, it should be initiated, and the document outlining the steps to be taken should be read, understood, and signed by the recipient. In most public jurisdictions, considerable time is given an employee for an improvement in job performance as based on a plan for action. Time spans or goals are written into the document for the attainment of specific objectives, in keeping with personnel policy. These procedures take time and often are completely frustrating because they represent, in many situations, delays in the administration of definitive action for these reasons: (1) They often are not taken seriously by the ineffective employee, (2) they "wear down" the supervisor to the point that often the supervisor believes it easier to tolerate the poor performance than to go through the innumerable steps called for by protocol, and (3) when completed, the action called for and the critical conclusions reached may not be supported by higher authority for fear, among other things, of an ethnicity backlash. To see a protocol through to the end—rehabilitation or termination—takes courage, patience, prompt application of all the procedural steps, and skill in accurate documentation.* Guidance from the personnel authority can be invaluable.

An astute supervisor will recognize a productive employee and will either enlarge the job, encourage the individual to take some courses, or motivate the employee to aspire to a position at a higher level. The last action may mean a loss to the current employer, but it will add some needed talent to the labor force at another institution. A good employee, contrary to Laurence J. Peter, can rise to a higher level of competence and should not be restrained or retained because of the loss that might result.

An error commonly committed in personnel management by supervisors who defer indicated corrective action is the granting of a step increase—either by failure to study the record, by having delegated something considered "routine" to someone else, or by not reading a paper submitted for signature—and following this false recognition of merit by an attempt at reprimand, suspension, or other negative move. Adverse action will not and cannot be supported shortly after an award, in a sense, was given. The inconsistency bespeaks poor supervision and a lack of continuous review of personnel.

A fact of life appears periodically. Employees do not equate general wage increases (GWI))—an across-the-board increase for all employees, particularly for white-collar workers when negotiations have led to a wage increase for union members—with step increases. The author had just announced to his OHS staff a GWI for all personnel. As soon as the meeting broke, one of the senior clerks came in wanting to know when her step increase would come through. Individual recognition surpassed in significance the addition of dollars to the paycheck.

GROWTH AND NURTURING OF PERSONNEL

In the ideal setting, with dedicated employees, work should be an experience in professional growth. It is the function of the OHS director to exercise all means to allow this maturation of the staff. Career development may not be too applicable to professionals in an OHS, but employee development is pertinent to the enlargement of one's technical or behavioral skills. The means to accomplish this goal might be attendance at conferences or workshops sponsored by various specialty societies, the National Institute for Occupational Safety and Health (NIOSH), educational resource centers, or continuing educa-

*A wise, experienced head nurse uttered the truth when she said that being a supervisor would never win one a popularity contest.

tion programs offered by innumerable colleges and universities.

The courses taken or the symposia heard need not necessarily be limited to technical matters but can encompass the improvement of personal skills in relating to patients, peers, or superordinates, the understanding of human behavior, sensitivity training, or improved methods in health promotion. Another mechanism lies in an educational enrichment program. Many community colleges conduct evening courses, sometimes on company premises, termed extension campuses, where managers might teach and where the employees find it convenient to learn without having to travel additional distances. As indicated earlier, if the course content relates directly to the employee's work, there is the possibility of having the tuition reimbursed by the company.

This kind of personal development is to be encouraged, not only because of the greater knowledge brought to the job by the employee and the benefit to the operation of the OHS, but also because the staff member feels better with the intellectual sustenance that has been provided and the pride taken in having learned.

One of the motivating factors that might play a role here is that with this external updating of information and improved capacity, the potential exists for upward mobility through job reclassification and thus an increase in salary.

Such an action, were it to be undertaken, might entail the preparation of a job description, if the position to which the employee is aspiring is new and does not represent a classification currently in existence somewhere in the company. Usually, the head of an OHS will be asked by the classifiers in the personnel department to prepare the new job description, and assistance will be provided in its drafting. The points to be covered in such a narrative should provide detail regarding:

Supervisory responsibilities—of personnel and operations or units
Functions performed
Knowledge of specialized subject matter required for various levels of position
Degree of work difficulty
Amount of technical specialization inherent in job
Complexity and variety of functions
Nature and extent of authority delegated
Nature and level of personal contacts involved in performance of the functions
Degree of supervision received
Level and nature of decision-making authority
Amount of initiative, originality, and judgment required in the resolution of new, but related, problems
Amount of responsibility for representing the unit supervised in relations with managers and administrators, scientific and technical personnel, customers, or the general public
Sites of performance of required functions
Knowledge required of pertinent data banks, information systems, and sources of available primary information
Preparation required of original documents, reports, abstracts, grant applications, technical manuals, or other written pieces
Minimum qualifications—in education, experience, and physical and emotional capacities (if different or unique)

As technology advances and is applied to the operation of an OHS, some existing job descriptions may have to be rewritten. The director of an OHS should anticipate that periodically a personnel audit will be conducted of the facility because of these changes. Procedures that once were considered highly complex might have been automated, computers might now prepare reports formerly done by personal calculations, or procedures that once represented innovative technical advances have become repetitive processes in no need of highly skilled supervision. Because of these changes, jobs might be classified downward, an upsetting procedure to both the medical director and the individual employee.

These disturbing decisions constantly should be anticipated, and the incumbent should be trained in additional or more skilled procedures or in computer applications so that the employee's skills will not necessarily be jettisoned in a reclassification action but elevated because of added worth. It is the wise director who will review the job descriptions semiannually to determine the presence of any mismatchings between the outline of the work on record and the actual set of functions being performed.

A mechanism that can be stimulative of professional growth is encouragement of staff members to publish. Every person in an OHS—semiprofessional and professional—can be motivated to report on some innovative program elements in which he or she has participated. Non-writers will be hesitant to undertake a task they have never participated in, but there can be no greater reward to them than to see their first publication. It will take patient guidance on the director's part, but the morale value cannot be measured.

One last element in the continued growth of an employee is the physical restoration or rehabilitation of a worker to improve or remove a physical impairment or limitation that has precluded upward movement on the employment ladder. An example of such a corrective measure was seen in a bright chemicalstoreroom attendant who was limited in his job by a poorly repaired cleft palate. With reconstruction and correction of the defect, a clear speech pattern resulted, and he was promoted to a middle-level administrative post.

DISPOSITION OF PERSONNEL

Individual staff members will leave an OHS, and each method of separation requires a personnel action to be initiated by the medical director. As various types of terminal pay must be settled, prompt notification of the action is needed. Termination of employment can be the result of any one of the following:

Voluntary termination or resignation
Discharge for cause of dismissal
Transfer
Voluntary retirement
Compulsory retirement
Temporary layoff
Indefinite layoff
Disability retirement
Job abandonment
Release during or at end of probationary period
Extended military leave
Investigatory leave
Medical separation
Expiration of appointment
Death from work-incurred injury
Death from other causes

Whatever the basis for the action, the necessary documents must be forwarded promptly to the personnel department.

BUDGET DEVELOPMENT AND PROGRAM COSTS

For which of you, intending to build a tower, sitteth not down first, and counteth the cost, whether he have sufficient to finish it?

St. Luke

Inherent in any departmental operation is the preparation and use of a budget that represents the resources needed to meet the established objectives of a health program, in keeping with the company's declared policy. The funds allocated to a staff or service unit represent overhead costs; therefore, the support is rarely generous and frequently is reflective of the organization's sales or profits. In good times, when production is high and increasing, the fiscal support will be larger to meet the need of greater hiring. In times of recession, there may be cuts in the dollars available, in the form of either an across-the-board reduction in total monies available to all departments or a need to release one or more employees. In certain sectors where income is determined by the taxes collected, the budget may undergo readjustment several times during a single year.

The OHS, like any function in a company, must prepare a budget, and frequently this exercise involves the development of such a plan for the next quinquennium. As it is relatively impossible to judge the activities to be undertaken in the future—because of potential production shifts, mergers, product obsolescence, new restrictive legislation, national preparedness, plant modernization, changes in manufacturing modes, public whims, replacement of lasting style by short-lived fads, and political shifts—planning may become strictly a blue-sky effort with guesses supplanting sound thought.

BASIC CONSIDERATIONS

It must be determined which temporal cycling is used by the company. Is the budget to be prepared for the fiscal year, usually July 1 through the following June 30? Or is the physical or calendar year the base of planning? Or, if the organization is an agency of the federal government, will the annual period begin October 1? Medical operations vary, as determined by the anticipated amount of seasonal illness, the number of expected new employees including summer workers, the need for new surveillance procedures, the aging of the plant population, the entry of women into nontraditional jobs, and the amount of research involving OHS personnel. This rising or falling of health care needs implies varying monthly expenditures so that no month may equal another in funds needed. These variations must be planned for so that at year's end there will be neither a shortfall nor an unexpended balance. The former will require subsequent trimming, and the latter may lead to an enforced lower fiscal request the following year.

METHOD OF PREPARATION

As determined by the size of the OHS, the budget will be prepared by the medical director in conjunction with the section heads. The initial phases of the framing of a fiscal base should be a cooperative effort, and as it is exemplified at all levels of governmental or industrial management, the unit head who requests budgetary increases must present, in writing, the justification for such expressed needs.

If the OHS is of a size that requires an administrator, then it will be the task of that person to solicit the sectional subsets of the budget and assemble them for review by the medical director. Irrespective of the OHS person preparing the initial draft document, it is sage counsel that can be offered by the fiscal officer or comptroller at all stages of budget development. Usually there will be one representative of that office who will be assigned responsibility for the OHS—and possibly other staff operations—who knows well what the true support expectations will be. Guidance from such a person will obviate the inclusion of glaring errors, miscalculations, or unrealistic requests. It is this individual who knows, in advance, what the allocations are most likely to be and will prevent the submission of a document that will be unrealistic or give evidence of a lack of substantive managerial skills. It is to this budget person that well-justified needs can be made known, and counsel will be given regarding the general tenor of the money supply and its distribution in the forthcoming year.

It seems that there are always certain managers who follow the principle of building excessive needs into a budget request, or "padding" or "adding fat," in anticipation of the standard cutting of a certain amount or percentage. Repeated efforts toward the grandiose soon make one suspect, and the cutting thereafter becomes a regular procedure by higher authority.

It has been seen to go both ways. The honest, lean projection can be sheared, and the excessive request may be accepted or even raised. It is difficult to make recommendations, for much depends on the professional or business relationship with the CEO, the general health of the organization, and the perception of the medical director as a producer *and* a manager. In many instances the budget may represent responses to specific needs expressed by the CEO, and incremental increases over the previous year will go by unquestioned. In essence, the budget is representative of the quality of OHS performance as viewed by both managers and labor. A quiet union, one satisfied with the medical service, may be a factor of tremendous worth to the company. An OHS that meets the personal needs of executives may have little difficulty in budget review. There is no good crystal ball.

CATEGORIES OF EXPENDITURES

Every budget puts on display a variety of categories for which expenditures must be planned. In a department where there are usually no accounts receivable, the budget becomes one of costs solely.* If consultative services are provided, as they are in rare instances, then there would be some income accruing the OHS and ultimately the company.

In most accounting systems, each category will be assigned a charge number so that expenditures can be correctly posted.

LABOR

Salaries
- Professional, paramedical, and support staff personnel; consultants
- Salary increases or job reclassifications (Plans must be made for periodic step increases, cost of living increases, wage raises through new contract negotiations, or reclassifications occasioned by skill changes in a job, for example, typist to word processor.)

Benefits
- Social Security or special retirement plan
- Disability and unemployment insurance taxes
- Group life, hospitalization, and medical care insurance plans
- Uniforms and laundry service (frequently a highly contested benefit)
- Meals, if furnished

MATERIALS

Capital equipment—clinical and administrative

Depreciation of equipment
- Maintenance service
- Repairs

Office supplies—consumable

Medical, nursing, and laboratory supplies—consumable

Industrial hygiene supplies—consumable

Printing—administrative and medical record forms, health education materials, OHS manual

Film or video tape rental, purchase of health education materials

Personal protective devices for staff members (hard hats, protective eyewear)

Personal protective devices for OHS visitors (hard hats, protective eyewear, protective clothing)

OVERHEAD

Rent, electricity, heating, air conditioning, gas, water (In some organizations, direct charges are made, in others there is a certain percentage charged for

*Savings can be demonstrated in such program elements as absenteeism control or counseling, provided there is fiscal quantification of workdays preserved, turnover decreased, and the like.

overhead, and yet in others, there are no such charges levied against the OHS.)

Telecommunications, postage, freight (A slight additional cost might be accrued if special postal-meter health-related cancellation slugs are used for all company mail. Freight costs may be included if the OHS wishes to exhibit at a national conference.)

Fire, theft, professional liability insurance

Building repairs, maintenance, alterations (In most companies, charges are made for estimates. Usually, these changes are more costly when done inhouse than by outside contractors. Decision may be made through the bidding process.)

Custodial service (Ideally, custodians should be full-time members of the OHS. Contract services frequently are inefficient, often negligible; waste-receptable emptying passes as custodial care.)

Data-processing time charge (only if totally dependent on a mainframe computer)

Specialized diagnostic and therapeutic instrument maintenance and/or calibration (needed to comply with certain federal/state mandates)

MEDICAL CARE

Special extramural examinations

Special immunization or case-finding programs (influenza or rabies vaccines, for example, or new medical surveillance procedures)

Blood bank (providing facilities, personnel, some supplies to community blood bank collecting blood from employees on company premises, using the OHS as the collection site)

Patient transportation—Taxicab or ambulance, to hospital, emergency service, physician's office, or home (For taxis, books of coupons might be the most expeditious and least costly form of payment.)

Optical dispensing (The costs of protective eyewear are back-charged to the individual employee's department, unless a prorated charge is deducted from the worker's paycheck, in addition to a partial departmental back-charge.)

CONTINGENCY FUND

Petty cash for emergency purchases (to meet a special need, to cover during a period of extremely delayed supply delivery, or to purchase an inexpensive item whose cost-accounting procedure would exceed by far the cost of the item itself)

Meals or company transportation for official visitors

STAFF DEVELOPMENT

Continuing professional education

- Travel and lodging
- Registration, course tuition, seminar fee
- Honoraria to invited speakers at staff meetings
- Materials for professional presentations (slides, exhibits, photocopied printed handouts)
- Professional monographs and subscriptions to journals

Staff retreats (for program review, overall planning, improved intrastaff communication)

Overtime, when required

RESEARCH

As determined by capability, feasibility of project, or use of new untested substances as constraints or motivating forces

ADDITIONAL CONSIDERATIONS

The potential exists constantly for changes in legislative mandates, either through new, more demanding enactments or through deregulation. The possibilities of additional acquisitions by the company may require either the establishment of an OHS of quality comparable to the one currently in the parent organization or even improvement in the latter if the newly added firm offers superior health care opportunities.

Contractual changes resulting from collective bargaining may require building in a new program element because the contested point was won by the labor representatives. It is wise to determine from the negotiating team if health issues will be introduced as possible additional benefits or merely as complaints with existing regulations. Any advance information can be helpful in the structuring of a budget for the activities required at the year's start, which can be strikingly changed by mandates appearing toward year's end.

Extreme caution must be exercised to avoid overruns in expenditures, for such inattention bespeaks poor management and, as mentioned previously, the OHS is to be as well-directed an operation as any department immediately connected with production. The medical director must be an astute manager, and the adherence to budgetary constraints is a measure of that skill.

To remain "in the black," reports must be obtained as frequently as possible, usually on a monthly basis. These documents must be scanned to determine which sections of the OHS are overexpending or underutilizing resources so that necessary adjustments can be made in sectional allocations throughout the year. It is desirable that all section heads be apprised of the currency of their shares of the budget so that they, at another level, become as managerially capable as those persons in the directorate. By the assignment of this kind of responsibility to unit chiefs, they acquire a truer feeling for some of the demands inherent in supervisory positions.

OPERATIONAL COSTS

It has always been a wish that medical directors of various OHSs could compare costs of operation between one medical organization and another. When attempts are made to match fiscal bases, it is found that rarely can a coupling of cost data be conducted. Bookkeeping systems differ vastly because of the variations in costing or charge-back customs.

However, progress can be seen if comparisons are made between time sequences either in a single year or among several years' experience. Naturally, geographic location will demonstrate a lack of parallel among professional salaries, and the level of staffing will elevate or lower the cost of operation. There are three methods of establishing a cost basis that can be used in temporal comparisons.

Perhaps the simplest is merely to take the figure representing the plant population and divide the year's expenditures for the OHS into that number of workers, to establish a *total cost for in-plant health care per person per year.* Data derived from workers' compensation costs are not included—only those expenditures made directly by or through the OHS.

A second manner of determining a cost planking is to use the total cost figure for a year and divide that amount by the number of visits made (or services rendered) to develop a *cost per visit* figure.

The last system requires the assistance of the comptroller, but it can be carried out and has been used successfully in certain manufacturing plants where the ultimate product is large and costly, such as an automobile. If the vehicle at point of delivery has cost $*XXXXX*, then it can be determined that for each unit made, the cost included $*YY* for OHS *in-plant* care.

Whatever the device used, comparisons can be made monthly or yearly, and changes can be requested at the next period of budget preparation, if indicated.

It may be necessary to defend or justify a budget request, and personal testimony or clarification may be required. Anonymous case histories of good preventive medicine—with cost savings—relay a strong message, as do well-prepared but uncluttered charts. Further, as the levels of review move up, some veiled material can be inserted that would have particular relevance to a member, or members, of the reviewing panel. An unidentified, yet personal approach may be extremely meaningful in an effort to justify the need for certain resources.

Two experienced medical directors have described systems of cost accounting that bear certain similarities. Collings [1] proposed the quantum equivalent technique (Q_eT), in which the basic concept is to define the equivalent quantity of work or total effort required for various medical services. To activate the method, certain data, readily available, must be obtained: (1) number of different services rendered in a given period and (2) the total expense dollars spent in the same time span.

With the participation of the medical staff, a ranking system was established through mutual agreement so that quantum equivalent values (Q_eVs) could be assigned to departmental activities. The executive periodic examination was selected as the base and was given the Q_eV of 100. Other services were assigned values, such as the following:

Preemployment regular examination	65
Occupational injury or illness without absence	70
Counseling	20
Immunization	10
Occupational injury or illness with absence	190

With these assigned values, the time spent per service can be determined. For example, as Collings has shown, in a 6-month period 306 multiphasic screening examinations were performed, and at a Q_eV of 75, the total Q_e units came to 22,950, or 3.22 percent of the 711,405 Q_e units of service provided. Further, some 4,527 preemployment regular examinations resulted in 294,255 Q_e units, or 41.36 percent of the total. The system highlights the procedures that consume the greatest amount of staff effort.

The cost of each Q_e unit can be determined. For instance, the expenses of one medical office during the same time frame came to $348,700 (1970 dollars). This amount divided by the total number of Q_e units (711,605) showed the unit cost to be $0.4902. From this point, one can cost out any particular activity. Executive examinations accounted for 11,100 Q_e units, or a total cost of $5,441.22.

In addition, the cost of a single service is derivable. As the executive examination was given the Q_eV of 100, then 100 × $0.4902, or $49.02 represents the cost of that particular service.

Comparisons in work output or program-element emphasis can be made among various medical facilities, demonstrating where program efforts are maximized or where functional deficits might exist.

Craig [2] utilized a similar system of assigning weighted values to various services. A value of 1 was assigned to an interview, and this figure was used as the base. Other assigned values comprised the following: treatment of an occupationally incurred condition, 7; treatment of a nonoccupational disorder, 3; periodic examination, 15; preplacement examination, 10; and other examinations, 5. The values assigned were in proportion to the additional costs attendant on the procedure or service. From these numerical values and the known costs (direct cost of the medical office plus the indirect cost), the total costs of various program elements can be determined. The resulting data allow not only both cost and activity comparisons among various health stations, but also a comparison between company-provided care and the services provided under contract.

These kinds of analyses were of extreme significance in the Tennessee Valley Authority (TVA) where health care would be required on-site in isolated areas where new construction was being undertaken. By providing medical facilities in trailers, permanent structures were not needed, and professional personnel from the organization could be assigned for the duration of the project in preference to contracting for costly care from local resources.

COST CONTAINMENT

OHS directors, like their colleagues in the community, hear complaints about the cost of medical care, for employees are not inarticulate in expressing their views concerning charges levied for either medical or surgical care and the frequently diminishing benefits or rising premium costs.* As the required deductible amount of a policy rises, so does the temper of the worker who has both a spouse and children.

Two issues present themselves for consideration. The first involves care received in the community, and this segment of therapy need not necessarily be viewed as outside the purview of the medical director. If it is feasible for an employee to review the options available in proferred care, guidance can be given regarding the conduct of care without hospitalization, the performance of certain surgical operations as ambulatory treatment rather than as inpatient procedures, the duplication of investigative services, and the like.

Much can be accomplished by *persisting, repeated* worker education in lifestyle change, preferably through behavior modification [3]. One must demonstrate with telling numbers the effect on the monthly cost of group health insurance premiums of the hazard-intensive practice of smoking and drug abuse, the presence of obesity, and the failure to exercise or maintain antihypertensive therapeutic regimens. As a practitioner who has interacted with patients for over half a century, no longer are feelings spared in discussing these self-destructive processes. The fear that someone might be offended by such efforts no longer should hold back the counsel, the caution, the honesty given us by the world's best epidemiologists. The true believer, to use the late Eric Hoffer's phrase, must convey the information relentlessly, backing the message with supportive clinical health-effect data whenever possible.

Also, when opportunity presents itself for a medical opinion, one need not fail to enlighten the worker that frequently professional restraint can be exercised, and second, or even third, opinions can be sought regarding advised elective procedures. If preoperative laboratory tests are needed, they can be accomplished by the OHS at considerably less cost than is seen on any hospital summary of charges, and the results can be relayed to the hospital or the reports can be carried by the patient.

As the private physician, frequently a surgeon, tends to recommend a rather protracted postoperative convalescence, the medical director can make contact with the practitioner and explain the actual job demands, physically and emotionally. In most instances the surgeon is unfamiliar with the job content and may be influenced by the patient's exaggerated description of the work requirements, and in many instances, the advised recovery period is unduly long. A frank clarification of the patient's work can usually bring about a shortening of the convalescent span, an earlier return to work, and a saving in costs.

Also, the various test batteries conducted as part of required examinations or surveillance protocols should be scrutinized to determine which procedures can be eliminated as not furthering the diagnostic potential. As an example, leukocyte differential counts might be eliminated unless it has been established that certain hematologic aberrations can be expected [4].

Lastly, the medical director should become involved in the negotiations concerning group health insurance with *both* the underwriters *and* the labor representatives. The director should know the medical needs of the workforce and should assist in the sculpturing of the benefit package and in interpreting the medical content or intent of the levels of coverage [5,6].

Platt [7], in his summary of a discussion on cost containment, tends to disparage most of the kinds of

*Health care expenditures for one company rose from $24,690,000 in 1978 to $37,168,000 in 1982, an increase of over one-half of the original cost. (See The numbers tell the story! *Newsletter,* The New York Business Group on Health, 3(9):7, 1983.

efforts alluded to in this discussion. He believes that a successful cost-containment program will comprise some or all of these elements: caps on public health expenditures and implicit limits on the quality and accessibility of health care provided at public expense, tighter governmental regulation of private health care expenditures, control of the physician supply, and modification of the fee-for-service reimbursement system for physicians and hospitals. He ends by observing that what we should not do is pretend that painless cost containment is an achievable goal.

Will the OHS, as one controlling mechanism, offer more care at the worksite? For the workers only? For their families? Some organizations are doing it. Will others follow?

Some observers have criticized the efficacy of our current "free-market" health care, maintaining that our various measures designed to improve the system—the Hill-Burton Act, Medicare, Medicaid, and health maintenance organizations (HMOs)—have served solely as patchwork efforts at reform [8]. Suggested as the solution is a unitary system, namely a national health service. With the innumerable factions unvalued, only time will provide the configuration of the future health care model.

REPORTS

The system of reporting events is age-old, for were it not for this mode of communication, there would be no role for the National Archives or, in large part, for the great libraries of the world. While the preparation of reports is rarely a task taken on with anticipatory pleasure, periodic announcements concerning the "state of the OHS" are necessary for a variety of reasons. Irrespective of the size of the occupational health operation, frequent summations of the activities of the unit must be submitted to the next level of authority. To whom in the organizational structure reports are forwarded is determined by the placement of the health function in the company.

OBJECTIVES

There is a broad rationale for timely reviews of the services provided by an OHS, and following are the objectives of a reporting system:

- To present the work accomplished in light of the population served.
- To offer a base for future comparisons at specified time intervals.
- To indicate progress, a plateau, or a decline in service.
- To show the personnel base that is carrying out the assigned functions.
- To depict the variety of services offered.
- To provide a data base for epidemiologic study of various entities: occupational disease, absenteeism, effects of specialized program elements (such as vision conservation), populations at risk, and so on.
- To show the takeoff point for planning.
- To give a rationale for budget requests.
- To create a mechanism for studying the effects of new laws, mandates, or regulations.
- To determine the success of both long-standing and innovative programs.
- To offer, through accompanying narrative, a means of putting flesh on the statistical skeleton, of allowing the data to come alive.
- To describe problem areas.
- To have an instrument for intramural and extramural public relations.
- To have available a device for acknowledging outstanding performance of certain staff members.
- To demonstrate, particularly in a research setting (university, think tank, mission-specific institute, library), that an OHS is similarly capable of investigative and published scholarship.
- To apprise higher authorities (CEO, industrial relations director, or other directors) of the "state-of-the-art" of the operations for which they have responsibility.

The ideal situation is one in which the report from the medical facility is allowed to stand on its own merits and dimension. By truncating it through conversion into a feeder report, it can lose its unique significance in the larger departmental review of activities. Some of the shine would be dulled were the information to be included with the number of breakfasts served in the cafeteria or a description of the quality of the custodial service.

USE BY RECIPIENTS

There are uses to which OHS reports can be put by the recipient, depending on current needs, the status of collective bargaining within the company, or the support tone of local media. These functions are the following:

- As a statement concerning the health of the labor force

As a base for comparison with data from other reporting facilities
As substantive material for publicizing good methods of operation
As an educational mechanism
As an assist in the determination of the fiscal, personnel, or equipment support pattern
As a clue (or clues) for needed research, either in-house or by contract
As a segment of a larger public relations thrust (house organ, local media, national advertising)
As continuing assurance that the OHS is a sound investment of overhead money

One cannot predict the ultimate use of documents emanating from an OHS, for a particular segment may be selected for broad distribution by an executive who has pride in the health-conserving efforts of the OHS.*

TYPES OF REPORTS

Regularly recurring or infrequently required reports generated by an OHS may be prepared in accordance with directives not only from the company but from the federal government, the state government, the municipality, the employer, granting or research-contracting agencies, and where indicated, trade associations. Such documents are primarily intramural, for distribution within the organization only, or extramural, with distribution to recipients outside the boundaries of the immediate plant. Commonly prepared reports are the following.

MANDATED BY THE FEDERAL GOVERNMENT

Department of Labor

Occupational Safety and Health Administration (OSHA) No. 200—Log and Summary of Occupational Injuries and Illnesses
OSHA No. 101—Supplemental Record of Occupational Injuries and Illnesses

In certain states, comparable reports are submitted to the state agency.

All report forms provide instructions for appropriate completion, submission, retention, and availability for inspection. Deaths usually are reported by telephone message.

Environmental Protection Agency (EPA)

Possible Substantial Risk Report: In compliance with Sec. 8(e) of the Toxic Substances Control Act (TSCA), such reports are to be submitted on materials manufactured, processed, or distributed commercially by the employer and will include "products, process or product research and development, raw materials, intermediates, by-products, effluents, emissions, waste products, and catalysts."

Consumer Product Safety Commission

Possible Substantial Risk Report: in compliance with Sec. 15(b) of the Consumer Product Safety Act (CPSA).

REQUIRED BY STATE AGENCIES

Department of Labor (Industrial Relations)

State counterpart of Log and Summary of Occupational Injuries and Illnesses, if required.

REQUIRED BY LOCAL AUTHORITIES

City or County Department of Health

Report of communicable disease.*
Report of animal bite, including information, if available, regarding animal behavior, owner of animal, nature of bite, and so on.

REQUIRED BY EMPLOYER

The reports of activities of an OHS required within an organization will vary greatly, as determined by company policy, the extent of familiarity of managerial personnel with the occupational health operation, the autonomy of the installation, the geographic location of the plant, the uniqueness of the health problems, the peculiar need for or dislike of frequent reports by the CEO, the networking of medical facilities between a corporate headquarters and outlying domestic and international facilities, and the need for cost data in charge-back procedures, if such a method of operation is customary.

Whatever the official policy may be, it is important

*As an example, during World War II, a manual on occupational medicine prepared by the author solely for use at a single port installation was distributed by the Army's Chief of Transportation to all ports of embarkation throughout the United States. (Medical Department, United States Army. *Preventive Medicine in World War II*. Washington, DC: Office of The Surgeon General, Department of the Army, 1969. Vol. IX, Special Fields. Pp. 123–124.)

*The Confidential Morbidity Report form is usually a state form but is to be submitted to the local health department. Certain reportable communicable diseases may be occupationally incurred such as anthrax, brucellosis, coccidioidomycosis, hepatitis A, B, non-A/non-B, leptospirosis, plague, psittacosis, Q fever, rabies, Rocky Mountain spotted fever, rubella, tetanus, tuberculosis, and tularemia, among others.

that the OHS director maintain a running statistical summation of the employee-patients seen and the services provided. It is not possible to predict when an exigent situation or need will arise for the immediate presentation of a set of data for planning, expansion, personnel utilization, or new contractual purposes.

It has been the author's experience that a monthly summation will meet whatever need manifests itself. A more frequent formal statistical presentation such as a weekly or daily set of totals rarely is required; besides, such figures are always readily derived from a monthly accounting. The report should contain several sections and the primary items suggested for inclusion are the following:

Patient caseload
Disposition of patients
Attendants providing services
Services provided
Specialized consultations
Special programs
Personnel in OHS
Changes in physical facilities
Changes in program
Special programs within sections of OHS
Visitors
Publications of OHS staff members
Attendance at professional meetings
Honors, awards, papers presented, commendations, and elections to office of staff members
Presentations to community groups
Unmet needs
Summary of trends and achievements
Future plans
Illustrations

The format for the annual report will not differ greatly; the statistical totals will represent a summation of the year's activities. A significant addition to, or component of, the annual submission would be an evaluation of the year's innovations or of ongoing programs whose continuance might be questioned. If longitudinal epidemiologic studies were concluded, an abstract of the project and its results should be included.

COMMENT

Every regularly recurring report that is prepared has an established distribution list. Apart from the managers—including department heads—to whom the report should be sent each month and at year's end, copies should be sent to other physicians within the organization who are located in plants or offices both in the United States and abroad. All section chiefs of an OHS should receive copies, not only to be apprised of the total output of the health facility, but also to see the result of their preparation of feeder reports. A technique that is useful and aids in elevating morale is the highlighting each month of the activities of a particular section of the OHS. By year's end, each unit will have been described, and the rotation can begin once again.

As part of the report, samples of health-education material should be included: brochures, posters (reduced in size and reprinted), newsletters, columns from the weekly or monthly house organ, and so on. If certain time-sensitive messages or notices have been distributed regarding special programs, health messages, precautions regarding epidemics, and the like, copies should be included. Interesting events or examples of the unusual might be related, provided discretion is used and the concerned individual(s) can be disguised. For example, when the author was associated with the OHS of the County of Los Angeles, many applicants were examined each day who hoped to see service in law enforcement. At that time and prior to contrary court rulings, sheriff's deputies had to meet a minimum height requirement of 5 ft 8 in. (172 cm). One young man who aspired to such a position was fearful that he was under the necessary height so he prepared the entire day and night prior to the examination by having himself "stretched." In order not to lose the presumed benefit of the lengthening, he had himself delivered to the OHS in the supine position on the bed of a station wagon and was rolled in by his friends almost with the rigidity of mummification. He did not fulfill the physical standard. This kind of illustration can lubricate an otherwise jejune document.

Finally, a regular reporting requirement need not imply that the writing be deadly dull. The reports submitted by Dr. Jeaffreson Lloyd, one-time medical director for a large British conglomerate, were masterpieces of literary writing, replete with humor, and not without retold relevant events that showed wherein he was outwitted or bested by a scheming employee. Those reports were extremely enjoyable and eagerly received in spite of their being single-spaced mimeographed copies, without the fancy dress of a binding, plastic covers, or attractive type fonts.

While writing for scholarly journals is not being discussed in any detail, some remarks are in order, for even the production of a report is an exercise in the respectful use of language. A plethora of new books on technical writing reaches the dealers' shelves every year, indicative of the fact that the disease of ill writing is still in need of a cure. Tagg [9] has observed that anyone who has ever had to edit someone else's writing or who has ever attempted seriously to teach others how to write or speak better must have heard the following hundreds of times: "Yes, but you know what I mean!" It is one of the great evasions. Tagg continued with this example. Once he pointed out to the author of a technical report prepared under contract with a government agency that he had written exactly the opposite of what he intended to convey. Undismayed, he nodded and said, "Yeah, but they'll know what I mean."

Tagg's piece on clarity in language concludes with these pithy statements: "I don't know what you mean until you've told me. I'll give you my thoughtful attention before I form a judgment about what you mean. And I will expect the same treatment from you. I will not try to hold you responsible for understanding more than I have said. I will try to write and speak in such a way that I can reasonably believe that you do know what I mean, because I have said it."

That reports must be clear on first reading needs no further exposition. The recipient of the material is busy, is flooded with paper, and to becloud the document he or she faces with fuzzy statements, current jargon, and time-fringed clichés is inexcusable, unpardonable, and insulting. Clarity—immediate clarity on reading—is mandatory. The cant and patois of medicine are bewildering and confusing, and their insinuation into a report will lead to rejection and, possibly, subsequent negative action. Pertinent to this discussion is the obfuscation encountered in another discipline. Kaufman [10] in his review of a work in sociology cited this sentence: "Thus, social-cultural linkage usually requires that the value orientation and the social structure of the change agent system and the target system are brought together in at least temporary closure." Each word, as a single entity, is understood, but when all are assembled, one simply does not know what the writer means.

In a lament by a cogent Britisher [11], Sir George Pickering is cited as questioning, for example, the educational value of the multiple-choice question, which, he feels, may test a candidate's fund of knowledge but does little to test the ability to present evidence, to argue from it, and to write lucidly about it. Further, he feels that if the present trends in medical education continue, it is inevitable that there will be a decline in the literacy and scholarship of the profession. One need only to read reports emanating from some contemporary practitioners' offices to form the belief that the decline is alive and flourishing.

The transition from speaking to writing frequently is undertaken without a change in format. What has been termed conveniently as Medspeak by Christy [12] will creep into the written report if one is not careful to expunge this occupational jargon. Christy offers some frightening archetypes: "He entered in a bad DKA." Translation: He had diabetic ketoacidosis. "How is this patient progressing?" "Zero delta." Translation to English: No change. "What are you giving the patient?" "Oids." What is meant is "—oids," and the translation is corticosteroids. Lastly, Christy targets on "sometimes," "occasionally," "quite," and "essentially," among other presumably clarifying modifiers. He points to the resident reading from a real-life laboratory report in which a statement is offered regarding the toxicologic findings in a case of overdose with multiple but unknown drugs—"Barbiturate level essentially normal." Christy asks, "Normal for a normal person? Normal for a person who has taken an overdose of barbiturate? Normal for a person who has taken an overdose of something other than a barbiturate? Or a little above or a little below 'normal' for any or all of the above? A triumph of Medspeak. Meaning is drained out, communication ceases to exist, thought wilts, action is paralyzed. The screen has screened. The young doctors are hidden and so is the laboratory. The attending is left alone to stare, helpless and immobile, at the nullity around him."

Without belaboring the need for clear understandable English in a report, one must ask also for a certain feeling and compassion as we move in the corporate areas of computers and the growing replacement of medical care offices by giant chains of hospitals, clinics, and governmentally designated facilities for health service. Exemplary of the requirement for compassion, even in a printed form, let one repeat the wording of a statement received by a friend who had to consult a physician in a two-man office in Edinburgh in mid-1983. The 5 × 8 inch slip gave the names, addresses, and telephone number of the practitioners, but carried no such indication of purpose such as "Statement," or "For professional services." After the date, it provided, in beautiful script, the following message: "H.N. MacPhail [and] W.T.K. Sellar present their compliments to Mr. C.K.—and beg to intimate that their fees for Professional Attendance amount to £5.00." That is class.

Lastly, for direction in the correct use of our language, one cites the "Ten Commandments for Technical Writers" [13]:

> Thou shalt remember thy readers all the days of thy life; for without readers all thy words are as naught. Thou shalt not forsake the time-honored virtue of simplicity. Thou shalt not abuse the third person passive. Thou shalt not dangle thy participles neither shalt thou misplace thy

modifiers. Thou shalt not commit monotony. Thou shalt not cloud thy message with a miasma of technical jargon. Thou shalt not hide the fruits of thy research beneath excess verbiage, neither shalt thou obscure thy conclusions with vague generalities. Thou shalt not resent helpful advice from thy editors, reviewers and critics. Thou shalt consider also the views of the layman, for his is an insight often unknown to technocrats. Thou shalt write and *rewrite* without tiring for such is the key to improvement. Amen.

DEPARTMENTAL MANUALS

It is desirable that each OHS have a manual of policies and procedures (MPP) wherein all material relating to the organization and operation of the facility can be collected and made available as a single compendium of reference. Frequently, numerous memoranda are issued on an ad hoc basis and rarely are collated either chronologically or by subject matter.

Nearly every corporate entity has an MPP that consolidates all of the instructional material in one or more volumes, so that the policies of the organization and the methods of implementing the stated principles can be a matter of common or at least accessible knowledge. In comparable vein, manuals are found in the armed services, and these documents may be strictly of a policy nature, or they may be technical, which implies greater use for training, guidance, or even the provision of specifications.

In many institutions, particularly since the birth of the space age, special technical writers have been added to various departmental staffs or coalesced into a single function, to prepare and annotate such documents. MPPs, in the overall company sense, provide all the information needed to carry out the mission of the organization, including directional material ranging from the functions of the board of directors to the requisitioning of stationery. Somewhere, in every social entity, there is a source of authority, be it a constitution, a set of bylaws, an operating manual, or a description of the details of a program that will serve as the ultimate guide for action by persons or leaders composing the responsible officership.

OBJECTIVES

An MPP is created, used, and updated so that there is, at all times, a current wellspring of action, recognized as "the word," for it bears the approval of the highest office in the chain of group responsibility. It is of particular importance that the medical arm of a company have a consolidated volume of directives or instructions, for within that health service there are personnel who operate exclusively under such medical directives, where the issues concerned can truly involve life or death. Such staff are representatives of the physician in charge, and they operate under his or her direction. While it is the medical director who is responsible for the health of the organization—certainly for the preventive, therapeutic, and rehabilitative care that is administered—the final individual who is responsible is the CEO, the president, the board chairman, the commanding officer, or in the event of possible untoward litigious action, one or all, in addition to the medical director. Nurses cannot carry out their functions independently unless there are written or published directives signed by a physician designated as the medical consultant to the company or by the full-time medical director. In substance, the MPP is important, it is needed, and it is used.

The objectives of preparing and having such a compilation of explanatory and directional material are many:

- To have in a single-source document, a statement of the policies of the company as they relate to the functions of the OHS.
- To provide information concerning the mission of the organization.*
- To indicate the personnel structure of the OHS, showing lines of authority and responsibility.
- To delineate the administrative roles, relationships, and functions of OHS personnel.
- To outline the program elements of the OHS and to assign responsibility for their conduct.
- To describe, in some detail, the technical (medical, preventive, nursing, instrumented testing, and other) procedures carried out daily in the OHS.
- To present the details needed in completing the administrative procedures required in both individual patient care and the conduct of the OHS as a whole.
- To indicate the responsibilities of the OHS in regard to its interactions with both official and voluntary health agencies and with the medical community at large.

*For newcomers to the staff of an OHS, a brief history of the company and of the OHS itself will provide a perspective when viewing one's new position in preventive health care and a better understanding of the background of the present plant's needs in human resources.

To describe in detail certain emergency medical care procedures required in the case of acute exposure of workers to toxic substances unique to the company or its production processes.
To relate the methods employed in staff development or in-service training or in the utilization of the OHS as field-training experience for students at an undergraduate, graduate, or residency level.
To depict the procedures needed in the conduct of research by the OHS, either by staff members or extramural institutions.
To familiarize staff personnel with the codes of ethical conduct as they apply to the OHS as a whole and as delineated by each professional discipline.
To orient new OHS personnel.
To establish uniformity of procedures.
To illustrate, in one document, the administrative, emergency medical care, and health education forms or publications used in the OHS.
To provide information regarding the occupational health hazards (toxic substances) present in the company, by operating unit.
To serve as an educational device for managerial or other concerned personnel of the organization, which will orient company executives to the operation of the OHS.
To serve as a text or reference for students undergoing field placement in the OHS.

TITLE OF THE MANUAL

As common to any publication, the title of the manual will vary in keeping with need, company policy or standardization, or perception of the medical director. Some titles that have been used follow:

Manual of Policies and Procedures of the Occupational Health Service
Medical Department Manual
Medical Manual
Procedural Manual of the Occupational Health Service
Medical Policy and Administrative Manual*
Nursing Policy, Procedure Manual and Medical Directives*
Medical Programs and Procedure Manual

While many organizations may operate without a detailed manual, most will have a document that will contain directives for OHNs who will have responsibility for care either in single-nurse units or on the second or third shifts of a company when physicians are not present. Many of these compilations may carry the designation of Medical Directives for Occupational Health Nurses or even the older, and now outdated, title of Standing Orders for Nurses.

CONTENTS OF THE MANUAL

Although program elements will vary with company policy, as established at corporate or local levels (for example, complete care for employees versus emergency medical care, level of sophistication or presence of innovative subsets of the primary program, the problems in potential toxicity unique to the company, geographic location, contract resulting from collective bargaining, among other variables), the following primary sections of a manual are suggested:

Statements by Chief Executive Officer (Company Policy) and Medical Director (Medical Consultant)
Table of Contents
General Introduction
Objectives and Program Components
Medical Examinations at Time of Employment
Periodic Medical Examinations
Medical Examination Components
Emergency Medical Care—Treatment Unit Procedures
Emergency Medical Care—Treatment Unit and Subdispensary Procedures
Ancillary Treatment Facilities
Subsequent Follow-up/Referral of Employees with Acute and Chronic Disorders
Special Programs
Counseling (Employee Assistance Program [EAP])
Industrial Hygiene
Health Education
Staff Development
Governance of OHS
Certification and Licensing
First Aid and Cardiopulmonary Resuscitation Training
Environmental Health
Radiography
Administration—Medical Records
Clinical Laboratory
Administration—Appointment System
Administration—Reports
Administration—Personnel Management

*Two concurrent manuals of the Allied Chemical Medical Services, courtesy of James A. Hathaway, M.D., former Director—Medical Affairs, Chemicals Company, Allied Chemical.

Administration—Supply and Service Management
Administration—Budget Preparation
OHS Safety
Research Activities
Field Training of Students
Relationships with Other Departments
Relationships with Other Agencies
Distribution

It is apparent from the suggested contents listed that not every OHS will have in operation all of the functions or programs indicated. An appropriate selection can be made for inclusion in the manual being developed.

PHYSICAL STRUCTURE OF THE MANUAL

Nearly all manuals in use currently are distributed in loose-leaf binders, mostly of the 2-inch- or 3-inch ring size, with custom printed tabs on the section separators. There may be four, five, or six tabs per set of divider sheets, depending on the number of words needed per tab. A greater number of tabs—they are available up to sets of 10—may allow inclusion of the full section title. The tabs may be of clear plastic or may be obtained in a color sequence such as red, green, yellow, blue, orange, brown, amber, pink, gray, and purple. The tabs extend ½ inch from the ledger sheets, and the dividers may or may not be reinforced with a plastic strip on the inside margin bearing the three punched holes.

Some early manuals were placed between fiberboard covers and bound with light-metal posts. Such a binding, however, made replacement of pages time-consuming, and the manual could not be opened so it would lie flat while in use.

Most binders are custom imprinted on the spine and front cover and have foam-padded covers. One type of less costly binder has a clear plastic envelope spine and front cover into which specially printed title cards can be inserted.

It is advisable that a standard printed blank sheet be used for the sake of uniformity that has, as a boxed heading, spaces for the title of the manual, the subject or title of the section, the section number, the page number, the date, and the number of the revision. Such a heading allows clarity in the numbering and dating of both new and revised pages. The system of continuous section numbers and pagination within a section allows ready access to the section in its place in the manual and ease in replacement, without disturbing the remainder of the manual.

SIGNATORIES OF THE MANUAL

To give the manual the weight of authority, it is advised that a brief statement appear at the immediate beginning of the manual over the signature of the CEO in which the philosophy of the company regarding occupational health can be given, with an additional comment concerning the approval and support for the OHS policies and procedures following. Such a paragraph or two should be prepared by the medical director for the CEO, which will provide precision in the statement.

On the same page, or just following the words of the first signatory, there should appear a brief statement, to be signed by the medical director or the medical consultant to the organization, to the effect that the content represents the official policies and procedures of the OHS, that they are in accord with the company-wide practice of occupational health, and that all staff of the OHS are obligated to follow the directives contained in the manual unless extraordinarily exceptional reasons for other action present themselves. In a sense, the two statements are two local parallels to the *nihil obstat* and *imprimatur* of church authority. In some instances, each section or chapter is signed by the head of the section concerned and countersigned by the medical director.

DISTRIBUTION

To whom should the manual be issued? The persons or offices following are the customary recipients of the manual:

Chief executive officer
Company officers (department heads)
Middle level managers, as needed
Medical director
OHS division and section heads
OHS physicians and OHNs
Personnel department—additional copies, as needed
Key personnel in contact with health-hazardous substances
Medical directors of other plants within the corporate structure
Corporate level officers, as indicated
Consultant physicians providing service on an ad hoc or contract basis.

Whether they receive the manual *in toto* or are issued selected sections only can be determined by the medical director. It might be that, in the preparation of the material, the sections can be grouped for field use, that is, one group of sections for personnel extramural to the OHS and one group strictly for use by staff of the OHS. If such a division is feasible, it might make distribution somewhat more difficult because of the element of needed selectivity. Forwarding whole copies is more easily accomplished, but much of the material would not be pertinent to a manager's operation because of the technical nature of many of the sections. The decision should be made locally as to the assignment of content—the entire binder or selected segments—and a record should then be made accordingly on the distribution list.

PREPARATION OF THE MANUAL

A final comment is in order regarding the actual preparation of a manual. If an administrator is part of the OHS staff, the function belongs to that office. In an OHS with several section heads, it has been found infeasible for several reasons to expect all of them to write the material germane to the operation of their sections. They often are unskilled in formal writing and will defer preparation, and deadlines will be passed without submission of any product. If the material is prepared, the styles of various writers will be so disparate as to require total rewriting for the sake of uniformity. Finally, because of workloads, the claim may be made that such unaccustomed work can only be accomplished after regular hours, and the issue then begins to involve discussions of overtime pay or compensatory time off.

To facilitate the compilation of the material, it has been found that a simple technique is the most effective in the preparation of the first draft. The section head or actual person involved with a procedure—technician, clerk, receptionist—is asked to listen to the material as it is being dictated to a secretary so that corrections or additions can be made during the process of construction. Also, this staff member is present as the resource person so that areas unfamiliar to the preparer of the manual can be explored immediately without recourse to an overly frequent use of the intra-office telephone. The responses will be fresh and can be used immediately.

On completion of the initial draft, the documents can be sent to the section heads for their comments, corrections, or additions. The total process is shortened in this manner, and even a lengthy manual can be produced in a reasonable period.

PREPARATION FOR RESEARCH

With the passage of safety and health legislation at all levels of government and with the increased number of academic departments concerned with worker and environmental health, there has developed a continuing need for further information regarding adverse health effects from occupational exposures. Even prior to the enactment of OSHA 1970, large companies involved in the manufacture of chemicals had added epidemiologists to their occupational health staffs. Significant intramural studies have been conducted over the years, but more recently, organizations have been asked by research teams from university centers to allow epidemiologic scrutiny of certain population groups presumably at health risk.

There has been a shift in policy within industry—not altogether voluntarily—to permit study of various segments of a labor force even to the point of publication of findings. As employees or their trade union representatives can request health hazard evaluations, such reviews are ordered in response, and the employer cannot refuse entry of the investigative team.

Certain preparatory steps are needed for such research. One does not purport in this section to discuss the principles of epidemiology, for they are available in specifically dedicated writings. Whether the study effort is epidemiologic, toxicologic, short-term, or long-term, an OHS can conduct certain activities that will facilitate a research project.

COMPLETENESS IN MEDICAL RECORDS

Although given emphasis in the discussion of medical records, the point must be reiterated that clinical documents or their computerized content are, or should be, one of the primary sources of data. Because of individual laxity of the professional staff member, the constraints of time or patient load in a busy OHS, the inability to express in writing known information, or the erroneous assumption that entries are made solely for the moment, the clinical record sorely lacks much important information regarding work exposures.

While the chronologic recordings in an OHS cover job-related injuries with almost a plethora of detail, the entries offer little in the area of early symptoms or objective findings relative to occupational disease. Rarely are environmental or industrial hygiene data correlated directly with clinical observations, and well-known OHS-visit recidivists are more likely to be given superficial care, with inadequate recording of complaints and treatment.

Because of this short-sightedness, an OHS staff must be reminded constantly of the importance and need of *complete, accurate, nonjudgmental* notations descriptive of the historic, occupational, clinical, therapeutic, and rehabilitative aspects of every patient visit. Even though such information may be obtained at the first of a series of visits, new exposures can ensue between visits, necessitating updating of the employee's history at each clinical contact.

SOURCES OF DATA

Information needed in a study is available from several sources, both in a plant and in related extramural institutions. The medical director's role in research is to know the sources and the person(s) responsible for record maintenance and to effect the contact of the investigating team with such individuals.

RECORDS

Company clinical records
- Identifying information
- Morbidity data
- Exposure data
- Environmental data
- Visitation rate
- Illness-absence information*
- Medical surveillance findings (biologic measurements)

Company personnel records (active employees and retirees)
- Identifying information
- Job titles
- Work locations
- Periods of employment
- Separations from service
  - Temporary
  - Permanent
- Personnel actions (promotions, transfers)
- W2 forms

Company safety records
Company industrial hygiene records
Mobile external medical surveillance units†
House organs
Trade unions/employee associations
State OSHA agencies
Company or underwriter health plan records
Social Security Administration
State registrar of vital statistics (death registries)
Cancer registries
National death index
Group life insurance underwriter

As determined by the quality of the data available at the plant, one or all of the above sources, internal or external, may be studied.

EPIDEMIOLOGY

Most of the research will most likely be conducted by epidemiologists, and while it may be belaboring a time-fringed point, a definition is in order. To clarify the issue as to what the nature of the discipline might be, Lilienfeld [14] reviewed previously published definitions and proposed a definition that would (1) summarize previous efforts at defining epidemiology; (2) be understandable to the nonepidemiologist; (3) be independent of the methods used by the epidemiologist; (4) not specify the type of disease being studied, that is, infectious or chronic disease; and (5) be applicable to any population selected for observation. His definition reads: "Epidemiology is a method of reasoning about disease that deals with biological influences derived from observations of disease phenomena in population groups." He further gave emphasis to the parallel of the definition with that expressed by Frost in 1936, which read that epidemiology at any given time was something more than the total of its established facts, for it included their orderly arrangement into chains of inference extending more or less beyond the bounds of direct observation.

Some epidemiologists are comfortable in industry, while others may find the environment strange and certainly different from some of their customary locales in academe or public health agencies. Reviews of epidemiologic activities in industry have been critical, and it is the purpose of this chapter to bring about more meaningful studies that utilize plant data. Stallones [15] has observed that most "routine"

*As indicated previously, insofar as possible, true illness-absence must be differentiated from absence attributed to illness.

†In some instances, mobile multitest vans will visit a plant and conduct instrumented testing procedures. Resulting data may be available only from workers themselves or their private physicians.

data systems do not provide information of research quality and often are not appropriate or sufficiently detailed to allow the testing of specific hypotheses. Yet, he believed that the monitoring of illness in employed groups can, and should, serve as a most valuable research source when viewed as a screening and detection mechanism. Baumgarten and Oseasohn [16] published a critique of articles appearing in English-language journals of occupational health, and while the comments refer to research design and methodology, the point is made that studies emanating from work groups do undergo severe scrutiny.

Enterline [17], in a classic review of various studies relating to the health effects of asbestos exposure, pointed out that in 11 such investigations the estimates of relative risk for respiratory cancer ranged from 1.2 to 9.2 because of a variety of faults in population selection, death certificate use, and lack of data concerning the level and duration of exposure. While medical directors may not have a primary role in the research design, they should be knowledgeable as to the sources and quality of the data being made available to the investigators and attempt to improve the information at the point of generation. Through the establishment of a company death register, some of the errors inherent in death certification might be obviated [18–20].

One of the points underscored in reviews of industry-located studies is the issue of level of exposure. The medical director or the industrial hygienist can provide some measure of accuracy for the epidemiologist if work contacts are classified in keeping with a rank order suggested by Greenberg and Tamburro [21]. The exposure index combines work history and job exposure categories, utilizing area-description codes that identify employment occurring in a particular building or area, independent of the job; in a particular job, independent of the building or area; or by both area and description. The chemical exposure rating is an ordered six-category ranking assigned to each area-description number for each calendar year:

Rating	*Level of Exposure*
0	*Absent from environment*(on leave, furlough, layoff)
1	*Lowest exposure*(includes exposure up to somewhere near 1 hour/day)
2	*Minimal exposure to low levels*(chemical in building—not handled; low vapor pressure and dust level; individual probably works on different floor)
3	*Moderate exposure*(works around the chemical, but exposure is minimal; individual is frequently exposed to little spills or leaks or infrequently—less than once/month—to large spills or leaks)
4	*Works in area subject to high occupational exposures*(normally exposure is minimal, but large spills or leaks occur once/month or more)
5	*Works in areas where level is high*(exposure levels in area are frequently high; might consider that some risk is involved if the chemical is extremely toxic)
6	*Intimate contact—skin or high inhalation* (includes individuals with daily and direct contact with the chemicals, such as poly cleaner in the old days and those who handled slurry)

ORIENTATION OF PLANT PERSONNEL

A study to be conducted in a plant requires preliminary arrangement, and usually this planning is carried out with a few representatives of the management staff or with representatives of organized labor. Word regarding such an undertaking rarely gets to the workers at large. It is the function of the medical director to orchestrate an orientation of *all* involved groups so that there will be understanding and cooperation. Such action is absolutely mandatory if interviews will be used in addition to the gathering of numeric data from the record sources indicated earlier.

A study may be requested by a single individual appealing to OSHA, by one trade union, by the OHS, and less frequently by the company management team. Word must be spread not only to prospective participants—study subjects and controls—but to all company employees. The first orientation must be of the OHS staff itself, because workers will be in contact with the medical, nursing, and technical personnel and will query them regarding rumors that already have begun to circulate. Unless the OHS staff is fully apprised of the research project, one or another might respond with a "I don't know a thing about it" and thus put out immediately a negative perception of something extremely worthwhile. The reaction is one of, "If they don't know what's going on, why should we do anything about it?"

The next two groups to be informed—to be given the objectives, the investigators, the methodology, the strategy, and the logistics—are the managers and the union or employee organization officials. The executives can be presented with the details at a staff meeting called regularly by the CEO, and the industrial relations director can be requested to arrange a meeting with union personnel in order "to meet and confer." The latter is of the utmost importance, for a research effort without the understanding and cooperation of labor will fail or be sabotaged. In worksite parlance, "Run it by us, Doc, and we'll consider it."

To do so is to make the leaders aware, so that they can respond knowingly to questions placed by their members. Further, it involves them as members of an advisory committee and gives them some of the dignity needed as leaders in their offices. Rarely, with an honest and forthright explanation will the group reject a proposal, for it does concern their health and, in many instances, that of their families.

In all such meetings, the actual research team—from principal investigator to interviewers—should be introduced, not only to present and make known the persons who will be concerned with the project, but also to identify the study as an activity of the OHS. Outsiders coming into a plant to conduct the noblest of research will be given a cold reception unless they have credibility. If there is confidence in the OHS, there will be confidence in the investigating team presented by the OHS leadership.

As the project proceeds, meetings with the same groups should be held periodically so that the progress of the research can be presented. Both supervisors and participants need updating so that the sense of contributing to a worthwhile effort can be retained. At the conclusion of the investigation, a final set of meetings should be held, both to draw the effort to a close and to have an occasion for the expression of gratitude to all employees who aided in the research undertaking.

Lastly, any study being solidified in the planning phase should be given publicity in the plant house organ. The same information—objectives, members of research group, methodology, site of interviews, and so on—should be given in a series of articles in either a weekly or monthly publication. The reason for repetition is that some individuals are ill, some are on vacation, and many may miss a single issue. Preparing the releases for the editor will prove helpful.

COMMENT

The medical director or the chief OHN can, and must, serve as a catalyst for research proposed by an extramural group. The task is the important one of bringing together the subjects of the investigation or the stewards of the records with the research team. A medical inquiry involves the health care arm of the company, and OHS leadership must be provided to ease the introduction of an outside group. The concept of research can be alarming to members of both management and labor, who probably have had no contact ever with either academicians or other investigative personnel, and most likely conjures up a variety of stereotypic images of "experiments," test tubes, laboratory animals, and "blood letting." To illuminate the scene and provide reality is the task of the OHS.

If the research is carried on by an epidemiologic team whose members are full-time employees of the OHS, some may be known to workers, but the same orientation should ensue.

OCCUPATIONAL HEALTH PERSONNEL—RELATIONAL AND ETHICAL ASPECTS

The personnel engaged in the practice of occupational health undergo both a surveilling and treating relationship with the employees of the organization, but they must differ in their behavior from that, for example, of the salesperson who has a short-term relationship only with a customer, for both the care staff and the workers are functioning in a relatively stable and permanent environment. It is true that all companies experience turnover, but in the main, OHS staff members are long-term associates, and their attitudes and behavior in the relationship with the patients are enduring and determining of the workers' return for future care.

In some business institutions, a pattern has been set by medical directors who view themselves as arbiters of all things involving people and who rigidly adhere to such ideas as the perpetual "rightness" of the company and the everlasting "wrongness" of the employees. The workers, in their eyes, are forever malingering, faking illnesses, defrauding the employer through repetitive injuries, and producing minimally. All workers are cheats, they believe, and this point of view is readily felt by the employees, so that a constant state of war exists between the health facility and the labor force. Such a situation is obviously counterproductive, and no preventive medicine programming will be successful, no matter how skilled and professional the plans may appear on paper. That there must be a humaneness in the operation of an OHS is a given.

THE WORK SETTING

Many factors are present that tend toward a dehumanization or depersonalization of the relationship between the healer or treater and the patient. The health policy designers have developed a vocabulary replete with terms such as health industry, cost effectiveness, delivery of medical care or producing a product, provider, consumer, recipient, customer, client, and financial transactions (for human interactions), among other designations convenient for a statistical, economic, or population fit, but inappropriate in the consideration of a human being's deep need for succor or support. A hospital in today's culture is a medical center or health care center, white uniforms are considered repressive or frightening, and first names are used ceaselessly in professional conversation with the elderly, who are yet to come around to the sport-shirt and jeans attire of many who allegedly are offering skilled care. True, the picture is changing, but most workers are conservative, adhere to long-established values, and do not understand the inroads made by electronic or computerized medicine when what they seek is understanding, compassion, and concern.

In a busy company, production deadlines have to be met, visits to an OHS are downtime disliked by the first-line supervisor, and the patients themselves no longer tolerate unforgivable delays occasioned by personnel who are "on their break," that great institution introduced during World War II, to be taken irrespective of employees waiting impatiently for care. At day's beginning in a full OHS, previously absent workers await certification for return to their jobs—particularly on Monday*—and the care given is hurried and the general tone is frenzied. Such rapidly paced contacts preclude the establishment of rapport, an essential quality in the offering and acceptance of care.

Many jobs require contact with oil, grease, and debris, often in confined, hot quarters, so that when visits are made to the OHS, the patients bear much occupational soil, are perspiring, and spread an aroma the staff may find repelling. Again, these are deterrents to an understanding relationship.

Patients themselves, because of personality deficits or perceived wrongs, become abusive, angry, rude, offensive, and frequently foul-mouthed. Impaired associations with superiors, occasionally with peers, are often projected onto OHS personnel, when actually the targets of employees' ill feelings are remote to the medical facility.† Individuals referred to an OHS for determination of physical fitness direct their feelings toward the examiners, who are only complying with a request, one that is made in keeping with company regulations.

Personnel in an OHS who have undergone a rapid, or too rapid, upward mobility, sometimes not as a factor of inherent skills but because local managers wish to establish good records in affirmative action, feel that the newly acquired position allows a behavioral expression of superordination and frequently alienate patients who were their former peers.* This behavior leads to resentment by the patients and requests for alternative practitioners within the OHS.

And there are certain members of an in-plant medical staff who have strictly a "9-to-5" mentality, who work solely for the income and for none of the psychic rewards that accrue from an effective occupational health practice format. They are, in some instances, the nurses who knit when patient visits are infrequent instead of leaving the facility to see how some of the workers fare at their work stations, following up on previous visits, or merely being available for questions or discussion. These staff members contribute little, are noncreative, and may actually attempt to subvert certain program elements, for they may mean more work.

Lastly, there are the attitudes carried over from the housestaff days with their accompanying derogation of some patients as "crocks," "spos," "gomers," "dirt bags," "turkeys," and "dirtballs" [22,23]. Such persons exist in industry and they do frequent the OHS, but each one has a problem that has not been resolved. Whether the person's difficulty can be diagnosed and treated, or whether the situation at home or work is insoluble, there is no place in a health care organization for such an unfeeling, deprecatory attitude. It was the author's experience some years ago to see, by request, such a group of patients at a large manufacturing installation to demonstrate the point that these employees were, in fact, people with problems. They were men and women who could not or would not work and who were unwelcome in the medical department because no one had identified the reasons for the recalcitrance. On close and persistent study, each one of the group was found to have a completely plausible behavioral reason for the picture presented, and when the problem was resolved, either immediately or soon, each returned to work. Many times the patients themselves are un-

*Rarely do employees return to work after an illness or convalescence from an injury on other days of the week. Might it not be better to return on Friday and have a brief recovery period before assuming the full load during a 5-day workweek?

†A young insulator, angered because of laxity in the provision by management of safeguards against the inhalation of asbestos fiber, became angry in a conversation with the medical director, yelled as to be audible throughout the OHS, slammed his hard hat noisily down a staircase, and stormed out of the building. The physician was the recipient of his displaced ire, for he could yell at him and not at the responsible executives.

*The grossest of pseudo-assumptions of status was seen in a hospital attendant who, while mopping floors, wore a stethoscope around his neck. The same pattern is encountered in operating room orderlies who go to lunch in restaurants adjacent to the hospital, fully clothed in surgical attire.

aware of the bizarre etiologies involved and, in some instances, actually do not want to continue the pattern in which they have found themselves.

THE ATTITUDE OF THE PHYSICIAN

So, what are the behavioral qualities of a good physician in industry? That the physician must be a respected human being is foremost, and this need was articulated well by Duttera [24]:

> My experience with patients tells me that they still place high value on a relationship with a physician who cares for them personally. They continue to value the touch of the healer's hand. In my community, when a new physician comes to town, the community will recognize his medical degree with great respect. But the first question about the physician that must be answered is what kind of human being he is. The question does not relate to the physician's technical ability but to what he is like when you talk with him. Is he concerned, or is he aloof?

The physician has to be *concerned* and involved with the patients, with *their* illness or injury, *their* anxiety or *their* stress, *their* families, *their* jobs, and the relationship of the presenting problem to those jobs. On many an occasion unrecognized opportunities for therapy and deepening of the practitioner-patient relationship are passed up because the professional person is more concerned with his or her own position or recognition than with the employee-patient. The following stories exemplify the opposite of care.

The author was taking a group of graduate students around the back lot of a major motion picture studio in Hollywood. The shops were visited, and many outdoor sets were seen. Accompanying the group was the company's medical director on a business visit from New York City. En route to a sound stage where a show was being filmed, the group passed the dispensary, and the wish was expressed to visit the facility. On entering the waiting room, it was difficult to determine how to make one's presence known, but on an interior wall there was an aperture not more than one-foot square, through which the OHN soon spied the visitors. On being invited inside, we saw a patient with a fairly extensive abrasion of his leg, which was propped up on a foot support. The ideal moment was there to have introduced Dr. W., all the way from the East, Professor F., and his students, and to have invited their opinion. In place of this desirable action, the nurse, obviously shaken, told the man she was busy, to get his things on, and to come back in the afternoon. With the dismissal went all the opportunity for improving relationships between the OHS and the employee.

In contrast was an event that took place in a dyestuffs plant in Manchester, England. The author was visiting the installation and in the company of the medical director, Dr. Thomas S. Scott, was walking down one of the streets of the factory. About halfway along, Dr. Scott asked that we cross over. A man, in full work garb and with clacking wooden shoes marking his progress, was approaching. We stopped, and Dr. Scott introduced Professor F. from California, and after some additional small talk, the man went on. When asked what the episode was about, Dr. Scott explained that the man was a union official on his way to a meeting, where, without question, he would mention meeting the visitor, which would not only heighten the man's own feeling of status but would help set a good tone to the conference.

The same kind of behavior—good and bad—is encountered with visitors to any OHS. When the director is showing the visitor about, it is always of interest to see if the director describes the activities of the unit or if the section chief is requested to "tell what you do in here."

A factor frequently forgotten by the occupational health physician is that the patient, as indicated in the early discussion of definitions, is a member of the health care team, possibly the most important member. The age has past when the physician's word was accepted unquestioningly and when the patient feared that the placement of pointed queries would anger the practitioner. As Kassirer [25] has commented, we have come a long way from the paternalism in medicine that excluded patients from discussions about their own health. In spite of the patients' rights movement and efforts to educate patients in medical matters, the practice of excluding the patient from decision-making persists.

Physicians in the plant setting are called on in two ways for opinions regarding medical care. Employees will come voluntarily seeking a point of view regarding a surgical procedure advised by a private practitioner, and the occupational health physician will counsel workers regarding diagnosis, surveillance, and treatment of job-related disorders. It may be that the physician's and the patient's wishes are discordant, and the employee is intimidated by the physician. Such patients, Kassirer [25] points out, must bear the burden of having been disenfranchised by their physician. One can only recommend a course of action to an employee, for it is the employee who must make the final decision and follow through to the point of actualization. Some patients find this procedure difficult, for they will often respond that they are laypersons and that they have come to the professional for counsel. As with informed consent, all the factors must be laid out for consideration and the patient's ultimate determination. Honesty is indicated, for patients can accept the fact that "a considerable body of medical information is fuzzy and uncertain" [25].

Also, patients are fully equipped to handle devastating news and should not be deprived of full disclosure. A 70-year-old unmarried woman with diabetes was recently informed of the diagnosis of bilateral breast adenocarcinoma with regional node involvement and pelvis, lumbar spine, and bilateral lung metastases. A warm, encouraging oncologist laid out the complete clinical picture, and it was accepted with hope. Rather badly affected were the patient's friends, who were considerably more shaken than she. A young married woman in her thirties was informed of her having leukemia in the period prior to the availability of current therapies. Her spirit improved and she felt better, for now she could make definitive plans with her husband for care of the children and settling of her "affairs," for the cloudiness of euphemistic messages had been dissipated.

Back to the physician and the patient. Sir George Pickering, Regius Professor of Medicine at Oxford over two decades ago [26], in his presidential address to the British Medical Association, stressed the view that the very core of medicine is formed from sympathy and understanding, and not from professional skill or scientific knowledge. He cited Wilfred Troller, who in consultation "always listened to what the patient had to say; he understood what the patient was trying to say; and he made it plain to the patient that he understood. Nine-tenths of the difficult patients that I see are difficult because their doctor has been unable or unwilling to appreciate their fears or peculiar problems, or has been unable to help allay or solve them." He continues by saying, "It is only by virtue of that rather intangible and neglected quality, his attitude of mind as expressed by devotion to his patient, the real ethos of medicine, that he becomes superior."

In a more current dating, Comstock [27] reports that patients prefer verbal demonstrations of caring from their physician rather than nonverbal caring behavior like touching, close positioning, or maintenance of eye contact. Patient satisfaction correlated highly with greeting the individual, telling the patient what will happen next, not discounting what the patient says, allowing the patient to talk, and providing closure to the interaction. Additional positive behaviors included the physician's use of open-ended questions, active listening, allowing questions to be asked, showing sensitivity to the patient's moods, and acknowledging the patient's socioemotional needs by responding to the expressed fears and anxieties.

One might ask why so much material is being devoted to communication with employee-patients. The explanation lies in experience, in that patients do not query their personal physicians, and they bring their concerns into the OHS for clarification of issues of diagnosis, treatment, and prognosis. Outstanding in personal memory is the employee who reported in one morning laden with syringes, needles, and insulin, who stated that his physician gave him all the equipment and medication, but no instructions as to the procedure of parenteral therapy. Careful training and practice followed in the OHS. Also recalled was a conversation with a health educator at the Cleveland Health Museum who stated that periodically she would mingle with exiting visitors and without identifying her affiliation would ask certain persons why they happened to come to the museum. On many occasions the response was to the effect that mother or father or someone was in the hospital nearby, and they wanted to find out what was going on with their loved one, for surgery was scheduled the next day.

While communication between the treater and the treated is improving, practitioners are busy, give brief, unsatisfying answers, and frequently still adopt an overseer-supplicant relationship with the patient. Two actions have been seen—the growth of the patient education movement, given birth and nurtured by personnel other than physicians, and the increased use of medical columnists and the American Medical Association (AMA) by persons seeking health information.* In a review of the work of the AMA's Department of Health Education, Douma [31] indicates that between 2,000 and 3,000 letters and telephone calls are received each month from the general public. While most of the inquiries came from people in educational settings, between 200 and 250 stem from persons with medical problems. When the callers were asked, "Have you consulted your own physician?" the responses were: (1) "I don't have a physician," or (2) "I'm afraid to bother my doctor." While trying to increase the number of "health-educated patients" and by referring people to their physicians,

*At times there has been acrimony between the givers of succor. Brachfeld [28] claimed that "To divert a patient toward the health educator or the 'patient-teaching' nurse may provide a lot of factual data but will make the patient who longs for the nurturing figure of the authoritative physician even more frustrated." Nurse Izzo [29] responded by doubting that the "figure" needs to be a physician, and Tabatabai [30] spoke more sharply by saying, "When physicians can put aside their arrogance and realize that most patients seek thoughtful, straightforward, and reasonably detailed information about their conditions, and not just comfort from the 'nurturing figure of the authoritative physician,' they may find that their communication problems, as well as patients' claims of 'complete ignorance' even though explanations have been offered 'time and time again,' will disappear."

Douma concludes that being the AMA's Ann Landers can be extremely frustrating, distressing, and yet satisfying and that "It is frustrating to be continually aware of the gap in understanding, distressing to hear the misguided wonderings of patients caused by their confusions and fears, but satisfying to perceive a spark of understanding and then know that the next telephone call will be to the personal physician."

Why does this gap in communication persist? Are we failing to train our medical students in the interpretation of clinical findings by giving them only a highly technical lexicon with which to work? Do they become tied of tongue when a patient needs clarification of a mouthful of medical jive? In a previous experience in the teaching of fourth-year medical students [32], the person who had presented the case history for discussion would be asked by the instructor, on completion of the total group review: "Doctor, you've finished looking me over. What kind of shape am I in?" Invariably, the student was unable to go into the role-playing mode, but would third-personalize the patient by saying, "I would tell him that he had. . . ." Then, the statement would be followed by, "Some arteriosclerosis of the coronary arteries, and that there was electrocardiographic confirmation in the S–T segment findings. . . ." When the persisting pseudo-patient demanded understandable words in place of technical jargon, the student would begin to perspire, turn red in the face, and would be unable to translate the material into the verbal stuff of clear conversation.

It is this failure that the OHS staff must pick up on, for comprehension of their health status is the workers' right, and until there is some ease of mind in this segment of their lives, job performance will be impaired. It may not always be easy, particularly when the medical director gets a call from an employee, as has the author many times, especially at night, that follows: "I didn't want to bother Dr. Mafoosky, so I thought I'd call you."

THE TONE OF COMMUNICATION

The response to a concerned or distraught patient cannot be one without hope. As the epidemiologists begin to identify closer etiologic ties between exposure to work materials and the development of malignant disease, the physician in industry will have more employee-patients *and* their families who place questions, seeking some element of encouragement or reassurance. And this exchange means a patient-physician partnership. Norman Cousins [33], who has reviewed the scene both as a patient and as a nonphysician faculty member in the Medical School at UCLA, puts it this way:

> When a physician tells the truth, he should be careful to do so in a way that does not deprive his patient of hope. Nothing he can do is more important than to enable the patient to be "potentiated"; that is, to make her feel that she has something of her own to contribute, that she is involved in the decision-making, and that she will be informed in a way that will enable her to make responsible choices. In short, he attempts to create a partnership.

Moser [34], in his discussion of psychosemantics (speaking to patients), cautions us equally: "How are we best able to help without adding an iatrogenic burden? A primary step is to state the message clearly, simply, concisely, devoid of equivocation, but with gentleness and kindness." He deplores demeaning the mature, well-educated patient by discussing the illness in soothing monosyllables that smack of intellectual condescension or by offering bland childlike generalities. Or the opposite, as implied previously, should the physician "cloak his answers in medical mumbo-jumbo which will leave the less perceptive patient confused and frightened." Also, Moser continues, that it is a grievous sin for the practitioner to "descend to sophistry and incant the catechism of Greco-Roman medicalese." The patient may sit and listen, not comprehending, but too proud to confess his "ignorance"—"as he conjures up frightening images built upon the few familiar phrases that do penetrate."

Cousins [35] further points the way when he writes, "The real issue is not whether the truth should be told but whether there is a way of telling it responsibly. Certainly it should not be allowed to become a battering ram against the patient's morale, impairing his ability to cope with the greatest challenge of his life."

In summary, we need no special "patient-educator" to provide the hope, the compassion that will carry the employee on to health or to death. This task is one equally shared by every member of an OHS and by the patient. As electronics spreads its flashing messages, and as pharmaceuticals reproduce their variants in greater number, let us not forget T. S. Eliot's [36] telling lines, "Where is the wisdom we have lost in knowledge?/Where is the knowledge we have lost in information?"

INVOLVEMENT OF THE FAMILY

Because members of a worker's family are usually remote to a plant site, they are not considered as useful agents in improving either the wage-earner's health or job performance. Over the years it has been the author's custom to invite to the OHS the spouse of an employee in whom certain medical problems have arisen or who is unable to verbalize information that could be important in the plan for health improvement. That entry of the spouse into the company's OHS can be arranged has been demonstrated, even in a work setting with high security limitations.

It is very helpful particularly in the case of a blue-collar male worker to meet the patient's wife, for usually she can articulate much more detail about an illness than can the patient himself. As indicated, she can provide considerable pertinent historical information regarding previous employers and work performed. With the spouse present, one can see and feel the depth of concern of a mate regarding the employee's illness, the severity of which the worker, in keeping with the macho ethos, has either denied or deprecated. It is possible to determine the strength of family support present in the case of serious illness and the intellectual level of the worker's wife, which usually surpasses one's expectation. Further, it is both fascinating and informative to see a rough/touch worker sit meekly by in one's office while an alert, sharp, no-nonsense woman tells her husband "what-fer," and he sits mute, without any of the belligerence that characterizes his usual in-plant behavior pattern.

The other advantage lies in the opening of communication pathways, for in the presence of a third and professional person, the worker's wife can now talk to her husband, saying things she was unable to utter at home. The situation is unusually helpful to all three—the worker, his wife, and the organization's physician.* That the family can be of inestimable help is given substance by Tumulty [37], who writes:

> The cooperation of the family in carrying out the program of management can be just as essential as the cooperation of the patient. If the family does not like the attitude of the physician, both he and the patient are in for an uphill fight. An exceedingly clever but inexperienced clinician may wipe out the advantages of a brilliant diagnosis and a sound plan of management for his patient simply by not bothering to bring the family into the problem in a thoughtful manner, for it is often the family that will have the strongest influence on the patient. It is wise to make an ally of the family from the very start.

Tumulty gives further strength to this concept in a practical vein when he adds, "If the family has been dealt with compassionately, if a reasonable understanding of what is wrong with the patient has been communicated to them, and if they comprehend what it is you are trying to do for the patient, the likelihood of such unfortunate consequences as law suits, refusal of autopsies, and so forth, will be negligible."

PROFESSIONAL MISADVENTURES

Errors are going to be committed in any busy OHS irrespective of the training given, the care exercised, or the quality of the supervision. However slight the incident, there must be a complete, detailed report made of the event in the patient's record, if an employee is involved and the episode was not merely limited to property damage. Certain items must be covered in the retelling, and Tumulty [37] reminds, "Regardless of the nature of the incident, there should be a frank, honest, and complete description of it in the patient's clinical chart, including an account of what was done to correct the error once it was recognized and a detailed description of the patient's physical state before and after the incident." Tumulty concludes by saying, "Any indication of a 'cover-up' can be legally mortal for the physician."*

*Most revelatory of experiences in having a wife share in her husband's medical/psychological welfare was when a physical scientist had reported to the author that he, aged about 33, would have his 7-year-old daughter go to bed with him when he would return from work. He thought that the practice, although not incestuous, was unusual and wondered if something should be done about it. His wife was asked to come by one day, and expectations were mixed. She had been the homecoming queen at a large southern university, married our handsome employee, and was the mother of the child in question. In place of being ushered into the author's office, she "swept" in, in a manner comparable to some of the Hollywood greats. She was a blinding picture of red and black, with a wide plaid shirt, a large hat, long gloves, and bedecked with jewelry at the neck, wrists, forearms, ankles, and dress front. The personality was totally out of phase with her beauty. Following a brief explanation regarding the wish to see her, she became extremely angry, berated the author endlessly, and continued at that pace and style for about 5 minutes. Finally, one was able to suggest to her to seek counseling, not only for her daughter's sake, but for the good of the entire family. No word was received until 6 months later, when an appointment was requested. She returned, dressed demurely in a simple dress, a watch the only jewelry, no hat or gloves, and for the first time, an earth-dwelling human being. After the opening pleasantries, she stated that she had returned to express thanks, tearfully, for the suggestion made previously regarding therapy. The daughter was now out of Daddy's bed, and relationships were restored between husband and wife. The difference in the spouse between her appearances in the two visits cannot be described adequately. From an exaggerated illustration out of *Women's Wear* or *Harper's Bazaar* or *Vogue* to the customary simplicity of a scientist's wife, she had coursed a long spectrum of growth phases. The spouse, in many cases, must be seen.

*Illustrative of such a situation was the case of a male employee who worked in a semiskilled craft position who presented one day with a laceration of the hand, claiming the wound to be job-related. Assuming the lesion to be

Needless to add, all details, irrespective of how trivial further description might be, should be provided, for careful documentation illustrates a usual high level of care and concern for the patient involved.

MEDICAL CARE OF MEN VERSUS WOMEN

As more women assume nontraditional jobs, the current high percentage of women in the workforce of 44.7 percent (1987) [38] will increase, implying greater use of an OHS. In a study involving a chart audit of 104 men and women [39] with particular reference to a quintet of symptoms, it was found that the physicians' workups were significantly more extensive for men than they were for women. The argument seems to be supported that male physicians take medical illness more seriously in men than in women.

If this finding can be extrapolated to the industrial setting, women workers may be erroneously interpreted as being typically hypochondriacal, while the men may be regarded as typically stoic. Such assumptions may lead to both inappropriate study and inadequate treatment. Misguided physicians may be inclined to be more cavalier in their care of injured women workers who are engaged in jobs equally as physically demanding for them as for men, but for which they are possibly less well prepared because of their smaller muscle mass. The precaution is included because of the shifting scene in heavy industry, with men occupying positions previously held exclusively by women and with women filling labor-intensive jobs.*

DRESS CODES

Rarely touched in the body of occupational medical literature is the matter of attire of personnel on duty in an OHS. Although referred to briefly in this chapter, the question of professional garb needs to be addressed. The author, having gone through medical school in an era long prior to the disruptive changes of the 1950s and '60s, has not shared the more youthful point of view that the uniform makes no difference in the physician-patient relationship. It is contended that other values tend to serve as the amalgam between the practitioner and the employee who is seeking care.

The issue was tackled directly by Kriss [40,41] following a comment by a student who was a member of a class requested to wear white coats in a session wherein two patients were to be presented. Not only did the student grade Kriss's performance, but added, "I would like to see the evidence that wearing of white coats by students is of any benefit to patients—isn't your request more to satisfy your own ego?"

Kriss pointed out that, truly, the white coat is only a symbol of an attitude, the latter being that the relationship between a physician and a patient is serious and purposeful, not social, casual, or random. Many times the issue has presented itself for discussion among OHS members, and for heated discussion at that. To be sure, the wearing of white, with its long history of development and perception [41] has undergone change, but lost in most of the verbal exchange is not only the seriousness and purposefulness of the physician-patient relationship, as pointed out by Kriss, but also the element of respect for the patient. The same kind of good occupational medicine can be practiced irrespective of the clothing worn, but workers expect a serious acceptance of their problems, and the customary clinical dress mode tells employees that the interchange has been prepared for in a comely manner.

---

one rather commonly encountered among shopworkers, the physician treated it according to fairly standard practice. The patient went on to die of clinically typical tetanus. As the worker was seeking care for a non-work-generated injury, he falsified the history. With such simplicity implied in the telling, the treating physician failed to tease out pertinent factors. The man had cut his hand on the protective wire of his rabbit hutch at home, thus sustaining the injury against which he should have been protected. The incident was reported in full detail to the CEO so that he would not have been found unprepared or unknowing by the inquiring media or a litigious family.

As another example, but with good precaution precluding disaster, the author was administering arsphenamine solution intravenously to army personnel early in World War II when that material was still the drug in use. The nurse handed over a filled syringe, but fortune shone, for it was asked that the original package be demonstrated. The syringe had been loaded with the complete content, sufficient for 10 injections. The nurse was terminated immediately, but the correspondence with the Secretary of War consumed weeks.

*Recalled also from World War II days was the woman welder who reported to the OHS that she had just been terminated from her job down on the pier while working on the preparation of an army transport for troop and material deployment. She had just begun her menses and wanted to lie down for half an hour. The foreman, unaccustomed to distaff workers, took the action he did, entirely oblivious to special needs. With OHS intervention, the decision was reversed.

The workers, as expressed earlier, can come in directly from a dirty job, but they would be somewhat taken aback to be faced with the casual, "laid-back" garb fancied by many of the younger practitioners—jeans, plaid shirts, jogging shoes. As indicated, workers have fairly conservative ideas, and they have rather rigidly followed dress codes of their own, although many are not formally documented but are adopted through tradition.

Most of the breaking away has been manifested by related personnel, especially nurses and clinical psychologists, many of whom wish to dissociate themselves completely from the medical model. Nurses in industry have been seen in civilian dress, in uniform, in uniform but without caps, or in a kind of uniform, but which has departed from the long-used white. Has the medical model become so distasteful that it must be jettisoned totally? Or is the action merely representative of the nurses' move toward total professional independence?

The point is reiterated that the clinical attire indicates concern for the patient and a devotion to the task at hand. One has always wondered about the response of hospitalized patients whose physicians visit at night or on weekends, dressed for golf or in dinner jackets. Does this action not depress a patient who is limited by the illness or injury from participating in the joys of an athletic, social, or theatrical experience? While physicians may believe that such visits show a dedication to the care of their patients, they could also indicate a poorly placed flaunting of their own state of wellness.

Further, many workers are older and are not accustomed to the dress displayed by the younger practitioner. With management-labor relationships stretched as they are in most installations, why should they be impaired even more so? There can be the erroneous equating of inappropriate attire with less than desirable medical care, and no amount of verbal substantiation of equality in that area will win over an employee whose first impression remains unchangeable.

Other points stressed by Kriss [40] bear repetition for applicability to the in-plant setting. He believes it is a mark of disrespect for one to smoke in the presence of patients, read a newspaper, or manifest any other unprofessional behavior. While many of his remarks are directed toward students, the precautions apply equally to physicians of an OHS. Particularly offensive is the ostentatious display of the *Wall Street Journal* on one's desk, giving further emphasis to the worker of salary differentials, as are audible telephone conversations a physician holds with a broker.

While expressing one's feelings freely, the issue might be carried to its fullest, in that, because of training the author received at the hands of one commanding general, the white coats should be buttoned fully at all times and not allowed to become winglike as though the wearer were in full flight. Besides, the pattern of complete buttoning aids in covering a particular unattractive, overhanging abdominal panniculus, especially indicated while endeavoring to motivate a patient toward weight reduction.

Paramedical personnel—technologists, technicians, exercise physiologists, aides, and the like—look better in white, using either short laboratory or clinical coats or the white uniforms of nurses, either in dress or slack format. In two OHSs with which the author was connected, female clerical personnel wore lightweight colored smocks that identified them with the OHS, serving as directional aids to perplexed newcomers, particularly persons referred for completion of their preplacement medical examinations.

In substance, then, the ruling out of casual wear is not a matter of biased rigidity but is an effort in demonstrating that the provision of care is seriously viewed, that the patient is respected, and that the spirit of medicine and nursing can be perpetuated in a manner that bears some of the long history of one's caring for one's fellow man.

MANNER OF ADDRESSING PATIENTS

Both the lay and professional print media have carried columns and letters concerning the manner in which patients are addressed by physicians and their staff members. The issue is of significance in occupational health, for misuse of one designation or another may disrupt a carefully built and balanced relationship with a patient.

From the physician's point of view, there will be a rather pleasant shock on first coming into a plant setting. Probably for the first time in his professional career, he or she will be called "Doc." The tender-sensed practitioner may resent this appellation, but underneath it is a feeling of warmth and some affection. The workers who are accustomed to seeing physicians in their private offices associate them with a different turf and, further, only see them intermittently. In the plant setting they will see physicians both in the OHS and around various worksites, where the feeling develops that "we are all in this together," subject to the same cultural norms and expectations, and where the physician is another worker who comes to the plant every day, the same as they.

In some companies, an interesting growth pattern is seen as the physician becomes better known and as there is acceptance of the professional as a person. The original designation is the formal "Doctor Jones," which in time becomes "Doc Jones," then "Doc," and penultimately "Doctor Joe," and finally, if there has been mutual acceptance and respect, and the physician is not of the stuffy variety, "Joe."

But, what about the opposite direction? As far back as 1975, Mosesson [43] pointed out that there is a correlation between the form of address and the structure of a medical relationship. Physicians who were interviewed varied in their rationales for use of the patients' first or last names. There was some agreement that an indiscriminate use of first names carries the risk of rebuff and embarrassment; especially has this practice been true with black patients, who for centuries degradingly were called by their first names, if not "Boy." It has been the author's policy consistently to use last names, with Mr., Mrs., or Miss, when addressing black patients, even after knowing them well, unless the relationship is so firmly founded that they know there is no lack of respect implicit in the use of the given name.

But the battle opened in print in early 1982, with one of the *JAMA*'s good contributions, under the rubric, "A Piece of My Mind," entitled "Hi, Lucille, This is Dr. Gold," the title telling all [44]. Inferiors, according to custom—children, menial workers, the elderly, and women—are addressed by the first name, stated the writer. What right has 30-year-old Dr. Gold to address 80-year-old Mrs. Silver in that fashion? She would have every reason to call him "Kid" or "Youngster" or "Boy," from her vantage point of 50 years' seniority. Conant [45] and Heller [46] do not favor the first-name usage, certainly on initial contact, and more recently, the lay press further articulated these feelings in a column in Los Angeles [47].

Thomas H. Middleton, the well-known essayist concerning correct usage of the language, writes of his experience in a physician's office [48,49]. With an acute injury, he was to be "squeezed" into a busy schedule. After completing the usual form and waiting 2½ hours, "the cute young receptionist in her cute starched whites said, 'All right, Tom. Come back to this room.'" For him, 30 years her senior, it indicated "a lack of manners and a presumptuous cutting off of respectful social distance."

The policy that seems a reasonable one for compliance in an OHS is to address each new patient—or each patient on first contact—by the last name, coupled with the conventional title of courtesy. If the employee requests a more informal relationship, he may say, "Just call me Charlie." If business relationships with department heads or other central staff members are frequent, a bilateral first-name basis will develop and will be followed in an OHS. At best, last names should be used unless there are requests or circumstances to the contrary.

In addition, a word is needed regarding the clerk or nurse whose task is to usher in patients and who consistently bellows down the hall or into the waiting area, "Smith!" or "Brown!" This kind of action will not win friends for the OHS. While there has been some exchange of notes regarding the use of "Dear" in medicine [50–53], it seems that "terms of endearment should be reserved for personal greetings between friends, not exchanges between patients and medical professionals" [52].

While not relating directly to forms of address, another element in the physician-patient relationship bears brief review. Well-known to all engaged in occupational health is the fact that each patient requires a different kind of attitude, affect, or persona on the part of the treating individual. The reason for mentioning this factor, important as it is in the occupational health arena, is that some members of the medical staff believe that all patients should be cared for in exactly the same manner. Whether the contact is effusive, reserved, jovial, deadly serious, rigidly unbending, or even abnegating, the reaction cannot be the same with all patients.

Some individuals require a response that is lighthearted, particularly if they are consistent visitors presenting with trivia, but nevertheless in need of support. Others, for whom every complaint spells dire disease and disaster, require a serious exploration and explanation of every problem. Still others will require a great deal of patience while they gather sufficient courage to verbalize the single, important concern that brings them in for consultation. The point is that the mix of a company's labor force demands flexibility on the part of the physician or OHN, and no one should manifest the same exterior to all patients, for there will be a lack of congruence, and retrofitting in human relationships is done only with difficulty and rare skill.

SMOKING IN THE HEALTH SERVICE

For several reasons, smoking should not be permitted in the OHS by either staff members or patients. Primarily the professional personnel should serve as role models in positive health behavior, and even if they smoke in designated staff lounges, the practice is readily detected through the permeation of the telltale smoke into clothing, drapes, and furniture. Filled ashtrays on OHS desks are no longer de rigeur. Patients need not be offered cigarettes as an anxiety-relieving gesture.

Further, solvents are used in clinical facilities, and the author has seen fires started in waste receptacles that contained solvent-saturated sponges.

Passive smoking (the inhalation of another person's exhaled smoke or sidestream smoke from a burning cigarette) has been shown to be productive of physiologic change, and many individuals are extremely sensitive to the combustion products.

Signs appropriately placed about the health facility will remind patients of the proscription.

ETHICS IN OCCUPATIONAL MEDICAL PRACTICE

The AOMA, in 1976, published its Code of Ethical Conduct for Physicians Providing Occupational Medical Services [54, 55], which has remained unaltered in the ensuing years. It follows in its entirety:

These principles are intended to aid physicians in maintaining ethical conduct in providing occupational medical service. They are standards to guide physicians in their relationships with the individuals they serve, with employers and workers' representatives, with colleagues in the health professions, and with the public.

Physicians should:

1. Accord highest priority to the health and safety of the individual and the workplace.
2. Practice on a scientific basis with objectivity and integrity.
3. Make or endorse only statements which reflect their observations or honest opinion.
4. Actively oppose and strive to correct unethical conduct in relation to occupational health service.
5. Avoid allowing their medical judgment to be influenced by any conflict of interest.
6. Strive conscientiously to become familiar with the medical fitness requirements, the environment and the hazards of the work done by those they serve, and with the health and safety aspects of the products and operations involved.
7. Treat as confidential whatever is learned about individuals served, releasing information only when required by law or by over-riding public health considerations, or to other physicians at the request of the individual according to traditional medical ethical practice; and should recognize that employers are entitled to counsel about the medical fitness of individuals in relation to work, but are not entitled to diagnoses or details of a specific nature.
8. Strive continually to improve medical knowledge, and should communicate information about health hazards in timely and effective fashion to individuals or groups potentially affected, and make appropriate reports to the scientific community.
9. Communicate understandably to those they serve any significant observations about their health, recommending further study, counsel or treatment when indicated.
10. Seek consultation concerning the individual or the workplace whenever indicated.
11. Cooperate with governmental health personnel and agencies; and foster and maintain sound ethical relationships with other members of the health professions.
12. Avoid solicitation of the use of their services by making claims, offering testimonials, or implying results which may not be achieved, but they may appropriately advise colleagues and others of services available.

The code is about as all-covering as any statement that can be universally applicable to all forms of occupational medical practice. Some comments are in order:

Principle 1: This principle is rightfully placed in a position of primacy, for it governs everything that is planned for, that is currently in operation, or that has been accomplished in the practice of occupational medicine.

Principle 2: Giving substance to this principle is the entire concept of continuing education, so that the practice evinced endures as a scientific undertaking, free of subjectivity and not subject to moral corruption.

Principle 3: This requirement demands that the program comprising the many subelements of occupational health be that scientific that only the truth will emerge when statements are made reflective of one's observations either of workers or of the work environment. Statements cannot deviate from the truth to meet pressured demands from certain sectors.*

*In another of the occupational health disciplines, the same adherence to the unbiased truth is emphasized: "Though we may work for management, labor, or government, our judgments must be consistent with the aims of industrial hygiene, not necessarily those of your employer." (Schinnpa, J. T. A new declaration of independence??? *Am Ind Hyg Assoc J* 41:A-4, Nov 1980.) The belief is voiced also by a British observer, not a physician, but one with close contacts with occupational physicians: "Some of the key strengths of the industrial medical officer are that he is a man of professional integrity with a greater loyalty to the profession than to himself or his company." (Garnett, J. Productivity, morale and occupational medicine. *Trans Soc Occup Med* 18:120, 1968.) The point is brought into relief by Amundsen, who writes, "No physician's professional allegiance can ever be solely to a specific individual or group (employees vs. employer). Instead, his obligation must be to those principles of medical practice which require an objective assessment of each patient's health status leading to conclusions and recommendations reflecting his best medical judgment." (Amundsen, M. A. Physician's allegiance. *J Occup Med* 19:589, 1977.)

Principle 4: In occupational medicine practice, particularly in relationship to two areas—in the adjudication of workers' compensation claims and in the acceptance by an employer of a demonstrated health-hazardous product or process—extraordinarily large amounts of money are involved. Claims can be fought unjustly, information can be withheld from workers and the public, and costly changes in manufacturing processes will not be made. The role of the physician is to apprise all concerned of the truth of a situation and make recommendations to right the wrong. Any other action is, in itself, unethical.

Principle 5: Although related to Principle 3, this element of conduct may enter into decision-making in different ways: what is good for the company is good for the country; not grounding certain pilots; the consistent declaration (as a private practitioner) of the work-relatedness of every alleged disease state, or the opposite if one is company-employed; different treatment of an executive; slanting of opinions to favor a patient,* and so on.

Principle 6: This body of knowledge is mandatory for a physician to practice sound, scientific, and knowledgeable occupational medicine. Without this familiarity with the work environment, the physician offers no advantage to a workforce whatsoever and is likely to be blind to a multitude of cause-and-effect relationships among the patients.

Principle 7: Of all this corpus on behavior, this principle is the one most often subject to noncompliance, not by the physician, but by those persons in the organization slurringly referred to as "personnel types." The nonprofessional executing the industrial relations or personnel function cannot understand the concepts of privilege or confidentiality, and consistently ask—even demand—the medical records of certain applicants or employees. The sole method of reversing this supposed need is dramatically to personalize the situation and suggest plant-wide distribution—for that is what happens occasionally with "rich" medical information in the hands of clerks—of the requester's own "juicy" file. The physician must remain adamant on this point, or the program will be lost, for no one will trust the OHS. Semper fidelis!

Principle 8: Some employers, in fear of sizable claims, will not permit findings on clinical or epidemiologic research to be given any distribution or to be published. However, as most persons now know, information regarding untoward health effects of certain work exposures, by law [56] must be given employees, and the physician is negligent if such material is not made known to the individuals at risk. While it may seem the cautious thing to do at first—to conceal important clinical findings—in the long run, the employer will be involved deeply both financially and morally, to wit, the case of asbestos-related disease. Over the years, trade associations have sponsored research, the results of which rarely find publication in journals. A timely correction of a process productive of harm will save much in the way of both health and compensation payments.

*The most blatant violation of the principle was seen during the Vietnam War when the following two letters came into our hands at an OHS, written by the same physician.

The first letter, regarding possible drafting into the service reads, "John Smith has been under our care since September, 1959, and has been treated for rheumatic fever. He has a systolic murmur which probably represents aortic valve disease and he is on a maintenance dose of penicillin for this. He has not had any decompensation but does have a definite valvular lesion. It is requested that this be taken into consideration at the time of his draft evaluation."

The other letter, regarding employment in law enforcement, reads, "John Smith came into the office on March 30, 1972 for an examination, reporting that he feels fine, plays handball regularly, and has not had any symptoms relating to his cardiovascular system or any other problems. Examination reveals a normal heart size and an electrocardiogram is perfectly normal and exhibits no sinus arrhythmia. A treadmill stress test was performed in which he accomplished 12 minutes and a pulse rate of 199, he had no ischemia and no arrhythmias and this is ample reflection of an excellent cardiovascular system. It would be my recommendation that he will be able to exercise in any way he desires without limitations or without danger of any complications. (Enclosure: Treadmill Stress Test)."

Principle 9: This principle parallels the essence of Principle 8. The significant words are "communicate understandably," implying that the uttering of medical jargon to a group of workers is not informing, teaching, or enlightening.

Principle 10: Consultants are available in all clinical specialities, in addition to epidemiology, biostatistics, toxicology, or legal medicine, among other areas. Their expertise should be sought *early,* either to prepare the appropriate design for study of a group or to evaluate a single employee-patient.

Principle 11: With the mandates regarding medical records, reporting of morbid and mortal episodes, cooperation with governmental health personnel can hardly be avoided. Most employers prefer to seek consultative assistance from private firms, such as industrial hygiene, so that citations can be avoided and corrections made without penalty. How much of the fear of contact with official agencies has been lessened since OSHA or the comparable state agencies have provided consultative help is not known. "Other members of the health professions" will include nearly everyone concerned with health as a legitimate, non-fadish, non-fraudulent undertaking. With the growth of "holistic" medicine, the "clinical ecologists," and the persuasive arguments offered to the laity, including expressed opinions of executives' wives, care must be exercised in establishing this type of relationship.

Principle 12: This guideline, in essence, implies strict professional behavior, avoiding the charlatanism of the old medical pitchmen, but does allow the time-honored customs of announcing the opening of an office, a geographic change, a description of services, addition of new partners, and the like.

The AOMA code is sound, and compliance with the "12 steps" will quiet critics and improve relationships with the medical and lay communities, employee organizations, and employers, in addition to allowing the physician untroubled sleep. Baum [57], in a single sentence, has restated the code in precis: "I wish to express my fervent and passionate commitment to life and to whatever I must do to protect and prolong it. As a physician I have always considered this my ethical and moral obligation in all situations." Finally, that the code is particularly fitting in a contemporary professional behavior is given solidity by King [58], who identified today's problems as "the manipulation of public opinion; the flexibility of moral standards wherever personal advantage is concerned; the identification of personal profit with philanthropic principle; and, of course, the appeal of hucksterism and humbug."

"I DO NOT KNOW"

Many persons engaged in occupational health practice believe, as do others, that it is wrong to admit a lack of knowledge in a particular area of thought or body of information. For some reason it is thought demeaning if the allegedly all-knowing practitioner in the health arts and sciences is without an answer to a specific question in the field with which one is familiar. Early on, when engaged at a nuclear energy research facility, preventive care was being given a great number of physical scientists at the doctoral level. It was commonplace for a chemist to inquire regarding the formula of a particular medication or the mechanism of the physiologic change involved in a constellation of symptoms. One learned then that the truthful answer of "I don't know" was perfectly acceptable provided it was followed by one of two responses: "But I'll certainly find out for you," or "Let's look it up." An immediate perusal of a textbook or specialty monograph told the patient that we were also scientifically concerned, and the joint seeking of the answer fitted the scientist's perception of handling a knowledge gap.

The same procedure has been followed over the years with all levels of patients, and on no occasion was the feeling ever detected that there was a sudden loss of respect or that the physician-patient relationship was impaired. Employee-patients are impressed when a question placed casually ends with forwarded documentation that provides a full explanation of the subject discussed. Such follow-up, simple as it is, can cement relationships between the OHS and the most recalcitrant of clients. No one is so knowledgeable that all answers are immediately at hand.

E PLURIBUS UNUM

In one of the cities in which the author had occasion to live, there was a restaurant that was extremely popular, for loud youngsters were tolerated and the menu combined both good food and junk food so as to please all palates. But there was a strange policy there that was carried out in this fashion: One young woman, the hostess, seated the customers at the table; a second attendant took the order; the salad was brought by a third person; the entree followed, being placed by a fourth waitress; the dessert and drinks came via another server; and, to top it all, the bill was presented by a person not seen previously.

Most likely it must have been felt by the management that such a protocol would lend for greater efficiency because of the specialization by course served. However, the feeling generated in the customer was that there was no *one* person to whom one could relate for the duration of the meal. Which person had responsibility for replacing the dropped fork or for filling the water glasses? There was no continuing relationship between server and served, so that by meal's end one still was a stranger in the restaurant.

The tale is told because in a busy OHS with two or more physicians, or with several nurses, there may be, for the sake of expediency, a wish to have patients seen promptly by any practitioner who is free so that the workers may be returned to work. The patient feels uncomfortable, for even though the clinical story is well documented in the record, the patient knows that this new person was not the one to whom the problem was related initially and that this stranger to the problem would have to be told or trained, in a sense, up to the level of the subsequent visit. In short, whenever possible, there should be a continuity in care, so that the same OHN or physician sees the patient throughout the duration of the illness or injury. The sense of fragmentation in care does not lead to total satisfaction for the patient.

THE PHYSICIAN AND THE FULLER LIFE

It is believed that the physician in industry needs to be a broad-scale person in interests, so that there can be areas of commonality with many of the people seen as patients. The practitioner who knows medicine solely and has limited all energies to its exercise may prove to be a pretty dull person to have around. During the years in medical school, because of the constraints of time and the curriculum, students lose contact with the arts and, in the main, with their involvement in practice and career building, frequently do not return to the sources of esthetic pleasure. While many practitioners are magnificent photographers, home craftsmen, musicians, lapidaries, and even poets, most physicians are without social concern, or ability, as Haskins [59] put it, to make effective choices among wide priorities.

If the physician truly wishes to help employees with some of the deeper causes of their troubles, there must be knowledge of the cultural background of the patients, their religious beliefs, their educational level, and sense of personal values or the philosophy that has been guiding them through life. Without this understanding, the finest recommendations that are offered may not be accepted or followed.

Harrell [60] says that the solution of problems facing us in health care in the next millenium will increasingly be moral and ethical rather than scientific, and their unraveling will require a broader, liberal, humanistic background in the education and training of the student, with more insight and perception on the part of the physician and greater sensitivity toward patients.

The point of a broad base is underscored by Stalley [61], a philosopher, who indicates that advice can be given only to the extent that human beings can share, or at least enter sympathetically into one another's values. One prefers to look to someone for counsel whose ultimate values are the same as our own; but we can also seek advice from someone who does not share our values if that person is able to understand and *enter imaginatively* into our goals (emphasis added). So advice-giving depends on the capacity of human beings to understand one another, by comprehending what it is like to be in a similar position and be able temporarily to make the other person's goals our goals.

In that interpretation lies the need for exposure to bodies of thought outside medicine so that we more quickly can reach that moment of truth, that moment in the preventing/healing process of desperately needed understanding. Many years ago in a brochure descriptive of the Menninger School of Psychiatry, its philosophy was epitomized in this description of the well-trained psychiatrist [62]: "... He should be a man of broad cultural interests and background, conversant with the principal social, scientific, literary and artistic developments of his own time and of the past." How different should be the well-trained occupational physician?

An additional point needs inclusion. Being a humanist in the practice of occupational medicine does not carry with it the image of a flaming liberal or a medical nihilist or anarchist, destructive of everything authoritative or established. Implicit in the concept was the seminal move in the Middle Ages away from the lockstep of theologic orthodoxy and its associated political despotism. The change represented a fresh and free attention to man, a return to the classics of antiquity, and the increased opportunity for contemplation and cultivation of the mind and spirit.

Consideration of the human being in such a light does not signify a less effective physician concerned more with the contemporary upsurge in string quartets than with the outrageous illegal usage of a new and proved health-hazardous work substance. Implicit in this mode of action is a deeply abiding sense of what is right, for what is right philosophically is usually what is right for the worker at risk. It means that the occupational physician has the fortitude to challenge the patently false letter from a private physician who alleges medical care of an employee who probably has not been seen professionally during the absence period being certified. It means forthright disagreement with the physician or the attorney who testifies to a job relationship for every symptom, syndrome, or miniscule finding presented by a dishonest claimant. And, lastly, it means providing the CEO with an occupational health philosophy that can bring good opinion and feeling to the company, the employees, and the medical group.

To meet with and be effective with the many different employees seeking support, ranging from a simple dressing to the resolution of a lifelong deep and abiding problem, one's vision must be broad and one's body of knowledge must course far beyond the boundaries of medicine. From this kind of productive interchange comes the deep psychic satisfaction that is anticipated long before entry into the grueling years of graduate preparation.

REPRISE

To stress the plea for a compassionate understanding of the workers of a plant, some brief quotations follow with the hope that they may solidify and illuminate what has come before in this section. They are offered alphabetically by author.

JOHN P. CALLAN, M.D. [63]
But therapeutic talk is more than a succession of words and phrases rattled off like a chemical formula. The sentences need to be administered with a tincture of compassion, balanced with sensitivity, and titrated with pathos if they are to work and become a communion of the suffering with the true spirit of medicine.

GEORGE L. ENGEL, M.D. [64]
The keystone around which medical care has evolved over the ages remains the interpersonal encounter between the patient and a physician. Regardless of how many other individuals may man the health care system or what aspects of care may be delegated to others, it is to a physician to whom the patient ultimately looks for decisions and by whom he expects his care to be directed. It matters not that the physician may in fact be operating within a group or as a member of a team; the nature of his encounter with the patient, brief or prolonged, superficial or intense, sensitive or aloof, may be the overriding determinant of whether or not he will even be in a position to apply his biomedical knowledge or his technologic skills, not to mention achieve success in so doing. Understanding the dynamics of the one-to-one, helper-helpee relationship is indispensable for the effective functioning of the physician.

RUSSELL V. FULDNER, M.D [65]
Ten injunctions for not-too-easy compliance:

1. Take the patient's history yourself, writing notes.
2. Apologize if you have kept him waiting.
3. Look receptive.
4. Listen; it is surprising how often the patient is right.
5. Try using these in your practice: your eyes, ears, hands, insight, and imagination.
6. If you give the patient a pamphlet, explain it.
7. Have every patient receiving active treatment telephone you at intervals.
8. Take an occasional look at your office, your staff, and yourself.
9. See the patient now who asks to be seen.

Do not follow the tenth injunction if you have disregarded the others:
10. Put malpractice from your mind.

L. J. HENDERSON, M.D. [66]
So far as possible, "do no harm." You can do harm by the process that is quaintly called telling the truth. You can do harm by lying. . . . It will arise also from what you say and what you fail to say. But try to do as little harm as possible, not only in treatment with drugs, or with the knife, but also in treatment with words, with the expression of your sentiments and emotions. Try at all times to act upon the patient so as to modify his sentiments to his own advantage, and remember that, to this end, nothing is more effective than arousing in him the belief that you are concerned whole-heartedly and exclusively for *his* welfare.

FRANZ J. INGLEFINGER, M.D. [67]
The medical profession is seen as dehumanized and deprofessionalized, adhering to the principles of the salesman rather than to those of the samaritan. Personal sympathy for the patient has been replaced by technologically efficient management of disease.

ALBERT R. JONSEN, S.J., PH.D. [68]
The work of curing is well financed, well manned and well publicized. The work of caring is poor in money, personnel, and public relations. Yet, increasingly, clinical competence is compromised by the poverty of the caring function.

IRVINE H. PAGE, M.D. [69]
Medical schools don't teach good manners to students and personnel. It's no wonder that they treat patients as though they're sides of beef. Every hospital needs an om-

budsman, someone older, perhaps an emeritus, someone to exercise common sense, humanity, warmth.

EDMUND D. PELLEGRINO, M.D. [70]
Physicians often fail to comprehend what the patient understands by the promise of healing; patients often fail to understand what the physician thinks he is promising. Physicians seem to be moving toward a restricted sense of the promise, emphasizing technical competence while patients seek technical competence plus compassionate help with the experience of illness as an assault on the person.

DAVID RABIN, M.D., AND PAULINE L. RABIN, M.D. [71]
. . . Open discussions in medical schools, societies, and journals could raise the consciousness of physicians that technologic advances do not render obsolete the need to express care and compassion.

GABRIEL SMILKSTEIN, M.D. [72]
I believe that physicians who commit themselves to the management of only highly technical procedures will be classified as biomedical manipulators.

PROGRAM INITIATION AND MANAGEMENT

It is common parlance among most medical practitioners that rarely, if ever, was any segment of the professional curriculum devoted to the management of an office or its staff. Only in more recent years has some of the teaching and have a few current publications endeavored to fill in this educational gap. Even in the post–OSHA Act training programs, little instruction has been given to future occupational health specialists in the area of program management.

While most of the managerial elements are reviewed in various sections, additional discussion is warranted in the area of "people" management. As Bullock and Stallybrass [73] have indicated, management is practiced at various levels of an organization: Top management is concerned with corporate strategy for the enterprise in the larger sense; middle management has functional responsibilities for production, accounting, finance, marketing, personnel, and the like; and operational management is carried out at the foreman or supervisory level.

The occupational health program directors may find themselves at the first or second levels and, it is hoped, rarely at the last level. The general scheme of management by objectives has been outlined previously. It is the intention in this segment to review some of the informal principles involved in staff management or leadership—the conveying of a sense of purpose, of worthwhileness, of social relevance to members of the OHS—so that whether the task at hand is thoroughly challenging and piquing of excited interest or is a repetitive clerical or test procedure, it is carried out with a feeling of valued contribution to the health of the workforce.

INITIAL PHASES OF DEVELOPMENT

Whether an OHS has just been mandated or a new director has been brought in to vitalize a stagnant program, the steps to be suggested are equally applicable. It must be remembered that a new health professional, given the assignment of creating a program that not only will respond to all legal requirements but also will meet the unique needs of the organization, comes to the company as an unknown. The newly employed medical director may have a dossier replete in experience, educational preparation, honors, and a fine, peer-based reputation, but to the officers and the employees, he or she is a stranger, whose merit must be proved. The process of acceptance—outside the walls of the medical unit itself—may take 1 or 2 years. The usual pattern of growth is one of acceptance of the director as a person, followed by acceptance of the program that has been designed and espoused.

DEMOGRAPHIC DATA
The newcomer, frequently an outsider and not a promotee from within, is often expected on Day 1 to don professional attire and begin to see patients. Such action can be defeating, for no body of knowledge regarding the company has been acquired. The demographic characteristics of the labor force must be learned, so that there is an awareness of these distinctions in the plant population:

Total number of employees
Number of employees by job family
Number of employees by department
Number of employees by job title
Ratio of male to female employees
Number of employees by 10-year age increments
Mean and median ages of workforce
Location(s) of employees—plant area, building, floor (if single high-rise structure)
Number of employees by ethnicity
Ratio of native-born to foreign-born employees
National or geographic source of workforce
Mean duration of employment
Duration of employment by 5-year increments
Turnover per year

Absenteeism percentage per year
Organizational structure
Structure of trade unionism and employee organizations

These data will provide an understanding of the population to be served, and when the mission and operations of the company are learned, with their attendant exposures and surveillance and control constraints, then a medical plan can be designed to respond to the organization's unique needs.

CREATION OF POLICY

The formulation of a policy, although touched on in the discussion of manuals, is the next logical step. At an early date, a written statement should be prepared for the signature of the CEO, which gives top managerial support to the occupational health program being developed. It should declare the purpose(s) or objectives of an occupational health program, the congruence of executive management, and the authority and responsibility given the medical director. With such a document in hand, the new health professional is ready to meet the personnel with whom there will be most interaction in the future.

MEETINGS WITH DEPARTMENT HEADS

Armed, in a sense, with authorization from on high, the new medical director is ready to meet the department heads. While no particular order is indicated in this early familiarization program, it is advised that one begin at the top and work down, for there are advantages in being able to say that one has already met the executive to whom a department head reports. One can rarely be refused audience, and the visit will bear greater authority and probably be more productive, for the department chief will not know what message might have been delivered about his or her functions.

It has been found useful to explore three areas after initial introductions are complete: the responsibilities or role of the department as it contributes to the company mission, recommendations regarding the new occupational health program to be structured,* and the existence of any personal medical problems.† Often the problems that are elicited are not personal but may involve the family and may not even be of a medical nature. But if one can be of referral assistance, the program is helped, and one will have unequalled executive support.

These interviews are important, for the acquaintance is two-way—the medical director has the opportunity of sizing up the executives, and they in turn can judge the qualities of the newly added physician. Many of the relationships established at the initial contact will prove enduring, warm, and productive.

MEETINGS WITH OHS PERSONNEL

Of equal need is a series of interviews with the OHS staff, many of whom will have had long periods of service with the company. It is essential that they be given the opportunity of meeting the new director in a one-to-one situation, so that each will learn something of the other. All staff members should be asked about their past professional experience and their current affiliation. The same approach should be used as with the divisional chiefs, in that they should be queried as to their recommendations regarding program updating or redesign, equipment needed, or reversal of past difficulties. It would be desirable that these interviews follow either a general explanatory staff meeting or a tour of the facility for introduction purposes to soften the usual anxiety that arises when a member of the OHS is asked to meet with the new director. To be derived from these interviews is some knowledge of the members' families, for personal and domestic problems will present themselves for solution during the director's tenure, and one should be prepared with some basic information.

PREPARATION OF A MANUAL

It is suggested that the OHS manual be developed as early as possible to provide staff members with program expectations and to familiarize department

*It has been the writer's experience that in offering recommendations, the department head will usually pour out all of the complaints held against the previous medical administration, which offers better leads in program planning than when asked for recommendations. The frequent response is, "Well, Doc, that's your business," and little comes forth. The practice of incision and drainage of feelings is extremely productive and can be conducted without impugning the faults of one's predecessor.

†The value of this intelligence—personal medical problems—was shown when the writer was conducting this kind of interview with the person second in command of an organization that the writer had just joined. The executive took out a current issue of *Time,* opened up to a news release regarding a pharmaceutical preparation just moving from the experimental to the production phase. "What do you know about this?" was the query. The response was, "Nothing, but I'll find out." The investigator was called, the details of the medication obtained, and the message delivered. The man was unaccustomed to such promptness and became the strongest supporter of the program, an action appreciated, for he had a majority of the workers in his departments, nearly all union members.

heads with the new effort in health conservation. This publication provides early visibility of the change in direction and gives staff solidity in the performance of their functions. As indicated previously, it should be prepared cooperatively with the section heads of the OHS.

LEARNING THE MISSION

It is at this point, provided there has been no plant accident, serious chemical leak or spill, or misadventurous loss of effluent, that one is ready to undertake a learning program of the plant's operations. Such an effort involves walk-throughs of all activities accompanied by the most knowledgeable supervisor, a review of departmental training manuals, and continuing receipt and reading of departmental publications.*

Following these preliminary procedures, an inventory of hazardous substances should be initiated, if not already undertaken by the industrial hygiene arm of the company or the OHS. Information is obtainable not only from various Material Safety Data Sheets (MSDS), but also from intracompany data and reports and from published and unpublished results of company-conducted or company-sponsored research. The material derived is readied for data bank storage.

By now, several activities have been solidified: familiarization with employee demography, company executives, and OHS personnel; declaration and distribution of an occupational health policy; partial preparation of a manual; familiarization with plant operations; identification of occupational health hazards; and storage of industrial hygiene data. At this point, the services and specialized programs described in other chapters can either be refined or introduced. The manual should be descriptive of the total program as envisioned,† thus providing goals for the OHS to seek and for plant managers to anticipate.

MANAGEMENT RESPONSIBILITIES

Vannevar Bush, the late eminent academician and engineer, considered management not only a profession, but also an art and a technique. But, more importantly, he felt that the central theme of any true profession is ministry to the people—not just a service, humbly rendered, but guidance, extended with pride and authority [74]. As there is guidance of patients in medical practice, so there should be equal ease in the guidance, support, direction, and motivation of a group. Unfortunately, this leap from interaction with a single individual to effective leadership of a number of employees is not made readily.

No aspect of contemporary medical education directs attention to the role of the physician as the operating head of an active health service. While certain practitioners have manifested the skills needed to serve as university presidents or chairmen of boards of directors, the rise to these positions has resulted essentially from a combination of inherent abilities in leadership and on-the-job training. In other professions—business, the military, engineering—there frequently is specific instruction in management; but in medicine, even though team membership is required in hospitals, clinics, societies, and the like, the physician must learn through trial and error, unless there has been recent learning through seminars initiated by societies dedicated to medical management.

Koontz and O'Donnell [75] have defined managing as the design or creation and maintenance of an internal environment in an enterprise, where individuals working together in groups can perform efficiently and effectively toward the attainment of group goals. The true manager stimulates and motivates the group—in this case, the OHS staff—in its meeting of the established objectives. Again, as pointed out [75], management includes the functions of planning, organizing, staffing, directing, and controlling (including evaluation and correction of deviations from the plan). The physician, as a technical specialist, may be totally unprepared to assume a managerial role either by training or personality skewing. This kind of misfitting has been seen on occasion in university medical centers where practitioners of considerable competence and broad acclaim are appointed department heads, and because of the lack of managerial skills, the department soon is plagued with internecine difficulties, personnel problems, and lowered effectiveness. Professional competence does not necessarily equate with leadership capability, and if the physician views himself solely as a medical specialist, then the OHS needs the assistance of an administrator. McDonagh [76] worded this idea well when he observed that if the physician does not manage, but assumes solely the role of the specialist, then the specialist will need a manager to plan, organize, integrate, and measure.

*In large organizations, in addition to the primary house organ, sizable divisions will have their own newsletters.
†Prospective program elements can be described, even though not as yet developed.

LEADERSHIP

While leadership is readily understood and more readily recognized, it is a rare attribute and frequently is seen or identified early in life. The quality is self-enhancing in that leaders, through their skills in bringing about understanding and cooperative accomplishment of a mission, are made even more capable through the successful attainment of a goal, for the sense of worth of all participants is heightened and reflects both on them and their leaders. A leader is both a person of influence as well as of action, and such qualities arise through an appreciation and understanding of human relationships [77].

Good directors are keenly aware of the principles of sound mental health and exercise this knowledge in the interactions with individual staff members and with the group as a whole. Every person needs recognition,* appreciation of the work accomplished, and evaluation of the quality of the job conducted. The merit increase often viewed by managers as the acknowledgment of commendable work performance has become an expected milestone and rarely serves as a personal reward for excellence. The latter comes from the words spoken by the leader and is nourished by the frequency and sincerity of the message.

In opposition to the giving of praise, often before other persons, the correcting of an employee must be accomplished without destructive impact. If there has been an error committed, the faulty action must be reviewed in private. The session can be an experience in growth, or it can be a conversion of an otherwise effective employee into a desultory, or even vengeful, worker, with the possibility of losing a person of considerable potential. A more heinous crime, of course, is the intemperate rebuking of an employee in front of others, especially patients. Such action is inexcusable, embarrassing to all within earshot, and productive of little except a denigration of the health program. Action of this nature reveals more of the unthinking supervisor than of the error-committing staff member.

Disciplinary measures, when indicated, must be taken in accordance with established company personnel policies, labor-management contracts, and ethical medical practice. Furthermore, the action must be timely and carried out privately unless the presence of an intermediate supervisor is needed or, in special cases, a witness or representative of a union or the personnel department.

The directors who have their own behavioral problems—impatience, unpredictability, temperamental outbursts or other mood swings, prima donna attitudes, arrogance, intolerance of another's race, creed, color, nationality, or idiosyncrasies, favoritism, inconsistency, procrastination, indecisiveness, or taciturnity [78]—will find these difficulties to be totally counterproductive in the creation of a dedicated workforce, and their display will result in a dispirited, disaffected, uncaring, disloyal, and even a sabotaging staff. With these qualities insinuated into a directorate, the solution is not merely to add an administrator, but to have the alleged manager obtain psychotherapeutic help. The personality aberrations mentioned can prove destructive of both the program and the people, and the hopes of the company concerning a consummate occupational health effort will be shattered.

The qualities most needed in a manager are sensitivity, warmth, conviction, and enthusiasm. Being attuned to situations and people will allow action to be taken before smoldering embers become a true flame. Directors who focus exclusively on their own tasks, oblivious to the emotional climate or feeling tone of the total OHS operation or the kinds of interactions between staff and clientele will soon be shaken by events that readily could have been averted simply by listening, inquiring, and rectifying.

Warmth is required, as in any group, to develop adhesion, a commonness of purpose, a dedication to the mission. Warmth means rapport and a sense of welcome and personal concern. The OHS is one unit in a company where the worker can come who is problem-beset and be counseled. A cold personality is infectious and may become the model for staff personnel who will feel that such aloofness is the professional mien, the industrial demeanor, or the better-than-thou-the-union attitude. For a program to succeed, a sense of managerial warmth must be experienced by all who serve in the department or seek its assistance.

Managers must believe in what they undertake to do and must carry out plans and actions with conviction and enthusiasm. Such a spirit can be emulated

*The most outstanding example of recognition, as recalled by the writer, was witnessed during World War II at the Oakland, California, Port of Embarkation. One of the functions at that installation was the preparation of army vehicles for overseas transport. On a bulletin board seen in the shop responsible for such materiel treatment was a clipping from a Bay Area newspaper bearing a photograph of General MacArthur in a jeep at an invasion site. The number of the vehicle was clearly discernible. Below the newspaper reproduction was a note by the officer-in-charge to the effect that John Jones checked the electrical system, Mary Smith had cleared the needed lubrication, Bob Brown had worked on the fuel lines, and so on, with every worker assigned to that jeep being named. Identification of these individuals and their collective contributions to the war effort was true recognition.

by the staff so that the program succeeds on the basis of its being right and courageously so. As discussed earlier, there will be occasions when a particular posture of management cannot be supported because it is opposite to the medical managerial sense of right. It will be difficult to manifest enthusiasm when a point of view is patently wrong or unjust. There cannot be enthusiastic support for something antithetic to personal or professional belief. The only action at those times is declaration of a firm rationale for one's opposing stance. Medical directors have been discharged for refusing to participate in wrongful arguments; if such is the necessary outcome, then the company does not deserve an ethical medical director.

FREE EXPRESSION

Leadership considers the feelings of people and allows for the expression of these feelings in both a formal and informal manner. At the time of hire, or when a new director joins an established organization, it should be made clear that all suggestions are welcome concerning improvement of service, alteration of method, betterment of facilities, and the like. The rather trite expression of an "open-door policy" should be given substance by behavioral evidence of a true willingness to hear new ideas. It is the staff members who face daily a variety of situations not shared by the director and thus are much more familiar with problems or interactions fraught with some difficulty.

Staff meetings should be held on a regular basis—weekly for section chiefs serving as an executive committee and monthly for the entire OHS. Agenda items can be introduced for discussion, with credit going to the person making the suggestion, unless propriety precludes identification. Problems should be reviewed and solutions reached, if not then, after appropriate investigation or consultation. Items that are so tabled must be reported on at a subsequent meeting, or constructive participation in future sessions will be abolished.

The concept of the staff meeting is carried to the fullest in the mode of the annual conference of health service personnel held by many of the large corporations, usually in conjunction with the yearly American Occupational Health Conference. These meetings include not only invited speakers who review topics germane to occupational medicine but also several hours devoted to discussion of problems present in the company's various OHS activities.

Whether the session includes a few staff members or representatives from various points abroad, there should be *free* discourse of a subject and not a series of declarations by the director indicative of preconceived positions. Single opinions rendered from the chair will negate every advantage offered by the discussion-group format. As indicated by the Canadian editorialist [77], "There is no problem, from writing a constitution for a nation down to designing a new office form, that cannot be solved by discussion around a table."

Probably one of the best descriptions of the ideal session headed by a manager was that of Kunetka [78], writing about Robert Oppenheimer during his Los Alamos period: "In meetings among his staff, Oppenheimer set the agenda, listened carefully, and gave leave to individuals to ramble, but always skillfully pulled together a dozen alternatives into a cohesive direction."

QUALITY CONTROL

In some medical organizations it is frequently assumed that because professional staff members have been trained adequately and have added some years of experience that the quality of the medical or nursing care is impeccable. At other levels, it may be assumed erroneously that the medical documentation or the relationships with departmental supervisors are consistently superior. Levels of performance do vary, and the company-mandated formal performance evaluations prepared annually are not sufficiently frequent in their completion to rectify a consistently impaired job of work.

Medical record notations must be scanned at intervals to determine that protocols of care are being followed, that no aberrant therapies are being prescribed, that there is adequate follow-up of patients, that the notations concerning patient visits are complete, and that they contain no judgmental comments that would represent the OHS badly were the record to be entered as evidence in court. This type of periodic review is necessary to avoid the continuation or perpetuation of repetitive and readily reversed errors of omission or commission.

In a similar vein, it is of worth to review one's clinical laboratory procedures by splitting samples and sending one of each specimen to an outside reference analytic facility for comparison.

Patients can be queried periodically by the medical director to determine if the clinical record entries match their memory of the examination/treatment procedures allegedly conducted.* This kind of secondary review is similar to the previously mentioned

*An employee who had been attended by a staff physician was referred to the writer, who was then serving as medical director at a particular facility. On reviewing the notations in the record, it was seen that there were comments regarding the presenting complaint, the current illness, the findings on examination, the conclusions

mixing with museum or theater attendees to determine their reaction to exhibits or performances and is a form of quality control. One cannot assume that the level of care is always the ideal.

PROBLEM SITUATIONS

If one practices medicine or nursing for any length of time, sooner or later something untoward will occur during an examination or treatment procedure. At no time should knowledge of such an event be kept intramurally within the OHS. The CEO should be notified immediately of an unexpected death, a needle broken and retained subcutaneously following an injection, an injury subsequent to a brief episode of syncope, or any episode that carries the potential of either investigative action by the print or broadcast media or a litigious move by the patient. The CEO must be prepared as quickly as possible for external inquiry so that explanations can be offered. It is not the intention to simulate the facts, but merely to have the company's representative sufficiently knowledgeable to respond to the usual interrogations.

RESPONSE TO CLIENTELE

TELECOMMUNICATIONS

A common cry with certain persons in industry is, "He never returns my calls." Unless one is consistently bombarded by telephone calls from sales personnel, which can be screened readily by secretaries, messages should be responded to early, for in many instances there is an element of immediacy that has generated the call. Messages coming in from supervisors usually are in need of prompt reply, for personnel action loses effectiveness if there is a delay between the incident giving rise to the call and the corrective action taken. A chronic postponement of call returns indicates both an arrogance and a lack of concern and is a measure of a disordered pattern of managerial behavior. In substance, it is thoughtless and impolite.

COMPLAINTS

A second area in which the measure of a manager is taken is in the method of responding to complaints. Any busy OHS will encounter complaints regarding staff personnel, the speed of providing attention,* the endless amount of report paperwork, waiting time, the scope of temporary work restrictions, and the like. A good manager listens to each complainer and assures the individual that the issue will be investigated and that the ultimate response will be forthcoming as quickly as possible.

As determined by the circumstances, no standard answer is given in that the client is always right or that yes, the OHS certainly erred, we made a big mistake, and fawningly promise it will never recur, and so on. The response must include, in some sense, the fact that we (the OHS management) can understand why you were (or are) upset, that we have looked into the matter, that such-and-such did take place, and that we regret that you were affected in the way that you were, and that every effort will be made to avoid recurrence.

After appropriate inquiry, the response must not derogate the individual complaining and must not falsely describe the OHS as a chronic wrongdoer because of time and caseload demands so that such actions "just cannot be helped." The OHS must be supported, yet it is stated that care will be taken to avoid similar experiences in the future. There is little point in having the accused OHS staff member face the originator of the complaint, for rarely does good result from such a confrontation. Whatever the explanation, the person at fault must be made to understand, in private, what was done in error. If the episode is one that could occur in any section of the OHS, then the complaint and the circumstances generating it can be reviewed anonymously at a general staff meeting.

The response to a complaint requires thoughtful handling and often can result in a better relationship with the individual at momentary odds with the OHS than was the bond before the voicing of the complaint.

USE OF CONSULTANTS

There may be times when consultants external to the company organization might be helpful. There might be need for assistance in the development of a new

reached, and the treatment prescribed. In the course of the scan, the remark was made, "And then Dr. X examined you?" The response was, "He didn't lay a hand on me. He just sat across the desk and wrote." Pursuit of the feigned procedure only met with denial by the physician, but continued backtracking disclosed other fractures of basic medical protocol. Burnout? Sloth? Senility?

*At an installation where both military and civilian personnel were served by a single OHS, complaints arose from each of the two groups. The uniformed clients felt that civilians were "being seen first," and the nonmilitary were certain that the "blue suits" were given preference. Neither group was right, for patients were seen in the order of arrival; but the beliefs were deeply positioned, and no effort at clarification ever eliminated the erroneous perceptions.

program or at times of reorganization, and their supportive arguments will aid in the presentation of the issue. It might be that an external review of the current program will highlight certain exceptional elements of the OHS effort and, in so doing, might uncover areas of deficit not realized by the medical director. Or there may be simply a need for the part-time services of a specialist for whom full-time employment is neither indicated nor feasible. The external assistance might come from a psychiatrist, cardiologist, radiologist, ophthalmologist, otolaryngologist, sociologist, or clinical psychologist. Lastly, the medical directors themselves are asked often to serve as consultants to other organizations either on an ad hoc basis or repetitively over an agreed-upon period of time.

In any consultative process, there is a meeting of two professionals, each with singular or different areas of expertise. The objectives of a consultation are (1) to define a problem clearly; (2) to indicate the available or unavailable bits of information; (3) to indicate certain experiences in previous or comparable situations faced by the consultee (extent of knowledge of the consultee or the practice or philosophy of the company); (4) to spell out specific problem points in the health activity of the company, in the resources available, in the consultee, in the immediate supervisor, or in previous consultations; (5) to specify precisely the type of consultative assistance being sought; and (6) to exchange, to teach, to learn.

In the consultation, the exchange must undergo preparation, so that all information is available and none that is possibly relevant is concealed. Such data must be presented even though it may underscore past errors made by the consultee. The material offered for review must be clear and understood. The consultant, on review of the issues, should not resort to denigration or deriding of the consultee's efforts, but should praise, whenever possible, what has been done and suggest or recommend future action. It was the mode of operation of the late, eminent Rockefeller Foundation scholar Alan Gregg [79], on reviewing medical schools around the world that were seeking foundation support, to avoid discussion of previous years' activities and say, merely, "Gentlemen, where do we go in the next 10 years?" Thus averted was any spotlighting of previous errors, faulty behavior, or unsound judgment.

Any behavior similar to that of a prosecutor is strictly to be eschewed, as is any action resembling entrapment, either overt or covert. Reports should be submitted promptly, and if a delay is anticipated because of information yet to be obtained, progress notes should be submitted. In essence, a consultant should be helpful, should instruct, should allow growth, and should be viewed as coworker whose goals are the same as the objectives of the consultee or the parent company—improved service, a more constructive preventive medical program, and better interrelationships with the plant's labor force. Studs Terkel [80], the recorder of life experiences, recalled the comments of a consultant: "The executive who calls me usually knows the answer to his problem. He just has to have somebody to talk to and hear his decision out loud. If it sounds good when he speaks it out loud, then it's pretty good. As he's talking, he may suddenly realize his errors and he corrects out loud. That's a great benefit wives provide for executives. She's listening and you know she's on your side. She's not gonna hurt you."

ADVISORY COMMITTEES

Each OHS should have an advisory committee that can serve both as a guide to the operations and as a receiver and conveyor of information. Such a group should be appointed by the CEO, on the counsel of the medical director, and most commonly comprises these members:

Representative(s) of top level management
Representative(s) of middle management
Representative(s) of operations management (foremen)
Representatives of unions, trades council, or primary labor negotiating bodies
Representatives of employee organizations
Representative of safety director's office
Representative of blue-collar workers
Representative of white-collar workers, nonunion
Representative of comptroller's office
Representative(s) of affirmative action office—women, ethnic groups or other minority workers, the "handicapped"
Representative of the workers' compensation office

The meetings of the committee should be held on a regularly established day at monthly intervals; should allow the attendance of all members to be counted as work time; should be chaired by a person elected by the committee; should expect regular reports from the OHS director, who serves in an ex-officio capacity; and should have an agenda distributed in advance and published minutes sent to all members after each meeting.

The creation of such a steering body provides both a sounding board for new occupational health ideas or programs and an opinion source for ongoing occupational health activities. Ideas are brought to the medical director for consideration or development through a conduit that might not otherwise be present. Also, complaints can be presented that might have appeared as formal grievances, thus defusing early certain issues that could readily assume undeserved proportions.

The writer had experience with an Occupational Health Advisory Committee and found it a uniquely helpful organizational concept. Appointment to the committee, particularly of nonmanagerial persons, gave a quantum of prestige to an otherwise regular job. The messages delivered to the OHS were forthright and nearly always on target and thoroughly constructive. Any OHS will benefit from the support given by a group of this composition.

PROGRAM MANAGER AND THE NEWS MEDIA

Soon or later there will be an event that attracts public attention, and because of attendant adverse health effects, representatives of the print and broadcast media will want to interview the OHS director. Certain errors, as pointed out by Roalman [81], are committed by managers when they face public criticism or inquiry. They follow:

The executive to be interviewed does not do his homework.
In all likelihood the top executive has not preceded the interview with a dry run.
The executive does not listen to the questions.
He does not say anything quotable during the interview.
He does not give the reporter any news.
He tries to shade the truth.
He tries to go off-the-record in his comments without the reporter's permission to do so.
He says things with a mistaken notion that he will be able to see the story before it appears in print and get a second chance to edit his comments.
The executive is unavailable for corroboration or follow-up after the interview is ended.
He does not follow through after the interview is over.

While the medical director may not be involved in the business of a multinational company, there is great likelihood that an accident will focus a reporter's attention on the one person most knowledgeable regarding human injury after accidental exposure to work-related toxic materials.

Bauder [82] has reviewed the relationship of the scientist to the news media and has added other counsel in connection with reducing the risks that arise during an interview or news conference:

Clear with the public relations officer of one's organization regarding (1) the news event or study triggering the interview and (2) any relevant institutional policy.
Avoid granting an interview covering results of a study not yet peer-reviewed or in print. Practitioners may be flooded with patients' calls and have no journal article to which to refer.
Identify the periodical or broadcast source seeking the interview to avoid reading one's comments in the shock headlines of a supermarket rag.
Determine the interviewer's motives—the antivivisectionists may be afoot.
News writing usually requires deadlines. Is the item headed for a feature that can wait, or is it needed now?
Face-to-face interviews are preferred over telephone queries.
Avoid compromising a patient's confidentiality for the sake of publicity.
During the interview, respond sparingly to questions as though one were on the witness stand.
Avoid "leaks" to the press.
Never lie for fear of losing credibility.
Employ simple, clear language.
Stay in the arena of normal scientific conservatism—for example, do not discuss marketing, but feel free to insert a little for its humanizing worth.
Make specific, rather than general, statements.
Do not oversell one's project.
It is helpful if one explains the high costs of research.
It is helpful to tape record the interview; it will facilitate getting a correction later if needed. If by telephone, record the permission.
If one feels trapped by a question to be avoided, obfuscate, or change the subject by "a deft, lateral arabesque."
Appear confident, but not arrogant.
Focus on the reporter, not the camera.
Do not wear, for television, boldly striped clothing or prints, and all black or white attire.

CLOSURE

The essence of effective management may be summed up in the definition provided by Thomas G. Spates [83], Professor Emeritus of Personnel Administration at Yale University:

> Administrative intelligence is defined as the knowledge, the skills, and the attitudes applied to help in the growth of individual personalities; to satisfy, not only their ma-

terial, but also their noneconomic and spiritual needs; to maintain mutually satisfying interpersonal relations among the members of each organizational group, to achieve the proper purposes of an organization by, through, and with its people.

REFERENCES

1. Collings, G. H., Jr. The quantum equivalent technique. *J Occup Med* 13:215, 1971.
2. Craig, R. L. Personal communication, March 16, 1981.
3. Pomerleau, O., Bass, F., and Crown, V. Role of behavior modification in preventive medicine. *N Engl J Med* 292:1277, 1975.
4. Shapiro, M. F., Hatch, R. L., and Greenfield, S. Cost containment and labor-intensive tests: The case of the leukocyte differential count. *JAMA* 252:231, 1984.
5. Collings, G.H., Jr. Examining the "occupational in occupational medicine." *J Occup Med* 26:509, 1984.
6. AOMA Occupational Medical Practice Committee. Scope of occupational health programs and occupational medical practice. *J Occup Med* 21:497, 1979. Sec. A11.
7. Platt, R. Cost containment: Another view. *N Engl J Med* 309:726, 1983.
8. Dickman, R. L., Ford, A. V., Liebman, J., et al. An end to patchwork reform of health care. *N Engl J Med* 317:1086, 1987.
9. Tagg, J. Wielding words to say something. *Los Angeles Times* V:2, Dec 14, 1983.
10. Kaufman, H. F. In a review of C. P. Loomis and J. A. Beegle, *Rural Sociology: The Strategy of Change. Am J Sociol* 63:242, 1957.
11. Lister, J. Training for what?—Winter of discontent. *N Engl J Med* 300:656, 1979.
12. Christy, N. P. English is our second language. *N Engl J Med* 300:979, 1979.
13. Shaw, E. W. Ten commandments for technical writers. *Science* 121:567, 1955. Copyright 1955 by the AAAS.
14. Lilienfeld, D. E. Definitions of epidemiology. *Am J Epidemiol* 107:87, 1978.
15. Stallones, R. A. Significance of data collection: Viewpoint—Academia. *J Occup Med* 21:204, 1979.
16. Baumgarten, M., and Oseasohn, R. Studies on occupational health: A critique. *J Occup Med* 22:171, 1980.
17. Enterline, P. E. Estimating health risks in studies of the health effects of asbestos. *Am Rev Respir Dis* 113:175, 1976.
18. Percy, C., Stanek, E., III, and Gloeckler, L. Accuracy of cancer death certificates and its effect on cancer mortality statistics. *Am J Public Health* 71:242, 1981.
19. Glasser, J. H. The quality and utility of death certificate data. *Am J Public Health* 71:231, 1981.
20. Rigdon, R. H. Reliability of data from death certificates. *N Engl J Med* 303:1422, 1980.
21. Greenberg, R. A., and Tamburro, C. H. Exposure indices for epidemiological surveillance of carcinogenic agents in an industrial chemical environment. *J Occup Med* 23:353, 1981.
22. Jiminy. A piece of my mind: Gomers. *JAMA* 243:2333, 1980.
23. Cato 6. A piece of my mind: Dirtball. *JAMA* 247:3059, 1982; Readers Respond to "Dirtball." *JAMA* 249:279, 1983.
24. Duttera, M. J., Jr. The healer's hand. *JAMA* 242:41, 1979. Copyright 1979, American Medical Association.
25. Kassirer, J. P. Adding insult to injury: Usurping patients' prerogatives. *N Engl J Med* 308:898, 1983.
26. Pickering, G. Manners makyth man: A plea for the importance of character in medicine. *Br Med J* 2:133, 1963.
27. Comstock, L. M. Cited in Patients prefer verbal sign of M.D. caring. *Intern Med News* 13:4, May 1, 1980.
28. Brachfeld, J. Do patients feign ignorance? *N Engl J Med* 302:817, 1980.
29. Izzo, M. Talking to patients. *N Engl J Med* 303:227, 1980.
30. Tabatabai, C. Talking to patients. *N Engl J Med* 303:227, 1980.
31. Douma, A. J. Informed patients and physician satisfaction. *JAMA* 243:2168, 1980.
32. Felton, J. S. Teaching preventive medicine by the group discussion method. *Arch Environ Health* 12:631, 1966.
33. Cousins, N. Potentiation and the patient. *Bull Am Coll Surg* 65:8, 1980.
34. Moser, R. H. In R. H. Moser and F. D. Adams (Eds.), *Diseases of Medical Progress: A Study of Iatrogenic Disease* (3rd ed.). Springfield, IL: Thomas, 1969. P. 812.
35. Cousins, N. A layman looks at truth telling in medicine. *JAMA* 244:1929, 1980.
36. Eliot, T. S. Cited in M. Lipkin, *N Engl J Med* 302:1209, 1980.
37. Tumulty, P. A. *The Effective Clinician*. Philadelphia: Saunders, 1973.
38. *World Almanac and Book of Facts 1989*. New York: World Almanac–Pharos Books, 1988. P. 152.
39. Armitage, K.J . Schneiderman, L. J., and Bass, R. A. Response of physicians to medical complaints in men and women. *JAMA* 241:2186, 1979.
40. Kriss, J. P. On white coats and other matters. *N Engl J Med* 292:1024, 1975.
41. Newgard, K., Walleigh, L., Rollow, B., et al. White coats. *Stanford M.D.* 14:24, Autumn 1975.
42. Blumhagen, D. W. The doctor's white coat: The image of the physician in modern America. *Ann Intern Med* 91:111, 1979.
43. Mosesson, B. What do you call a patient? (To his face) *Med Dimens* 4:44, June 1975.
44. Watkins, L. B. "Hi, Lucille, this is Dr. Gold." *JAMA* 247:2415, 1982.
45. Conant, E. S. Addressing patients by their first names. *N Engl J Med* 308:226, 1983.
46. Heller, M. E. Addressing patients by their first names. *N Engl J Med* 308:226, 1983.

47. Parachini, A. Doctors: Familiarity breeds contempt. *Los Angeles Times* V:1, Feb 1983.
48. Middleton, T. H. Take my word: Breach of last-name barrier. *Los Angeles Times* V:3, June 29, 1983.
49. Middleton, T. H. Addressing the first name custom. *Los Angeles Times* IV:15, Dec 26, 1984.
50. Calmes, S. H. What *Dear* really means. *JAMA* 248:2321, 1982.
51. Janis, M. Dear. *JAMA* 249:2459, 1983.
52. Clowney, D. L. Dear. *JAMA* 249:2459, 1983.
53. Calmes, S. H. Dear. *JAMA* 249:2459, 1983.
54. Committee on Ethical Practice in Occupational Medicine (AOMA). Code of ethical conduct for physicians providing occupational medical services. *J Occup Med* 18: cover, 1976.
55. Schuman, B. J. Physicians and patients in the occupational setting: The rules of the game. *JAMA* 244:2417, 1980.
56. Public Law 91-596, Sec. 21c(1) and (2).
57. Baum, B. L. L'Chaim! *Arch Intern Med* 139:921, 1979.
58. King, L. S. In a review of N. Harrison. *Humbug: The Art of P.T. Barnum.* Boston: Little, Brown, 1973. *JAMA* 226:1125, 1973.
59. Haskins, C. P. Science and social purpose. *Am Sci* 61:653, 1973.
60. Harrell, B. T. The doctor as a humanist. *S Afr Med J* 53:701, 1978.
61. Stalley, R. F. The Role of the doctor: Technician or statesman? *J Med Ethics* 6:19, March 1980.
62. *The Menninger School of Psychiatry.* Topeka, KS: The School, 1955. P. 3.
63. Callan, J. P. Therapeutic talk. *JAMA* 244:2202, 1980. Copyright 1980, American Medical Association.
64. Engel, G. L. "The best and the brightest": The missing dimension in medical education. Copyright © 1973 by Alpha Omega Alpha Honor Medical Society, reprinted by permission from *The Pharos,* volume 36, page 129.
65. Fuldner, R. V. The buttoned-lip syndrome. *JAMA* 244:1195, 1980. Copyright 1980, American Medical Association.
66. Henderson, L. J. Physician and patient as a social system. *N Engl J Med* 112:819, 1935.
67. Ingelfinger, F. J. Medicine. *Saturday Rev* 3:25, Nov 1, 1975.
68. Jonsen, A. R. Society looks at clinical competence. *Am Coll Physicians Bull* 17:19, March 1976.
69. Page, I. H. cited in I. H. Page, Not one man, but many. *JAMA* 244:1765, 1980.
70. Pellegrino, E. D. Being ill and being healed: Some reflections on the grounding of medical morality. *Bull NY Acad Med* 57:70, 1980.
71. Rabin, D., and Rabin, P. L. Isolation of the ill physician. *N Engl J Med* 307:1650, 1982.
72. Smilkstein, G. Primary care commentary: I can take off my shoes, too. *JAMA* 241:1272, 1979.
73. Bullock, A., and Stallybrass, O. (Eds.). *The Harper Dictionary of Modern Thought.* New York: Harper & Row, 1977. P. 366.
74. Bush, V. *Science is Not Enough.* New York: William Morrow, 1967. Pp. 51, 68–69.
75. Koontz, H., and O'Donnell, C. *Principles of Management.* Cited in T. J. McDonagh, The physician as a manager. *J Occup Med* 24:99, 1982.
76. McDonagh, T. J. The physician as a manager. *J Occup Med* 24:99, 1982.
77. On being a department head. *R Bank Can Monthly Letter* 48:1, Aug 1967.
78. Kunetka, J. W. *City of Fire: Los Alamos and the Birth of the Atomic Age, 1953–1945.* Englewood Cliffs, NJ: Prentice-Hall, 1978. P. 58.
79. Gregg, A. Personal communication to the author.
80. From *Working: People Talk About What They Do All Day and How They Feel About What They Do,* by Studs Terkel. Copyright © 1972, 1974 by Studs Terkel. Reprinted by permission of Pantheon Books a division of Random House, Inc.
81. Roalman, A. R. Ten sometimes fatal mistakes top executives make in press interviews. *Management Rev* 64:51, July 1975.
82. Bauder, M. S. The scientist and the news media. *N Engl J Med* 308:1170, 1983.
83. Spates, T. G. *Administrative Intelligence: Our Greatest Need for Good Success.* (Lecture delivered while a visiting lecturer at California Institute of Technology, February 23, 1956.) Pasadena, CA: The Institute, 1956. P. 2.

APPENDIX 13-1
A LETTER

It is voiced frequently that feeling and compassion have left the occupational medical scene. As stated in this chapter, the family of the employee must be involved. When the goals of an OHS are expressed, they will become known to the immediate relatives. The following is a letter received by the author when high-risk personnel were being examined, with the protocol including an exercise test using the bicycle ergometer. Only the names have been changed; the remainder is the original.

Dear Dr. Felton:

Today your staff will do the exercise part of my husband's physical and this is a plea for him in our name. Maybe John will pass everything with flying colors and because of that he will consider himself healthy and find no reason to stop smoking.

I'll give you three very valid reasons why he should. Five of us Jones' love him more than life itself. Sally our ten-year old offered her Christmas this year if he would "just stop smoking by going to the Shick Center." Our four children know the pitfalls of smoking, they've seen the diseased lungs, emphysema films, and statistics on family night at the five day plan which helped him for six weeks.

John's brother 42, has had two coronary occlusions, his first at 33. His sister is on digitalis in her 40's.

Most of all—I really do love him and to think one sentence from you or your staff might be his turning point. I hate to think there might be 6–8 years I wouldn't have him to love and spend my life with him. It's not I can't accept him for what he is but then he wasn't born with a cigarette in hand or worst yet watch him die with terminal cancer as I have so many times in my profession.

Thank you for your time and consideration.

Yours truly,
Mrs. John J. Jones (16 years)
also Jane Jones, R.N.
Tom 14, Harry 13, Sally 10, Mary 9

14. LEGAL RESPONSIBILITIES

Law: an ordinance of reason for the common good, made by him who has care of the community.
St. Thomas Aquinas

Prior to the passage of the landmark Occupational Safety and Health Act of 1970, legislative efforts aimed at health protection of the worker were created at the state level but were lacking in enforcement strength. With various health departments being assigned responsibility for determining compliance with the legislation, little was done to implement the mandates. There was great permissiveness between the agency guardians and the employers so that industrially incurred injuries and illnesses were considered the price one paid for doing business. Fines were not placed on erring companies, and the costs of the safety and health infractions were usually cared for through the workers' compensation system. The days of litigation were still to come.

PERTINENT PUBLIC LAWS

Because of public pressure, several federal enactments came from the Congress that were to change the policy of laissez-faire in the protection of worker health. While the increase in supportive production for World War II did focus attention on better safeguards in manpower conservation, the efforts were directed primarily toward minimizing absenteeism rather than reducing worker morbidity and mortality. All of the public laws that are germane in the arena of occupational safety and health have requirements to be met by health service and safety personnel. The primary mandates of the several acts that impinge on in-plant programs will be indicated.

OCCUPATIONAL SAFETY AND HEALTH ACT OF 1970 *(PUBLIC LAW 91-596, 91ST CONGRESS, S. 2193, DECEMBER 29, 1970, EFFECTIVE APRIL 28, 1971)*

The purpose of the Occupational Safety and Health Act of 1970 was delineated as follows:

Sec (2)(b) The Congress declares it to be its purpose and policy . . . to assure so far as possible every working man and woman in the Nation safe and healthful working conditions and to preserve our human resources—

1. by encouraging employers and employees in their efforts to reduce the number of occupational safety and health hazards at their places of employment, and to stimulate employers and employees to institute new and to perfect existing programs for providing safe and healthful working conditions;
2. by providing that employers and employees have separate but dependent responsibilities and rights with respect to achieving safe and healthful working conditions;
3. by authorizing the Secretary of Labor to set mandatory occupational safety and health standards applicable to business affecting interstate commerce, and by creating an Occupational Safety and Health Review Commission for carrying out adjudicatory functions under the Act;
4. by building upon advances already made through employer and employee initiative for providing safe and healthful working conditions;
5. by providing for research in the field of occupational safety and health, including the psychological factors involved, and by developing innovative methods, techniques, and approaches for dealing with occupational safety and health problems;
6. by exploring ways to discover latent diseases, establishing causal connections between diseases and work in environmental conditions, and conducting other research relating to health problems, in recognition of the fact that occupational health standards present problems often different from those involved in occupational safety;
7. by providing medical criteria which will assure insofar as practicable that no employee will suffer diminished health, functional capacity, or life expectancy as a result of his work experience;
8. by providing for training programs to increase the number and competence of personnel engaged in the field of occupational safety and health;
9. by providing for the development and promulgation of occupational safety and health standards;
10. by providing an effective enforcement program which shall include a prohibition against giving advance notice of any inspection and sanctions for any individual violating this prohibition;
11. by encouraging the States to assume the fullest responsibility for the administration and enforcement of their occupational safety and health laws by providing grants to the States to assist in identifying their

needs and responsibilities in the area of occupational safety and health, to develop plans in accordance with the provisions of this Act, to improve the administration and enforcement of State occupational safety and health laws, and to conduct experimental and demonstration projects in connection therewith;

12. by providing for appropriate reporting procedures with respect to occupational safety and health which procedures will help achieve the objectives of this Act and accurately describe the nature of the occupational safety and health problem;
13. by encouraging joint labor-management efforts to reduce injuries and disease arising out of employment.

Responsibility for compliance was given both employers and employees, and particularly pertinent to these writings was the emphasis given the institution of new, and the perfection of existing, programs that would provide safe and healthful working conditions.

Subsequently, certain standards were promulgated by the Department of Labor through the work of the assistant secretary of labor for occupational safety and health, as based on recommendations provided by the secretary of the Department of Health and Human Resources, as developed by the director of the National Institute for Occupational Safety and Health (NIOSH). The reports required by the act have been indicated previously.

Of prime significance in the act is the section referred to generally by industry as the General Duty Clause, which follows:

SEC. 5.(a) Each employer—
(1) shall furnish to each of his employees employment and a place of employment which are free from recognized hazards that are causing or are likely to cause death or serious physical harm to his employees;
(2) shall comply with occupational safety and health standards promulgated under this Act.
(b) Each employee shall comply with occupational safety and health standards and all rules, regulations, and orders issued pursuant to this Act which are applicable to his own actions and conduct.

The reason this segment of the law is important is that Occupational Safety and Health Administration (OSHA) compliance officers may cite this clause during a field inspection in the absence of a specific OSHA regulation. The initiation of a proper occupational health program is the responsibility of the chief executive officer (CEO), the plant manager, or the head of an operating unit, in cooperation with the company's medical director. It is to be remembered that although the NIOSH criteria documents do not carry the full empowerment of law, the material contained in them is used by OSHA representatives as a resource in regard to federal government reviews of plant medical programs.

Surveillance Specifications

For the ease of use and as a ready reference, the OSHA medical and environmental surveillance specifications must be abstracted and collated. In developing cross-reference tables, certain data should be presented for easy visual scan, so that identifying information and frequencies of observation can be determined readily. The following primary headings in Table 14-1 should prove helpful, if such material is not available through a computerized system, as provided by courtesy of Harry Burr, Hilton Head, South Carolina.

Additional notes can clarify the various mandated

TABLE 14-1. *Environmental and Medical Surveillance Specifications*

Part A Environmental surveillance specifications

Worker exposure [or substance]

Exposure code no. (a number cross-referenced to Part B to indicate the required medical procedures)

Status [of the standard, i.e., permanent, proposed, or criteria document]

Regulation or criteria document number

Threshold limit value (TLV)

Ceiling level (CL)

Action level (A)

Required frequency of industrial hygiene monitoring

Sampling and analysis methods

Employee or representative may observe monitoring

Recordkeeping
- Notice to OSHA required
- Retention
- Access—to whom available

Part B: Employee medical surveillance specifications

Worker exposure

Exposure code no.

Regulation or criteria document no.

Medical procedures (mandated or recommended)

Examination frequency by physician

Laboratory and other procedures

Employer medical records
- Maintenance by source
- Retention by source

Required communication by employer
- To physician
- To employee

Required communication by physician
- To employer
- To employee

SOURCE: Burr, H., personal communication. 1980.

surveillance actions and allow the primary tables to remain clear and uncluttered. An individual occupational health service (OHS) can abstract from such a major table those exposures pertinent to local operations and create more brief working tables.

Preparation for Inspection

Hammond [1] prepared guidelines for a chemical plant anticipating an OSHA inspection. As exposures would be greatly multiplied in such a plant, as the potential for citation is increased, and as health and safety concerns usually exceed those of most other installations, compliance in advance of the site visit would be both a wise and an educational activity.

The guidelines [1] follow, although not necessarily in the order of activation:

Have an inventory list of all chemicals used in the plant.

Know what amount of material is handled, where it is stored, and in what departments it is used.

Have in your office files the text of every precautionary label and directions for safe use for all chemical substances.

Have Material Safety Data Sheets for each substance used.

Know how and why a substance creates a hazard under conditions of storage, handling, and usage.

Inform employees of hazards by training courses and periodic retraining.

Know how potentially exposed employees feel about conditions in working areas where they are handling and using chemicals.

Have on file air sample results for general work areas. Know when retests are required. If personal exposures are needed, be familiar with this requirement.

Know and have on file exposure criteria for each substance.

Have on file exposure time weighted average for 75 percent of exposed workers if possible.

Know route substance is absorbed (skin, eye, lung) or otherwise how it might cause harm.

Know what special control measures or work practices are provided.

Know what personal protective equipment is available in case of emergency and for regular work conditions.

Know where a physician and emergency help may be reached.

Know what biologic tests have been used to evaluate employee exposure to certain chemicals and where this means of monitoring is applicable.

Be informed of management's, including local supervisor's, attitude toward OSHA inspectors.

Try to develop and instill into others a healthy respect for OSHA and its authority.

Know how the plant rates in the area of illumination. Are there any rooms or spots where illumination is below standard?

Are there emergency washing and first-aid facilities in work places where corrosive chemicals are stored, handled or used?

Are the workrooms furnished with approved signs required by OSHA?

Make sure that management understands the advantage of having a constructive closing conference with an OSHA officer after a plant inspection.

Ask for an "extended" conference at the proper time if it might serve to your advantage.

State Plans

Some states have found it advantageous to create their own OSHA under Sec. 18 of the Occupational Safety and Health Act, preempting the federal authority in those jurisdictions. When such action is taken, the plan must be "at least as effective in providing safe and healthful employment and places of employment as the standards promulgated under section 6 [of the Act]." The states executing their own plans will vary within time, available tax funds, political ideology, and extent of pressure of certain interest groups.

Questions that arise regarding compliance with OSHA mandates should be reviewed with the appropriate federal or state office, as determined by the agency responsible for the current plan in occupational safety and health.

FEDERAL MINE SAFETY AND HEALTH ACT OF 1977 *(PUBLIC LAW 91-173, AS AMENDED BY PUBLIC LAW 95-164, 95TH CONGRESS, 1977; PUBLIC LAW 95-239, 95TH CONGRESS)*; BLACK LUNG BENEFITS REFORM ACT OF 1977; *AND* BLACK LUNG REVENUE AND REFORM ACT OF 1981 *(PUBLIC LAW 97-119, 97TH CONGRESS)*

It was declared in the Federal Mine Safety and Health Act that "the first priority and concern . . . in the coal or other mining industry must be the health and safety of its most precious resource—the miner . . . and that there is an urgent need to prevent death and serious physical harm . . . and occupational disease." Further, under Title II of the act, it was the purpose to provide, to the greatest extent possible, that the working conditions in each underground coal or other mine be sufficiently free of respirable dust concentrations in the mine atmosphere so that each miner should be able to work underground during his entire adult working life without incurring disability from pneumoconiosis or any other occupation-related disease* during or at the end of such period.

Chest radiographs are mandated at the time of employment and again 3 years later if the worker is still so engaged. If there is evidence of pneumoconiosis (category 1, 2, or 3 simple pneumoconiosis or complicated pneumoconiosis—International Labor Organization [ILO] classification), a third roentgenogram will be taken 2 years following the second study. The roentgenograms shall meet certain specifications of the secretary of Health and Human Services, and are to be supplemented by such other tests as deemed necessary by the secretary.† Through use of a standardized report form and the ILO system of classification in the interpretation of radiographs demonstrating the pneumoconioses, relative uniformity has been attained for all mines and their employed coal miners.

It is pointed out specifically in the Black Lung Benefits Act of 1972, Sec. 4(f) that claims for disability benefits will not be denied solely on the basis of radiographic findings but that all relevant evidence will be considered, including, where indicated, blood gas studies, x-ray examination, electrocardiogram, pulmonary function studies, physical performance tests, and medical history.

In 1974, following a suit brought by a coal operators' association, the constitutionality of the Black Lung Benefits Reform Act of 1977 was upheld by the U.S. District Court for D.C. [2]. The belief, as established by Congress, was supported that the act was essential to the implementation of effective occupational disease legislation. The retroactive operation of the statute and of various liberal medical and evidentiary standards was needed to ensure that thousands of victims of coal workers' pneumoconiosis were provided adequate benefits.

By 1979, changes regarding the chest radiographic examination of miners were effected through rules and regulations published in the *Federal Register,* Vol. 43, No. 148, for August 1, 1978. Specifications were outlined regarding both the radiographic equipment and the technique of exposure, film processing, and viewing of films to ensure roentgenograms of high quality. Reference should be made to the cited regulations by those facilities concerned with the examination of miners "employed *in* or *at* any . . . underground coal mines . . ." (emphasis added).

Chest radiographs should be interpreted initially by a "B" reader, who is described in the regulations as follows: "Proficiency in evaluating chest roentgenograms for roentgenographic quality and in the use of the ILO-U/C classification for interpreting chest roentgenograms for pneumoconiosis and other diseases shall be demonstrated by those physicians who desire to be 'B' readers by taking and passing a specially designed proficiency examination given on behalf of or by ALOSH* at a time and place specified by ALOSH." Of current B readers, most are radiologists, while several specialists in occupational medicine also have taken and passed the examination. All interpreters, when viewing films under the Federal Coal Mine and Safety Act, must have immediately available for reference a complete set of the ILO-U/C International Classification of Radiographs for Pneumoconiosis, 1971.†

Significant abnormalities other than pneumoconiosis encountered by the physician first to interpret and classify the roentgenogram (cardiomegaly, tuberculosis, pulmonary malignancy) must be communicated to the personal physician indicated by the miner on the miner's identification document, previously submitted.

FEDERAL TOXIC SUBSTANCES CONTROL ACT *(PUBLIC LAW 94-469, 94TH CONGRESS, S. 3149, OCTOBER 11, 1976)*

The essence of the Federal Toxic Substances Control Act (TSCA) is the protection of human health and the environment by requiring the testing of, and necessary use restrictions on, certain chemical substances. It is declared in Sec. 2(b)(1) that adequate data should be developed with respect to the effect of chemical substances and mixtures on health and the environment and that the development of such data should be the responsibility of those manufacturers or processors producing or handling such materials. While control authority is exercised, it should not impede unduly or create unnecessary economic barriers to technologic innovation. It is the intent of the Congress that the administrator of the Environmental Protection Agency (EPA) act reasonably and

*The Black Lung Benefits Reform Act of 1977 enlarges the definition of pneumoconiosis to include any other respiratory and pulmonary impairment arising out of employment in or around the nation's coal mines.

†The radiographs must be of acceptable quality, taken by a qualified person, interpreted by a qualified radiologist, and free from any belief that fraud was involved. (Goldsmith, F., and Kerr, L. E. *Occupational Safety and Health*. New York: Human Services Press, 1982. P. 250.)

*Appalachian Laboratory for Occupational Safety and Health, Box 4258, Morgantown, WV 26505.

†This set may be obtained from the International Labor Organization Occupational Safety and Health Branch, CH 1211, Geneva 22, Switzerland.

prudently in carrying out the mandates of the legislation in consideration of the environmental, economic, and social impacts of such action.

Of particular importance is the requirement that new chemicals be subjected to a premanufacture review program before being allowed into the United States. TSCA requires the chemical industry to notify EPA before making or importing a new chemical into the United States for a commercial purpose. A "new" chemical substance is one not included in the TSCA inventory, compiled by EPA, which lists existing substances already in U.S. commerce [3].

Of pertinence to an occupational health program is Sec. 8(e) of TSCA, which requires that any person who manufactures, processes, or distributes in commerce a chemical substance or mixture and who obtains information that reasonably supports the conclusion that the material presents a substantial risk of injury to health or the environment shall immediately inform the administrator of EPA of such knowledge unless it is a certainty that such information has already been forwarded. Included among the materials on which to report, in addition to those manufactured, processed, or distributed commercially, are products or processes involved in research and development, raw materials, intermediates, byproducts, effluents, emissions, waste products, and catalysts.

Information to be included in a report comprises the following*:

Title of report: Possible Substantial Risk Report TSCA 8(e)/CPSA 15(b)†
Date of report
Date information obtained
Name of material(s) potentially implicated
Related to health, environment, consumer product
Situation: concise description, including medical description of symptoms if health-related or technical description of environmental hazard
- Names of persons affected
- Geographic location affected
- Nature of occurrence, circumstances, quantities, and ambient conditions involved
- Other involved personnel who may have pertinent information
- Risk information known to EPA/CPSA (yes/no/not sure
- Other relevant data and information
- Names of person(s) initiating report, job title, location, telephone numbers

*Report content provided through courtesy of James A. Hathaway, M.D.

†See next section on Consumer Product Safety Act (CPSA).

A copy of the completed report should be returned to the originator and should carry the date of forwarding to TSCA or CPSA.

It should be pointed out that certain categories of products are exempt from TSCA, as they are regulated under other federal laws. They are tobacco, nuclear materials, firearms and ammunition, food, food additives, drugs, cosmetics, and pesticides [3].

The information to be submitted to EPA regarding a new chemical must be forwarded at least 90 days before marketing such a product and will include

All available studies on the health and environmental effects of the chemical
Its common or trade name
Its chemical identity and molecular structure
Proposed uses and estimated amounts to be produced or imported for each use
Methods of disposal
Workplace exposure
Byproducts

FEDERAL CONSUMER PRODUCT SAFETY ACT *(PUBLIC LAW 92-573, 92ND CONGRESS, S. 3419, OCTOBER 27, 1972, AND AS AMENDED IN 1976 AND 1978)*

Sec. 15(b) of the Federal Consumer Product Safety Act (CPSA) requires that every manufacturer of a consumer product that is distributed in commerce and every distributor and retailer of such a product who obtains information that reasonably supports the conclusion that such a product either fails to comply with an applicable consumer product safety rule or contains a defect that could create a substantial product hazard* shall inform the Consumer Product Safety Commission of failure in compliance, unless it is known that the commission has been informed previously [4].

The report form suggested in the previous section will provide the pertinent information.

ATOMIC ENERGY ACT OF 1954 *(AS AMENDED); NUCLEAR REGULATORY COMMISSION AUTHORIZATION ACT OF 1978 (PUBLIC LAW 95-601, 95TH CONGRESS)*

Under the rules and regulations of the U.S. Nuclear Regulatory Commission (Title 10, Chapter 1, Code of Federal Regulations—Energy, Part 19), certain

*As outlined in Sec. 15(a)(2) of the CPSA, a substantial product hazard is a product defect that (because of the pattern of defect, the number of defective products distributed in commerce, or the severity of the risk) creates a substantial risk of injury to the public.

Estimated whole body exposure range (rems)*	Number of individuals in each range
No measurable exposure	
Measured exposure less than 0.1	
0.1 to 0.25	
0.5 to 0.75	
0.75 to 1	
1 to 2	
2 to 3	
3 to 4	
4 to 5	
5 to 6	
6 to 7	
7 to 8	
9 to 10	
10 to 11	
11 to 12	
12 +	

FIGURE 14-1. *Example of form to summarize exposure to radiation in personnel monitoring report. rem = Roentgen-Equivalent-Man, the quantity of any ionizing radiation that has the same biologic effectiveness as 1 rad of x-rays; 1 rem = 1 rad × RBE (relative biologic effectiveness). A rad (acronym for Radiation Absorbed Dose) is a unit of measurement of the absorbed dose of ionizing radiation and corresponds to an energy transfer of 100 ergs per gram of any absorbing material (including tissues). The biologic effect of 1 rad varies with the kind of radiation to which the tissue is exposed.*

procedures must be executed regarding radiologic working conditions. The workers concerned are those persons engaged in activities licensed by the commission and controlled by a licensee, one authorized to operate a production or utilization facility or to possess power-reactor spent fuel in an independent spent-fuel storage installation.

Each licensee must post current copies of the regulations in Parts 19 and 20 of the code cited above. Further, all persons working in or frequenting any portion of a restricted area—an area with controlled access for purposes of protection from exposure to radiation and radioactive materials—must be informed of the storage, transfer, or use of radioactive materials or of radiation in the areas. Also, these workers must be instructed in the health protection problems associated with exposure to such materials or radiation. The instruction will include the precautions or procedures needed to minimize exposure, the functions of protective devices,and the reporting of unnecessary exposure.

The individual worker is to be given all radiation exposure data, and each notification and report is to be in writing and must include identifying information (name of licensee, name of employee, and the social security number), the exposure information, and the statement, "This report is furnished to you under the provisions of the Nuclear Regulatory Commission 10 CFR Part 19. You should preserve this report for further reference." On termination of employment or assignment to work involving radiation, the worker is to be furnished with a record of the measured exposure undergone or an estimate of such exposure.

Under Part 20—Standards for Protection Against Radiation—the licensee must report immediately any whole-body exposure of an individual to 25 rems or more of radiation; exposure of the skin of the whole body of 150 rems or more; or exposure of the feet, ankle, hands, or forearms of 375 rems or more. There will be notification within 24 hours of comparable exposures at levels of 5 rems, 30 rems, or 75 rems. The regulations specify also the reporting requirements for the release of radioactive materials in concentrations exceeding specified limits.

Personnel monitoring reports are required during the first quarter of the year following the calendar year of the report and should include a summary of exposure as shown in Figure 14-1.

Certain states under agreement with the Nuclear Regulatory Commission have assumed responsibility for radiation control and have issued regulations comparable to the federal rules cited above, as provided to state administrative or health and safety codes. The governing legislation should be sought for local compliance.

EMPLOYEE PROTECTION

The Committee on Scientific Freedom and Responsibility of the American Association for the Advancement of Science (AAAS) has identified certain public laws that contain employee-protection sections. In these sections, employers cannot take adverse action against employees who assist in carrying out the regulatory purpose of the legislation, as exemplified by their notifying responsible officials, either of legal violations or possible hazards regulated by the legislation [5].

Such sections are included in

Occupational Safety and Health Act of 1970 (Public Law 91-596, Sec. 11c)
Federal Water Pollution Control Act Amendments of 1972 (Public Law 92-500, Sec. 507)
Safe Drinking Water Act of 1974 (Public Law 93-523, Sec. 1450)
Toxic Substances Control Act of 1976 (Public Law 94-469, Sec. 23)
Resource Conservation and Recovery Act of 1976 (Public Law 94-580, Sec. 7001)
Clean Air Act Amendments of 1977 (Public Law 95-95, Sec. 312)
Federal Mine Safety and Health Act of 1977 (Public Law 95-164, Sec. 105(c))
Nuclear Regulatory Commission Authorization Act of 1978 (Public Law 95-601, Sec. 10)

The sections cited offer a means of appeal for employees who have been discharged or otherwise retaliated against for undertaking action to ensure that their organization complies with the regulation.

PERTINENT LEGAL GUIDELINES

Many other issues have led to the development of precedents through case law, which carries essentially the same weight as legislation at the federal or state levels. Some of the guidelines may have been articulated in various documents promulgated by professional associations or in published reviews of certain court rulings.

INFORMED CONSENT

While some discussion of the doctrine of informed consent was undertaken in the discussion of medical records, elaboration of needs and the principles of practice is indicated. There is no question that court decisions have increased the work burden for physicians. Further, as the legal requirements differ in various states, it has been difficult to formulate guidelines by which prudent practice and compliance can be conducted [6].

A definition is in order. According to Miller [7], the doctrine of informed consent may be defined as the duty of a physician, before treating a patient, to explain the procedure to the patient and to warn him/her of any material risks or dangers inherent in or collateral to the therapy, so as to enable the patient to make an intelligent and informed choice as to whether to undergo such treatment [8].

As each new court decision is derived, the status of the law in a state can be subject to change. A few principles, derived from many jurists' opinions as of 1974 [6], may aid the physician in his or her disclosure to a patient:

Physicians may tailor the extent of their preoperative warnings to the particular patient to avoid the unnecessary anxiety and apprehension that such appraisal might arouse in the mind of the patient.
A consent to a surgical procedure is effectual if the consentor understands substantially the nature of

the procedure attempted and the probable results of the operation.

A physician is required to disclose to the patient all information relevant to a meaningful decisional process.

Beyond minimal disclosure, a physician must also reveal to the patient such additional information as a skilled practitioner of good standing would provide under similar circumstances.

A physician need not make disclosure of risks when the patient requests that he or she not be so informed.

Whether a practitioner is under a duty to warn a patient of the possibility of a specific adverse result of a proposed treatment depends on the circumstances of the particular case and of the general practice with respect to such cases followed by the medical profession in the locality. (In another ruling, it was stated conversely that a physician's duty to disclosure is not determined by medical custom and practice.)

The topics importantly demanding a communication of information are the inherent and potential hazards of the proposed treatment, the alternatives to that treatment, if any, and the results likely if the patient remains untreated.

In emergency situations when the patient is incapable of consenting, the physician should, as current law requires, attempt to secure a relative's consent, if possible.

The physician's duty of disclosure applies only to the duty to warn of the hazards of a correct and proper procedure of diagnosis or treatment and has no relation to the failure to inform of the hazards of an improper procedure.

The duty of a physician to make full disclosure is one that arises from the physician-patient relationship, being owed to the patient him- or herself and not to the spouse or other members of the family.

When informing the patient regarding relatively complicated surgery, the physician must, in addition, disclose the known risks of death or serious bodily injury.

It is the physician's duty to make reasonable disclosure of the consequence of treatment and of the dangers within the physician's knowledge that are incident or possible in the proposed treatment. The physician is not under obligation to describe in detail all of the possible consequences of treatment. To make a complete disclosure of all facts, diagnoses, and alternatives or possibilities that might occur to the physician could so alarm the patient that it would, in fact, constitute bad medical practice.

When a physician is silent and makes no disclosure whatever, the physician has failed in the duty owed the patient, and the patient is not required to produce expert medical testimony to show that the physician's failure was contrary to accepted medical practice.

The physician-patient relationship is of such a confidential and vital nature that an affirmative duty requiring full disclosure of the facts of the medical case does exist and that silence in this regard may be sufficient to infer a constructive misrepresentation.

Some of the conclusions given above may, at any time, be changed through appellate decisions in a particular jurisdiction. While certain informed-consent decisions involve procedures or treatment not usually provided in an OHS, certain therapeutic actions may be undertaken in an in-plant service that would require the physician to adhere to the doctrine of informed consent.* Some of the procedures serving as a basis for suit have included the following [9]: bromsulfophthalein, removal of callus, removal of cyst, drug therapy, removal of foreign body, reduction of fracture, and tooth extraction.

In recent years, the professional standard approach—the standard of practice among physicians—has been considered less and less relevant in informed-consent law. It has been shown that even if the patient can establish the lack of informed consent, the patient cannot recover unless it can also be proved that the physician's failure to inform was a proximate cause of the injury sustained [10,11]. Most courts currently favor an "objective" test—"whether a reasonable person in the patient's position would have undergone the proposed treatment if he had been adequately informed" [7]. With this test, the patient's testimony, if offered, is relevant to the issue of proximate cause, but such testimony neither is necessary nor controlling [7].

While mandates for the execution of the process of informed consent may have led to greater legal compliance in the area of patients' rights, the level of patient understanding has most likely not changed [12,13]. Comprehension must be the goal, and lengthy forms must be studied and recast to provide better insight for the patient being informed.

Negative opinions have been strong regarding the

*An employer who provides total care to employees or to employees and their dependents would have broader need for disclosure because of the greater variety of therapeutic procedures offered and conducted.

need for such physician-patient communication. One such point of view reads [14]:

> Informed consent is a legalistic fiction that destroys good patient care and paralyzes the conscientious physician. It hedges the experimental situation with barriers that cannot be surmounted. It is not applicable, even by definition, to a large segment of the involved population. The term has no place in the lexicon of medicine. The integrity of the physician continues to represent the most effective guarantee of the rights of the patient and of the experimental subject. However, for this to remain valid, the medical profession must augment its concern for the moral values of its members.

Consent is needed for a broad variety of procedures, a few of which apply to an OHS. Appropriate forms should be devised for the explanation, reading, comprehension, and signature of the concerned employee-patient and signature of a witness in these issues: minor surgery, sigmoidoscopy, needle biopsy, research, nonstandard treatment, refusal of treatment, disposal of amputated members, and clinical photography.

Further, an entry in the clinical record should reflect a summary of the discussion with the patient and the patient's responses, comprehension, and agreement. A note stating that "Consent form signed" is insufficient. Of additional worth is having the patient write a sentence in the record that he or she has read and understood the content of the consent form and sign the statement.

Informed consent can be summarized as follows, as derived from a California Supreme Court landmark decision previously cited [10], *Cobbs* v. *Grant*, 8 Cal 3d 229 (1972):

> In sum, the patient's right of self-decision is the measure of the physician's duty to reveal. That right can be effectively exercised only if the patient possesses adequate information to enable an intelligent choice. The scope of the physician's communications to the patient, then, must be measured by the patient's need, and that need is whatever information is material to the decision. Thus, the test for determining whether a potential peril must be divulged, is its materiality to the patient's decision [15].

REFUSAL OF TREATMENT

Infrequently an employee-patient will refuse the treatment proferred by a member of the OHS professional staff. This action may be based on the individual's belief that the treatment offered places one at undue risk or that the person providing treatment is judged incompetent, or it may stem from religious beliefs. While it has long been accepted, in keeping with one's right under the Constitution to privacy and free choice, that a mentally competent person has the right to refuse medical treatment, even if it means a fatal outcome, such a rejection on the part of the injured worker runs afoul of provisions under workers' compensation legislation. In most jurisdictions the refusal of treatment, if deemed unreasonable, leads to denial of benefits. The question of when compensation should be suspended because of refusal, for example, of a recommended surgical procedure is an extremely difficult and delicate issue to resolve.

This act is considered to be misconduct, and the problem that remains for decision is whether this conduct should bar the receipt of benefits. The test for determining the unreasonableness of refusing treatment by or through the employer is to weigh the chance of improvement through treatment against the risk entailed [16].

The grounds on which refusals have been held to be reasonable, in one jurisdiction, have been (1) the tender of treatment was inadequate, (2) the employee relied in good faith on medical advice (from another practitioner), (3) the proposed treatment was too dangerous, (4) the proposed treatment was ineffective, and (5) the refusal was innocent [17].

Refusals that have been found to be unreasonable have included (1) fear without substantiation, (2) desire to avoid loss of earnings, (3) personal preference for one's own physician or method of treatment, and (4) religious objections. Most decisions that have been rendered indicate that the act of refusal bars compensation only to the extent to which it caused, continued, or aggravated the disability [17].

Contrarily, if a risk does exist in therapy, or there is the possibility of attaining no improvement or even worsening the condition subsequent to surgery, the courts have consistently ruled that the injured worker cannot be forced to choose surgery in order to obtain benefits [16]. Exemplary of some findings in favor of the worker have been refusals of corrective surgery for a hernia or a protruded intervertebral disc. In arriving at a decision, the court considers the age of the worker, the physical condition, previous experience with surgery, and the statistical record of the success of such surgical procedures—deaths versus cures. In substance, supporting a claim for benefits after refusing emergency care through an OHS would be difficult to substantiate as reasonable in today's medico-legal-industrial culture. Although most cases today involving refusal of treatment concern terminal illness and the use of living wills [18], which lie outside the purview of occupational medicine, counsel might be sought by concerned relatives employed by the organization.

Under no circumstances should the physician undertake invasion of a worker's privacy (bodily intrusions for recommended therapy) when treatment is refused by the patient. As indicated before, such an action should not be initiated, even though it is recognized as being lifesaving. The procedure to be followed is to document the offer of care and its refusal and have the clinical notation in the record signed by the injured worker and witnessed and signed by a third person. The question may arise in a company that employs the mentally retarded: Can such a person consent to necessary treatment? Although this issue belongs more appropriately under the discussion of informed consent, permission for the conduct of a procedure must be sought from the guardian, if there is such a person, or from a parent if the employee is a minor. One must keep in mind the long-standing legal principle, "Every human being of adult years and sound mind has a right to determine what shall be done with his own body" [19]. Here the mind is presumed not to be sound, but that does not alter the need for consent by a responsible party. Further, in the case of an employed minor, if the minor refuses treatment, even though parental permission is given, one should not proceed in the face of the child's vehement refusal [19]. In substance, as concluded by Fiscina [20], a patient's right to privacy, and consequently the right to refuse treatment, may be preserved and applied even when the individual is incapable of exercising it directly. By applying the principle of "substituted-judgment," some courts have permitted the indirect exercise of this right by a duly authorized person acting on the incompetent patient's behalf.

The same has been summarized succinctly by Gaylin [21], who commented, "Every competent adult is considered to be the master of his own body. He may treat it wisely or foolishly. He may even refuse lifesaving treatment, and it's nobody else's business. Certainly not the state's; that is the law of the land."

CARE OF MINORS

Although the authorization of the examination of, or care for, employees who are minors has been alluded to previously, emphasis must be given the need for proper permission. Opportunities for summertime employment will bring persons under 21 years of age into work situations, subjecting them to both the medical examination process and the potential of traumatic injury. Infrequently youths under 18 years of age will be hired. In a case cited by Rosoff [22], a 17-year-old boy, without parental consent, submitted to a vaccination that was a condition of his employment. The court ruled that the procedure was properly authorized on the basis that he was capable of appreciating the nature and consequences of a simple medical procedure such as a vaccination.

In another cited case [23], the court, implying that a 20-year-old patient would have been capable of giving an effective consent, found the "physician liable for going beyond an authorized operation without giving the patient an opportunity to decide on the extension." In most instances the courts have determined that the effectiveness of a minor's consent should not relate solely to the age standard alone, but intellectual maturity and understanding should be considered as well. While the requirement of parental consent has been adhered to closely in nonemergent situations involving young persons, it has been relaxed when the minor was over 15 years of age and the medical procedure was for the patient's benefit. Unsettled is the question of the minor misrepresenting his or her age as older than the true chronologic age. Proof should be sought, however, by checking a driver's license or other evidence of birth date.

As indicated earlier, the age of majority has been subject to new interpretation by reason of emancipation—by marriage and cessation of parental support or by becoming a parent. Stated previously was the need to learn of local statutes regarding emancipation and consent for treatment. The issue attains reality when a minor employee, for example, presents with a sex-related infection. Confidentiality should be maintained, and the law has respected the wishes of minors in keeping certain "sensitive information" from their parents [24]. As the law has been ambiguous on this point, ethical rather than legal considerations are given primacy.

The issues at hand are two, only one of which is germane in an OHS setting. The first concerns the physician's liability for battery if a valid consent is not obtained. The second relates to the practitioner's right to compensation for services not authorized by a person with legal capacity to make a binding contract [24].

Parents may refuse care for a minor employee. Most of the cases reaching litigation involved elective surgery; however, if the minor has sustained life-threatening injury and treatment of the minor is unauthorized, a court order can be secured. Such a patient most likely would be better served in a local hospital and should be transported there as expeditiously as possible. The question of consent has probably faced the hospital authorities with greater frequency than the personnel of an OHS and could be handled with greater knowledge.

For the conduct of examination it is desirable that a form be signed jointly by the minor and the parent or legal guardian, in which consent is given for the conducting of all aspects of the preplacement evaluation, such as taking blood specimens, obtaining radiographs, giving immunizing injections, and the like.

Some organizations have consent for treatment granted by a parent or guardian at the time of employment of a minor so that minor emergency care may be instituted when needed in the future. Such a form to be signed, authorizing care of the minor, would carry the phrase, "while he or she is in the employ of. . . ."

GOOD SAMARITAN ACTS

It has been common experience in many companies with in-plant medical services that individuals other than employees, while on plant premises, may become ill or may sustain an injury. Usually without any question, care will be provided by OHS personnel. These persons include visitors, vendors, delivery personnel, job applicants, students, inspectors, and consultants. Are such health care staff members protected legally, if for some reason the treated individual decides to sue?

Although, in the past 20 years, Good Samaritan laws have been enacted by every state legislature, the District of Columbia, and the Virgin Islands [25], variations exist. Such laws eliminate the right of victims under common law to secure redress for their injuries; the "good samaritan" is granted either absolute or qualified immunity from suit.

When the American Occupational Medical Association (AOMA) Committee on Occupational Medicine Practice was queried on this issue, they replied that the question was complex and that an opinion should be obtained from the company counsel or an attorney should be retained to interpret the statutes or case law in the various states where there might be organizational installations. To be considered are the plant location, the presence of in-plant health care services versus a private provider, the proximity of community care, the standard of care, and the company's position regarding professional liability coverage [26].

In most instances, care was received gratefully, and there has been little negative repercussion. When the patient provides the name of an employer or a private physician, a summary narrative forwarded to one or the other, or both, would be of value and would indicate a continuing interest. The few cases on which there have been rulings have ordinarily met with decisions favorable to the provider of care.

PROFESSIONAL LIABILITY—MEDICAL MALPRACTICE

Physicians employed by industrial or commercial firms have been involved, although infrequently, in suits charging medical malpractice. While the decisions have differed, there has usually been a question of the relationship of the practitioner either to the employer or to the plaintiff who is a fellow employee.

According to Holder [27], the company physician has been held to be an "independent contractor" and not an employee. In light of this interpretation, the employer generally is not liable for the physician's negligence as long as reasonable care was used in selecting the physician. The rule follows the common law principles of agency under respondeat superior,* in which a physician's employer is held liable only when circumstances are such that the employer controls the way in which physicians treat their patients.

However, it has been held generally that when an organization provides medical care gratuitously, the doctrine of respondeat superior does not apply, and the company has no liability for the physician's malpractice. The practitioner is an independent contractor because the company has no right to control its physicians professionally or to tell them how to treat their patients. Most of the decisions concerning company-employed physicians have involved alleged negligence in the care provided, most being workers' compensation actions. Holder [27] indicates that generally the employer is found to be liable if due care was not used in the selection of the physician and the latter was demonstrably incompetent. The Federal Employer's Liability Act has been interpreted in more modern decisions to indicate that a railroad may be liable for injuries to its employees arising from the negligence of a physician, but this construction has not been accepted universally.

It might be helpful to clarify "What is malpractice?" Warshaw [28], at the height of the so-called malpractice crisis, observed as follows:

> New knowledge and technologic advances have proliferated high risk procedures with increased chances of complications and failure. People, fully aware of these advances, have demanded their application with increasingly unrealistic expectations so that when a good result is not achieved or side effects occur, it is automatically attributed to error or neglect. Yet, unquestionably, poor medical practice does exist. Avoidable errors are being made, and professional and governmental efforts to discipline medical practice have so far been largely ineffectual.

*Let the superior answer; let the principal answer for the acts of his or her agent.

Vaccarino [29] describes malpractice in this manner: For all intents and purposes, malpractice is ordinary negligence or carelessness, and by legal definition, it is an unintentional act. One cannot form the intent to commit an act of ordinary negligence. One may be intentionally careless, but such an act is outside the definition of ordinary negligence or malpractice and would be categorized as willful and reckless misconduct. If one cannot form the intent to commit an act of ordinary negligence, it is logical then that one cannot, by an act of the will, prevent ordinary negligent conduct. An act of ordinary negligence will occur with statistical surety in a random fashion in all our daily lives and can be prevented only by diligent conduct—the practice of good medicine.

Some of the suits germane to this discussion have involved preplacement medical examinations. In *Beadling* v. *Sirotta* [30], a patient undergoing radiography as part of the examination sued the radiologist, claiming that the report was erroneous. The court held that the roentgenologist had to defend the suit even though the report had been prepared for the plaintiff's prospective employer and not at the request of the plaintiff or for therapeutic purposes. The court stated that "where physical health is a factor in the determination of qualifications, the worker has the right to have the state of his health diagnosed with reasonable care and reported with reasonable accuracy and correctness." It was held that the physician-patient relationship was readily implied and did exist, with duty on the part of the radiologist "to exercise reasonable care in the examination and diagnosis he was called upon to make."

The essence of the case lies in the need for the physician to be as careful in examining a prospective employee as one is in any examination, to be as thorough as is warranted, and to report to the applicant any condition that is disclosed for which treatment or some course of action appears advisable. The fact that the examiner will not treat the patient or that the cost is covered by the prospective employer does not exempt the physician from those responsibilities. It was suggested that examiners retain, in their own files, records of the examination in a manner comparable to their retention of records in their regular practice.

A variation in views of jurists is seen in *Lotspiech* v. *Chance Vought Aircraft* [31]. An employee was examined at work, the protocol including chest radiography, and she was told by the nurses on duty that if any abnormal findings were encountered she would be informed. Three years after termination of employment she was told by Air Force physicians that her chest x-ray showed active tuberculosis, and a rereading of the old films revealed far-advanced tuberculosis, while the interpretation made at the time consisted of "negative for pulmonary pathology; cardiac shadow within normal limits." The plaintiff brought suit against the former employer and its physician for failing to inform her of the presence of the disease.

The court ruled that the relationship between the plaintiff and the physician was not the usual one and that the latter was employed only to determine whether she was qualified to do the work for which she applied. It is questionable if the situation were to be repeated today that the court would find for the defendant.

Another ruling further illuminates the variation in opinions concerning malpractice on the part of in-plant physicians. In a case brought before the Pennsylvania Superior Court [32], it was ruled that a full-time, salaried plant physician is an employee and therefore not susceptible to a malpractice suit by a fellow employee. The physician worked full-time for the company, was paid a fixed salary, was forbidden to engage in private practice, received the same fringe benefits as other supervisory employees, and had his hours and days worked controlled by the company. The argument that he was an independent contractor was rejected by the court, and the determination whether plant physicians and others in similar circumstances, exercising independent professional judgment, should be liable for their negligence must be left to the legislature, as it was concluded. In an Ohio case of 1972, *Proctor* v. *Ford Motor Co.* [33], it was ruled that a full-time, salaried physician is protected under the immunity provisions of the workers' compensation laws. Were the statute not to apply, the physicians' employment must be both casual and not in the ordinary course of business. Where the immunity rule holds, workers' compensation would be the exclusive remedy for incidents of medical negligence arising in this context [33].

Although pertinent to full-time, salaried physicians in universities, hospitals, or HMOs, Curran [34] concluded, in a review of malpractice liability and the immunity rule insofar as the Commonwealth of Virginia was concerned, that it would be best for all if the legislature of the commonwealth removed sovereign immunity and adopted a clear and equitable form of liability. Until all jurisdictions interpret their laws in parallel, there will be decisions involving both the immunity rule and the concept of the independent contractor, a state most unsettling to the occupational physician.

As a final point of interest, particularly to physicians engaged in freestanding occupational medicine clinics, is the classification of the specialty among those of highest risk, hence more costly premiums. Some underwriters place occupational medicine in class VII in a nine-point scheme, while others designate such practitioners as class VI in a seven-point gradation with "industrial" as the parenthetic modifier. These classifications do not separate out physicians practicing occupational medicine as a form of medicine.

PREVENTION OF MALPRACTICE LITIGATION

Morris [35] lays some groundwork for the use of medical liability suits in the past decade or two:

> It is a popular belief among patients today that almost all doctors are making enormous amounts of money, refuse to make house calls, play golf on Wednesdays, drive expensive cars, own yachts, hunting lodges, and apartment houses. Once thought of as "the old country doctor driving through the rain all night to sit beside a sick patient," he is now thought of as a "super-successful businessman." This, perhaps subconscious attitude on the part of the patients makes them more willing to sue their doctors and makes juries more willing to return a verdict.

Compounding this attitude are the impersonalization of medicine, poor public relations—often physician-generated—lawsuit-prone personalities, and the increased delegation of care to allied medical personnel with increased risk of wrongdoing [34]. So, in light of this negative environment, what can the physician do to avert suits claiming negligence or incompetence?

Aluise [36] has provided some guidelines useful as preventive measures against the possibility of a suit for malpractice:

Every patient should be treated in keeping with the precepts of good medical practice, which implies the degree of care, judgment, and skill exercised by physicians and other health professionals in similar circumstances.

No practitioner should render a judgment, initiate treatment, or carry out a medical procedure that exceeds his or her qualifications. Seek consultation if the issue is in doubt.

Obtain a radiographic examination whenever a patient presents a real or suspected injury to a bone or joint.

Do not use clinical judgment solely as a basis for an important diagnosis when reliable diagnostic laboratory aids are available.

Avoid overoptimistic outcomes, and do not promise or guarantee cures.

Do not, under any circumstances, criticize the care of a patient by another health professional in the presence of the patient or a family member.

Obtain a written "informed consent" for any procedure that is "nonroutine," such as a surgical operation, blood transfusion, or x-ray therapy.

Maintain complete and proper medical records that describe what was done and when it was done. Make no erasures in, or alterations to, the original entry.* Avoid entering any admission of fault or judgmental comments regarding the patient's personality or behavior, such as "malingerer," "trouble-maker," or the like.

Determine that all diagnostic and therapeutic instruments and equipment are safe to use and are in proper working order. Drugs, anesthetic agents, oxygen, and all medications must be stored safely, avoiding obsolescence, accidental mixing of chemical agents, and erroneous labeling.

Be tactful, considerate, and professional toward the patient and members of the family. Explain all procedures and the reasons for their conduct. Good rapport is mandatory.†

Other caveats that serve prophylactically include the following:

Make no perjorative or even a slightly questioning remark or careless comment regarding the care given a patient by another, to an employee, assistant, or colleague, which can be misconstrued as improper care. Likewise, caution all associates that no comparable comments are to be made.

Be sure to note in detail in the patient's record any rejection of offered treatment or recommended diagnostic test procedure or examination, be it in person during consultation, by telephone, or by letter.

*Also, give no evidence of squeezing in words around existing entries, a change in slant, pressure, or uniformity of handwriting, or the use of two or more inks or two typewriters to make one entry [37].

†Morris [38], who has defended many physician-clients in malpractice litigations, has observed, "If you will take the time and trouble to build the rapport and keep the rapport high, most patients will ride through a bad result and not sue. But if the rapport breaks down, you are in trouble. It is no small accident that we see repeater defendant doctors. . . . They are malpractice-suit–prone because they have had bad personalities with patients, and they do not build and keep the rapport high." Cousins [39] substantiates this point with the observation, "The better the relationship between physician and patient, the smaller the probability of legal action . . . the chances of lawsuits increase in direct proportion to the distance between physician and patient."

Communicate all information that is implied in "informed consent," but be absolutely certain that it is understood. One must never assume that because the message is clear to the physician that it is clear to the patient. If devices are to be worn, be sure full instructions are given in their use [40].

Note in the record that certain alternative serious conditions were considered diagnostically, and document the fact that the patient was informed about self-care and the means of recognizing any deterioration in his or her condition [41]. Document all evidence of *good* medical practice.

Note in the record all broken appointments or discontinuance of treatment before prescribed date of completion.

Do not abandon a patient. If there is ongoing treatment and the physician anticipates a period of absence from the OHS, inform the patient and arrange for continuing care by an associate.

Avoid diagnosing, prescribing, or instructing over the telephone, as it is medically and legally dangerous. If a judgment must be rendered, be certain that one makes a complete record of all the facts.

If in the physician's professional judgment certain information—in the obtaining of informed consent—is felt better to be withheld (for example, the resulting fear and apprehension would increase the operative risk), then the reasons for therapeutic nondisclosure should be recorded. It may strengthen the rationale for such action if the responsibility is shared with another physician, who should be present at the time of securing consent.

Keep up not only with the literature pertinent to occupational medicine but also with recent legislation, administrative regulations, and judicial decisions relating to standards, contested OSHA citations, workers' compensation rulings, and malpractice litigation.

In the conveying of information, all of the patient's full range of resources, emotional and physiologic, must be considered and utilized. As Norman Cousins [42] has commented, truth can be communicated with moral artistry, or it can be dumped on a patient like a truckload of bricks. He cites an example of how not to inform a patient. A specialist entered a hospital room where the patient and his family were waiting to learn of the results of exploratory surgery. The physician was "explicit to the point of brutality" when he said, "Your kidneys have crapped out; your liver has crapped out. Well, that's the way it is." Cousins pointed out that if any hope had been entertained before the specialist arrived, it was totally expunged by the time he left.

One specific recommendation, as offered by Roth [43], relates to the record of written prescriptions. He suggests that the ideal system for prescriptions is a serially numbered book with four copies per prescription: one for the dispensing pharmacist, a second for the patient's record, a third for a separate prescription file (in case of warning or medication recalls), and a fourth to be retained in the book. This method, he feels, provides insurance against a variety of legal dilemmas, including malpractice suits. The essence of the issue of avoidance of malpractice claims lies in good, continuing, caring communication with the patient that allows for timely airing of grievances, accurate and complete record-keeping, obtaining of necessary "informed consent" for all but regular, standardized non-life-threatening procedures in examination and treatment (except as infeasible during dire emergencies), prudent attitudes toward previous providers of care, understanding of the difficult or litigation-prone employee-patient with extra effort to meet his or her emotional needs, ready consultation or referral, a physically "safe" OHS, and above all, an ongoing interest, sympathy, and warmth with all patients [44].

A comment is needed regarding liability for negligence of staff assistants. As physicians rely on OHS personnel to perform certain simple diagnostic or therapeutic procedures, there may be instances of negligence when paramedical persons are engaged in such activities. The rulings have not been that clear. If the physician allows an assistant to perform functions for which the individual is not adequately trained, the physician may be held liable for any resulting injury to a patient. The same liability may hold even if the assistant is qualified and an injury is incurred either through a negligent act or a negligent omission.

In a hospital setting—and an OHS may be comparable—a physician may be held liable for the institution's employee if the latter is a "borrowed servant" or "agent" of the physician. This situation may eventuate when, for example, the physician exercises supervision or control over a specific hospital employee [45,46].

It must be stated that a physician who is sued for malpractice truly never "wins," even though the court may rule in favor of the practitioner. Patients, or the public through the print and broadcast media, remember the suit without necessarily recalling the decision. The whole procedure is costly and wasteful of time and of the energies of the physician involved, diverting effort from his or her usual responsibilities. The tasks attendant on such a suit include the gathering of records, taking of depositions, issuing and responding to interrogatories, and time spent with counsel in preparation for trial, all in addition to the actual time spent in court, both waiting and testifying. The institution of a malpractice suit represents an attack on the medical judgment and integrity of a health professional, and one cannot avoid the emotional effect of such a challenge. Pending the outcome of the case, there is loss of peace of mind, increase in anxiety and tension, and probably less effective professional practice [47]. Knowledge of such a suit in an industrial plant setting, because of networking, augurs ill for the acceptance of care from the OHS in which the defendant is a staff member.

By way of summation, Byrne [48], a general practitioner in England's National Health Service, pointed out some common legal pitfalls subject to encounter in practice, which are readily transferrable to the OHS setting:

Visit the patient; do not rely on information given over the telephone. "It should be remembered that the doctor is expected to make the diagnosis and not the patient or his relatives" [48].
Be wary of patients who cry "wolf" for years, for an acute "unpleasant condition" can arise in the individual who has had "nothing wrong" over a long time span.
Examine the patient.
Use an ophthalmoscope, but refer a patient promptly to an ophthalmologist if there is *any* question of serious disease (local or constitutional).
Order radiographs in all cases of suspected fracture.
Avoid injudicious lavage of the ear canals.
Use the clinical laboratory.
Communicate *all* details of treatment to the physician or hospital assuming follow-up care, particularly when continuity of care by a single practitioner is not possible.
Exert extreme care in the writing of prescriptions, indicating the correct medication and refill instructions.

THE RIGHT-TO-KNOW

At the time of writing, the federal government and some 30 jurisdictions [49,50] including states and some cities, have enacted right-to-know laws governing chemicals with which workers are in contact. The essence of the legislation is the requirement that employers make known to their employees the names and hazards of toxic substances in the workplace. Efforts are being made to have a weaker OSHA regulation preempt the state right-to-know laws, and presumably the issue will have to be resolved in the courts, as unions and some of the states have filed suit to challenge the federal regulation [51]. Differences are to be found in the number of substances or industries covered. For example, the New York law covers 57,000 substances in contrast to the 600 under the proposed federal regulation, and whereas the OSHA edict relates only to manufacturing, the state laws are broader, extending to agriculture, construction, and many other industries.

Involved, as Ashford and Caldart [52] express it, is the democratization of the workplace and the mandatory sharing of information between management and labor or, actually, the transfer of information. To have a right to the information, the manufacturer or employer must be required or obligated to provide the information.

The movement for the right to know has grown, in spite of administrative efforts to offer a diluted standard. Bingham [53] speculates on the reasons for the success of the demand for such laws. She believes that a growing sophistication on the part of the public regarding health, an increased awareness that "inside the factory" becomes "outside the factory" (often into homes as demonstrated by toxic waste dumpsites), and the political savvy of health and safety coalitions play a part. It remains a fact that the most effective means of achieving ultimately worker and community knowledge regarding hazardous work materials is through the efforts of many local coalitions of public health activists, labor unions, and even some business leaders toward eliminating ignorance of toxic chemicals [53].

In California, the Hazardous Substances Information and Training Act (California's SB 1874 on General Industrial Safety Order [GISO], 5194, [signed September 19, 1980, for implementation in 1982] to become Division 5, Chapter 2.5 of the California Labor Code) requires that employers make available to their workers Material Safety Data Sheets (MSDSs) or other information they have about any substances that employees may use or to which they may be exposed if these materials are listed in the NIOSH Registry of Toxic Effects of Chemical Substances (RTECS). The objective of the act, in conjunction with a companion General Industry Safety Order (GISO) 3204 developed to ensure workers access to their medical and exposure records, is to focus employer and worker attention on the prevention of job-related illness. The legislation aims at ensuring that workers have the information and training necessary to avoid exposure to toxic substances [54].

Further mandated by California's right-to-know law was the establishment of a list of hazardous substances, and all substances included in the list require MSDSs. The materials included were those that appeared in publications promulgated by several sources: International Agency for Research on Cancer (IARC), EPA, CAL/OSHA (list of airborne chemical contaminants), California Food and Agriculture Code list of restricted materials, and the California Hazard Evaluation System and Information Service (HESIS) hazard alerts [55]. The manufacturer of any substance (or a mixture containing a substance at a certain percentage appearing on the list) must prepare and provide an MSDS to anyone who purchases the material or within 15 working days to anyone who requests an MSDS. Any seller of a list substance must also provide purchasers with an MSDS.

The information to be provided is subdivided into scientific information, technologic information, and legal information. The scientific information refers to data regarding the nature and consequences of exposure to toxic materials and is divided further into ingredients information, exposure information, and effects information.

Training programs have been instituted so that workers will understand the information being conveyed to them. Samways [56], concerned with health and safety education for a large corporation, has indicated that in the selection of instructional methods and media one must bring the learner as close as possible to learning and practicing the behavior that is to be the end product. A lecturer, she believes, is probably least effective in teaching employees how to handle hazardous chemicals safely. A lecture with slides would be better, while a videotape demonstration would be even better still; a combination of some didactic instruction, a demonstration, practice, and the provision of supporting job aids and pictorial reminders would be the best method of all. Simulated situations should be included.

Santodonato [57] has designed a program to meet the requirements of a right-to-know law. He developed an outline for a typical program, as follows:

Substance identification
  Formula
  Synonyms and trade names
  Chemical abstracts service (CAS) and NIOSH registry numbers (RTECS)
Chemical and physical properties
Permissible exposure limits
  OSHA
  American Conference of Governmental Industrial Hygienists
  NIOSH
Use of the chemical
Major manufacturers and distributors of the chemical
Health hazard information
  Routes of absorption
  Effects in experimental animals
    Short-term exposures
    Long-term exposures
    Effects in humans
    Signs and symptoms of exposure
    Effects of short-term exposures
    Effects of long-term exposures
  Health effects of special concern
Inflammability and reactivity
Emergency and first aid procedures
Special protection information
Spill or break procedures
Sources of additional information

Further, a program evaluation checklist has been provided by Santodonato [57] that lists the program elements most needed for success and compliance with local legislation:

The right-to-know program must have top managerial support.

There should be documentation (possibly as part of the health education section of an OHS manual) descriptive of the program, the methods of conduct, and the aspects exceeding minimum criteria.

A directive should be issued establishing the right-to-know program with sufficient funds and staff support (technical specialists and administrative and support personnel).

A system should be developed for informing managers of program activities.

Responsibility and authority for the program should be given an appropriate (technically and attitudinally) person.

Records must be maintained indicating activities completed, preferably using forms adaptable to computerization.

The program must be integrated into the total occupational health and safety program.

That the program can be part of the general effort in health education seems logical.

Compliance with a right-to-know law cannot be considered apart from regulations allowing access to medical and exposure records.

If the state OSHA authority has published materials descriptive of a worker's rights to a healthful and safe workplace, such as the publication promulgated by CAL/OSHA—*How to Protect Your Health and Safety on the Job, a Worker's Guide,** they should be made available through the company's occupational health or safety activity.

*A brochure of 48 pages, published by CAL/OSHA Communications, San Francisco, October 1983.

DUTY TO WARN THIRD PARTIES

Most OHSs will provide counseling services. In some situations these program elements will be offered through a company's employee assistance program. There will be occasions when material emerging from a counselor-client relationship indicates serious danger of violence to a third party. Should the intended victim be warned, thus fracturing the "complete candor and trust [that] are considered essential elements of the therapist-patient relationship" [58]?

The case that posed the dilemma to the medical community, particularly mental health specialists, was *Tarasoff* v. *Regents of the University of California* [58]. A student in therapy on an outpatient basis with the student health service told his therapist that he wanted to kill a girl living in Berkeley. The psychologist requested the campus police to detain him, which they did, but they released him when he appeared rational. The student discontinued therapy and 2 months later killed the young woman, neither she nor her family having had any warning. The parents sued the university regents, the campus police, and the therapist employed by the university for failure either to warn the young lady or to have the patient confined. On appeal, the Supreme Court of California reversed the lower court's action—dismissal of the parents' complaint—ruling that a therapist who determines or should have determined that a client presents a danger to a third party has a duty to warn that party. A second case cited concerned not murder but the suicide of a client, involving the principle of potential self-inflicted harm.

The court in *Tarasoff* v. *Regents of the University of California* held that the therapist, when learning that a client presents the possibility of serious violence to another, is obliged to use reasonable care in protecting the intended victim. The responsibility could be discharged, the court maintained, in one or more of the following ways: (1) warn the victim or others who could apprise the victim of the danger, (2) notify the police, or (3) take whatever other steps were reasonably necessary.

The case, as Curran [58] observed, had already become infamous among mental health programs in California and among college student health programs throughout the country as it progressed through the various levels of the state's trial and appeals courts. The parents had brought suit for damages against the university, the therapists (the psychologist, another therapist, and the assistant director of the department), and campus police, as university employees and as individuals. In suing the director of psychiatry, the plaintiffs sought not only general money damages for negligence in his failing to warn the girl and her parents and to detain the student, but exemplary or punitive damages—assessable in huge amounts as multiples of the general damages or in any amount as determined by the jury—for "malicious and oppressive abandonment of a dangerous patient."

The Supreme Court in its reversal of the lower court's decision held for general damages against all the therapists and the two directors of psychiatry and against the university as their employer for "breach of the duty to warn Miss Tarasoff." The claim for exemplary damages was dismissed, action against the police was dismissed by virtue of their statutory immunity, as was the suit against the therapists for failure to confine the patient under a commitment order, also because of statutory immunity. However, the Supreme Court implied that had there not been the immunity, the actions would have had merit.

The decision met with considerable criticism, and Cooper [58] has pointed out that definitive guidelines on balancing the confidentiality of the therapist-client relationship with the failure to take action to prevent a patient's potentially harmful acts and thus incurring liability to a third party have not been established. Further, Cooper admits that simple and authoritative methods of resolution have not been formulated. However, she offers these suggestions: First, the therapist should evaluate the client's previous behavior. Were previous threats carried through, or was any action taken to further the threatened activity? Secondly, how would the patient respond to the therapist's direct and knowing effort to impose controls? The therapist should be able to show that one acted on a reasonable belief that the behavior warranted the warning of the third party. Finally, the therapist should endeavor to limit such disclosures to those reasonably necessary to avert potential danger. To avoid a total negative impact on the therapist-client relationship, the specialist should "discuss frankly with the patient the therapist's duty and position on this aspect of their relationship" [58].

This case and its discussion have been reviewed at length because an OHS is not unlike a student health service, and even though a long period of therapy is not undertaken at the worksite, the same kind of behavioral information can emerge in the short-duration contacts a therapist may have at a plant. Murder and suicide have occurred *on* plant premises in addition to actions of employees in the community, so that the problem is real and the same kind of dilemma will present itself. At best, in keeping with the suggestion of Cooper, the therapist should confront the client with the former's societal responsibilities and take informed action in keeping with his or her view of the seriousness of the threatened behavior. Also, such discussion should be documented.

One point not mentioned heretofore that was highly inconsistent with the appropriate maintenance of records was the fact that in *Tarasoff* the director of psychiatry asked for the return of the psychologist's letter to the police and required that all copies of the letter be destroyed. Such behavior, apart from compliance with court orders directing that action, is unconscionable and may lead to serious legal or judicial inquiry.

The issue of disclosure was summarized in an opinion of the American Medical Association's (AMA) Judicial Council [59]. After confirming the confidentiality of the physician-patient relationship, the exception was stated as follows:

> The obligation to safeguard patient confidences is subject to certain exceptions that are ethically and legally justified because of overriding social considerations. Where a patient threatens to inflict serious bodily harm to another person and there is a reasonable probability that the patient may carry out the threat, the physician should take reasonable precautions for the protection of the intended victim, including notification of law enforcement authorities. Also, communicable diseases and gunshot and knife wounds should be reported as required by applicable statutes or ordinances.

EMPLOYMENT EQUALITY OF THE PREGNANT WORKER

In light of the increasing number of women in the labor force, attention has been focused on the pregnant worker and her employment status. Legal protection for pregnant workers and new mothers arose at the federal level with the passage of the Pregnancy Discrimination Act in 1978. The legislation amended the section of the 1964 Civil Rights Act that prohibited discrimination on the basis of sex, so that the definition of sex includes "pregnancy, childbirth, or related medical conditions" [60]. In essence, women in these categories are to be treated identically to other employees in regard to their disability benefits.

Some persons find equating motherhood with disability or illness to be offensive. Health professionals in a company will be asked regarding the ability of a pregnant woman to perform a certain job or certain tasks. Rarely can an employer force a pregnant worker to go on leave if she can still perform in her job. As other employees on disability leave can return to their jobs, so can the new mother. The pregnant employee is entitled to all the pertinent fringe benefits such as disability, sick leave, and health insurance coverage [60]. Health insurance must cover pregnancy-related conditions, inclusive of abortions. However, the employer is not so obligated unless the life of the mother is endangered by carrying the fetus to term or complications have arisen because of the abortion.

If the woman is unable temporarily to carry out her assigned job, she is to be treated as are other temporarily disabled workers. She may have her job modified or her assignment changed, or she may be granted disability leave or leave without pay. If she is assigned to another job because of potential hazard or inability to perform in her regular position, the employer can reduce her pay to that of the new job.

While companies previously had established certain time limits for the postpartum return to work, now the return is based exclusively on the new mother's ability to return to the job. The job must be held open pending return unless the employer is notified that the worker does not intend to return. Seniority is unaffected by the pregnancy, as is credit for vacations or a pay raise. Pregnancy cannot preclude hire if the applicant can perform the major functions required in the job. Also, the applicant cannot be rejected because of any preference, real or imagined, on the part of coworkers, customers, or suppliers [60]. If an employer grants travel or education leaves, so shall a request for child care be granted.

The issue of pregnancy is important to a physician in industry, for counsel will be sought regarding a pregnant woman's ability to carry out certain tasks or to work in certain environments that may be hazardous to her or her unborn child.

MISCELLANEOUS LEGAL CONSIDERATIONS

MOUNTED ELECTROCARDIOGRAMS

The question of the legality of electrocardiograms that are mounted prior to interpretation has been raised. It is advised that a sounder principle would be to have the cardiologist evaluate the full tracing and mark the sections that should be mounted and retained in the patient's record [61].

CLINICAL PHOTOGRAPHY

If a physician takes a photograph of a patient for the clinical record or for use in teaching, and the patient observes the physician taking the photograph and fails to object, consent is implied. Patients who do not wish to be photographed, in whole or in part, have an obligation to object. However, if a photograph is to be published, even though the patient may not be identified, consent of the patient must be obtained. It would be more prudent to obtain a signed consent irrespective of any possible publication [62].

REFILLING OF PRESCRIPTIONS

The Federal Food, Drug and Cosmetic Act provides that prescription drugs

> . . . shall be dispensed only (i) upon a written prescription of a practitioner licensed by law to administer such drug, or (ii) upon an oral prescription of such practitioner which is reduced promptly to writing and filed by the pharmacist, or (iii) by refilling any such written or oral prescription if such refilling is authorized by the prescriber in the original prescription or by oral order which is reduced promptly to writing and filed by the pharmacist. The act of dispensing a drug contrary to the provisions of this paragraph shall be deemed to be an act which results in the drug being misbranded while held for sale (21 USC 353).

The AMA has indicated in a policy position that the prescribing physician should designate the number of refills the patient is to have. Also recommended is the nonrefilling of any prescription that fails to indicate the number of refills or that is labeled "p.r.n." or "ad lib." The 1970 Controlled Substance Act, in addition to classifying drugs according to their potential for abuse and dependence,* includes restrictions on the timing and number of refills:

Prescriptions for drugs in schedule II—cannot be refilled.

Prescriptions for drugs in schedules III and IV—cannot be filled or refilled more than 6 months after the date of issue of the prescription and authorizations for refill are limited to five.

Prescriptions for drugs in schedule V—may be refilled only as expressly authorized by the prescriber on the prescription. Without authorization, the prescription cannot be refilled.

The controlled substances acts of the various states contain similar, if not more restrictive, provisions governing refills [63].

MARATHON PARTICIPATION

With the increased interest in physical fitness, organizations may sponsor or include as an activity in family day programs 5- or 10-kilometer runs. It might be necessary to have the runner sign an assumption of risk statement. An example of such a document is the following:

> In consideration of the acceptance of my entry, I, for myself, my executors, administrators, and assignees, do hereby release and discharge the XYZ Company and any individual associated with the organization, for all claims of damages, demands, actions whatsoever in any manner arising or growing out of my participation in said athletic event. I attest and verify that I have full knowledge of the risks involved in this event and I am physically fit and sufficiently trained to participate in this event.
>
> ____
>
> Runner's Signature Guardian
> (if participant is under 18)

SPECIAL ASBESTOS WORKERS' COMPENSATION PROGRAMS

To provide workers who have sustained asbestos-related disease with workers' compensation temporary disability and medical benefits promptly without their having to have liability determined through lengthy litigation delays, California established an Asbestos Workers' Account in late 1980. Other states may resort in the future to similar enactments. As physicians in an OHS may be participating medically in establishing a worker's entitlement to benefits, familiarity with one jurisdiction's requirements might be helpful.

Payments from the Asbestos Workers' Account as advances on workers' compensation temporary disability and medical benefits will be furnished a worker for injury resulting in asbestosis if the following conditions occur [64]:

The asbestos worker demonstrates to the account that, at the time of exposure, the worker was per-

*The schedules of controlled drugs follows: *Schedule I substances:* drugs without medical use in the United States and have a high potential for abuse, e.g., heroin, LSD, peyote, etc. *Schedule II substances:* drugs with a high abuse potential with severe psychic or physical dependence liability, including certain narcotic, stimulant, and depressant drugs, e.g., opium, morphine, codeine, phenmetrazine (Preludin), secobarbital, etc. Prescriptions are to be written on official triplicate forms. *Schedule III substances:* drugs with less abuse potential than substances classified I and II and include compounds containing limited quantities of certain narcotic drugs in combination with non-narcotic substances, e.g., glutethimide (Doriden), Paregoric, Tylenol with Codeine, etc. *Schedule IV substances:* drugs with an abuse potential less than substances listed as III, e.g., chloral betaine (Beta Chlor), meprobamate (Equanil), chlordiazepoxide (Librium), flurazepam (Dalmane), etc. *Schedule V substances:* drugs with an abuse potential less than substances listed as IV, but still sufficient to warrant control, such as medications generally used as antitussives or antidiarrheal preparations.

forming services and was acting within the scope of prescribed duties in an occupation that subjected the worker to asbestos exposure.

The asbestos worker demonstrates to the account that he or she is suffering from asbestosis.

The asbestos worker is entitled to compensation for asbestosis as otherwise provided for in this division.

The findings of the account shall not be evidence in any other proceeding.

The account shall require the asbestos worker to submit to an independent medical examination.

As the litigation of the thousands of cases pending will continue for years, the account will aid those claimants who present definitive evidence of asbestos-related disease.

INTENTIONAL TORTS AND CRIMINAL ACTIVITY

The increase in litigious action may readily involve occupational health personnel. A case involved a transsexual pilot whose employment had been terminated when the individual underwent a sex change operation *(Ulane* v. *Eastern Airlines).* The earlier decision dealt with the question of employment discrimination because she was a woman [65]. Other cases, however, remain in which it is alleged that certain of the defendants committed intentional torts, actions of a person causing injury to another. The significance to occupational health is that the actions are directed personally against the top-level managers of the company, including the medical director of the organization. Also to be noted is the fact that company liability insurance and personal malpractice or errors and omissions insurance will not provide coverage. In essence, as Goerth [65] points out, persons sued for an intentional tort may have to provide their own legal defense as well as pay any damages awarded by a judge or jury.

In the case cited, the intentional torts claimed to have been committed included defamation of character, intentional infliction of emotional distress, and interference with the expectancy of employment. By naming company individuals as defendants, pressure is put on the company to settle because of the added costs of providing legal defense for its employees. These costs can be high for the employer, for its liability insurance carrier may refuse to provide a defense when the allegation involves intentional torts. Pressure is put on the individuals to encourage early settlement, particularly if they suspect that the employer may be unwilling to cover the costs of defense and awarded damages.

The *Ulane* v. *Eastern Airlines* case exemplifies strikingly, Goerth indicates, the vulnerability of employers and key managers, including occupational health professionals in employment decisions. It gives further emphasis to the need for hiring strictly on the basis of the ability to carry out the tasks of the job in keeping with the physical requirements of the position.

A more serious development has been the filing of criminal charges against a company and five of its executives when a worker at the small Film Recovery Systems, Inc., specializing in the recovery of silver from used film, died of acute cyanide poisoning. After investigation, the state of illinois charged the corporation with manslaughter, and the five executives were charged with murder and, if convicted, could receive prison terms up to 40 years [66].

The workers were neither warned of the hazards involved in the process nor protected against them. The employees spoke almost no English, and the skull and crossbones warning symbols had been scraped off the drums of cyanide material.

In a second case undergoing investigation wherein a worker died of silicosis, also a situation without warning of the hazard or provision of protective devices or controls, the company officials are held as criminally responsible. The cases point to a developing trend toward criminal prosecution for deaths stemming from worksite or public safety and health violations. No longer are corporations or their officials immune from such charges. Philip Scaletta, a Purdue business law professor, cited by Liancianese [66], indicates that corporation prosecutions will become more frequent in the future because of society's increasing distrust of business and the determination to make corporations more responsible for their actions.

If these actions continue, they may bring about the long-delayed use of consultative assistance from occupational health professionals in all areas of environmental evaluation, clinical surveillance, hazard communication, personal protection of workers, and engineering control of life-threatening substances or operations.

Almost in the same vein of societal concern is the comment made by Curran [67] in his review of the 1979 passage of the Massachusetts Patient's Bill of Rights: ". . . The time has come to change hospitals from remote citadels ruled by kings and knights in white armor to more commonplace community facilities where the language is understandable to patients and families and their concerns prevail over unnecessary and repressive technical or managerial interests."

REFERENCES

1. Hammond, J. W. Guidelines for a chemical plant in preparation for an OSHA inspection. *Med Bull* [Exxon] 34:252, 1974.
2. News Release USDL 74-85. Washington, DC: Office of Information, U.S. Department of Labor, Feb 25, 1974.
3. *The Toxic Substances Control Act: Protecting People and the Environment from Dangerous Chemicals.* Washington, DC: Office of Toxic Substances, U.S. Environmental Protection Agency, 1980. P. 10.
4. *Compilation of Laws Administered by the Consumer Product Safety Commission.* Washington, DC: The Commission, 1982. P. 25.
5. Notice of legal protection for employee rights. . . . *Am Ind Hyg Assoc J* 40:A-28, 1979.
6. Simonaitis, J. E. *Cases on Informed Consent.* Chicago: American Medical Association, 1974.
7. Miller, L. J. Informed consent: I. *JAMA* 244:2100, 1980: II. *JAMA* 244:2347, 1980.
8. *Sard* v. *Hardy,* 397A 2d 1014, 1020 (Md 1977). As cited in L. J. Miller, Informed consent. *JAMA* 244:2100, 1980.
9. Simonaitis, J. E. *Law of Informed Consent.* Chicago: American Medical Association, 1974.
10. *Cobbs* v. *Grant,* 502P 2d at 11. As cited in L. J. Miller, Informed consent. *JAMA* 244:2100, 1980.
11. Healey, J. M. Informed consent: Disclosing the risks of refusing treatment. *Conn Med* 44:673, 1980.
12. Baker, M. T., and Taub, H. A. Readability of informed consent forms for research in a Veterans Administration medical center. *JAMA* 250:2646, 1983.
13. Robinson, G., and Merav, A. Informed consent: Recall by patients tested postoperatively. *Ann Thorac Surg* 22:209, 1976.
14. Laforet, E. G. The fiction of informed consent. *JAMA* 235:1579, 1976.
15. *Guidebook to Laws Governing the Practice of Medicine by Physicians and Surgeons* (3rd ed.). Sacramento, CA: State of California Department of Consumer Affairs, Board of Medical Quality Assurance, 1981. 8.2B Informed Consent. P. 54.
16. Goerth, C. L. R. Questions of consent. *Occup Health Saf* 51:39, Apr 1982.
17. Ziskind, D., Jr. Refusal of treatment: Legal effects under the Workmen's Compensation Act of California. *J Occup Med* 4:314, 1962.
18. Elliott, J. More support for refusing medical treatment. *JAMA* 243:506, 1980.
19. Isele, W. P. Medical treatment of a mentally impaired person or a minor: Who may consent? *JAMA* 245:778, 1981.
20. Fiscina, S. F. *Medical Law for the Attending Physician: A Case-Oriented Analysis.* Carbondale, IL: Southern Illinois University Press, 1982. P. 155.
21. Gaylin, W. Cited in M. M. Freed, Quality of life. The physician's dilemma. *Arch Phys Med Rehabil* 65:109, 1984.
22. *Gulf & Ship Island Railroad Co.* v. *Sullivan,* 155 Miss. 1, 119 So. 501 [1928]. Cited in A. J. Rosoff, *Informed Consent.* Rockville, MD: Aspen, 1981. P. 189.
23. *Tabor* v. *Scobee,* 254 S.W. 2d 477 (Ky. 1951). Cited in A. J. Rosoff, *Informed Consent.* Rockville, MD: Aspen, 1981. P. 187.
24. Rosoff, A. J. *Informed Consent.* Rockville, MD: Aspen, 1981. Pp. 187, 207.
25. Sullivan, B. Some thoughts on the constitutionality of Good Samaritan statutes. *Am J Law Med* 8:27, 1982.
26. Clinical occupational health inquiry [Good Samaritan Laws]. *J Occup Med* 23:82, 1981.
27. Holder, A. R. Law and medicine: Liability of company for ship's surgeon. *JAMA* 215:1381, 1971.
28. Warshaw, L. J. The malpractice problem and the occupational physician. *J Occup Med* 19:593, 1977.
29. Vaccarino, J. M. Malpractice: The problem in perspective. *JAMA* 238:861, 1977.
30. *Beadling* v. *Sirotta,* 71 N.J. Super. 182, 176A. 2d 546 (1961), 39 N.J. 34, 186A. 2d 680 (1962). Cited in L. J. Warshaw and J. V. Thornton, Malpractice liability in pre-placement examination. *J Occup Med* 7:353, 1964, and Five malpractice pitfalls in routine physicals. *Hosp Phys* 5:137, 1969.
31. *Lotspiech* v. *Chance Vought Aircraft,* 369 S.W. 2d 705, Texas, 1963. Cited in I. R. Brand, Malpractice. *Mod Med* 34:232, May 9, 1966, and A. R. Holder. Creation of the physician-patient relationship: Part I *JAMA* 230:278, 1974.
32. *Babich, et al.* v. *Pavich, M.D. et al.,* No. 1459, Apr. I, 1978 (Pa. Super., filed Sept. 28, 1979), *appeal denied* Jan. 29, 1980, and *Babich, et al.* v. *Pavich, M.D., et al.,* No. 1459, Apr. 1, 1978, slip op. at 6 (Pa. Super. Sept. 26, 1979). Cited in F. Speaker, Court rules company doctor immune from malpractice. *Pa Med* 83:16, Dec 1980.
33. *Proctor* v. *Ford Motor Co.,* 302 NE 2d 580 (1972). Cited in J. D. Blum, Growing Legal Liability in Corporate Health Clinics. In R. H. Egdahl (Ed.), *Background Papers on Industry's Changing Role in Health Care Delivery.* New York: Springer-Verlag, 1977. P. 168.
34. Curran, W. J. Malpractice liability and immunity of full-time salaried physicians. *N Engl J Med* 303:1406, 1980.
35. Morris, R. C. The rise of medical-liability suits. *JAMA* 215:843, 1971.
36. Aluise, J. J. *The Physician as Manager.* Bowie, MD: Charles Press, 1980. Pp. 168–169.
37. Roth, R. Avoiding malpractice: Tips for young doctors. *Mod Med* 40:46, Jan 24, 1972.
38. Morris, R. C. Cited in Why 127 patients said . . . "I'm going to sue you!" *Resident Staff Phys.* 16:41, Nov 1970.
39. Cousins, N. A piece of my mind: Unacceptable pressures on the physician. *JAMA* 252:351, 1984.
40. *Crosby* v. *Grandview Nursing Home,* 290A 2d 375,

Maine, 1972. Cited in AMA Office of the General Counsel, Leading cases. *JAMA* 232:654, 1975.

41. "Malpractice is social, medical problem, not legal one." *Intern Med News* 13:6, Feb 18, 1980.
42. Cousins, N. Malpractice backlash. *Saturday Rev* 7:18, May 1980.
43. Roth, R. In review of D. J. Flaster. Malpractice: A guide to the legal rights of patients and doctors. *N Engl J Med* 309:1591, 1983.
44. Bergen, R. P. How to avoid malpractice claims. *JAMA* 211:2233, 1970.
45. Hoppe, W. G. Physicians' liability for negligence of office assistants and hospital employees. *JAMA* 238:1485, 1977.
46. Ladimer, I. Liability of the "extended" doctor. *Mod Med* 37:226, March 24, 1969.
47. Bernzweig, E. P. *Legal Aspects of PHS Medical Care.* Washington, DC: Bureau of Medical Services, Public Health Service, U.S. Department of Health, Education, and Welfare, 1966. Part C, Principles of Malpractice Prevention, Sec. 1, General. Pp. 35–36.
48. Byrne, J. G. Some common legal pitfalls in general practice. *Practitioner* 210:813, 1973.
49. Hazard Communication; Final Rule. 29 CFR Part 1910, Nov 25, 1983.
50. McElveen, J. C., Jr. Despite pre-emption threat, local right to know laws increase. *Occup Health Saf* 54:20, Jan 1985.
51. Three states join in suing OSHA on hazard regulation. *Occup Health Saf Letter* 14:1 Jan 8, 1984.
52. Ashford, N. A., and Caldart, C. C. Framework provides path through right-to-know law. *Occup Health Saf* 52:11, Oct 1983.
53. Bingham, E. The "right-to-know" movement. *Am J Public Health* 73:1302, 1983.
54. CAL/OSHA Fact Sheet. *Workers' Right to Know: Hazardous Substances Information and Training Act.* Sacramento, CA: CAL/OSHA, Apr 22, 1981.
55. *The Director's List of Hazardous Substances.* San Francisco: CAL/OSHA Communications Unit, Aug 1985.
56. Samways, M. C. Informing those with a need to know. *J Occup Med* 24:387, 1982.
57. Santodonato, J. Design and implementation of a workers' right-to-know program. *Am Ind Hyg Assoc J* 42:666, 1981.
58. *Tarasoff* v. *Regents of the University of California,* 551 P 2d 334 (Cal 1976). Cited in A. E. Cooper, Duty to warn third parties. *JAMA* 248:431, 1982, and discussed in W. J. Curran, Confidentiality and the prediction of seriousness. *N Engl J Med* 293:285, 1975.
59. Recent Opinions of the Judicial Council of the American Medical Association. Confidentiality: Physician-patient relationships. *JAMA* 251:2078, 1984.
60. Goerth, C. R. Pregnant workers have discrimination protection. *Occup Health Saf* 52:22, Oct 1983.
61. Smith, W. B. Questionable legality of ECG mounted prior to interpretation. *JAMA* 213:2088, 1970.
62. Simonaitis, J. E. Photographs of patients. In Medicolegal Rounds, Questions and Answers. *JAMA* 229:844, 1974.
63. Anderson, B. J. Prescription refill without authorization by physician. *JAMA* 231:1394, 1975.
64. Statutes [of the State of California] of 1980. Chap. 1041, sec. 1—added to the Labor Code, Part 1, Division 4, Chap. 11, Art. 1, Sec. 4406(a)(1) to (4).
65. Goerth, C. R. Top Eastern executives face intentional tort claims of Ulane. *Occup Health Saf* 53:23, June 1984.
66. Lancianese, F. Criminal charges loom over workplace fatalities. *Occup Haz* 46:43, Dec 1984.
67. Curran, W. J. Massachusetts Patients' Bill of Rights: Cabbages, kings, sausages and laws. *N Engl J Med* 301:1433, 1979.

APPENDIX 14-1
FEDERAL LEGISLATION INVOLVING HAZARDOUS MATERIALS

Date	*Acronym*	*Act*
1899	RHA	River and Harbor Act
1906*	FDCA	Federal Food, Drug and Cosmetic Act
1947*	FIFRA	Federal Insecticide, Fungicide and Rodenticide Act
1952	DCA	Dangerous Cargo Act
1952*	FWPCA	Federal Water Pollution Control Act
1953*	FFA	Flammable Fabrics Act†
1954	AEA	Atomic Energy Act
1956*	FWA	Fish and Wildlife Act
1960*	FHSA	Federal Hazardous Substances Labelling Act‡
1965*	SWDA	Solid Waste Disposal Act
1966	MNMSA	Metal and Non-Metallic Mine Safety Act
1969	NEPA	National Environmental Policy Act
1970*	CAA	Clean Air Act
1970	PPPA	Poison Prevention Packaging Act†
1970	WQI	Water Quality Improvement of 1970
1970	RSA	Federal Railroad Safety Act of 1970
1970	RRA	Resource Recovery Act of 1970
1970	OSHA	Occupational Safety and Health Act
1972	nCA	Noise Control Act of 1972
1972	FEPCA	Federal Environmental Pollution Control Act
1972	HMTA	Hazardous Materials Transportation Act
1972	CPSA	Consumer Product Safety Act
1972	MPRSA	Marine Protection, Research and Sanctuary Act
1972*	CWA	Clean Water Act
1972*	CZMA	Coastal Zone Management Act
1973	ESA	Endangered Species Act of 1973
1974*	SDWA	Safe Drinking Water Act
1974	TSA	Transportation Safety Act of 1974
1974*	ESECA	Energy Supply and Environmental Coordination Act
1976	TSCA	Toxic Substances Control Act
1976*	RCRA	Resource Conservation and Recovery Act
1977	FMSHA	Federal Mine Safety and Health Act
1977	SMCRA	Surface Mine Control and Reclamation Act
1978	UMTCA	Uranium Mill Tailings Control Act
1978	PTSA	Port and Tanker Safety Act
1980	CERCLA (Superfund)	Comprehensive Environmental Response, Compensation, and Liability Act of 1980

*Revised/Amended
†The responsibility for implementing these acts, in addition to the Refrigeration Safety Act of 1956, was transferred to the Consumer Product Safety Commission.
‡Later amended to Federal Hazardous Substances Act.
SOURCE: Paustenbach, D. J. The need to educate engineers in occupational safety and health: A proposal for schools of engineering. *Professional Saf* 29:15, Dec 1984.

549408

15. HEALTH CONSERVATION

The object of this paper is to excite the public attention to the subject. Myself and my pupils have personally and carefully inspected the state of the artisans in most kinds of manufacture, examined the agencies believed to be injurious, conversed on the subjects with masters, overlookers, and the more intelligent workmen, and obtained many tables illustrating the characters of the disorders prevalent in the several kinds of employ. It will be remembered that the subject is new.

Charles Turner Thackrah

Out of this nettle, danger, we pluck this flower, safety.

William Shakespeare
King Henry IV, *Part I*

I have done the deed, Didst
thou not hear a noise? . . .
Whence is that knocking?
How is't with me, when every noise
appals me?

William Shakespeare
Macbeth

Blessed are the eyes which see the things that ye see.
Luke 10:23

. . . I have met a number of industrial doctors who were devoted to the interests of their employers to the point of indifference to the welfare of the workers, but I have met only one industrial nurse of whom that could be said.

Alice Hamilton, M.D.

INDUSTRIAL HYGIENE

Although Thackrah's observation was written over a century and a half ago, the points of communication and newness were made. Industrial hygiene (IH) was given birth only as late as the decade preceding World War II. The growth of the chemical industry and the passage of the Occupational Safety and Health Act of 1970 gave great stimulus to the development of the specialty, and by the 1980s, the number of industrial hygienists had increased more rapidly than had those members of the other occupational health professions.

While no attempt will be made to offer any discourse on the technology of IH, certain elements will be reviewed that touch on the relationship of the occupational health physician to the hygienist and that, if followed, will allow the total effort of worker protection to succeed.

ROLE OF INDUSTRIAL HYGIENE

Before reviewing interprofessional relationships or the specificity of certain skills not readily subsumed under the usual concept of IH, a brief summary of the specialty should be presented.

DEFINITIONS

The American Industrial Hygiene Association (AIHA) in its statement "Definition, Scope, Function, and Organization" [1] offered the following definition:

> Industrial Hygiene is that science and art devoted to the recognition, evaluation and control of those environmental factors or stresses, arising in or from the work place, which may cause sickness, impaired health and well being, or significant discomfort and inefficiency among workers or among the citizens of the community.

Important in that clarification is the inclusion of the community residents, for it emphasizes the fact that IH is not exclusively limited to the confines or the premises of the industrial operation, for effluents or waste may affect nonemployees living in the vicinity of the plant.

A second definition [1]:

> An Industrial Hygienist is a person having a college or university degree or degrees in engineering, chemistry, physics, or medicine or related biological sciences who, by virtue of special studies and training, has acquired

competence in Industrial Hygiene. Such special studies and training must have been sufficient in all of the above cognate sciences to provide the abilities: (1) to recognize the environmental factors and stresses associated with work and work operations and to understand their effect on man and his well being; (2) to evaluate, on the basis of experience and with the aid of quantitative measurement techniques, the magnitude of these stresses in terms of ability to impair man's health and well being; and (3) to prescribe methods to eliminate, control or reduce such stresses when necessary to alleviate their effects.

ACTIVITIES

Following recognition and evaluation of an adverse environmental factor or stressor, corrective measures are carried out that may include one or more of the following [1]:

Prescription of corrective procedures, when necessary to protect health, is based on past experience, knowledge and the quantitative data available. Among control measures most frequently used are: (1) isolation of a process or work operation to reduce the number of persons exposed; (2) substitution of a less harmful material for one which is more dangerous to health; (3) alteration of a process to minimize human contact; (4) ventilation and air cleaning to provide an atmosphere safe for human occupancy; (5) reduction of exposure to radiant energy by shielding, increasing distance and limiting time; (6) wet methods to reduce emission of dust to the atmosphere such as in mining and quarrying; (7) good housekeeping, including cleanliness of the work place, proper waste disposal, adequate washing, toilet and restroom facilities, healthful drinking water and eating facilities, and control of insects and rodents; (8) personal protective devices, such as special clothing and eye and respiratory protective equipment.

The terms worker, workplace and community, as used in this discussion, are hereby defined: A worker is a person engaged in any occupation or vocation. A workplace is any building, structure, excavation, site, device or area in which work is done. A community is the environs of one or more workplaces.

Hendricks has summarized in two writings [2,3] the broader functions of a hygienist:

- Program activities for the occupational health service (OHS):
  - Advises medical staff on IH matters.
  - Develops liaison with other company departments on items of IH concern.
  - Coordinates IH with long-range plans for other company operations.
  - Compiles and reviews information on environmental health matters and reports to the medical director and managers.
- Program activities for the plant or other operations:
  - Serves as IH advisor.
  - Conducts IH studies:
    - Plant surveys and studies.
    - Atmospheric sampling.
    - Analytic determinations.
    - Physical measurements.
    - Analysis of biologic samples.
    - Statistical studies.
    - Development and application of toxicologic data.
    - Correlation of environmental and medical data (through use of computerized systems).
  - Provides technical information and consultation on environmental health problems.
  - Works with engineering and other groups in developing control methods and installations.
  - Cooperates with safety and sales departments.
- Other program activities:
  - Participates in the activities of technical and professional organizations.
  - Maintains university connections.
  - Attends scientific meetings.
  - Maintains liaison with governmental agencies and other agencies concerned with environmental health and related matters.

Hendricks [3] observes that all other factors being equal, the success of an IH program will depend to a great extent on good relationships and communication; the program should

- Have free access to managerial personnel in various company areas.
- Be able to enlist the support of various technical and operating groups.
- Be informed and aware of long-range technical plans of the company.
- Establish good working relationships with governmental regulatory groups.

POSITION OF INDUSTRIAL OR OCCUPATIONAL HYGIENE

The placement of IH in the organization scheme has varied. It has been the responsibility of the OHS; it has been a freestanding activity, with or without the presence of a medical program; and, rarely, it has had a position of primacy, frequently under the rubric of Environmental Management or a comparable designation. When the press of the Occupational Safety and Health Administration (OSHA) legislation first impacted on industry, many industrial hygienists were employed, and training programs were developed to meet the new need. The mandated demands placed on IH considerable responsibility in effecting programs that would bring the companies into compliance with the multitudinous standards that early were promulgated. With some deregulation, however, certain employers felt that the intensity of the initial IH effort could be lessened, and a number of occupational health specialists were released.

Recognized, however, are the facts that IH was an American creation and that the goals of the occupational environmentalist must be the goals of the company, for the health (or ill health) of the worker has finally been spotlighted by the attention of both the public and some elected officials.

The position of IH in a company pattern will vary, as indicated, in keeping with numerous variables, including location, type of industrial operation, the pertinence of certain promulgated standards, the leadership, knowledge, or strength of the medical director, the strength and experience of the hygiene leadership, and the views of the corporate executive body.

In most instances, IH has been an element or division of the OHS, and this placement is ideal if the communication and relationship between the physicians and nurses and the hygienists are good, productive, ongoing, supportive, and collaborative. If there is no working rapport between medicine and IH, then positioning in the OHS will not foster a better IH program. Also, if the physician is totally unknowing as to the role and capabilities of IH, then a joint association will not be assistive to the hygienist.

But today's training programs in occupational health are providing physicians with nearly the same curricular content that is given students in IH, so that they can speak a common language and work cooperatively toward mutually understood objectives. Further, the sharing of the total curriculum gives hygienists a clinical background so that they will be able to function comfortably with physicians and nurses and will not be limited to the chemistry, physics, and engineering mainstays of an IH practice. With this kind of background—an understanding of occupational disease, employee placement, counseling, rehabilitation, and industrial sociology—the hygienist becomes a true working member of the occupational health team and is placed logically within the occupational health structure.

In those organizations where a corporate position has been created for environmental management, there must be close interrelationships between occupational health and IH for the total mission of health protection to prevail. Often, the goals of the two specialties are not seen as congruent end points, and strong dissension erupts, which eventually can prove destructive. Such fractures may result when a behaviorally oriented practitioner attempts to work with a materials-and-methods–directed engineer. Whatever the placement of the professionals, it is the employee's health that is the joint focus and the merged allegiance.

The issue was faced some years ago by King [4], a Britisher, occupational hygienist and academician, who commented that although history was a poor teacher, it could explain certain attitudes and reactions. He traced a developmental chain in that many years ago gross disease was being uncovered in industry by a few interested physicians. Such activity was followed at a time of general social progress by limiting the disease through individual care of the workers and crude environmental control. Radiographic and biochemical techniques aided in diagnosis of the disease at a preclinical stage. Then came the involvement of physicists, chemists, toxicologists, and engineers, who acted initially as ancillaries to the physician insofar as the presence or absence of disease was the criterion used. Slowly there evolved the discipline of IH, with the professionals acting in their own right. Some of the physicians fell in with the changing pattern and in their own companies became hygienists rather than physicians. Others, continuing with the study of disease, fell between the two emerging groups. With the realization that good environmental control is the only true preventive of most industrial illness, medicine, as King viewed it, became more the long stop in detecting the worker who may have escaped protection, rather than the primary means of control. The balance began to shift.

In recent years, various formulas have been designed to reconcile the two concepts. One view still widely held then, but rarely voiced, was that, at best, the hygienist was a technician to the occupational health physician. Next, there was a vague "partnership," with the senior partner understood but, as before, not verbalized. Then, more recently came the suggestion of equality in England's National Health Service. King [4] pointed to the equal partnership between health physics and occupational physicians, which this writer experienced extremely comfortably for an 8-year span. One other view was that IH, being primarily an engineering discipline, was essentially freestanding.

In substance, King concluded that, in his contact with managers, physicians, engineers, and hygienists on real, not theoretic exercises, these considerations rarely arose and each contributed his or her part. Any general formula of supremacy, he felt, would fail in the majority of its applications, is unnecessary and undesirable, and must involve waste on one side or the other. "A built-in dominance of one side may lead to a downgrading of the other in status, ability and effectiveness" [4]. Where, then, is IH? The placement is made that allows the best in a mutual activity aimed at the elimination of work-associated disease, dysfunction, and disability.

BROADENED ROLES

The "right-to-know" mandates governing the transmittal of information to employees concerning potentially hazardous work exposures have enlarged the role of the traditional industrial hygienist. The creation of large IH staffs has required the attainment of managerial skills by the IH director. The weakening of the once strong federal OSHA legislation has obligated IH professionals to be heard locally, regionally, and nationally in an effort to retain the worker's protection afforded by the ideal codification of 1970.

These kinds of roles are new to practitioners whose primary activities have comprised environmental study, instrumented measurement, and report preparation. For some persons whose professional lives were spent within the limits of a plant or plants as interpreters of the work-worker interface, the conversion to communicators, managers, spokespersons, and witnesses at hearings has not been easy. A new element of social responsibility has entered into the profession. That roles are being modified was given voice in a workshop devoted to a review of occupational health engineering control technology [5]. From the discussion of professional skills there emerged identification of several new skill requirements. While the recognized subject areas of chemistry, physics, engineering, biology, toxicology, and facilities design were identified as warranting *greater* emphasis today relative to the past, writing, verbal communication, and managerial planning were ranked *very great to very much greater* among today's emphases and requirements. Field sampling, field testing, and analytic laboratory skills were viewed as deserving less emphasis in today's practice. The need for communicative skills has been voiced in several arenas. The vice-chairman of the Monsanto Company [6], speaking to industrial hygienists, told them that they must inform managers how they can protect profits, in "language that people with budget authority can understand." He sought further communication when he said that it was their responsibility as professionals to stand up and be counted when they see unreasonable restrictions being put on workplace practices. And as they have the obligation to tell the company that employs them that it is not operating in a responsible way, they have an equal responsibility to make sure that the company is not penalized unnecessarily by overregulation. Managers, thus, are asking the hygienist to be vocal and to be heard, whether it is by the company or by the regulators. The end result of well-directed communication, he concluded, was managerial support and a matching effort by executive officers to educate themselves—a resulting mosaic that will protect the goal of the organization and satisfy the concerns of the worker.

In a discussion of the establishment of a career hierarchy at IBM [7] in IH, the types of skills needed to be an effective employee were the following:

Work content skills
- Equipment calibration
- Sampling devices
- Statistics
- Analytic equipment
- Ventilation design

Functional skills
- Writing
- Presenting
- Negotiating
- Listening
- Organizing
- Persuading
- Leading
- Problem solving

Adaptive/self-management skills
- Initiative
- Risk-taking
- Reliability
- Persistence
- Diplomacy
- Optimism
- Enthusiasm
- Decisiveness

Immediately, there is a sense of need for skills not usually associated with the accepted set of professional tasks. Emphasis is given communication *and* listening skills. Further, the hygienist, irrespective of the level of experience, is given the responsibility of training. As the hygienist moves from entry level to well experienced, the teaching/training assignments move from occupational health training of employees to educational programs for managers, other hygienists, medical environmental planners, and safety specialists [7]. In defining career plans, the behavioral aspects of the profession are weighted heavily.

Another top manager [8] gives as a basic function in IH the communication of information regarding health risks and the programs combatting such risks, which requires "the ability to translate often complex technical data into comprehensible laymen's language, and the diplomatic skill to elicit concern and cooperation."

Also, from academe there comes under the title "What the Young Industrial Hygienist Needs to Know to Advance" [9] a summary of opinions elicited from former graduate students and practicing peers. Universally, irrespective of the site of practice, IH was seen as a profession where communication was of the utmost importance. The hygienists must relay understandably information concerning the prevention of adverse health effects to a spectrum moving from relatively unskilled production workers to research investigators. They must be able to communicate effectively with professional associates—persons with whom they must work and to whom they report. Every activity requires the preparation of a written report, and the product must be literate and well organized and the conclusions expressed in a clear, concise, and effective manner [9].

Smith [9] offers a comment whose content has been experienced by all of us in graduate education when he states that many industrial hygienists are technically competent but are woefully inadequate in written expression. Many graduates, regardless of the school granting the degree, practice what he would call innovative spelling. He elaborates: "At some point in their background they have decided that phonetic spelling is adequate, and [they] do not concern themselves with the niceties of correctly spelling each word. The same observation applies to their grammatical habits, and it is not uncommon to find every grammatical rule known being violated or ignored."

Lastly, Smith points up the need of good communication to upper managerial personnel who are the decision-makers, to their own professional superiors, and to such others as representatives of organized labor, government agency persons, reporters in both the print and broadcast media, and the general public.

Other areas of personal involvement, which were not necessarily taught in school, included the principles of management, labor-management relationships, corporate policies, financial practices, and basic principles of accounting. These areas are in addition to such ancillary informational needs as air pollution, safety, and liquid and solid waste disposal.

Why are such skills as communication or speaking up at the appropriate moment given such emphasis here, when little consideration is given the technical phases of IH practice? The latter is a given in the professional world, while the abilities to communicate or relate are skills not usually taught to industrial hygienists and commonly are not inherent in an individual.

Hygienists are members of the occupational health team, and their ability or inability to obtain cooperation or alienate plant personnel will reflect directly on the total occupational health effort. The hygienist represents the health effort in the field, and arrogance, abruptness, talking down, or failing to explain will all come back to both company and occupational health managers and may negate or defeat every well-intentioned effort toward health protection.

The plea is made, therefore, to visualize IH as an interpersonal relationship, not merely the placement of monitors, the recording of electronic readouts, or the entry of environmental data into a computer. It can be a highly personalized activity, one that motivates workers into a better health behavior pattern. As it has been said so many times since Benjamin Franklin offered the comment when signing the Declaration of Independence, we must all hang together, or assuredly we will hang separately.

The broader professional was described some years back by Schulte [10] in the Cummings Memorial Lecture, when he viewed the industrial hygienist as an involved social scientist and not as a disinterested professional. He pointed up the need for currency in such areas as law, psychology, communication skills, public relations, and sociology and asked that greater emphasis be given the social aspects of the specialty.

As our culture and the nature of our industrial society change, the concern of the hygienist in the greater issues is desperately needed.

ETHICS

Closely tied to the issues just discussed is the matter of professional ethics. The American Academy of Industrial Hygiene has issued its Code of Responsibility for Professional Practice of Industrial Hygiene, and it follows in its entirety:

A. *PURPOSE*

This Code provides a standard for ethical conduct as the Industrial Hygienist strives to accomplish his goal of protecting the health of the worker, improving the work environment, and upgrading the quality of environmental health in general. He has the responsibility to practice his profession in an objective and impartial manner following recognized principles of Industrial Hygiene, recognizing that the lives, health and welfare of the public are dependent upon his professional judgment.

B. *PROFESSIONAL RESPONSIBILITY*

1. To objectively and impartially apply recognized scientific methods and interpret findings factually.
2. Maintain the highest level of professional integrity and qualification by keeping abreast of current developments in Industrial Hygiene.
3. Promote an understanding of the purpose and functions of Industrial Hygiene as a professional discipline.
4. Exchange scientific knowledge for the benefit of society and the profession.

C. *RESPONSIBILITY TO THE WORKER*
   1. To approach the basic goal of Industrial Hygiene with responsibility and scientific objectivity.
   2. To maintain an objective attitude toward the evaluation of health hazards regardless of external influences, realizing that the health and welfare of worker is dependent upon the Industrial Hygienist's professional evaluation and judgment.

D. *RESPONSIBILITY TO EMPLOYERS AND CLIENTS*
   1. Act as a faithful agent or trustee in the application of sound industrial hygiene principles for the improvement and maintenance of healthful working environments.
   2. Be a loyal employee, respect confidences, advise honestly and objectively all findings, and avoid all circumstances where a compromise of professional judgment or conflict of interest may arise.
   3. While the Industrial Hygienist owes the highest degree of fidelity to his employer or client, such fidelity must remain subservient to his ultimate responsibility for those whose lives, health and welfare depend upon his professional judgments, decisions and practice.

E. *RESPONSIBILITY TO THE PUBLIC*
   1. To report factually on health matters of public concern.
   2. To state only professional opinions founded on adequate knowledge and honest convictions, while serving as a witness before a court, commission or tribunal.
   3. To express opinions publicly only when based on facts, and never to express opinions for personal publicity or gain.

F. *RESPONSIBILITY TO OTHERS*
   1. To promote professional development and advancement for colleagues, co-workers and associates.
   2. To promote and encourage the exchange of scientific knowledge for the development of others.

While most of the responsibilities listed are met without difficulty, it is the behavioral ethics given in C2 and D3 where the greatest pressures will be brought to bear—the "external influences." When a hazardous situation is uncovered and is in need of reversal or control, several issues present themselves—cost, public relations, and labor relations. Pressure may be brought on the hygienist to downplay the findings, to remain quiet regarding levels of offending materials, or to report the results of the study verbally only. The situation requires considerable strength in the selection of the appropriate action. Is the information to be retained as directed? Should the issue be pushed until managerial understanding and support are obtained? Should one, as the law dictates, make the findings known immediately to the workers at risk? To whom goes the allegiance? When assuming a new position once with a large county government, the writer was asked by a trade union president, in a public forum, to whom his allegiance would go. Expecting that the response would be dichotomized, he was astonished to hear that the allegiance would be to medicine—not to management or labor. The implication was that what was sound medically would be the guiding ethic, irrespective of the label of the affected person or group. There were no further questions.

The point was underscored by Sheriff [11] when he wrote in strong, understandable language:

> By believing our code of ethics only applies to our research, and its accuracy, we do ourselves a gross disservice. How could we possibly feel we haven't compromised our code of ethics when taking a weak initial position just because we expect opposition! Because the compromise occurred before anything was presented, we somehow think that it's alright? Why do we believe that our ethics doesn't require us to defend our findings—only present them? Why do we believe it's only our manager's fault if industrial health hazards aren't corrected? How many times have we heard it said—or said it ourselves—"I just present the facts, it's up to someone else to defend them!"
>
> I can assure you with such an approach we will become known as a profession of sample takers and lab techs! If we don't support our findings and defend them, our personal as well as professional ethics can—and should be—questioned.

The decision-making process is not an easy one, as indicated. And there will be the voice of labor frequently muddying the scene by declaring loudly that a certain operation is "killing people" when all factual, scientific information cannot support such a contention. So the decision must be made, adhered to, communicated, and supported until corrective action is taken. Otherwise, living with one's self and one's behavior becomes difficult. Industrial hygiene, like occupational health in general, has the goal of averting work-related illness. This concept must remain as the objective, and by assuming a strong positive position, the industry, the company, the workers, and the hygienist are all protected.

REPORTS

Completeness and exactitude in an IH report are mandatory, for the document may be entered as evidence in a hearing or trial, and embarrassment can be avoided if the report contains accurate information and carefully drawn conclusions and recommendations.

Certain information must be included in an IH report that will provide all the particulars of an environmental evaluation—be it descriptive of the study of an acute exposure with resulting morbidity or of a regularly recurring review of an operation free of mishap to the workers involved.

The needed data for inclusion in a report follow:

Introduction
- Person(s) requesting the study
- Person(s) conducting the study
- Worksite studied
- Hazard(s) investigated

Evaluation procedures
- Methods of detection or analysis
- Instruments used
- Calibration status of instruments
- Analytic laboratory procedures

Analytic results
- Location where samples were obtained
- Types of samples (atmospheric, work materials, etc.)
- Hazard factor(s) involved (toxic dust, fume, radiation, etc.)
- Standard(s) (Threshold Limit Value—Time-Weighted Average [TLV-TWA], Threshold Limit Value—Short-Term Exposure Limit [TLV-STEL], Biological Exposure Index [BEI], OSHA Standard, Criteria Document Recommendation, etc.)
- Quantitative levels found (ppm, mg/m^3, dBA, etc.)
- Conditions at time of sampling (normal operation, ventilation off, machine running at maximum rpm, unusual weather conditions, etc.)

Sketch of worksite showing sampling points (if applicable)

Interpretation of results
- Statement(s) regarding degree of hazard

Recommendations for control of hazardous operation
- Environmental control(s)
- Protective equipment to be worn
- Medical control(s) (surveillance, on-site emergency care, report mandates, etc.)
- Emergency care of spills, leaks, and so on

Summary of evaluation

In keeping with the nature of the problem, the report might vary, so that not all topics listed above necessarily will require coverage or description. Even the sequence of the sections might be altered. As to format, tabulation of numerical findings will allow greater ease in reading. Needless to say, notes taken in the field or calculations attendant upon the findings should be entered into a single field notebook and not made on pieces of paper that either might be lost or give indications of loose scientific organization. Further, the notes might be used in court and, like the final report, might be entered in evidence.

Reports should be prepared quickly, for a long delay in the submission of important information will attenuate the worth or necessity of the study, and particularly, if corrective action is needed, it should be taken promptly and with the appropriate managerial or fiscal support. Procrastination of preparation of the document may affect adversely an entire IH or occupational health effort.

It is advisable that each report carry a brief summary that will convey the essence of the evaluation to the lay managers, so that action will be initiated without burdening executive personnel with a great amount of technical detail. The use of simple language will always prove helpful and lead to more immediate cooperation. Finally, the report should be delivered in person to the individual requesting the study so that questions can be answered or unclear material clarified.

INTERNAL ACTIVITY REPORTS

As every section of an OHS is responsible for reporting its activities periodically, IH, if it is part of an OHS, must maintain a running account of time expenditure. The list that follows provides categories for the assignment of professional time. In certain situations where departments might be backcharged for IH studies, the time allocation will serve as a basis for accurate cost accounting.

TIME ALLOCATION IN IH FOR STATISTICAL RECORDS

Site visits
- On-site evaluation
  - Identification
  - Measurement
- Off-site activities
  - Conferences, seminars, literature search, education (hazard communication), presentations to line managers and employees, procurement of occupational histories
  - Site-visit follow-up (return visits)

Preparation of reports

Professional activities
- Initiation of new projects (evaluation of plans, research, participation in epidemiologic studies)
- Professional meetings
- Teaching
- Reading (monographic and periodic literature)

Telephone communication
- Incoming inquiries
- Outgoing calls

Staff meetings

Supervision of IH staff

Travel time

SAFETY DATA INFORMATION

Typical of any industrial establishment is either the introduction of new work materials or the initiation of an additional operation that requires the use of substances bearing brand names but no description of the ingredients. Needed in the preparation of a Material Safety Data Sheet (MSDS) is knowledge of the ingredients and certain data regarding the physical, explosive, or health-hazard characteristics of the product. To obtain such information, if it is not readily available through library sources, technical files, or data banks, one can communicate with the manufacturer and either request an MSDS or send a letter, comparable to one that has been used, reading in general as follows:

Dear Sir:

The Industrial Hygiene Department at this activity is responsible for protecting the health and hygiene of military and civilian personnel in carrying out functions relating to the operation of the ______Shipyard. To do this effectively, we need the cooperation of all companies supplying chemical compounds and materials to the activity. To ensure that we have the latest information on the hazards of your chemical products, we are requesting that you supply the data on the enclosed forms. We are required to treat information concerning proprietary product composition as confidential, and I can assure you that the information provided will be utilized only for the protection of the health and safety of the personnel at this activity.

Should you find it necessary to withhold the exact formulation of these products, we would appreciate receiving a list of ingredients with an approximate percentage of the composition. For example, if the exact formulation of the material is:

Methylene chloride	50.0%
Methyl ethyl ketone	35.0%
Toluene	14.5%
Benzene	0.5%

an acceptable completion of the enclosure could be:

Methylene chloride	Over 40%
Methyl ethyl ketone	20–40%
Toluene	Less than 25%
Benzene	Trace or impurity

Your cooperation would be greatly appreciated in replying at your earliest convenience.

Sincerely,

Medical Director

Little difficulty is usually experienced in obtaining the required data, provided certain constraints are recognized and appreciated, that is, proprietary information.

MALPRACTICE IN INDUSTRIAL HYGIENE

While normally a malpractice action against an industrial hygienist is rarely undertaken, Keane [12] has offered some comments regarding the concern in IH of such litigation. He indicates that subsequent to a suit for negligence where the plaintiff has lost, countersuits have been filed against both the plaintiff and the plaintiff's attorney. The idea was suggested that such countersuits would discourage legal actions of this type.

Keane warns that before such a retaliatory suit is undertaken, one should be aware of the risks involved. Action for malicious prosecution will hold only if the defendant was prosecuted unjustly solely for reasons of malice or harassment, if there was no reason to believe the defendant negligent, if the defendant was ultimately exonerated, and if the initial suit caused damage to the defendant.

It is interpreted that with the plaintiff's suit being filed ordinarily with the hope of receiving monetary compensation for the alleged injuries, such pecuniary motivation does not amount to "malice." The essence of Keane's conclusion is that, as demonstrated through case law, a countersuit for malicious prosecution must await the exoneration of the safety and health professional in the preceding negligence or malpractice action and that the professional must show that "the injured person's suit was actuated by malice and brought without probable cause" [12]. In practice, these requirements are rarely proved, and one is left without legal remedy. The cost of processing such a suit is substantial, and this fact, in itself, must be weighed against the extraordinarily small chance of success.

SOURCES OF INFORMATION

CONSULTANTS AND ACCREDITED LABORATORIES

Not all companies have in-house IH personnel or a capability to conduct their own environmental evaluations. Two listings are published periodically that indicate sources of consultative assistance. One comprises the names, addresses, telephone numbers, and specialties* of industrial hygiene consultants, and the

*The specialties are the following: air pollution, audiometry, biologic monitoring, ergonomics, expert witness, industrial hygiene—comprehensive plant studies and/or analyses, occupational medicine, product safety—labeling, radiologic control, respirator protection, safety specialist, toxicology, training instruction, ventilation, waste disposal, water pollution.

second provides the names, addresses, telephone numbers, names of the directors, and the analyses conducted by accredited laboratories. These laboratories have been accredited under the Laboratory Accreditation Program of the AIHA. As proficiency testing is an integral part of the accreditation program, this protocol is fulfilled by the participation of the laboratories in the National Institute for Occupational Safety and Health (NIOSH) Proficiency Analytical Testing (PAT) Program. This program includes analysis of bimonthly samples for lead, cadmium, zinc, asbestos, silica, and organic solvents. The solvents provided on a rotating basis include carbon tetrachloride, benzene, trichloroethylene, *p*-dioxane, toluene, and chloroform. For accreditation, laboratories are required to analyze all materials in the PAT Program, which they analyze as part of their standard analytic operations.

WALL CHARTS

Certain commercial sources make available, in most instances at no cost, wall charts that might prove helpful.

Medical Reference Chart A

Available from Health Evaluation Programs, Inc.; 808 Busse Highway; Park Ridge, IL 60068.

This chart cross-references the legal mandates and the frequency of conduct of recommended clinical and laboratory tests to evaluate worker exposures.

Industrial Hygiene Reference Chart B

Available from Health Evaluation Programs, Inc., as given above.

This chart cross-references the training programs required, the routes of entry, the harmful effects, the personal protective equipment needed, the sampling equipment to be used, and the analytic methods to be employed in worker exposure.

OSHA Concentration Limits for Gases

Available from Foxboro Analytical; Wilks Infrared Center; P.O. Box 449; South Norwalk, CT 06856.

This chart provides users of infrared spectrophotometers with adjustable, long path-length gas cells, assistive calibration information enabling one to make ambient air determinations of many materials.

Air Monitoring Filter Selection Guide

Available from Millipore Corporation; Laboratory Products Division; Bedford, MA 01730.

This chart summarizes relevant information for monitoring, such as filter types, NIOSH analytic methods, and OSHA exposure limits.

Charcoal Tube User Guide

Available from MDA Scientific, Inc.; 808 Busse Highway; Park Ridge, IL 60068.

This chart provides, for a great number of substances, the OSHA or American Conference of Governmental Industrial Hygienists (ACGIH) TLVs (the latter when different), the recommended sampling rates, and other data concerning this sampling method.

Hazardous Waste Classifications

Available from Laboratory Safety Supply; 3430 Palmer Drive; Janesville, WI 53546.

This chart provides lists of hazardous wastes by name and the number assigned by the Environmental Protection Agency (EPA), in accordance with Appendix VIII of 40CRF Part 261.

Chemical Hazards Chart

Available from Laboratory Safety Supply, as given above.

This chart is of assistance in the safe handling and storage of chemicals, by providing, for over 500 substances, their toxicity; whether they are irritant, corrosive, carcinogenic, flammable, or explosive; their reactive characteristics; their vapor density; and TLVs.

Guide to Air Sampling Standards [a brochure]

Available from SKC West, Inc.; P.O. Box 2805; 2021-G West Commonwealth; Fullerton, CA 92633.

This combined guide and catalog lists by substance the NIOSH/OSHA air sampling standards, including sample volume, rate, time, and the analytic method.

ENVOI

To return to humanitarianism in IH, it is helpful to envision these characteristics in the professionals who interact with employers, peers, and workers, as attributed to the eminent Leslie Silverman in an obituary written shortly after his death in early 1966 [13]: He "will be remembered by his students and colleagues for his extraordinary fund of scientific and engineering knowledge which he shared with them with courtesy, patience, and generosity; for his inexhaustible vigor in scientific investigations; and for his keen wit, which made every association with him a delightful experience. He was a warm friend who responded unfailingly to requests for his counsel and assistance. . . ." May all occupational health professionals manifest these qualities as they endeavor to improve the working environment as part of the effort of conserving health.

OCCUPATIONAL SAFETY AND INJURY PREVENTION

In only a few corporate situations is occupational (industrial) safety a responsibility of the medical director, but a knowledge of the offerings of the safety professional is mandatory for a cooperative effort in preventing accidents and their attendant injuries. "While every professional group with a tradition of attainment resists outside influences as an incursion into its sovereignty," as Booth [14] has put it, one feels obligated to include more than mere mention of occupational health's most closely associated discipline.

A primary reason for inclusion of the basic tenets of accident prevention in a treatise on plant occupational medicine lies in the occasional difficulties in communication and cross-appreciation of skills in installations where both safety and medicine serve the same work population. This bilateral lack of recognition of worth has led to ineffectiveness in lowering the accident frequency and has precluded a sound joint activity in the conservation of an installation's human resources.

Kilian [15] has observed that far too often there existed a lack of understanding and communication between the safety engineer and medical directors as to the causes of, and responsibility for, specific types of work-related morbidity. The same bilateral lack of understanding would frequently characterize the degree and expected duration of disablement. The physician trained to see patients as individuals and not as members of a larger workforce would be inclined to be unsympathetic to the tendency of some safety engineers to see illness and injury solely in terms of lost-time records and compensation cost. The safety director, in turn, sometimes could feel that the physician was either uninformed about the industrial environment or did not appreciate the great cost of injuries and illnesses or the amount of human suffering that the safety practitioner was able to prevent.

Unfortunately, some of this antithesis in viewpoint persists in certain establishments where highly specious return-to-work mechanisms are used that allow the healing or convalescing injured employee to come back to the worksite prematurely and to be assigned to a sinecure position to minimize the time lost. These are spurious efforts, and while an *early* return to one's *regular* position is rehabilitative, a temporary placement in a "make-work" situation is neither honest nor good for the employee; he or she feels uncomfortable as a pawn in a numbers' game. The physician in industry tries to be as accurate as possible in judging the length of healing time and in avoiding a premature return. The in-plant practitioner does not overextend needlessly a period of convalescence. Assignments to "library work" or other ill-befitting temporizations are anathema to good morale, and physicians do not enjoy being pressured into joining in this kind of record manipulation. Fortunately, this practice is beginning to diminish as cooperation between the two disciplines increases and as given union by the Occupational Safety and Health Act of 1970.

THE NEED FOR ACCIDENT PREVENTION

The prevention of accidental injury—or death—has been of concern to both employers and the public, for injuries can result in a loss of life or, more frequently, some permanent disablement, which can readily upset a family's fiscal base. With most industrially incurred injuries there is a loss in salary, for workers' compensation pays possibly two-thirds or less of one's regular wage. Injuries sustained at home or from recreational activities may require use of sick leave and, if prolonged, leave without pay.

As a loss of manpower is disturbing to a company, an accident prevention program must necessarily extend beyond the demands of a job to the employee's home, community, and leisure-time activities. That there are innumerable opportunities for personal injury are readily seen. The level of premature mortality has been studied by the National Center for Health Statistics and is expressed as years of potential life lost (YPLL), involving all persons who die between their first birthday and 65 years of age. While "accidents and adverse effects," or termed more recently "unintentional injuries," remained the leading cause of premature loss of life, they did undergo the largest percentage decrease, 8.5 percent of all causes, between 1980 and 1981 [16]. Data for 1971 placed all accidents in the third level of cause of death, and at that time, with 113,336 deaths, there were 4,030,340 years of potential life lost [17]. Job-related injuries and illnesses declined in 1982, falling to 7.7 per 100 full-time workers from the 8.3 of the previous year [18]. In 1972, the incidence rate was 10.9 per 100 full-time workers. There were 3.5 lost workday cases in 1982 and 4.2 nonfatal cases without lost workdays in the same year. The incidence rates for 1982 were 58.7 per 100 workers for occupational injuries and illnesses and 57.5 for injuries alone. The average number of lost workdays per lost-workday case was 17 days [18]. The actual number of work-related deaths in the private sector in 1982 was 4,090, and nearly 30 percent resulted from car and truck accidents. There were 4,750,000 injuries sustained at work in 1982.

Another system of recording injuries was instituted by NIOSH in conjunction with the Consumer Product Safety Commission (CPSC), which was a monitoring of all patients presenting with occupational injuries who were treated at a sample of 66 hospital emergency services [19]. From data submitted and extrapolated to a crude national estimate, it was determined that 3.3 million occupational injuries were treated in hospital emergency services in 1981. The salient characteristic of that reporting system was its ability to provide more current statistics than other modes of surveillance.

In 1981, at the hospitals reporting, lacerations represented 25.4 percent of the injuries seen, with abrasions, contusions, and hematomas second at 23.6 percent, and sprains and strains in the third position at 19.5 percent. Injuries to the fingers were highest at 25.3 percent of the total, followed by injuries to the face (14.2 percent) and trauma sustained on the trunk (13.2 percent) [19].

Baker and her coworkers [20] reviewed the deaths resulting from work-related injuries during a 1-year period in Maryland. Of 148 who were killed, all but two were men, and 41 percent involved transportation vehicles. Handguns accounted for 11 percent of the deaths, and head injuries were the most common cause of death. Interestingly, the majority of the deaths involved either hazards not covered by the Occupational Safety and Health Act of 1970 or workers in categories excluded by law from this regulation but whose responsibility for protection lies with the Department of Transportation.

For the period 1979 through 1981, Kraus [21] studied the occurrence of homicides at work, finding an average annual rate of 1.5 per 100,000 workers. Workers at highest risk were police, security guards, and persons in occupations having frequent public contact involving an exchange of money, particularly in late afternoon or evening hours.

Other injuries and deaths occur not at the worksite but among wage earners engaging in recreational activities. Potential workers are hurt or killed—for example, adolescents aged 9 to 16 years who sustained injuries ranging from lacerations to paraplegia from riding minibikes, motorcycles, or go-carts [22]. In 1978, there were 824 deaths from pedal cycling (mostly bicycles) [23].

Some 10,000 people in 1974 were estimated as engaging in hang-gliding, and Krissoff and Eiseman [24] reported on eight cases of nonfatal injury, all involving fractures, with one person sustaining burns requiring bilateral below-elbow amputations from contact with concealed high-tension lines. There were four fatalities among other sky sailors, one a 28-year-old man who was hang-gliding during a lunch break from work. From 1964 to 1974 there were 16 fatalities among balloonists [25]. Even among the military (navy), occupational injuries were tabulated in various reporting regions at 5.4 to 58.7 per 1,000 per month, with nonoccupational accidents producing rates of 1.5 to 29.7 per 1,000 per month [26].

Considerable study was undertaken some years ago by Waller [27–30] in the relationship of chronic medical disorders to traffic accidents. He concluded that there is an increased accident risk associated with several chronic conditions, including alcoholism, cardiovascular disease, epilepsy, diabetes, and mental illness. In about 50 percent of the accidents resulting from heart attacks, the driver had no previous knowledge of the illness. The relationship between drunk driving and accidents showed that 50 to 75 percent of all severe accidents and fatalities involved the use of alcohol, a finding to be confirmed in the ensuing decades.

In another review of 99 fatal motorcycle crashes [31], blood alcohol levels were determined for 62 drivers. Measurable amounts were found in two-thirds, and one-half had illegally high concentrations of 100 mg/100 ml or more. The high blood alcohol levels were encountered most commonly in the age group of 20 to 34 years. When the state of California was presented with the proposal of using privately owned motorcycles on official business on a reimbursement-for-mileage basis to affect fuel savings, the Board of Control rejected the suggestion. In a previous study, the California Highway Patrol pointed out that the injury cost for motorcycles was 16.1 cents per mile, in contrast to that of automobiles of 0.59 cents per mile, traceable to the discrepant costs of medical care and disability payments to injured motorcycle operators [32].

Finally, another measure of the problem, and a factor to be reckoned with in prevention and training, is the finding that workers generally influence disproportionately high injury rates during their first year on a new job or when working for a new employer. Almost all age and sex groups demonstrate this difference [33]. Some variations of these findings are given in a study of automobile-related injuries by the American Medical Association (AMA) Council on Scientific Affairs [34]. Fatality rates per 100 million passenger miles are highest for persons 16 to 29 years of age, and in that group the rates are more than twice as high for males as for females. Also, the fatality rates for the elderly, oddly enough, are almost as high as they are for the young group. Injuries in older persons were more likely to be fatal. Alcohol-impaired drivers are responsible for 25 to 35 percent of crashes causing serious injuries and for about 6 percent of all crashes. The driver's probability, or relative risk, of sustaining a fatal accident rises dramatically as the blood alcohol concentration increases.

DEFINITIONS

Adequate reason is seen for the creation of programs aimed at the reduction of accidents and accidental injuries, not only in the workplace, but also in the community, for injuries occur there that cause time-loss of employees. Although it might be contended that the employer is not concerned with the activities of workers after quitting time, it is apparent that accidental happenings in the home, on the highway, or in the recreational arena can remove the employee from the job for the period of hospitalization or for convalescence from the injury.

THE PROGRAM DESIGNATION

As with most social undertakings, titles change as disciplines develop and become more sophisticated, as research broadens understanding and brings to light more basic truths, or as current technologies demand newer differentiations of labor with their recast supervisory and support systems. Initially designated "safety"—later termed "industrial safety" to distinguish it from flight safety, marine safety, and farther along, "occupational safety"—other variations of the central theme appeared, such as "accidental prevention," and as additional functions were added, the labels of "loss prevention," "loss control," or "risk management" came onto the scene, particularly among casualty insurance underwriters.

To define the last terms first, "loss prevention" is viewed by Boylston [35] as management action that is directed toward preventing, reducing, or eliminating business risks. In further dissection of the concept, "loss prevention management" involves the application of proved professional managerial techniques and skills to (1) identification of existing or potential risk exposures; (2) analysis of identified exposures; (3) development of effective, feasible exposure controls; and (4) management of a loss prevention program.

Of the loss prevention techniques and procedures used to identify properly the risk exposures, one conducts (1) facility design reviews; (2) new or altered procedure, facility, or equipment audits; (3) job safety and health analysis; (4) annual safety, health, and fire prevention audits; (5) regularly recurring facility, area, group, and shift inspections; and (6) regularly recurring equipment inspections [35]. It is seen instantly that there are areas of overlap, some functions customarily being carried out by an OHS, and others being subsumed under the total responsibility of IH.

The assignment of functions is determined by the organizational structure, the presence or absence of related disciplines, and frequently, the strength or sophistication of a particular unit in contrast to the capability of an associated unit. Where no OHS exists within a plant structure, the prevention of loss through illness will be assumed by a safety section or director. As mentioned previously, in several large companies, safety is a function of the corporate medical director, and while the goals may be identical, the mode of reaching the goals will differ.

RESPONSIBILITY

In a small organization, the safety program is headed by the chief executive officer (CEO), with other responsibilities being delegated to the supervisors. In larger companies, this function is given to a special assistant to the CEO, a vice-president, or the personnel director, but it is the heads of the various operating divisions who have the responsibility for the detailed safety program in their own units. To be successful in preventing accidents and injuries there must be strong support by the top managers. If they are cavalier in their attitudes relative to the safeguarding of human lives, there will be laxity on the parts of all personnel who are on the reporting ladders, and safety will be relegated to a position of unconcern. It is the immediate supervisors who interpret the philosophy of the CEO and who demand good work practices of their employees through behavioral example, training, analysis, review, and the institution of corrective action. As the accident record—good or poor—reflects on the management of a department, the unit heads usually are emotionally involved with the performance of their personnel and demand improvement from their supervisors. It is they who have the closest knowledge of the work processes and are able to initiate corrections, improve the morale of a work group, or identify the reasons for a series of recurring injuries. It is at the first level of supervision where effective safety direction is given and retained.

In large concerns there are safety directors whose sole responsibility comprises the functions enumerated previously. Assisting the director in most organizations is a safety committee, a group of employees appointed to aid and advise management on matters of worker safety. It is composed of top executives, supervisors, workers, and the safety director, and it is advised that the medical director, or a staff physician representing the director, serve on the committee. The appointee should be one who provides care for injured employees, who would have direct knowledge of the types of injuries and the workers sustaining them, and who would have some insight into the behavior dynamics, that is, an interest in ferreting out the reasons for the trauma and its causative events.

The committee usually includes workers who are familiar with a plant's operations and, in a review of a month's or a quarter's injuries, could contribute knowingly to the group's discussion. Through the committee's deliberations, hazardous conditions can be identified, faults in work procedure recognized, and corrective measures recommended. Through a group effort, the stimulus needed for the maintenance of safe working conditions will emerge [36].

Minutes resulting from the meetings should be prepared and distributed to all department heads. These minutes serve as good openers for a supervisor's early-morning "tailgate conference" on safety. At one installation, material concerning the accident/injury record was printed on the obverse of a report that listed all punitive actions taken against plant workers. The anger resulting from a reading of the adverse personnel actions fully negated any salutary effect that might have been produced initially. Issues so antithetic should not be mixed.

CONCEPTS

Abercrombie [37] has offered a working lexicon of terms important in a safety program, and some of these definitions are given so that common understanding might result.

Accident: An unplanned and sometimes injurious or damaging event that interrupts the normal progress of an activity and is invariably preceded by an unsafe act or unsafe condition or some combination thereof.

Accident analysis: A critical examination by one or more qualified persons of the information developed in an accident investigation for the purpose of identifying its causal factors and prescribing measures designed to prevent its recurrence.

Accident prevention: The application of countermeasures designed to reduce accidents or accident potential within a system, organization, or activity; programs directed toward accident avoidance.

Attitude: A semipermanent cluster of human emotions, feelings, and cognitions about a situation, thing, or idea. An attitude may or may not manifest itself in overt behavior, depending on such factors as intensity (its positive or negative direction with reference to the zero or neutral point), opposing or conflicting forces, the value system applied to a particular situation, motivational forces, timing, and other influencing or controlling forces. An attitude may produce a predisposition toward behavior in certain ways depending on its intensity, assuming the forces of all other behavior-influencing factors are equalized.

Carelessness: A catchall term used to describe inattention or indifference as a causal factor leading to an accident. *Its use should be avoided in favor of a more specific and detailed identification and explanation of the human error involved.*

Certified Safety Professional (CSP): An individual who has met all of the requirements for certification by the Board of Safety Professionals and who recognizes and assumes responsibility to the safety profession for maintaining (1) professional competence by remaining abreast of the technical, administrative, and regulatory developments in a chosen field and (2) professional integrity that reflects the highest standard of ethics in relations with clients, associates, and the public.

Injury, cumulative: A term used to describe any physical or psychological disability that results from the combined effects of repeated injuries or illness in the workplace. Although each injury or illness may be minor at the time it occurs, the cumulative effect over time can lead to claims for physical or psychological disabilities such as coronary heart disease, hypertension, ulcers, stroke, cancer, arthritis, or neuropsychiatric problems that may be interpreted as compensable under workers' compensation laws. Also called gradual injury, long-term disease process, or repeated trauma.

Injury, disabling: A work injury that results in death, permanent disability, or inability of the injured worker to return to work on the day following the injury [38]. Often called lost-time injury.

Injury, minor: An injury where no lost time or major medical costs are involved.

The American Society of Safety Engineers (ASSE) [39] has delineated the functions of the safety professional as "an individual, who, by virtue of his specialized knowledge, skill and educational accomplishments, has achieved professional status in the safety field." Further, the ASSE has elaborated on the scope of the position as follows [39]:

> Safety professionals are engaged in hazard identification, hazard evaluation and hazard elimination or mitigation to an acceptable level in all aspects of human endeavor.

In this context, a hazard is any condition or action which presents an exposure to danger or harm to people, property or the environment.

The safety professional may serve as an engineer, as a manager or as a consultant in every aspect of the planning, organization, direction, operation and control of an endeavor. In performing these functions, the safety professional must draw upon the specialized knowledge in the physical and social sciences. Knowledge of engineering, physics, chemistry, statistics, mathematics and principles of measurement and analysis is integrated in the evaluation of safety performance. The safety professional must have a thorough understanding of the causative factors contributing to accident occurrence and combine this with knowledge of motivation, behavior and communication in order to devise methods and procedures to control hazards. Knowledge of management principles, theory of business and government organization is essential to apply the safety professional's specialized knowledge to the work, home or leisure environment.

The ASSE further points out that today's safety professionals are engaged not only in occupational safety, but in "fire protection, traffic and transportation safety, industrial hygiene, product safety, system safety and public safety" [39].

SAFETY AND OCCUPATIONAL HEALTH COOPERATION

A fused functioning of the two disciplines of safety and occupational health is vital in the conduct of an injury-preventing program. The most readily initiated joint effort is in cross-referrals. Much information is elicited from the just-injured worker who is being given care in the OHS. If the safety director, or a representative of that office, has not been made aware of the occurrence, notification should be carried out as soon as possible, particularly if more than one person has been injured from a single untoward event. While immediate questioning of a seriously injured patient is not a prudent or judicious undertaking at the moment of first contact, some information will be obtained from fellow workers that will be both helpful and needed by the safety office. Full cooperation should be manifested at all times.

When an industrial hygienist, occupational physician, or occupational health nurse sees glaring infractions of safety principles at a worksite, involving behavior, equipment, or the use of personal protective devices, this information should be conveyed to the safety authority. In the same vein, the safety professionals who are "in the field" and encounter exposures potentially productive of occupational disease should notify the medical arm of their findings. The retention of information by either office is counterproductive in the prevention of both injury and illness.

There have been members of an OHS who have felt that pertinent information regarding accident causation has been the sole property of the health service and should not be shared. As an injury in a plant moves the patient and the episode into the public domain, there is no break in confidentiality when historical material is given the safety director. If a nonoccupational disorder has been partially related to or causative of the injury, discretion must be used. In most instances, the relaying of diagnostic information is not necessary. As in placement, statements can be made that are administratively useful without compromising the privilege of the personal information, which is critical to the physician-patient relationship.

Finally, the OHS should welcome frequent visitation from the safety director's office staff. The better each staff knows the other, the more effective will the total occupational health and safety effort prove to be. In fact, a desk should be made available in the OHS for the safety representatives to facilitate either the accident record review or the interview with the patient or the member of the OHS staff.

KNOWLEDGE OF SAFETY EQUIPMENT

While the use of devices that are physically protective of workers or that provide barriers between them and hazardous processes or operations is the working knowledge of the safety professional, the physician in industry should be familiar with the wide assortment of these kinds of mechanisms. This lore is not unrelated to the total concern of worker health and safety, for an awareness of the various accident-preventive products allows physicians to be much more knowingly conversant with their clientele at the worksite. Further, opinions will be solicited regarding the efficacy of certain devices and the indications for particular kinds of respirators. A broad classification and listing are offered below, as provided in part by *Occupational Hazards* [40], which includes devices used in or for

Fall protection
Fire protection
Housekeeping and sanitation
Machine and tool safety
Material handling
Noise control
Personal protection
  Arms and hands
  Body

Eye protectors
Foot protection
Head and face protection
Plant engineering
Signs, identification

OHS ROLE IN ACCIDENT PREVENTION

The primary stanchion in support of occupational health is prevention, and the activities of the occupational health professional staff must be extended to the preclusion of industrially incurred injuries. While the more dramatic and visual means of directing workers' attention to the need for safe work practices may be undertaken by the safety personnel, the occupational physician and nurse can aid greatly in elucidating the nonphysical, nonequipment causes of accidents. Studies concerning some of the behavioral determinants of accidents go back several decades to the seminal investigations of Flanders Dunbar [41–43]. The classic observations of Hirschfeld and Behan [44–46] carried out among Detroit auto workers demonstrated that the physical disturbance manifested by the injured employees resulted from the psychological need for a solution to personal problems. Because of this dynamic, relationships with treating physicians were impaired, and efforts at physical restoration became countertherapeutic.

Enelow [47] picked up on the concept when he indicated that the chain of events called "the accident process" was a result of a complex matrix of interacting psychological, physiologic, social, and physical environmental factors. Some of them, he felt, were unavoidable, while others resulted from a failure to recognize the complexities present or to deal with them appropriately. There seems to be a continuum seen among persons sustaining accidental injury. Most people incurring an injury are susceptible to psychological complications only when faced with special circumstances—a life crisis or a severe emotional stressor. Some are unusually subject to the development of such complications, while the psychological state of others makes them especially vulnerable to accidental injury. Some of the factors encountered are depression, dependency, immaturity, aging, alcoholism, and the sociopathic personality.

Well discarded by now is the concept of accident-proneness, which once implied that there was a personality configuration that led to the sustaining of injuring. Today, we encounter many workers who are injury recidivists or accident repeaters who are not similar among themselves but who seem to experience an excessive number of injuries.

It is at this point that the treating physician or nurse can gently explore with the injured employee some of the recent life stressors that have been impinging themselves upon the patient. Frequently, there can be teased out a mounting pressure that finally had to be released through the action of the "accident process." Counseling, or just talking with the patient, may bring about a spontaneous alignment in the patient's mind of paralleling life problems and injuries. Referral to a mental health professional may obviate future trauma and even save a life.

The focus cannot be on the wound; it must be on the worker as a total entity. Many professionals are inclined to see the lesion only and lose sight of the complex series of events behind each employee's traumatic events. That this has been the concern of legislators was seen in the Occupational Safety and Health Act when it was directed that there be "research in the fields of occupational safety and health, including the psychological factors involved . . ." [48] and also ". . . research into the motivational and behavioral factors relating to the field of occupational safety and health" [49].

NIOSH has complied with this mandate and has engaged in research aimed at the recognition and control of job-related hazards, emphasizing the behavioral aspects of industrial accident problems and efforts at remediation [50]. The investigative activities have comprised three areas: (1) human elements in accident risk at work and psychological strategies for improved job safety, (2) management-oriented approaches to work safety, and (3) workplace environmental exposure limits and behavioral safety requirements. More recently there has been concern with the development of guidelines in the delivery of health-risk messages that will increase worker understanding and responsiveness [51].

Psychological testing was used in studying personality factors such as emotional stability, activity level, and impulsiveness, in addition to other factors—expressions of workers' attitudes toward their jobs, safety consciousness, supervisor/manager concern for work safety, and needs for job improvement related to safety, among others. Behavioral safety guidelines resulted from one study and were formulated into action statements, a few of which follow [52]:

Organizations should have as part of their philosophy a commitment to safety.

Whenever possible, self-paced work should be designed into work operations, as opposed to machine-paced work, thus lowering stress response, fatigue, and the probability of error, accident, or both.

Proper responses to emergencies should be defined and practiced to the point of being overlearned.

To instill safe work practices in a worker, the supervisor or other superordinate of a work establishment should reward safe job behaviors when they occur and be sure that unsafe practices go unrewarded.

While these statements are within the purview of supervisory personnel, they give the occupational health professional a glimpse into the concerns of the behavioral scientist as they relate to job-generated injuries. Occupational health personnel must remain acutely sensitive to the roles of personal or environmental stressors in accident causation, and being frequently the first prolonged human contact of the injured worker, apart from bystanders or witnesses, they will obtain a greater insight into the relationship of personality factors and individual needs to self-destruction. Exhortations and condemnations will serve no part in reversing the experience of accident repeaters. Warm understanding and counseling or extended professional help may be the only step toward the ultimate avoidance of injury-creating work practices.

SAFETY IN THE OHS

While there is participation in the general plant safety program by medical directors and their staffs, there must be detailed attention to the prevention of accidents and injuries within the OHS itself. The physical plant—offices, reception areas, diagnostic and treatment facilities, storage rooms—can present hazards that may be productive of morbidity of either OHS members or employee-patients.

The following listing may be used to review regularly the premises and their potential for injury causation.

OFFICES

Containers: empty containers removed to storage or disposed of.

Cutting and pointed equipment: guards on paper cutters; knives in drawers; pushpins boxed.

Electrical equipment for staff use (coffee makers, microwave ovens): training in use; posted on-off schedule.

Electrical outlets and wall switches: intact and free of bare wiring.

Electric wiring: cord insulation damage; shock-free; three-prong plugs for grounding; adequate for heavy equipment use; taped where required; no overload.

Files: return of drawers to closed position; bolted to walls.

Fire alarms: knowledge of location and use.

Fire drills: frequency of training.

Fire exits: clear; locations posted.

Fire extinguishers and hoses: appropriate to area; training in use; periodic testing and inspection for ensured operation.

Floor: nonslip; free of tripping or slipping hazards, spills, and defects.

Furniture: needed repairs requested and broken furniture removed; protection from sharp, protruding edges.

Illumination: appropriate to need.

Liquids: appropriately bottled and capped and stored (cleaning fluids).

Office machines (photocopiers, paper shredders, printers, calculators, typewriters, video display terminals): lifting by authorized personnel only; adequacy of training in use; isolation of hazardous parts.

Partitions: adequately positioned and fixed.

Placement of workers regarding skin response to toxic materials (carbonless copy paper, solvents, dyes, cleansers).

Smoking: no-smoking areas enforced or total abolition of smoking by both staff and patients; ashtrays in smoking areas (if smoking permitted); wastebaskets used as trash receptacles and not as ashtrays.

Space allocation: overcrowding; impaired ventilation; adequacy of ingress and egress.

Sprinkler system: adequacy; inspection and testing.

Staircases: clear; handrails; illuminated.

Step stools or ladders: availability; periodic inspection.

Storage area: adequate for need; flammables contained.

DIAGNOSTIC AND TREATMENT AREAS

Drawers: returned to cabinets.

Eye protection: of staff during certain treatment procedures.

Respiratory protection: of staff during certain patient contacts.

Floors: as in office areas.

Gas cylinders: adequately secured.

Glassware: disposal of broken glass containers.

Gloves: availability to staff, including custodians.

Laboratory equipment: wiring; temperature controls; proper disposal of specimens, broken glassware, and used reagents; safety shower, if deemed necessary.

Lifting of patients: authorized personnel/equipment only.

Lockers: separate facilities for street clothing and contaminated work clothing.
Mirrors: placed as to avoid drain stoppage or flooding by shed hair.
Physiotherapy equipment: wiring, temperature controls, adequacy of aide training.

RESTROOMS AND CHANGE FACILITIES
Showers: adequate drainage and protective ledge to avoid wetting of restroom floor and slippage.
Skin protection: approved lotions or creams between handwashings.
Smoking: placarding and enforcement of no smoking.
Sterilizer, autoclave: insulation; precautionary placarding.
Wash water: not above 105°F (40.5°C).

RESPIRATOR FITTING AND USE

*MEDICAL CLEARANCE CRITERIA FOR USE**

Standards prepared by both OSHA and the American National Standards Institute (ANSI) require the use of respirators in those work environments presenting respiratory hazards such as particulates, vapors, and gases, exclusive of nuisance dusts. A hazardous environment has been defined as one from which an individual cannot escape unprotected within half an hour without irreversible health effects or that has the potential for sufficiently severe eye or respiratory irritation that would preclude escape without injury.

The examining or "local" physician must determine if a worker can wear a respirator and function safely with it in place, an evaluation separate from fit-testing, to be discussed later. It is hoped that those criteria will aid the physicians in their judgment.

The potential usage outcomes following determination are the following:

1. The worker is cleared for use of the employer-supplied respirator with no restrictions.
2. The worker is exempted medically from use of the employer-supplied respirator.
   a. The worker is exempted additionally from use of all types of respirators.
   b. The worker is exempted but may use a type of respirator recommended by the physician.
3. The worker is cleared for use of the specified respirator, but with limitations.

Certain questions must be answered by the physician in reaching a judgment:

1. Can the worker fit and adjust the respirator indicated for use?
2. Can the worker achieve and maintain a good seal of the mask to the face?
3. Can the worker detect a seal or respirator failure?
4. Can the worker tolerate extended respirator use?

The types of respirators in current use are the following:

- Air-purifying respirators (inhaled air purified through a filter/sorbent cartridge)
  - Inhalation (depends on negative inhalation pressure to preserve integrity of the seal)
    - Half-mask
    - Full-mask
  - Powered (depends on positive pressure in the mask to exclude contaminants and not on an intact seal)
    - Half-mask
    - Full-mask
- Atmosphere-supplying respirators (inhaled air supplied from a clean source)
  - Self-contained (air tank, full-mask)
  - Air-line
    - Half-mask
    - Full-mask

Table 15-1 outlines the medical criteria as they might adversely affect the use of the various types of respirators.

The relationship of the criteria given to respirator use follows:

Facial hair: Precludes a good mask-to-face seal. Forcing hair removal may not be feasible; an alternative is the use of a powered air-purifying respirator. As normal facial hair growth can interfere with the seal, daily shaving should be mandated, and workers should be monitored for compliance.
Prominent cheekbones, depressed cheeks or temples: Interfere with the seal; the powered air-purifying respirator would be a reasonable alternative device.
Deep skinfolds, creases,or scars: As with prominent cheekbones, above.
Abnormal chin configuration: May interfere with seal around the chin.
Vision correction: Contact lenses are prohibited in the industrial environment. Spectacles with temples cannot be worn with full-face masks. Special glasses without temples, with a mount assembly,

*The criteria outlined here have been developed by Robert Estrada, M.D., and are reproduced with permission.

TABLE 15-1. Medical Clearance Criteria for Respirator Use

		Adverse effect by type of respirator					
		Mask		Air purifying		Atmosphere supplying	
Question number*	Medical criteria	Full	Half	Inhalation	Powered	Tank	Air-line
	Anatomic Factors						
2	Facial hair—beards, sideburns, growth stubble	X	X	X		X	X
2	Prominent cheekbones, depressed cheeks or temples	X	X	X		X	X
2	Deep skinfolds, creases, or scars	X	X	X		X	X
2	Abnormal chin configuration	X	X	X		X	X
2	Dentures Full or partial Worn at work?	X	X	X		X	X
	Vision correction						
2	Eyeglasses	X		X		X	X
4	Contact lenses	X	X	X	X	X	X
2	Facial deformity or surgical resection of supporting tissue or bone	X	X	X		X	X
2	Irregular skin surface, such as healed acne scarring	X	X	X		X	X
	Facial palsy						
2	Asymmetry	X	X	X		X	X
3	Decreased skin sensation						
4	History of contact dermatitis from mask materials	X	X	X	X	X	X
2	Tympanic membrane perforation	X	X	X	X	X	X
3	Impaired olfactory sense	X	X	X	X	X	X
1	Impaired range of motion or dexterity in use of upper extremities	X	X	X	X	X	X
	Physiologic Factors						
	Cardiovascular disease						
4	Angina					X	X
4	Severe or uncontrolled hypertension	X	X	X		X	X
4	History of myocardial infarction	X	X	X		X	X
	Pulmonary disease						
4	Chronic obstructive pulmonary disease	X	X	X		X	X
4	Asthma	X	X	X		X	X
4	History of pneumothorax			X			
	Pneumoconiosis	X	X	X		X	X
4	Profuse perspiration	X	X	X	X	X	X
	Personal habits						
2,4	Tobacco or gum chewing						
2,4	Expectoration						
2,4	Nose blowing						
2,4	Scratching						
2,4	Allergic rhinitis or rhinorrhea	X	X	X	X	X	X
4	Miscellaneous limiting conditions such as convulsive disorders, diabetes, etc.	X	X	X	X	X	X
	Psychological factors						
4	History of claustrophobia, vague complaints of mask discomfort, anxiety	X	X	X	X	X	X

*Question numbers refer to the four questions listed on p. 419.

are available for fitting in the mask, but are not satisfactory. Further, the bridge of the spectacle frame may interfere with the nosepiece of the half-face mask.

Facial deformity or surgical resection of supporting tissue or bone: As with prominent cheekbones, above.

Irregular skin surface: As with prominent cheekbones, above.

Facial palsy: The problem is dual, in that the resultant asymmetry may not permit a good seal, particularly with speaking or change in expression, and the user may not have tactile awareness of seal failure on the affected side.

Contact dermatitis from mask material: If determined by history, effort should be made to find a nonoffending brand. If none is available, the worker should be excluded from respirator use.

Tympanic membrane perforation: There is a risk of inspiration through the perforation. A respirator may be worn if a completing occluding ear-protective device is used. The worker must be monitored for compliance. If the insert fails, the worker should not be required to use a respirator.

Impaired olfactory sense: The worker would be unable to detect a seal or respirator failure in the case of substances whose presence is normally detected by smell.

Impaired range of motion or dexterity in use of upper extremities: The worker would be unable properly to fit the respirator, contraindicating the use of all respirators.

Cardiovascular disease: Angina contraindicates the use of equipment requiring tanks or air lines, but inhalation respirators can be considered. Severe hypertension or a recent myocardial infarction also would contraindicate the use of all devices except powered air-purifying respirators.

Pulmonary disease: Workers with significant disease must be exempted from use, particularly if the work involves contact with fibrogenic dusts. Persons with mild to moderate disease—forced expiratory volume to forced vital capacity ratio (FEV/FVC) greater than 50 percent—might be permitted use, particularly individuals who have been reasonably comfortable with a respirator in the past despite diminished lung function. A history of pneumothorax may not be important, since inhalation negative pressures are probably not significant, even with increased exertion and loaded filters.

Profuse perspiration: The discomfort resulting tends to discourage respirator use. Further, the wearer may be tempted to remove the mask momentarily in a hazardous atmosphere in order to dry off.

Personal habits: Chewing movements may compromise the seal. Persons who expectorate frequently may remove the mask, thus endangering themselves. Workers with these habits must be monitored.

Allergic rhinitis or rhinorrhea: The worker is uncomfortable with a mask and may remove it periodically.

Miscellaneous limiting conditions: If a worker with a convulsive disorder or diabetes is in poor control, there is risk of collapse in a hazardous environment.

Claustrophobia: A worker with a history of such fear of confinement may find it impossible to wear a respirator for a prolonged period. This factor alone is of extreme importance and should not be deprecated.

The physician must evaluate three elements—the worker, the work, and the respirator. It is difficult to establish immutable criteria, for a disease state is neither fixed nor equal in intensity among all workers, and workers vary in their ability to function with what might be an individual impediment. Also, some persons may become anxious because of a diminished capacity in communication. No one should be deprived of employment because of the mandated use of respiratory protection, and workers who cannot use a respirator should undergo placement in a job not requiring this form of personal device. Concerned and perceptive judgment is required of the clinician asked to evaluate the worker.

FIT-TESTING

As the fitting of respirators to prospective users usually is conducted concurrently with a preplacement medical examination, it is important that OHS physicians and nurses be familiar with devices used in industrial respiratory protection. While for some decades the Bureau of Mines tested and approved a great variety of respirators, presently the Testing and Certification Board (TCB), Division of Safety Research, NIOSH, in Morgantown, West Virginia,* was established to assure users that certain devices and instruments used for the control and evaluation of occupational hazards met certain minimum performance requirements needed to protect the health and safety of workers. The functions of the TCB include (1) the publication of certification requirements; (2) the testing and certification of products or

*Located at 944 Chestnut Ridge Road, Morgantown, WV 26505. An approved device will carry a legend reading: NIOSH/MSHA Approval No. TC ____. In many jurisdictions it is illegal for an employer to allow a worker to use a respirator that has not been approved by NIOSH.

devices meeting those requirements; (3) the publication of lists of certified products; (4) the survey of manufacturers' plants to determine the acceptability of their quality assurance programs; (5) the sampling of products from the open market and the testing of them for continued conformance to certification requirements; and (6) the conduct of research in the development of new test methods and requirements for product improvement, where necessary for the assurance of worker protection [53]. Devices that are certified are listed in *NIOSH Certified Equipment List,* published periodically.

To ensure the maximum amount of respiratory protection, approved respirators will be selected, fitted, used, and maintained in accordance with the provisions of the American National Standard Practices for Respiratory Protection (ANSI) Z 88.2-1980, American National Standards Institute. The devices that are certified include the following:

- Atmosphere-supplying respirators
  - Self-contained breathing apparatus (SCBA)
    - Closed-circuit SCBA
      - Compressed or liquid-oxygen type
      - Oxygen-generating type
    - Open-circuit SCBA
      - Demand type
      - Pressure-demand type
  - Supplied-air respirators
    - Hose mask
      - Hose mask with blower
      - Hose mask without blower
    - Air-line respirator
      - Continuous-flow class
      - Demand type
      - Pressure-demand type
    - Combination air-line respirators with auxiliary self-contained air supply
- Air-purifying respirators
  - Vapor and gas-removing respirators
  - Particulate-removing respirators
  - Combination particulate, vapor, and gas-removing respirators
- Combination atmosphere-supplying and air-purifying respirators

It must be indicated early that personal protective devices such as respirators are *not* a substitute for engineering control in hazard elimination. There are several drawbacks: (1) Respirator use does nothing to reduce or eliminate the hazard; (2) their failure in use leads to an immediate exposure to the hazard; and (3) respirators may become ineffective without the user's awareness of the change. Only when it is infeasible to provide engineering controls is it necessary to protect the worker by means of a respirator from contact with a variety of airborne and respirable toxic materials.

Several qualitative tests can be performed to ensure fitting of the respirator to the individual worker. The fitting of the device is only part of a training program mandated by OSHA that required, irrespective of circumstances, an opportunity to handle the respirator, proper fitting, a test of facepiece-to-face seal, and a long familiarizing period of wear in normal air. The requirements originate in ANSI Standard Z88.2-1980, with details given in section 7.4.

For details regarding respirator fitting tests, reference can be made to a NIOSH technical report, *A Guide to Industrial Respiratory Protection,* by John A. Pritchard of the Los Alamos Scientific Laboratory, published in June 1976, wherein both qualitative and quantitative testing are discussed.

The qualitative tests are generally adequate for determining the fit of a respirator before entering a hostile atmosphere. They are easily completed, are not time-consuming, and require only a modest amount of equipment. For the testing of respirators at the time of *initial* selection of a brand that fits best, the quantitative fitting tests are preferred and are mandatory in keeping with the lead and arsenic standards. Also, the Nuclear Regulatory Commission requires quantitative fit tests for respirators used as protection against radionuclides. The details are available in the NIOSH document by Pritchard.

Occupational health personnel should know of the quality of the respirator maintenance program, although the function normally is one undertaken either by the industrial safety staff or by tool crib personnel at points of respirator issue. The program includes inspection for defects, including leak check, cleaning, disinfection, repair, and storage. A poorly maintained or cleaned group of respirators will lead only to nonuse or limited use, with the associated potential of hazardous exposure. While many blue-collar workers will tolerate considerable occupational soil of their clothing or skin, they will be extremely wary of a respirator that they believe has been worn by another employee and that has not been restored to a near-immaculate state.

In keeping with OSHA requirements (1910.34), it is stated that "after inspection, cleaning, and necessary repair, respirators shall be stored to protect against dust, sunlight, heat, extreme cold, excessive moisture, or damaging chemicals. . . . Routinely used respirators may be placed in paper bags." Complete cleaning systems for respirators are commercially available.

In summary, as provided by OSHA [54], the minimal acceptable requirements for a respiratory program are as follows:

Written standard operating procedures governing the selection and use of respirators shall be established.
Respirators shall be selected on the basis of hazards to which the worker is exposed.
The user shall be instructed and trained in the proper use of respirators and their limitations.
Where practicable, the respirators should be assigned to individual workers for their exclusive use.
Respirators shall be regularly cleaned and disinfected. The devices issued for the exclusive use of one worker should be cleaned after each day's use, or more often if necessary, and the respirators used by more than one worker shall be thoroughly cleaned and disinfected after each use.
Respirators shall be stored in a convenient, clean, and sanitary location.
Respirators used routinely shall be inspected during cleaning. Worn or deteriorated parts shall be replaced. Respirators for emergency use such as self-contained devices shall be thoroughly inspected at least once a month and after each use.
Appropriate surveillance of work area conditions and degree of employee exposures or stress shall be maintained.
There shall be regular inspection and evaluation to determine the continued effectiveness of the program.
Persons should not be assigned to tasks requiring use of respirators unless it has been determined that they are physically able to perform the work and use the equipment. The local physician shall determine what health and physical conditions are pertinent. The respirator user's medical status should be reviewed periodically (for instance, annually).
Approved or accepted respirators shall be issued when they are available. The respirator furnished shall provide adequate respiratory protection against a particular hazard for which it is designed in accordance with standards established by competent authorities.

Selection of Respirators

It is necessary, of course, that only certified respirators be used, as listed by NIOSH in its periodic publication [53]. The list covers all types of self-contained breathing apparatus, gas masks, and respirators and provides for each device the following information:

Approval number
Manufacturer (to whom approval issued)
Model number(s)
Respirator type
Facepiece type
Number of cartridges
Type of respiratory protection (for example, organic vapor, chlorine, sulfur dioxide, hydrogen chloride, ammonia, methyl amine, dusts, metal fume, radon daughters, asbestos-containing dusts and mists, abrasive blasting, pesticides)

Facial Hair: Effects on Respirator Use

As indicated, a problem in the use of respirators has arisen with the increased and persisting custom of wearing moustaches and beards. With the freedom felt by nearly all persons in their selection of hairstyle, clothing, and use of various adornments, any regulation regarding facial hair will be viewed as an infringement of personal rights. However, experience has demonstrated the difficulty in fitting respirators on workers who are not clean-shaven.

To study the issue, Skretvedt and Loschiavo [55], at two DuPont plants, fit-tested 37 male employees, who were tested both qualitatively and quantitatively. Of the group, 67 had fully grown beards of varying lengths, shape, density, and texture. The bearded subjects consistently failed the protocol of qualitative fit-testing. On the quantitative test procedure using half-mask respirators, the bearded workers had a median fit factor of 12 (8-percent leakage).* In contrast, clean-shaven employees demonstrated a median fit factor of 2950 (0.03-percent leakage). Bearded subjects manifested an average 246-fold drop in protection. With full-facepiece respirators, the bearded men showed a median fit factor of 30 (3 percent), while with the same device on clean-shaven subjects, the median fit factor was 10,000 (0.01 percent). It was concluded that the presence of a beard greatly increases the leakage through the face seal of the respirator and that such leakage should not be permitted when workers are required to wear respirators. The caveat is given greater strength in the current ANSI Standard Z88.2-1980 (section 3.58), which states, "A respirator equipped with a facepiece shall not be worn if facial hair interferes with valve function." In another section (7.31) in the same standard: "A person who has hair (stubble, moustache, sideburns, beard, low hairline, bangs) which passes between the face and the sealing surface of the facepiece of the respirator shall not be permitted to wear such type of respirator."

In other experiments, it was shown that only a 2-day's growth of beard decreases the protection of a

*A fit factor of 1 indicates that a respirator is providing no protection.

respirator by about 50 percent, and a growth of 8 days reduces it nearly to zero because of the loss of pressure inside the facepiece caused by the facial hair. In one jurisdiction (California's General Industry Safety Order 5144—Title 8, California Administrative Code), it is stated specifically, "Respirators shall be inspected before each use and shall not be worn when conditions prevent a good gas-tight face seal" [56]. There should be periodic retesting in all users, bearded or not. In one other study relating to test-fitting it was demonstrated among clean-shaven users that, with the passage of time, better respirator fits were obtained, indicating, perhaps, that time allowed more experience in the use of the device [57].

The issue of enforced shaving has been tested in the courts. A machinist, a Sikh, who had been working for a petroleum company in California for several years, claimed that he could not abide by the new company policy that required shaving by respirator users [58]. His religious beliefs prohibited the shaving of any body hair. An effort was made to find a job equivalent in pay to that of a machinist and that did not require wearing a respirator. None could be found, so the worker accepted a transfer to a janitorial job that paid 17-percent less than the original position.

The trial court found that the employer had in good faith tried to accommodate the religious belief but that further accommodation would have caused the company undue hardship. Three coworkers who refused to abide by the shaving requirements were terminated, and the plaintiff was suspended, but each was offered an alternative position. A promise was made that if a respirator were developed that would prove safe for his use, he would be returned to his job. The policy was adopted by the company to come into compliance with CAL/OSHA standards, and if the plaintiff worked without protection, the company would have risked liability for violation of the standard.

Holt [59], after discussing suits involving alleged discrimination because of facial hair rules, cautioned that employers reviewing or preparing a no-beard policy should ensure that it is

Justifiable and reasonable.
Properly worded.
Adequately posted and that employees are notified by letter.
Considerate of religious dictates.
Part of a well-managed, comprehensive respirator program.
Enforced consistently and not arbitrarily.

Single-Use Respirators

While dust or dust/mist (half-mask) disposable respirators are usually selected and distributed through channels other than the OHS in a plant, it should be known that some employees erringly will use them as protection against a variety of extremely toxic substances. The one-time-use respirator is approved only for protection against dusts and mists with a permissible exposure limit (PEL) of not less than 0.05 mg/M^3, including asbestos. These devices are of light weight and can be contoured to the structures of the face. Breathing and communication are readily conducted.

A knowledge of the limitations of use of such respirators is mandatory. Irrespective of the length of exposure time or the concentration of the material, there are innumerable toxic substances that contraindicate the use of this type of respirator. For such a listing see *3M Brand Gas and Vapor Respirators—Reference and Selection Guide.**

It must be pointed out, in closing the discussion of respirator use, that the Board of Directors of the American Conference of Governmental Industrial Hygienists (ACGIH) [60], on behalf of its professional industrial hygiene members, unanimously endorsed continuation of the current OSHA policy to require employers to use feasible engineering controls, work practices, and administrative controls to prevent employee exposures above permissible levels. In endorsing engineering controls as the preferred mode, it was indicated that personal protective equipment, including respirators, may be used as alternatives only when other methods were not adequate, were not feasible, or had not as yet been installed. The membership agreed with the board's resolution, and a letter went forward on May 31, 1983 to the OSHA Docket Officer, over the signature of Morton Corn, Ph.D., former Assistant Secretary of Labor (OSHA).

MEDICATIONS AND SAFETY

As innumerable employees have been prescribed medications, usually without specific inquiry as to the functions or physical requirements of the patient's job, it is wise periodically to review the drugs currently being used. This evaluation can be conducted during any visit of an employee to the OHS. While the question regarding prescribed medicines is commonly included in the history questionnaire por-

*Available from Occupational Health and Safety Products Division/3M, St. Paul, MN.

tion of a preplacement examination protocol, there is seldom a follow-up in later work years.

Workers' age, screening discovering treatable chronic disorders, tensions appearing in the domestic or work settings, and reversing therapeutic regimens are outlined by workers' personal physicians. It is wise, therefore, to know if beta-blockade has been instituted, if antihistamines are used with frequency, if tranquilizers (major or minor) are depended on, or if any prescribed medicament is being taken that in any way may affect wakefulness, equilibrium, mentation, vision, other psychomotor performance, or even intellectual capability.

When there is admission of medication use by ingestion, inhalation, or even injection or transdermal absorption, a notation should be entered in the employee's record, including the counsel given regarding precautions or job modifications. What might be safe utilization of therapy at home could easily become imprudent or hazardous at work. Package inserts challenge the comprehension of most lay people, and the occupational physician or nurse can be practicing a large quantum of preventive care by investigating both medication practices and specific sensitive responses to drugs.

SAFETY OFF THE JOB

OHS personnel can be highly effective in assisting an employee who is experiencing a number of accidentally incurred injuries at home, while engaged in construction, repair, hobbies, recreation, or driving. As such episodes may, and frequently do, lead to worktime lost, scrutiny of the medical record and frank discussions with the employee may bring to light causative behavior of which there might be no awareness.

Many companies have instituted off-the-job safety programs because the injuries sustained are costly—health insurance payments, downtime, substitute workers, disability pay and so on—and are disruptive to both the production protocol and fellow workers. The OHS can participate in such programs through health education and counseling efforts.

HEARING CONSERVATION

That noise as a problem to humans is not new is given substantiation in the decree issued by Julius Caesar in 44 B.C. that ordered, "Hence forward, no wheeled vehicles whatsoever will be allowed within the precincts of the city from sunrise until the hour before dusk. Those which shall have entered during the night and are still within the city at dawn must halt and stand empty until the appointed hour." [61]. Even Ramazzini, in his discourse on the diseases of coppersmiths, commented on work-area noise as being productive of hearing loss and recommended the use of cotton in the ear canals [62]. One of the earliest efforts at mass audiometry was the testing conducted of nearly 35,000 persons by the Bell System at the New York and San Francisco World Fairs [63].

With the first work claims of noise-induced hearing loss generated in the years following World War II, the attention of both legislators and workers' compensation administrators was directed to a new occupational illness rarely scheduled in existing state acts.

LEGISLATIVE BACKGROUND

Prior to the 1970 passage of the Noise Pollution and Abatement Act of 1970 (Title IV of Public Law 91-604), the position had been taken that noise abatement was either a local or state concern, with certain exceptions involving occupational health, noise associated with aviation, and, to a lesser extent, highway transportation. Before the passage of the Occupational Safety and Health Act in 1970, the only controls enforceable by the federal government over workplace noise were those requirements spelled out in the standards of the Walsh-Healy Act, involving solely places of work holding contracts with the United States government. The 1970 enactment extended to virtually all industrial establishments the mandate for protection of workers' hearing from noise [64].

The passage of the Noise Control Act in 1972 gave to EPA the task of identifying and regulating the manufacture of consumer products that account for a significant amount of the noise produced in this country. This action led to maximum limitations on the noise levels produced by trucks, buses, air compressors, motorcycles, and other machine sources. In short, the act applied to community noise.

Following hearings held by the Subcommittee on Resource Protection—conducted because Congressional attention had been directed more toward other aspects of the environment—the 1972 statute was amended, and The Quiet Communities Act was passed and signed into law in late 1978. The bill increased financial and technical assistance to the states and local communities, emphasizing noise reduction around airports and highways [61].

By early 1981, the Hearing Conservation Amendment to the Occupational Safety and Health Act was promulgated [65], which covers all employees except persons engaged in construction or agriculture. Later that year there was a partial lifting of the administrative stay, and the effective date was deferred to allow time for evaluation of many requests for clarification and petitions for stay [66]. Eventually, the final rule became effective April 7, 1983, and the baseline audiograms mandated by the amendment had to be completed by March 1, 1984 [67,68]. However, in a suit brought by the Forging Industry Association against the Secretary of Labor [67,68], the U.S. Court of Appeals for the Fourth Circuit struck down the amendment. The appellate court determined that OSHA had "exceeded its authority by adopting a rule which required employers to protect their workers from hearing loss that could be caused by noise sources outside the workplace" [69]. The decision has no direct effect on compliance with state noise standards.

In spite of the decision, OSHA has been enforcing the Hearing Conservation Amendment, and rehearings are being sought [69]. The amendment and its requirements are cited in the material that follows because it is believed that the decision will be reversed eventually and because the content of the standard composes a rational and complete hearing conservation program, which can serve as the model for worker protection against the particular hazard of noise at the place of employment.

CURRENT HEARING CONSERVATION MANDATE

The Hearing Conservation Amendment comprises the following primary required components: monitoring, audiometric testing, audiogram evaluation, hearing protectors, training, and recordkeeping. Some of the details follow [70].

MONITORING

The Hearing Conservation Amendment requires employers to monitor noise exposure levels in a manner that will accurately identify employees who are exposed to noise at or above 85 decibels (dB) averaged over 8 working hours, called an 8-hour time-weighted average (TWA). The exposure measurement must include all noise within an 80 to 130 dB range and must be taken during a typical work situation. This requirement is performance-oriented, since it allows employers to choose the monitoring method that best suits each individual situation.

Under the revised amendment, employees are entitled to observe monitoring procedures, and they must be notified of the results of the exposure monitoring of their workplace. The method used to notify employees is left to the discretion of the employers.

Instruments used for monitoring employee exposures must be carefully checked or calibrated to ensure that the measurements are accurate. Calibration procedures are unique to specific instruments. Employers have the duty to ensure that the measuring instruments they are using are properly calibrated. They may find it useful to follow the manufacturer's instructions to determine when and how extensively to calibrate.

AUDIOMETRIC TESTING

Audiometric testing not only monitors the acuity of an employee's hearing over time, but also provides an opportunity for employers to educate employees about their hearing and the need to protect it. The important elements of an audiometric testing program include baseline audiograms, annual audiograms, training, and follow-up procedures. Audiometric testing must be made available to all employees who have average exposure levels over an 8-hour period of 85 dB. And the audiometric testing program follow-up should indicate whether hearing loss is being prevented by the employer's hearing conservation program. A professional audiologist, an otolaryngologist, or a physician must be responsible for the program. Both professionals and trained technicians may conduct audiometric testing. The professional does not have to be present when a qualified technician is conducting testing, however. The professional responsibilities include oversight of the program and the work of the technicians, review of problem audiograms, and the determinations as to whether referral is necessary.

There are two types of audiograms required in the hearing conservation program: baseline and annual audiograms.

Baseline Audiograms

The baseline audiogram is the reference audiogram against which future audiograms are compared. Baseline audiograms must be provided within 6 months of an employee's first exposure at or above an 8-hour TWA of 85 dB. Where employers are using mobile test vans to obtain audiograms, baseline audiograms must be completed within 1 year after an employee's first exposure to workplace noise at or above a TWA of 85 dB. Where mobile vans are used and employers are allowed to delay baseline testing for up to a year, after 6 months their employees exposed at or above 85 dB must be issued and fitted with hearing protectors to be worn until the baseline audiogram is obtained.

Testing to establish a baseline audiogram shall be preceded by at least 14 hours without exposure to workplace noise. (Hearing protectors may be worn to meet this requirement.)

Baseline audiograms taken before the effective date of the amendment are acceptable baselines in the program if the professional supervisor determines that the audiogram is valid.

Annual Audiograms

The annual audiograms must be conducted within 1 year of the baseline. It is important to test hearing on an annual basis to identify changes in hearing ability so that protective follow-up measures can be initiated before hearing loss progresses. Annual audiograms must be compared with baseline audiograms to determine whether the audiogram is accurate and to determine whether the employee has lost hearing ability (that is, if a standard threshold shift [STS] has occurred). STS is defined in the amendment as an average shift in either ear of 10 dB or more at 2000, 3000, and 4000 Hz. An averaging method of determining STS was chosen because it diminishes the number of persons falsely identified as having STS who are later shown not to have had a change in hearing ability. Annual testing may be conducted at any time during the work shift.

AUDIOGRAM EVALUATION

If an STS is identified, employees must be fitted or refitted with adequate hearing protectors, shown how to use them, and required to wear them. Employees must be notified within 21 days from the time the determination is made that their audiometric test results showed an STS. Some employees with an STS may need to be referred for further testing if the professional determines that their test results are questionable or if they have an ear problem of a medical nature that is thought to be caused or aggravated by wearing hearing protectors. If the suspected medical problem is not thought to be related to wearing protectors, employees must be informed that they should see a physician. If subsequent audiometric tests show that the STS identified on a previous audiogram is not persistent, employees whose exposure to noise is less than a TWA of 90 dB may discontinue the wearing of hearing protectors.

A subsequent audiogram may be substituted for the original baseline audiogram if the professional supervising the program determines that the employee's STS is persistent. This substitution will ensure that the same shift is not repeatedly identified. The professional may also decide to revise the baseline audiogram if an improvement in hearing has occurred, which will ensure that the baseline reflects actual hearing thresholds to the extent possible.

HEARING PROTECTORS

Hearing protectors must be available to all workers exposed to 8-hour TWA noise levels of 85 dB or above. This requirement will ensure that employees have access to protectors before they experience a loss in hearing. Hearing protectors must be worn by (1) employees for any period exceeding 6 months from the time they are first exposed to 8-hour average noise levels of 85 dB or above until they receive their baseline audiograms in situations where baseline audiograms are delayed because it is inconvenient for mobile test vans to visit the workplace more than once a year; (2) employees who have incurred STSs, since these workers have demonstrated that they are susceptible to noise; and (3) employees exposed over the permissible exposure level, an 8-hour TWA of 90 dB or above.

Employees should decide, with the help of a person who is trained in fitting hearing protectors, which size and type of protector is most suitable for their working environment. The protector selected should be comfortable to wear and offer sufficient attenuation to prevent hearing loss.

Hearing protectors must reduce adequately the severity of the noise level for each employee's work environment. The employer must reevaluate the suitability of the employee's present protector whenever there is a change in working conditions that may cause the hearing protector being used to be inadequate. If workplace noise levels increase, employees must be given more effective protectors. The protector must reduce employee exposures to at least 90 dB and to 85 dB when an STS has already occurred in the worker's hearing. Employees must be shown how to use and care for their protectors and must be supervised on the job to ensure that they continue to wear them correctly.

TRAINING

Employee training is extremely important. When workers understand the reasons for the hearing conservation program's requirements and the need to protect their hearing, they will be better motivated to participate actively in the program and to cooperate by wearing their protectors and taking audiometric tests. Employees exposed to TWAs of 85 dB and above must be trained at least annually in the effects of noise, the purpose, advantages, and disadvantages of various types of hearing protectors; the selection, fitting, and care of protectors; and the purpose and procedures of audiometric testing. The training program may be structured in any format, different parts being conducted by different individuals and at different times, as long as the required topics are covered.

RECORDKEEPING

Noise-exposure measurement records must be kept for 2 years. Records of audiometric test results must be maintained for the duration of employment of the affected employee. Audiometric test records must include the name and job classification of the employee, the date, the examiner's name, the date of acoustic or exhaustive calibration, measurements of the background sound pressure levels in audiometric test rooms, and the employee's most recent noise exposure measurement.

Although no method or timetable is mandated for the retention of sound-room certification and audiometer calibration records, it is advised that they be retained. In a litigious society one cannot predict the need for a particular document.

ADDITIONAL DETAILS

Some additional clarification [66] of the Hearing Conservation Amendment may be helpful.

Cost

The program shall be provided at no cost to employees. The total cost of the hearing conservation program as outlined in the amendment was estimated to be $254 million per year, or $53 per worker per year.

Audiometric Testing

Technician. The technician performing the testing must be certified by the Council of Accreditation in Occupational Hearing Conservation (CAOHC) or must have demonstrated satisfactorily competence in administering audiometric examinations, obtaining valid audiograms, and properly using, maintaining, and calibrating audiometers. The technician must be responsible to an audiologist, an otolaryngologist, or qualified physician, as indicated previously. A technician who operates microprocessor audiometers does not need to be certified.

Instruments. In the event that pulsed-tone audiometers are used, they shall have a tone on-time of at least 200 milliseconds.

Self-recording audiometers shall comply with the following requirements:

1. The chart on which the audiogram is traced shall have lines at positions corresponding to all multiples of 10-dB hearing level within the intensity range spanned by the audiometer. The lines shall be equally spaced and shall be separated by at least ¼ inch. Additional increments are optional. The audiogram pen tracings shall not exceed 2 dB in width.
2. It shall be possible to set the stylus manually at the 10-dB increment lines for calibration purposes.
3. The slewing rate for the audiometer attenuator shall not be more than 6 dB/sec, except that an initial slewing rate greater than 6 dB/sec is permitted at the beginning of each new test frequency, but only until the second subject response.
4. The audiometer shall remain at each required test frequency for 30 seconds (± 3 seconds). The audiogram shall be clearly marked at each change of frequency and the actual frequency change of the audiometer shall not deviate from the frequency boundaries marked on the audiogram by more than ± 3 seconds.
5. It must be possible at each test frequency to place a horizontal line segment parallel to the time axis on the audiogram, such that the audiometric tracing crosses the line segment at least six times at that test frequency. At each test frequency the threshold shall be the average of the midpoints of the tracing excursions.

Test Rooms. Rooms used for audiometric testing shall not have background sound pressure levels exceeding the following:

Octave-band center frequency (Hz)	500	1000	2000	4000	8000
Sound pressure level (dB)	40	40	47	57	62

The measuring equipment must conform at least to the type 2 requirements of the American National Standard Specification for Sound Level Meters, S1.4-1971 (R1976) and to the class II requirements of the American National Standard Specification for Octave, Half-Octave, and Third-Octave Band Filter Sets, S1.11-1971 (R1976).

Biologic and Acoustic Calibration of Audiometers. Before operation each day, the audiometer should be checked for functional accuracy by testing a person with known, stable hearing thresholds and by listening to the output of the instrument to ensure freedom from distortion or unwanted sounds. Audiometer calibration shall be checked acoustically, at least annually.

Age Corrections in Audiograms. If it is desired, and the procedure is *not* mandatory, to correct an audiogram so that the contribution of aging to the change in hearing level can be accounted for, the procedure and age correction tables to be used may be found in the NIOSH Criteria Document titled, *Criteria for a Recommended Standard . . . Occupational Exposure to Noise.*

Miscellaneous Notes

While the Hearing Conservation Amendment solidified guidelines regarding the protection of workers' hearing, there has been voiced opposition because of either the cost or the permissiveness. One of the primary objections has been directed toward the use of ear protectors in place of the installation of engineering controls at the point source of noise generation [71]. The amendment allows area monitoring, the employers being allowed to choose the method best for their particular situation. But such monitoring is not always appropriate; personal monitors should be used if area samples prove inadequate. In settings where workers are highly mobile, where tasks are dissimilar, when a large component of impulsive sound is contained in the exposure, or where there is considerable variation in the sound level, area monitoring is more difficult and not befitting desired accuracy [71]. Training requirements spelled out in earlier versions have been revoked, the minimum standards now calling for training of employees exposed at or above the action level in the (1) effects of noise; (2) purpose, advantages, disadvantages, and amount of noise reduction of various protectors; (3) selection, fitting, and care of ear protectors; and (4) purpose and procedures of audiometric testing.

PROGRAM ELEMENTS

Even though the Hearing Conservation Amendment provides the detail needed in the institution and operation of a hearing conservation program, certain segments can bear elaboration. The American Occupational Medical Association (AOMA), through its Noise and Hearing Conservation Committee, comprising experts in otology and industrial audiology, published guidelines for the conduct of a hearing conservation program [72]. Five elements compose the program, specifically measurement of the exposure, use of hearing protection, audiometric testing, education and training, and assessment of program effectiveness. In essence, the guidelines were paralleled, but in greater length, by the Hearing Conservation Amendment.

MEASUREMENT OF THE EXPOSURE

While the environmental measurement is ordinarily a function of the industrial hygienist, the physician must be aware of the technical aspects and validity of sound evaluation. Exposure to noise may be measured by use of an audiodosimeter or by a sound level meter (SLM). Verification of the results obtained by the audiodosimeter can be accomplished by means of the SLM. The instrument requires calibration before and after each reading, and there must be a permanent record made of all data. The microphone must be placed in the employee's so-called hearing zone, which has been defined as a 2-foot diameter sphere surrounding the worker's head. For organizations desiring hard-copy records of sound levels, AC line or battery-powered strip-chart recording instruments are available for use with a SLM that will provide records for permanent filing. When noise is to be analyzed in detail, a magnetic tape recorder can be used. Multichannel recorders are utilized frequently, linked to a number of analyzers, to allow study of measurements made at different locations [73].

The personal audiodosimeter will indicate the time-weighted exposure to noise above a predetermined limit, usually at about 85 dBA (decibels using the correction factor from the "A" weighing network, which brings the dB reading to the sound level approximating the responses of the ear). Exchange rates are specified, permitting an increase in intensity if there is a reduction in exposure time; for example, a typical exchange rate would be between 3 and 5 dBA for a 50-percent reduction in exposure length [73]. The personal dosimeter is worn by the worker not restricted to confined areas, such as airport ramp employees or personnel who move about in chemical plants. Many dosimeters are equipped with alarm systems, which register when a cumulative exposure has exceeded an established threshold or when an instantaneous sound level reaches a danger point, such as 115 dBA. These devices are portable, lightweight, and battery-powered and will show actual cumulative doses or a percentage of a determined limit.

Whereas the original personal audiodosimeter employed a memory cell that recorded and stored noise exposure information and at day's end required removal of the cell and readout by a desktop device, the current model uses microprocessor electronics and a hybrid random access memory (RAM). The instrument, still small and portable, functions as a 24-hour data logger and records, in 1-minute increments, the average sound level for the full 24 hours of operation. The data are accessed either through a printout or a computer interface and a desktop computer of several choices. Once accessed, the data allow construction of the time history profile and sound level histogram. A built-in liquid crystal display permits immediate availability of information, the operating time in hours and minutes, the time when the maximum level has occurred, and the time when the first greater than 115-dB event has taken place. The dosimeter can also function as a SLM.

USE OF HEARING PROTECTION

Although hearing protectors (sometimes referred to as ear defenders or, more colloquially, earplugs when insertable) have been employed for decades, at times with exactitude in fitting and at times with gross ear/device mismatching, insufficient attention has been given their dispensing or their care and use. There are several varieties of aural, supra-aural, circumaural, and enclosure devices to be selected for wear by all employees regularly exposed to worksite noise at levels and durations shown to be detrimental to hearing. The reference standard in attenuation is ANSIS12.6-1984, "Method for the Measurement of the Real-Ear Attenuation of Hearing Protectors."

Before fitting and issue of protectors, a history should be obtained of auditory problems such as infections, otorrhea, excessive ceruminosis, or previous difficulty in the use of these devices. An otoscopic examination should be carried out to determine the existence of any disorder contraindicating the use of such aids. Because of the availability of both disposable and permanently issued varieties, there are few clinical conditions that would preclude the use of one of the many types in common usage. There are advantages and disadvantages among the various protectors, and the choice may rest with the kind of exposure. For example, inserts are generally more protective against high frequencies, while muffs defend the wearer more effectively against low frequencies of sound. Programs more likely will succeed when the worker is given a personal choice of the device to be worn [72].

Always to be remembered is the temporary nature or expedient of personal hearing protective devices (PHPDs), engineering methods or devices being consistently the choice in hazard control.

*AURAL DEVICES**

These protectors fit into the external auditory canal and remain in situ without additional support, and as protective efficiencies were indicated previously, their specifications may include 40 dB attenuated at 4000 Hz, but only 15 dB below 1000 Hz. The types available are formable, which are disposable; preformed, which are reusable; and custom-molded. Irrespective of the kind of protector used, the instructions provided by the manufacturer must be followed.

Formable Protectors

Because they are made of pliable material that can be inserted, formable protectors conform to the configuration of the external auditory canal without requiring individual fitting or sizing of the device. The fact that they are considered disposable implies that once used they should be removed and discarded. With each new exposure, a new pair should be used; thus, a worker may use several sets in a day, requiring a plentiful stock on hand. They are made of a wax-impregnated cotton and are individually packaged, and both they and the hands of the user must be clean before insertion. It is claimed that by filtering out the higher frequencies, normal speech and desirable sound—warning signals, for example—can be heard readily. A second variety of individually packaged protectors is made of a polymeric foam and requires compression before placement in the canal. Through expansion, or return to the precompression state, it will conform to the unique structure of the individual's external auditory canal. Some reuse of this device is possible.

An earlier product, bulk-produced and available as a pocket pack or from a dispenser, is eardown, or acoustic wool. While resembling cotton, it should not be considered the same, for it has the advantage of sound attenuation and allows air and moisture to pass through, obviating any sense of pressure or vacuum. It has been suggested by manufacturers that if dispensers are used, that they be placed in time-clock areas, at locker room exits, at every entrance to a noise area, and throughout operating areas to maximize their availability and to increase compliance with the ear-protection segment of the hearing conservation program. One dispenser is recommended for every 25 to 30 workers.

Preformed Protectors

Preformed aural inserts are fabricated usually of soft silicone or other plastic material and are produced in different configurations. The so-called individually fit protector is available in a range of five sizes, and the different-size inserts are usually color-coded and are marked for ready identification. Often, a small finger-graspable projection is attached to the protector to facilitate insertion. Nearly every manufacturer of the "individually fit" aural inserts has available fitting devices (to measure size) with spherical simulators of the inserts in the five sizes mentioned previously.

These protectors are available also as a corded device, which not only precludes losing one of the two

*Much of this material is taken from Mellard and Geier [74].

inserts but also makes on-the-job use by an employee immediately visible to the supervisor.

A second type of preformed protector allegedly fits all users, but nevertheless comes in different sizes. These inserts have two to five flanges, coursing from the smallest at the front to the largest at the back or external end. If the fit does not seem right, the wearer can snip off the flanges or discs until comfort is attained with the plug in place.

The third of this variety is the ear valve, which consists of a sound chamber embedded in soft silicone rubber. With a high-frequency impulse noise, a sensitive mechanism within the chamber closes but permits the sound of low-frequency speech to be heard. They are not advised for use in an area where noise is constant or steady state.

At one installation, small pressure-sensitive labels are issued at the time of fitting with the hearing-protective device, for placement in the hard hat. The label allows entry of the type and size of the device issued initially, and its use is recommended, for it expedites replacement of the protectors.

Custom-Molded Protectors

Custom-molded protectors are custom-fitted by trained personnel using a moldable material (a special material plus a catalyst) that is placed in the ear canal and pressed to fit the particular configuration of the employee. The material is allowed to remain in place while hardening occurs and then is removed for complete "setting." Some of the devices need a sealant or a coating. One form utilizes a dental-quality acrylic and a thermal acrylic canal. The attenuation claimed by one manufacturer varies from 34.4 dB at 1000 Hz to 41.0 dB at 8000 Hz. A variety is available that fits the canal only and not the external ear, and the two protectors are connected by a flexible cord.

SUPRA-AURAL DEVICES

Supra-aural protectors, also called canal caps, seal the ear canal without requiring insertion into the ear and thus presumably are more comfortable to wear. The caps are connected by a headband, which maintains a slight pressure to keep the caps in place. The banded caps are color-coded to distinguish the right from the left, and they can be worn with a face shield over the band over the head or below the chin, between a hard hat and a sweatband, with long hair, with a welding hood and safety glasses, or with a respirator in place. In the interest of certain users, the device can be worn without disturbing the hairdo or the cap worn on flight lines. The attenuation with canal caps ranges from 22 dB at 500 Hz to 42 dB at 8000 Hz [74].

A variation of the banded caps is a combination of safety glasses and caps with the caps affixed to the temples of the spectacle frame. When not needed, the ear pods may be swung out, away from the temple pieces, into a standby position.

CIRCUMAURAL DEVICES

Circumaural protectors are ear muffs that cover the entire external ear and are maintained in position by a padded spring headband. The muffs usually are oval-shaped, and the band can be worn over the head, behind the head, or under the chin.

To conform to the shape of the wearer's head, plastic ear seals or cushions are placed around the ear cup, and they are filled with acoustic down, foam, or a liquid. Liquid allows a more comfortable conformation to the head but may not be possible for use in extremely cold weather.

The content of the ear cup itself usually consists of material that absorbs sound, and it may be acoustical down, a foam pad, or both. In addition to being worn by means of the spring headband, the ear muffs can be mounted directly onto a safety cap (bump cap), a hard hat, or a hard hat with a face shield, or they can be worn in combination with a welding helmet/hood. Further, communication systems can be built into noise-attenuating headsets to improve communication in high-noise areas, utilizing either a telephone or a two-way radio.

ENCLOSURES

Although not used with the same frequency as other protective devices, helmets provide head protection and attenuation of high-frequency noise. Wearers object to the weight, heat, and general bulkiness of this device.

COMMENT

A summary of the advantages and disadvantages of ear inserts versus earmuffs, according to Mellard and Geier [74], are listed in Table 15-2.

Continuing educational programs are needed to maintain effective, knowing use of PHPDs.

It was believed by Berger [75] that the attenuation provided by a single PHPD might be inadequate and that double protection might be required. It is recognized that the overall attenuation offered by two protective devices is not equal to the sum of the individual attenuation of each protector because of the bone-conduction flanking paths and the acoustical-mechanical interaction between two such closely spaced devices. It was shown experimentally that double hearing protection—ear inserts plus ear muffs—may provide the additional reduction of noise needed in extremely high noise-level environments.

Riko and Alberti [76] have indicated that while

TABLE 15-2. Advantages and Disadvantages of Ear Plugs Versus Ear Muffs

	Ear plugs	*Ear muffs*
Advantages	Low initial cost Compact size Can be carried on person Easier sound localization Easily used with other equipment	Low replacement rate Easily monitored Individual fitting not critical No increase in ear infection
Disadvantages	High replacement rate Requires personal dexterity Requires otoscopic screening Increased probability of ear infections High loss rate Attenuation dependent on fit Difficult to monitor	High initial cost Bulky size and weight Increased discomfort because of headband tension Increased temperature buildup in warmer climates Ear seals deteriorate with use, decreasing attenuation Difficulty in use with other equipment

PHPDs are affordable and readily available, many questions remain regarding their effectiveness. Laboratory verification has been difficult because the human head cannot be simulated with a model in light of hair and bone effects, variations in anatomy of the ear, and bone conduction hearing. PHPDs reduce only air-conducted sound, and in practice, the reduction of sound theoretically possible is not actually achieved. The attenuation encountered in the work setting is much less than expected from the manufacturers' specifications, attributable to such reasons as acoustical degradation, poor maintenance, and misuse of the devices.

Over 400 workers were tested, using the various currently available PHPDs. Of the findings it was learned, for example, that foam-sponge inserts and flanged air-filled plugs provided good attenuation, whereas the personally molded plugs resulted in such a scatter of attenuation scores as to make them unsatisfactory for use. Problems in use were identified: inappropriate fitting, poor maintenance, and deliberate abuse of the devices. The seal between the head and a muff would be broken; the muff was not fitted over the ear; the temples of safety eyewear broke the seal; the cushion was old, and a good seal was not possible; plugs often were seated improperly or were too small; and finally, almost no one was aware that because of anatomic differences, a user might require a different size plug in each ear. The personally molded devices were in poorest condition—distorted, cracked, or trimmed.

It was found, also, that while a worker with normal hearing could relearn vital industrial sounds with the PHPDs in place and that speech discrimination was not affected, in the hearing-impaired employee, the device significantly degrades the ability to discriminate speech. If the individual was not fluent in English, the negative effect was increased 10 to 15 percent.

Riko and Alberti [76] noted further that little noise reduction takes place with protectors in the low-frequency range. The net effect of the protector on a person with a typical high-frequency noise-induced hearing loss is not only to lessen the overall level of sound getting to the ear but also to create an even greater high-frequency loss. They concluded that hearing conservation programs require these elements: enforced use of PHPDs in noise-hazardous areas; promotion of the program by a key person; communication among all staff levels, including administrators; and the availability of a variety of effective protectors. Until engineering controls become universal, the use of PHPDs can preserve hearing—but this fact must be accepted by both managers and workers and must be taught, reinforced, and supported repeatedly.

AUDIOMETRIC TESTING

As indicated previously, audiometry is a mandated element of a hearing conservation program. Several aspects deserve consideration such as the environment for audiometry, the audiometric technician, the audiometer, and recordkeeping.

The Environment for Audiometry

The Hearing Conservation Amendment requires that background sound pressure-level measurements be made at the following octave bands—500, 1000, 2000, 4000, and 8000 Hz—and that the date of measurement be recorded. For reliable audiometry the environment for testing must be quiet and nondistracting. The test environment, as indicated by Singer [77], must meet the requirements given in the ANSI 53.1-1977 "American Standard Criteria for Background Noise in Audiometer Rooms," while the required octave-band sound-pressure levels are more liberal, the suggested levels cannot exceed 27 dB at 500 Hz, 30 dB at 1000 Hz, 35 dB at 2000 Hz, 42 dB at 4000 Hz, and 41 dB at 8000 Hz.

There are limits established also for acceptable

outside noise levels for test rooms, and it is suggested [77] that a safety factor of at least 10 dB be subtracted from the attenuation data reported by the manufacturer because (1) measurements made and reported by manufacturers are obtained under extremely controlled conditions not prevalent in field-testing situations, (2) ambient noise levels fluctuate, and (3) a safety factor is considered part of good planning for continuing and future use of a test facility. The allowable outside noise levels for audiometry rooms vary, as determined by the type of room used—a single-wall room (small or large) or a double-wall room. The permissible octave band levels, per ANSI 53.1-1977, as cited by Singer [77], are the following: 34.5 dB at 125 Hz, 23 dB at 250 Hz, 21.5 dB at 500 Hz, 29.5 dB at 1000 Hz, 34.5 dB at 2000 Hz, 42.0 dB at 4000 Hz, 41.0 dB at 6000 Hz, and 45.0 dB at 8000 Hz. The attenuation increases as the environment changes from a small single-wall room to a standard single-wall room to a double-wall room.

The examination rooms are .available as single units with single-wall enclosure or double-wall enclosure; suites comprising a conjoined single-wall control room and a single-wall examination room; suites comprising a combined double-wall control room and a double-wall examination room; suites including a joint double-wall examination room with a single-wall control room; and the last with three 4-inch thick acoustical walls between the two rooms.

Each unit is available in a variety of sizes, but thought must be given the more than occasional claustrophobic worker who might find a unit with inside dimensions of 3 ft 4 in. × 3 ft × 6 ft 6 in. extremely uncomfortable. Because of the constraints of the Hearing Conservation Amendment, an adequate testing area should be selected, not to be determined by the space available but by the need for the most accurate audiometry and the least anxiety-provoking facility. It is recommended that the testing unit be a prefabricated enclosure purchased from a manufacturer who provides performance criteria. No "homemade" booth can be depended on to meet the rigid standards of quality hearing acuity measurement. The credibility of a hearing conservation program will be seriously questioned by employees who are tested in an environment that fails to exclude high levels of ambient noise.

Audiometric Technician

While the Hearing Conservation Amendment refers to trained or certified audiometric technicians testing under professional supervision, CAOHC has indicated that such persons are now designated as occupational hearing conservationists (OHC) [78]. The course leading to certification as an OHC (after passing a practical and written examination) has been outlined by the CAOHC and includes the following topics [78]:

- The technician's own limitations in the program
- The technician's responsibility as an OHC
- The responsibilities of the other members of the hearing conservation team
- The parameters of sound as they relate to audiometric testing
- Basic anatomy and physiology of the ear
- The concept of compensable hearing impairment in state compensation legislation
- The concept of the federal Occupational Safety and Health Act legislation
- Types of audiometric instrumentation (manual and self-recording)
- Performance check and calibration of audiometric instruments (biologic and electroacoustic [in concept])
- Care of instruments
- Pure-tone threshold-testing techniques
- Basics of recordkeeping
- Personal hearing protection (selection, fitting, and achieving compliance)
- Employee education programs in hearing conservation
- Principles of noise measurement and control

The course consumes 20 hours, and recertification is required quinquennially on completion of a course lasting a minimum of 8 hours.

The Audiometer

The advance in electronics technology has made possible a broader range of choices in the selection of an audiometer. While the instruments course from a rather simple screening device to the most sophisticated microprocessor audiometers, several factors should be considered in the selection of an instrument, with cost-effectiveness as the basis for choice. The elements to enter into the appraisal include (1) the number of employees exposed and in need of testing, including workers in job rotation; (2) time per test*; (3) available technical personnel; (4) labor cost of personnel; (5) available funding; and (6) potential duration of program.† Manufacturers claim

*The distance of the test facility from the worksite will determine the amount of additional time needed in travel. While this item is not test time, it is chargeable to overhead and is not a direct labor item. Backup of waiting employees is costly.

†The program could change if engineering controls were universally feasible and instituted.

that although the initial cost of a microprocessor audiometer is perhaps five to six times as costly as a manual instrument, the individual cost per audiogram, when the number of examinations per year is around 500, is nearly 50 percent less.

If a plant population is large, group audiometers accommodating four, six, or eight persons might be considered, although such a facility impersonalizes tremendously the conduct of the examination. Other costs, above the initial investment in instrument and hearing rooms, include such entities as audiogram cards, medical record forms, instrument service, printer paper, printer ribbons, and an audiometer calibrator, when preferred to biologic calibration.

The audiometers presently available are manual, automatic, and microprocessor or audiometric computer [79]. As indicated previously, the instrument must conform to the ANSI Standard Specifications for Audiometers for limited-range, pure-tone audiometers. The manually operated instrument requires that the technician provide the test tone and that the test subject indicate the instant of hearing the tone either by raising a finger, visible through the window, or by pressing a switch that activates a response light. The point or level at which the tone is heard is entered on the audiogram card.

When an automatic audiometer is used, the examiner depresses a control held in the hand, which activates a recording pen that marks automatically the response on the audiogram within bracketed ranges. The microprocessor—the technology having recently changed from integrated circuits to chips—has the tones presented as in manual audiometry, but in addition to recording the responses, the instrument stores the information and produces a hard-copy printout. When interfaced with a computer, the results can be stored and retrieved not only for review of an individual's threshold but also for compilation of an entire group of test findings. Software is available for direct storage, even up to 100 tests per day. Some computerized instruments require storage of test results on a tape cassette, which in turn requires interface with the computer and makes retrieval of a single subject's results rather time-consuming.

The advantages of completely automatic audiometric computer testing have been summarized [80] as follows:

Easy operation—obviates rigorous training of operator.
High quality of hearing test data results, assuring validity, reliability, and worker acceptance.
Tests are accurate with first testing, limiting the collection of unacceptable data. (Failure rates have been shown to be less than 5 percent [81]).
Change to a manual mode can be accomplished for verification.
Minimal calibration and repair.
Extremely reproducible data.
Formats data in standard electronic data processing layout for faster processing and reporting.

Audiometers differ in their frequency range, some having a minimum test level of 125 Hz, others beginning at 250 Hz or 500 Hz. Most instruments course to a maximum frequency of 8000 Hz. The time per test will vary from 3 to 8 minutes and about half of some 14 brands will include validity checks [79].

History Relating to Hearing
Before any hearing test is carried out, a specialized history should be obtained and recorded. Irrespective of the format of the questionnaire that is designed to meet this need, the following areas should be explored after notation of identifying information:

History of ache or pain in ear—right or left ear, and date
History of running or draining ear—right or left, and date
Treatment received, if any
Loss of hearing in family members
Frequency of colds
History of ear or throat surgery—mastoidectomy, tonsillectomy, and adenoidectomy
Use of firearms (at work or recreational, frequency, type by gauge, ear protection worn)
History of injury to ears
Significant past noise exposure—job, employment period, hours per day; tools, engines, machines used
History of head injury with or without unconsciousness
Tinnitus before first exposure to noise
Tinnitus after first exposure to noise
Tinnitus currently a symptom
Use of ear protectors—type
Current exposure to noise—job, date of first exposure, hours per day

Precautions in Audiometry
Certain basic principles govern hearing testing and should be followed [78].
Manual Audiometry
The subject is seated so that the operator and any manipulation of the dials cannot be seen, yet the examiner is so positioned that the operator can observe facial expressions.
The operator places the earphones on the subject.
To be avoided is the establishment of a rhythm in

setting the dials that would allow a timed anticipation of the next tone.

A pure tone signal is not to be prolonged, for there can be auditory adaptation or a decrease in threshold sensitivity, productive of an erroneous threshold elevation.

Instructions should be explicit.

Self-Recording (Automatic) Audiometry

Constant visual monitoring of the recording excursions is essential.

It should be determined that the examinee's attentiveness or alertness remains throughout the test.

Calibration is performed to check the accuracy of the instrument. Biologic calibration is conducted daily. Every 1 to 5 years, an exhaustive calibration is run by the manufacturer or an instruments distributor, checking for harmonic distortion, tone-envelope characteristics (rise and decay times, overshoot, and "off" level), and unwanted sounds from the test earphones or other sources.

Records of calibration are to be maintained—date, type of instrumentation used in calibration, and measurement data—for 5 years, or even longer, as determined by the nature of the plant's operations, the workers' compensation claim history, and the findings on continuing audiometry.

Miscellaneous care factors: Headphones are not to be removed by pulling on the wires, the cords must not be coiled, audiometers must be used regularly, the test area is to be free of dusts, and rubber headset cushions are to be checked for softness (if the rubber has hardened, replacement is necessary).

Whenever possible, these behavioral aberrations are to be identified so that testing can be rescheduled for more valid results: drug use, alcohol use, marijuana use, uncooperative behavior, malingering, fear, and clowning [82]. If behavior persists and there is a variability in response, referral should be made to an audiologist.

Recordkeeping

While the Hearing Conservation Amendment has spelled out the periods of retention of hearing test results,* background noise measurements, and work exposure levels [83], the format of the records was not delineated. As determined by the type of audiometer used, the record displays will vary. In manual audiometry, printed audiogram cards are available from manufacturers of audiometers for hand entry of the hearing levels (intensity levels or pressure levels) found on testing at the various pure-tone frequencies from 125 to 8000, expressed as hertz (Hz), or the number of times the pressure variations occur in a second. Hand entries are made separately for each ear, both color and an X or O differentiating one from the other. While human beings generally can hear sound from 20 to 20,000 Hz [84], it is not essential to test in the full range of acuity. The frequencies that are tested include the spectrum of speech. Audiometry in the upper frequencies is important, for it is in this range that noise-induced hearing loss occurs. In practice, an individual displaying a 15-dB hearing level in most frequencies is considered as having a hearing loss [85].

When an automatic audiometer is used, the record cards are supplied by the manufacturer. When the microprocessor audiometer is utilized, a complete printout is available immediately. Irrespective of the record form that is employed, comparison must be made of the current hearing levels with the reference or baseline audiogram. The ideal record form will allow serial entries so that the display of sequential audiograms—or numeric values—will indicate readily any change in hearing acuity. The Department of Defense has developed a series of forms for use in hearing conservation programs covering four record entities: (1) Noise Survey, (2) Reference Audiogram, (3) Hearing Conservation Data, and (4) Biological Audiometer Calibration Check. The records, except for the last of the series, are available in carbonized, prepunched, multiple form packets and carry detailed instructions for completion on the reverse of the form.

EDUCATION AND TRAINING

To have an effective program and one that is accepted, it is necessary that the participants understand the objectives and the methods of attaining those objectives through implementation. As indicated previously, employees exposed to TWAs of 85 dB and above must be trained at least each year in the following areas: (1) the effects of noise; (2) the purpose, advantages, disadvantages, and attenuation of various types of hearing protectors; (3) the selection, fitting, and care of protectors; and (4) the purpose and procedures of audiometric testing [83]. The Hearing Conservation Amendment is permissive in the structure of the training format, and various segments could be offered at the most propitious times; for example, audiometric procedures could be reviewed prior to audiometric testing.

Some additional elements in training required in a state program [86] include making available to af-

*Noise exposure measurement records are to be retained for 2 years. Audiometric test results, including measurements on the background sound pressure levels in audiometric test rooms, calibration dates, examiner's name, and employee's most recent noise exposure measurement, must be maintained for the duration of employment of the affected worker.

fected employees copies of the pertinent article from the General Industry Safety Order and posting a copy in the workplace of the same directive. Also, the involved employees shall be given the same informational materials relating to the standard as are supplied to the employer by OSHA. Further, the employer shall provide, on request, all materials related to the training and education program to the chief of the state occupational safety and health program and the director of NIOSH.

It is recommended that personnel intimately related to the hearing conservation program be given the responsibility of training, rather than having the company training or employee development unit undertake such a technical task. The program must be understood and *felt* as a needed component in the preservation of worker health, and it must be presented by representatives of the OHS and the safety directorate. Professional trainers, while adept at programs involving communication, morale, interpersonal relations, personnel actions, report preparation, and the like, often are seen mouthing technical phrases whose meaning is not completely clear. The workers are sensitive to this lack of comprehension, and the program can quickly lose its credibility when in the hands of unrelated personnel.

If the organization lacks capability in graphic art, audiovisual materials can be obtained from commercial sources on a loan, purchase, or rental basis.

Lastly, training must be conducted for both managerial and hourly personnel. The formats will differ, but without bilateral exposure, there cannot be complete involvement.

EVALUATION

Periodically the audiometric data obtained in testing must be reviewed to determine the effectiveness of the entire hearing conservation program. The analytic findings must be communicated to both supervisory personnel and the workers to ensure continuing cooperation. Every person involved is entitled to this body of knowledge, for employees do not enjoy participating in an activity that avoids feedback. The assurance that hearing is being preserved is needed by everyone, and if there is evidence to the contrary, worker assistance will be of immeasurable aid in isolating the operations or operators in performance default.

As an example of an evaluative effort, Pell [87,88] initially (1973) and Pell, Dear, and Karrh [89] subsequently (1982) studied the effectiveness of a hearing conservation program based on the use of PHPDs and all of the other program elements indicated in this section. They demonstrated that a successful program can be cost-effective at less than $20 per worker per year, in contrast to extremely costly engineering and administrative controls. The diversion of resources, they believe, to meet unnecessary compliance requirements by infeasible engineering controls utilizes scarce capital and expertise for unjustifiable, nonproductive costs. While these statements are at variance with the then (1980) OSHA compliance hierarchy that required engineering controls first, both built-in and retrofit; secondly, administrative controls; and lastly, personal hearing protection, the use of PHPDs, when backed with strong activity in audiometric testing, training and monitoring of employees wearing the devices, medical surveillance, and ongoing education and training programs, will preserve workers' hearing. The studies are cited primarily as methods for evaluation.

Royster and Royster [90], in addition to monitoring audiometric test data, looked at changes in potential workers' compensation costs. Of 7,000 employees reviewed, the potential compensation cost per $1,000 of compensation payable per employee dropped from $25.20 to $15.80. In the state where the study was conducted, the maximum compensation payable for a total bilateral hearing loss due to occupational noise exposure was $25,000. On this basis, extrapolating data from serial audiograms, there was a potential savings of $1,645,000—a decrease in the total potential compensation cost from $4,410,000 to $2,765,000. While other factors enter into such a study, the potential drop in cost is enticing to an employer of an industrial noise-exposed population.

NOISE-INDUCED HEARING LOSS AND WORKERS' COMPENSATION

DEFINITIONS

In the determination of hearing impairment, certain definitions should be remembered, as provided in the second edition of the AMA's *Guides to the Evaluation of Permanent Impairment* [91]. *Permanent hearing impairment* is a reduced hearing sensitivity outside the range of normal. Hearing is to be evaluated after maximum rehabilitation is achieved and when the impairment is nonprogressive. *Permanent binaural hearing impairment* is the disadvantage caused by a bilateral impairment sufficient to affect the individual's efficiency in the activities of daily living (ADL). The *estimated hearing level for speech* is the simple average of hearing threshold levels (HTL) at the four frequencies of 500, 1000, 2000, and 3000 Hz [91].

EVALUATION OF MONAURAL HEARING IMPAIRMENT

If the average hearing level of the four frequencies is 25 dB or less, no impairment is presumed to exist in one's ability to hear everyday sounds under everyday listening conditions. If, however, the average of the four HTLs exceeds 91.7 dB, the impairment is considered 100 percent for hearing everyday speech. For every dB that exceeds a 25-dB loss, there is assigned 1.5 percent of monaural impairment, to a maximum of 100 percent, which is reached at 91.7 dB [91].

EVALUATION OF BINAURAL HEARING IMPAIRMENT

The range of binaural hearing impairment is not so wide as the audiometric range of human hearing. Impairment does not begin at audiometric zero, presumably the average normal HTL. Binaural hearing impairment is determined using the following formula [91]:

$$\text{Binaural hearing impairment} = \frac{5 \times \text{\% hearing impairment of better ear} + \text{\% hearing impairment of poorer ear}}{6}$$

From this formula are derived the percentage values for impairment to be found in *Guides to the Evaluation of Permanent Impairment* [91, pp. 156–157]. A second table [91, p. 158] converts the percent binaural hearing impairment to percent impairment of the whole person. Some rules apply in the extremes. If the HTL at a given frequency exceeds 100 dB or is beyond audiometric range, the level is considered as 100 dB. If the HTL is better than normal at a given frequency, the level is taken as 0 dB.

This material is included to meet other needs of OHS personnel, for it is recognized that few are engaged in disability evaluation. There are long-service workers who will have had extensive noise exposures prior to the institution of a hearing conservation program. They will seek counsel as to whether they should file a claim for noise-induced hearing loss. With the definitions of impairment in mind, counsel can be given in keeping with the methods of calculation cited. Also, existing levels of impairment can be shared with a worker in an effort to retain the worker's cooperation in following the mandates of the conservation program. By now, the old pride manifested by stationary engineers or tunnel workers in their loss of hearing, as a stigma of their trade, is probably gone, fortunately.

BASIS FOR COMPENSATION

In the present workers' compensation system, the end result of adjudication is a decision that it has been established, or not, that the individual has a work-related hearing loss caused by, or aggravated by, the employment [92]. In general, a hearing loss is considered occupational in origin if (1) the medical findings are compatible with the effects of the occupational noise to which the worker has been exposed, (2) records exist that demonstrate that the exposure to the noise level at the workplace was sufficient to have caused the hearing loss, and (3) the evidence supports the occupational causation, rather than a nonoccupational cause, of the loss.

MOBILE HEARING TEST UNITS

Throughout the United States personnel in commercial audiometric vans can visit a plant and conduct complete audiometry on a worker population, in compliance with current mandates. These visiting, certified testing-and-evaluation programs teams will come on site, conduct audiometry in mobile, heated and air-conditioned vans that have acoustically insulated sound booths. Depending on the size of the van, 4 to 12 persons can be accommodated simultaneously, and facilities are usually available for both manual and microprocessor testing. The rate claimed for a six-person van is 36 tests per hour.

Examples of the kinds of computerized reports that result from such group audiometry are the following [93]:

Yearly management summary report of employee hearing status from "most recent" audiometric test on record based on worst ear speech frequency range average
Yearly management summary report of employee hearing status from "earliest (or baseline)" audiometric test on record based on worst ear speech frequency range average
Employee name lists
Audiometric status and change report
Employee name list with OSHA "standard threshold shift" OSHA report

If desired, as an option, individual letters can be prepared for employees giving the results of the hearing tests.

Some of these extramural organizations offer complete hearing conservation programs comprising not only on-site audiometric testing but also performance of sound level surveys, provision of recommendations regarding engineering controls, calibration and repair of company-owned instruments, employee education, and data management.

Before seeking an outside facility, study should be conducted of the cost-effectiveness of such a program. Further, a decision may depend on the credibility of the plant OHS versus that of an outside group. If there is confidence in the company's medical arm, the effectiveness of a hearing conservation program may be increased by use of OHS staff personnel. If the addition of a hearing conservation program will diminish the scope of other preventive health activities, then extramural assistance might prove basically sound. As is often found with building alterations, printing, and the like, outside services are less costly than in-house labor.

In any event, before contracting with an external firm for on-site testing, references should be sought from other plant medical directors regarding experience with the testing team, the validity of their results, and the quality of their interpersonal relationships with the test subjects.

Glorig [94], long identified with quality in hearing conservation programs in the work setting, has issued this editorialized warning:

> Now that our Federal regulators have issued the regulations concerning hearing conservation in industry, "Will there be a genuine interest in conserving human hearing?" Or will industry in general be interested only in compliance with the regulation? The past has adequately demonstrated that mere compliance most often falls short of altruistic goals.
>
> In the shadow of these regulations there are many hastily organized and ill-conceived hearing conservation service companies. As is frequently the case, professionals, semi-professionals and non-professionals see an opportunity to get in on the financial bandwagon. Many groups feel that a hearing conservation program consists of an occasional noise measurement in dBA with a simple sound level meter, plus annual hearing measurements done by poorly trained personnel in inadequate test environments are all that are necessary to comply with the new OSHA regulations. This is far from the truth. Gathering data and storing the information will produce little if any good for anyone, least of all the employee. Information gathering should be the basis for action; action with respect to the individual and action concerning the effectiveness of the hearing conservation program.
>
> Properly organized programs and analysis of the data should include essential information on the effectiveness of ear protection and noise control procedures, quality of audiometry and potential liability. Service programs that offer less than this bare minimum are doing industry a severe injustice. Industry should investigate the qualifications of each offerer of such services. The price for services is by no means the deciding factor. Seeking such services on a bid basis is fine, but be sure your specifications include the proper essentials of a quality program. You run the chance of not being in compliance, but most of all you endanger the hearing health of your employees. . . .
>
> The present OSHA regulation is a reasonable and workable regulation. Our Federal regulators should be complimented for a job well done. It took a long time to come to fruition, and now that it is here we should get to work and conserve human hearing—a very precious commodity.

USE OF CONSULTANTS

One should not hesitate in referring employees to a consultant if the findings on audiometry or the test results plus examination of the ears indicate a problem for diagnosis and resolution, the solution of which lies beyond the capabilities of OHS staff members. Certain otologists have been active in occupational hearing conservation programs, as have some audiologists. If the question of causality is unanswered, a professional review is indicated, and an occupational association may be established or contradicted. If coexistent auditory disease is suspected, a specialist examination is indicated.

Those audiologists who have tested workers claiming a work-relationship of their hearing loss will usually submit a lengthy and highly informative report that should include consideration of the following entities [95]: identifying information; description of occupation; history; relevant past history; present complaints; examination; diagnostic tests and results; diagnoses; industrial causation; recommended treatment; disability; review of physician's reports; summary and conclusions; date of evaluation; references and attachments; audiologic analysis; pure-tone audiometry (including air conduction and bone conduction) and speech audiometry; tabular analysis and comparison of previous audiometric results.

SIGNALING DEVICES FOR HEARING-IMPAIRED PERSONNEL

Various instruments are available for the hearing-limited worker, in the form of wake-up alarms, multipurpose signaling devices, and warning devices. Information regarding such units can be obtained from the National Institute for the Deaf* or the Alexander Graham Bell Association for the Deaf, Inc.†

*Located at the Rochester Institute of Technology, One Lomb Memorial Drive, Rochester, NY 14633.

†Located at 3417 Volta Place, N.W., Washington, D.C., 20007.

VISION CONSERVATION

Even though there was much early work in ophthalmology, concern regarding workers' eyes and ophthalmic injuries became manifest only before World War I when the National Society for the Prevention of Blindness* published a booklet, *Eye Hazards in Industrial Occupations*. As the National Safety Council edged into its seminal years, eye protection was given more attention in an effort to reduce eye loss from trauma.

In a 1913 report of the Wisconsin Industrial Commission [96], it was related that during a 15-month period, 24 of 366 workers sustaining eye injuries lost their sight completely, 7 incurred permanent visual impairment, and 335 experienced a period of disability of 8 days or more. It was believed that 70 percent of the injuries could have been prevented by "the use of eye glasses or goggles." Protective devices were available but were not worn with frequency.

With the advent of World War II and the need for vision-screening devices to expedite the determination of visual skills of the innumerable workers entering war production plants, interest heightened in what was then termed industrial ophthalmology. As Dr. Hedwig Kuhn [97] put it, "Prior to World War II, the field of industrial ophthalmology was limited and vague, never having been sharply defined or crystallized." The components of a full vision-conservation program were assembled, aided by both industrial and academic research. While many of the elements of these programs have not endured, most medical and safety facilities have persisted in the reduction of eye injuries and the provision of corrective/protective eyewear.

OBJECTIVES

The purposes of a vision conservation program in work establishments can be identified as follows:

To eliminate, as much as possible, injuries to the eyes from mechanical processes through use of protective eyewear.

To provide the maximum visual acuity in keeping with the needs of the job through the use of corrective lenses.

To minimize visual fatigue by providing adequate contrast of work materials and background.

*Currently the National Society to Prevent Blindness.

To minimize injury to other body parts by improving visual acuity.

To place job applicants and incumbents in jobs appropriate to their level of visual skills, ranging from maximal vision to amaurosis.

To minimize product wastage.

To reduce damage to costly equipment.

To protect workers' eyes against the hazards of horseplay (skylarking) initiated by fellow employees.

To minimize localized physical fatigue through the issue and use of corrective/protective eyewear that provides near or middle-distance segments in the superior portions of the lenses, averting acute repeated extension of the cervical spine.

To ensure accurate color discrimination by workers in jobs requiring such skill.

To ensure the capability of reading and distinguishing visual warning signals, labels on service lines, and the descriptions of ingredients accompanying bulk shipments of hazardous materials.

To permit assignment of employees to driving or other control positions of heavy mobile equipment—hoists, cranes, ladles, trucks—who manifest maximal depth perception and good peripheral vision.

To allow identification of all physical or chemical hazards to the eye.

To acquire the information permitting development of a joint list of eye hazards and the kinds of personal or environmental protective devices needed to prevent worker injury.

To establish a baseline of workers' acuities for comparison in cases of future eye injury.

To identify visual functional disorders or anatomic or physiologic variants requiring professional referral, diagnosis, and correction.

To provide a base for health education efforts targeted toward proper eye protection, first aid in emergencies, and frequent reexamination of the eyes and determination of visual skills.

To determine the illumination levels needed in different work areas.

To allow control of contact lens usage, its appropriateness, and concurrent need for eye protection.

To identify industrial operations or areas in need of adjacent emergency eyewash facilities.

To meet OSHA requirements.

VISION REQUIREMENTS SURVEY OF PLANT OPERATIONS

To establish a program in vision conservation, it is necessary that a body of information be developed that will identify the visual requirements of all jobs. Forms for the recording of data can be created locally or may be obtained from certain commercial sources. From the results assembled, a profile can be prepared to aid in the placement of a job applicant or an employee being transferred to a different position. The survey can be conducted by an industrial hygiene technician, a safety analyst, an optometric technician, or, if need be, an occupational health nurse. The person(s) conducting the survey should have some familiarity with the visual needs of jobs, the usual working distances involved, the need for special lenses or lens segments, and the modes of correction and protection. It would be particularly helpful to have as one member of the survey group an individual who is familiar with the physical properties and biologic effects of chemicals subject to splash or spray, for the style of protective eyewear frame for this problem will differ. The following information should be obtained through walk-through inspections, review of job descriptions, interviews with first-line supervisors, study of MSDSs germane to the operations, and review of industrial eye-injury records:

Job title
Department
Class of operation
Eye protection requirements (impact, glare, harmful radiation, splash hazard, fume hazard, frame style, time of use/need)
Special color vision requirements
Remarks
Visual demands (distant visual acuity [binocular], near visual acuity [binocular], muscle balance, binocular vision, depth perception [stereopsis], color discrimination, visual fields)

Elaboration or additional analysis of some of these items follows:

Distance or distances from eyes of worker to point of operation—fixed or changing (relates to acuity)
Motion of work—slow or rapid, rotation, vertical or horizontal, fixed or intermittent (relates to muscle balance)
Size of central working area (relates to stereopsis)
Type of visual attention required—fixed or changing, casual or concentrated, detailed or gross
Colors to be perceived and discriminated
Foot candles of illumination at work—point and surrounding area—direction of light, reflected or direct glare, contrasts
Color of light source and work area (functional area painting)
Types of working surface—glossy or nonglossy, slightly or grossly uneven, angle of working surface, position of eyes in relation to work (looking down, ahead, up) (related to need for occupational bifocals or trifocals)
Eye hazards—flying objects, particles of dust, fumes or vapors, splashing chemicals, molten metal, type of radiation

Implicit in this analysis is the need for identification of any unusual eye performance, for example, the demands made on the melter in a steel mill, the so-called optical pyrometry, or on the inspector in quality control.

The individual elements of required vision are seen in Figure 15-1, along with the method of deriving a visual requirements profile, against which can be matched the visual skills of the worker, obtained either by screening or professional examination.

The results of the survey, preferably maintained as a card index—computerized for display if the medical facility has the capability—should be retained in the occupational optometry section or ophthalmic dispensing service for ready access by the eye care professional or optical technician.

In the development of the survey, it may be necessary to classify jobs or job families differently from systems usually employed by personnel authorities, for the purpose differs. It has been suggested that the "visual job families" developed by Purdue University [98] be used, a classification that establishes six basic occupational groupings separated by their vision requirements:

Clerical and administrative work—desk work and use of office machines.
Inspection and close machine work—inspection of small items, machine operations with close working distances, and assembly of small parts.
Operation of mobile equipment—operation of moving vehicles, such as trucks, cranes, high lift trucks, and the like.
Machine operation—Operation of machines at arm's length distance but not requiring extremely close work, such as lathes, drill presses, spinning machines, and the like.
Laboring—unskilled work involving carrying, cleaning, loading, digging, and comparable operations.
Mechanical and skilled trades work—technical work, such as that performed in radio repair, carpentry, engine repair, plumbing, or electrical installation.

A total should be reached of employees by *age group* (because of different needs in vision correc-

1		2		3		4		5		6		7	
Distant Visual Acuity (Binocular)		**Near Visual Acuity (Binocular)**		**Muscle Balance**		**Binocular Vision**		**Depth Perception (Stereopsis)**		**Color Discrimination**		**Visual Fields**	
20/10	A	20/10	A	No Marked Imbalance Permissible	A	Required	A	105%	A	Required	A	Good Field Required	A
20/15	B	20/15	B					90%	B				
20/20	C	20/20	C			Not Important	B	75%	C				
20/30	D	20/30	D										
20/40	E	20/40	E										
20/50	F	20/50	F	Not Important	B	One-Eyed Person Adequate	C	60%	D	Limited Requirements	B	Fair Field Acceptable	B
20/70	G	20/70	G					45%	E				
20/100	H	20/100	H			No Vision Required	D	Less	F	Not Required	C	Not Important	C
20/200	I	20/200	I										

1	2	3	4	5	6	7
C	C	A	A	A	A	A

FIGURE 15-1. *Individual elements of required vision (primary visual skills) and example of resulting profile for one job.*

tion), by *number who wear glasses* (needed in the establishment of a policy regarding issue of prescription safety eyewear), by *number requiring specialized vision correction* (need for special occupational versus dresswear glasses), and *number requiring magnifying instruments or special illumination* [98]. This information will be helpful in both the preparation of and justification for the budget of a vision conservation program, particularly one involving the issue, maintenance, and replacement of prescription safety glasses.

In the planning phase of a survey, the intent, conduct, and use of the study should be explained well in advance not only to managerial and supervisory personnel, but to designated trade union representatives. To have an unidentified group appear in a shop area without previous clarification of purpose, especially a group comprising persons making notes after observing workers, can be extremely upsetting. In addition to descriptions of the impending survey in the plant house organ and discussions during safety meetings or "tailgate conferences," a card providing the objectives of the study—in easily understood language—can be given to those persons in jobs undergoing review.

DETERMINATION OF VISUAL SKILLS

Vision screening, as indicated earlier, is an essential component of both the preplacement and periodic health examinations. In place of the more complex instruments of the private ophthalmologic office, a portable precision, stereoscopic device is used that allows a rapid determination of the following primary visual skills:

Visual acuity for near and distance (monocular and binocular vision)
Lateral phorias for near and distance
Vertical phorias for near and distance
Depth perception
Color discrimination
Peripheral vision

Several instruments are commercially available that include tests for all of these skills:

OPTEC 2000 Vision Tester, manufactured by Stereo Optical Co., Inc., 3539 North Kenton Avenue, Chicago, IL 60641.
Ortho-Rater, manufactured by Bausch & Lomb, Optics Center, 1400 North Goodman Street, P.O. Box 450, Rochester, NY 14692.
Sight-Screener II, manufactured by American Optical Corporation, 14 Mechanic Street, Southbridge, MA 01550.
Titmus II and 2C Vision Testers, manufactured by Titmus Optical, Inc., Petersburg, VA 23804-0191.
VS-II Vision Screener, manufactured by Keystone View, Division of Mast Development Company, 2212 East 12th Street, Davenport, IA 52803.

Score cards for recording the findings on vision testing are available from the equipment manufacturers, and the data are convertible to the Snellen notation system.

The devices can be operated by a technician after brief training. The test findings can be compared with the profiles obtained from the study of various jobs, aiding in appropriate placement. Employees with unusual findings at considerable variance with previous levels of acuity should be referred to the occupational optometrist or an ophthalmologist. Infrequently workers will present refractive errors or eye disorders unfavorable for correction of the subnormal vision, and such findings call for prompt referral, review, diagnosis, and recommendation regarding placement.

An example of the newer vision test devices that incorporate a microprocessor is the Besserman Microprocessor Test System.* The tests are self-administered by the subject, and the unit includes a controller and a viewer. A visual instruction panel guides the subject in the operation of the device through the battery of tests indicated for the other screeners, exclusive of visual fields. There is an automatic printout, with an integral printer built in. The instrument is available in three models (700V, 800V, and 800VC), and the second allows connection with additional vision testers or an audiometer. If new programs are required for updating of test procedures, a new insertable module will meet that need. The 800V model will transmit data to a computer for storage, and the 800VC model will, in addition, store 100 tests in its memory.

The problem of illiteracy or written language differences can be overcome through use of most screening instruments, but if the Snellen chart is the sole test device, other charts can be employed that do not require a reading skill. Turnbull[99] has developed a chart showing birds, animals, body parts, and inanimate objects. The Massachusetts Vision Test Chart†

*Manufactured by the American Health Sciences Corporation, 4811 North 7th Street, Phoenix, AZ 85014.
†Manufactured by Welch Allyn, Inc., Route 321, Skaneateles Falls, NY.

displays Snellen's test symbol "E" in four different positions.

Although the screening devices test for color perception, a practical test can be given that demonstrates results most vividly to a candidate applying for a position as electrician, telephone repairman, or any other job requiring a high level of skill in color identification. Two bundles of color-coded wires can be prepared—one with the thin, multicolor-coded copper wires, and the second with the single, color-coded heavier gauge wires used in electrical conduits. The subject will appreciate the additional testing, for it involves actual work materials and bears more meaning to a worker than the pseudo-isochromatic plates included in the test targets of most of the screeners.

It is reiterated that the purpose of vision screening obviously is for accurate job placement, and it is only with a knowledge of a job's visual demands that matching can be accomplished.

TONOMETRY

At the Second National Conference on Glaucoma Detection and Treatment [100], it was stated that in spite of the efforts of eye specialists and primary care physicians, of professional organizations and service clubs, of paramedics and volunteers, glaucoma stubbornly remains as one of the few forms of preventable blindness. The OHS can readily include glaucoma detection as part of its vision conservation program, if such a program element is consistent with its policy of preventive medicine, budgetary base, and staffing table.

Although the Schiotz tonometer must be used by physicians, the devices employing the principle of applanation can be operated by trained technicians. An applanation tonometer—unlike the Schiotz instrument, which requires anesthetization of the cornea and conjunctiva and direct contact with the eye—measures intraocular pressure by sensing deflections of the cornea in reaction to a puff of pressurized air. The measurement is converted to millimeters of mercury, and the result can be seen as a digital readout.

With the ease of operation, many employees can be tested in a short period of time. It must be pointed out, though, that intraocular pressure is not a totally reliable standard for identifying persons with glaucoma [100]. Tonometry misses approximately one of three persons with glaucoma because the intraocular pressure is not elevated at the time of the test. Those individuals not understanding the limitations of the procedure may be assured erroneously that they are free from glaucoma. The person who is under treatment for the disorder may believe that there has been a "cure" because of the test result—as with patients with hypertension and diabetes—and that no further treatment will be required. Conversely, through tonometry, many persons with a slight elevation in pressure at the time of the test are in no immediate risk of developing glaucoma. Elevations encountered at the time of testing, however, followed by referral to an ophthalmologist have saved the vision of innumerable people. In summation, tonometry is encouraged as part of the program, but with the understanding that the procedure is not diagnostic; an elevated pressure requires further evaluation, and a normal reading is not justification for refraining from regular eye examinations or for disregarding previous findings [100].

In consideration of cost-effectiveness of screening, an OHS can concentrate its efforts on high-risk groups, in which the yield of glaucoma suspects would be predictably greatest—the elderly, blacks, persons with a family history of glaucoma, individuals with diabetes or hypertension, and people who are extremely myopic or who have other vision difficulties. As in any screening program, follow-up is mandatory.

An excellent guide for glaucoma detection in industry—a complete program outline with sample communications—is entitled *Glaucoma Detection for Business and Industry.**

REPORT TO EMPLOYEE OF TEST RESULTS

If a vision examination has been conducted as a separate test entity for purposes of special assignment or job change, by reason of aging of the subject, or because of special complaint regarding vision, notification of the test results can be done by computer printout or by a printed card.

PROTECTIVE EYEWEAR

The occupational vision (or occupational optometry) section of an OHS may offer limited services or may provide a full service as determined by unique needs, geographic location, the extent of community ophthalmic capability, or even, on occasion, the terms of a negotiated union contract. The use of pro-

*Available from the National Society to Prevent Blindness, 500 E. Remington Road, Schaumberg, IL 60173.

tective eyewear has been mandated by OSHA in parallel with the particulars given in ANSIZ87.1-1979.

In some occupational health activities, an optometrist may be a full-time staff member as, for example, in the medical facility of one of the armed services where both military and civilian personnel are given care. In this situation, refractions might be conducted so that the employee is provided immediately with a prescription for corrective/protective eyewear. In most industrial installations, however, the employee in need of corrective safety glasses is asked to bring in a current prescription from an eye specialist.

It was reported by the medical director of one telecommunications company [101] that because of the extreme cost of refractions by local ophthalmologists, he established his own company-based eye-examination program for protective eyewear. Three optometrists were employed for this purpose, each spending one day per week in the medical department. The initial equipment cost of $20,000 was amortized within 2 years.

PROCUREMENT/DISPENSING PROTOCOL

The conduct of a program of procurement and dispensing of occupational eyewear involves several procedures, for which there must be the necessary space, instruments, and equipment, not only for the issue of spectacles, but also for their maintenance and repair. The steps needed toward the proper equipping of workers are the following.

Patient Service

1. Verification of authorization for issue.
2. Determination of worker's eye protection needs.*
3. Verification of prescription in keeping with visual requirements of the job.
4. Measuring worker for frame size.
5. Preparation of order form for transmittal to optical manufacturer.
6. Completion of clinical record, that is, notation of prescription and frame specifications.
7. Verification of frames and lenses on receipt from manufacturer.
8. Notification of employee of receipt of glasses.
9. Fitting of eyewear.
10. Rendering of instructions regarding maintenance of spectacles.
11. Preparation of cost accounting form.
12. Completion of entry in clinical record of service rendered.
13. Notation of service in daily statistical record.

*As determined by the visual requirements survey and classifications to be described presently.

General Service

1. Maintenance of stock items and parts for issue of plano glasses.
2. Replacement of parts and adjustment of safety eyewear after initial issue and use.
3. Maintenance of liaison with local ophthalmologists and optometrists.
4. Interpretation to employees of visual requirements.
5. Courtesy adjustment of personal eyewear, as convenient.

Equipment

To execute such a service, devices such as a heating cone, frame warmer (sand), vertometer, and a stamping machine or label maker (for personal identification of glasses) are needed. For maintenance of glasses, pliers and adjusting tools are required, and if company policy permits a choice of frames in place of one standard frame for all workers, a sample set should be available to allow selection.

Program Precautions

Certain problems will arise that may require resolution or clarification. It has been customary in some companies to have plano glasses issued through a tool crib. This practice is defeating, for the proper fit—temple length, interpupillary distance, individual adjustment—cannot be obtained. Further, workers do not wish to wear protective devices requiring skin contact that have been worn by others, for they fear contracting any of a variety of illnesses. Also, safety glasses returned after a brief use will not be cleaned appropriately or maintained. A user will attempt self-adjustment, which will change the alignment of the frame, and the glasses will not fit the next borrower. The worker will not wear the glasses if they do not fit, so the eyes will not be protected. Those persons unaccustomed to wearing glasses may find safety eyewear an encumbrance and discard the spectacles. Malfitting frames, temples, or temple ends (spatula or cable) may irritate the skin and cause abrasions, further causing the worker to "go without." Do-it-yourself repairs and adjustment should be forbidden. In essence, then, if the OHS provides an optical service, it should include issue and maintenance of plano glasses as well as prescription eyewear.

Many employees attempt elaborate rationalizations for the issue of tinted safety glasses in place of their personal purchase of sunglasses. Many heated arguments can ensue when the worker is refused glasses that are truly not needed in the job. The ophthalmic dispenser, representing the OHS, must be adamant in adhering to the policy established for the use of tinted lenses. On occasion, even a supervisor will deviate from the classification of need and will authorize their issue, which complicates further the need to follow the instituted lists of recommended eye protection devices. Safety eyewear is costly, and abuse can add considerably to a budget. A variant of this theme is the employee who requests a second pair on the ruse that the initially issued glasses were lost. The additional spectacles were actually wanted for a spouse or friend, and some employees are sufficiently brash as to make the fact known.

There may be requests for photochromic lenses; if they are authorized, and being absorptive, they are approved for outdoor use only. They do not meet OSHA standards, however. Special-tint glasses for certain jobs, such as welding or glassblowing, will be needed.

Workers must be motivated to bring in scratched or pitted lenses and frames that are cracked, so that replacement can be effected. In the area of motivation, one of the most negative factors is the supervisor who fails to wear safety eyewear in a worksite demanding of eye protection. If the leader does not comply with the mandates, why should the worker?

The placement of cleaning stations throughout a work area will aid in the maintenance of the glasses and encourage their constant use. These stations may include spray bottles of silicone liquid that can be used to clean both glass and plastic lenses and that will prevent steaming or fogging of the glasses. Also available for use are dispensers of soft silicone-treated, nonwoven lens cloths; untreated soft lens cloths for plants where silicone should not be used (electronics, communications, paint); and silicone-treated tissues.

The issue of cost is handled in various ways by different employers. Some companies require that workers pay for safety glasses at their basic cost price and will arrange for wage deduction. Other organizations ask that employees pay for one-half of the cost, and still other companies will issue the safety glasses at no cost to the user. No recommendation can be made, except that payment for safety equipment by a new employee who has not been working for a considerable length of time may prove to be a hardship, unless some terms of extended payment can be reached.

Record Maintenance

A daily record must be maintained of the ophthalmic services provided, and irrespective of the format of the daily/monthly statistical summary, the following activities should be recorded:

Number of employee visits
Number of screening examinations
Number of tonometric examinations
Number of plano safety glasses fitted and issued
Number of prescription safety glasses received and verified
Number of prescription safety glasses fitted and issued
Number of clear safety glasses fitted and issued
Number of tinted safety glasses fitted and issued
Number of spectacle adjustments, repairs, parts replacements
Number of consultations, other
Number of safety spectacles received from terminees
Number of total replacements of safety spectacles

If the ophthalmic unit serves both military and civilian personnel, the first group will require additional services, such as:

Number of refractions
Number of regulation spectacles issued
Number of contact lens examinations
Number of contact lenses ordered
Number of contact lenses dispensed
Number of contact lens progress examinations
Number of contact lens insertion and removal visits

Further statistical entries will be made if ophthalmic services are provided from a mobile unit in addition to the activities at the central OHS.

CLASSIFICATION OF HAZARDS AND INDICATED EYE PROTECTION

The National Society to Prevent Blindness has established some preliminary caveats in its analysis of operations and listing of recommended protective devices [102] as follows:

The general recommendations regarding eye protection devices are applicable, but not limited to, agribusiness, construction, manufacturing, and service industries.

Eye hazards not covered specifically must be analyzed by the company's management to determine the appropriate devices required by current federal and state laws and regulations.

Visitors and frequenters must wear eye protection devices as required in areas being visited.

The final selection of eye and face protection devices is the responsibility of management and safety specialists.

The selection of eye protectors must be made in relation to other types of personal protective devices, such as respirators, ear muffs, or helmets, that are worn concurrently.

Table 15-3 illustrates the method to be used for the classification of hazards and matching protection [102]. The devices recommended are illustrated in *A Guide for Controlling Eye Injuries in Industry* [102] to facilitate identification and selection.

In listings utilized by the Department of the Army, positions in the two civilian personnel series, classification of enlisted personnel, and warrant and commissioned officers are given with their vision standards and need for eye protection. Table 15-4 shows samples selected at random as a model for local adaptation [103]. The Department of the Army [103] uses a listing of eye-hazardous areas in this manner: location (area and building number), operations, potential exposures, protective equipment, medical examination, and frequency of examination.

VARIETY OF SAFETY SPECTACLES

While goggles will be issued through other company channels, prescription and plano safety spectacles, as indicated previously, will be a function of the ophthalmic vision unit of an OHS. The types available for fitting and issue include the following [102]:

Safety spectacles with spatula temples
Safety spectacles with comfort cable temples (convertible temples are available, permitting change from spatula to cable, or vice versa.)
Safety spectacles with full cup side shields and spatula temples
Safety spectacles with full cup side shields and comfort cable temples
Safety spectacles with semi-flat side shields

The lenses available for use in safety eyewear include

Heat-treated crown-glass
Laminated crown-glass
Chemical hardened crown-glass
Plastic

Special safety eyewear includes absorptive lenses needed in operations involving exposure to infrared and ultraviolet radiation; cobalt blue lenses for furnace and certain viewing operations, as in the determination of temperatures and conditions of the melt in steel manufacturing; didymium lenses that eliminate most of the yellow sodium flare and that are particularly useful in the electronics and glass industries, in laboratories, and in all work where sodium flare is present (without additional specification by the prescriber, they provide a scratch-resistant surface; if the same characteristic is wanted with CR-39 lenses, it must be requested specifically), and certain yellow lenses that can reduce the diffused reflected light from haze by absorbing the blue of the spectrum and thus improve contrast.

It must be mentioned that if an employer is not desirous of having an ophthalmic service in-house, an in-plant optician service can be obtained at no cost through some of the manufacturers of safety eyewear.

By way of finale regarding protective spectacles, the mandate of the Occupational Safety and Health Act of 1970 places the burden of enforcement of their use on the employer. The specific regulations read as follows [104]:

Part 1910—Occupational Safety and Health Standards, Section 1910.133, Eye and Face Protection
(a) General
1. Protective eye and face equipment shall be required where there is a reasonable probability of injury that can be prevented by such equipment. In such cases, employers shall make conveniently available a type of protector suitable for the work to be performed, and *employees shall use such protectors.* No unprotected person shall knowingly be subjected to a hazardous environmental condition. Suitable eye protectors shall be provided where machines or operations present the hazard of flying objects, glare, liquids, injurious radiation, or a combination of these hazards.
2. Protectors shall meet the following requirements:
   (i) They shall provide adequate protection against the particular hazards for which they are designed.
   (ii) They shall be reasonably comfortable when worn under the designated conditions.
   (iii) They shall fit snugly and shall not unduly interfere with the movements of the wearer.
   (iv) They shall be durable.
   (v) They shall be capable of being disinfected.
   (vi) They shall be easily cleanable.
   (vii) The protectors should be kept clean and in good repair.

LASER PROTECTION

As observed by Sliney [105], the probability of hazardous exposure to lasers is almost always a remote one. The pencil beam of most lasers is so small, he points out, that the entry into a pupil of 2 to 7 mm is unlikely unless an attempt has been made at direct exposure or the attitude in the work area is one of extreme carelessness. When workers who fail to follow precautions or who do not wear eye protection see that they sustain no injury, there can result an overconfidence and a lack of credibility in the health and safety professional who seeks maximum guarding against adverse effects. Special glasses or lenses are available and must meet the standard established in ANSIZ136.1-1980, Safe Use of Lasers.

A laser protective eyewear program has been initiated at the Los Alamos National Laboratory and

TABLE 15-3. *Classification of Eye Hazards and Matching Protection*

Operation	*Eye hazard*	*Eye protection devices recommended*
Carpentry	Flying nails and stock kickback, chips, dust	Safety spectacles equipped with attached side shields (for severe exposure, ADD face shield)
Chemical handling	Splashing and/or spilling	Chemical goggles (for severe exposure, ADD face shield)
Foundry		
Chipping and grinding, core and mold making	Flying chips, sand, and parting compound	Safety spectacles equipped with attached side shields or goggles (for severe exposure, ADD face shield)
Heating and pouring metal	Splashing and sputtering molten metal	Safety spectacles equipped with attached side shields (for severe exposure, ADD face shield)

TABLE 15-4. *Vision Standards and Need for Eye Protection for a Sampling of Personnel Positions*

Job title	*Vision standard**	*Eye protection*
GENERAL SCHEDULE POSITIONS		
Biological aid	5	Yes
Chemist	3	Yes
Detective	5	No
International economist	1	No
WAGE GRADE POSITIONS		
Aircraft brake repairman	4	Yes
Blacksmith	5	Yes
Compositor, hard, paste-up	4	No
Electrical inspector	3	Yes
ENLISTED PERSONNEL		
Cannon crewman	6	Yes
Graves registration specialist	1	No
Hawk fire control mechanic	5	Yes
Orthopedic specialist	1	Yes
WARRANT OFFICER		
Aviation technician	3	Yes
Chief engineer, coastal vessels, 1200 HP	2	Yes
Field artillery radar technician	3	No
Forensic chemist	3	No
COMMISSIONED OFFICERS		
Armor	5	Yes
Conventional munitions material management	1	Yes
Military judge	1	No
Telecommunications center	4	No

*There are six recommended job-vision standards, ranging from the requirements for clerical occupations, through machine operation, to unskilled labor.

SOURCE: *Occupational and Environmental Health—Occupation Vision.* Technical Bulletin 506. Washington, DC: Headquarters, Department of the Army, Dec. 15, 1981.

has been described by Winburn [106]. Laser personnel, as defined by the ANSI standard—"those who work routinely in laser environments. These individuals are ordinarily fully protected by engineering controls or administrative procedures, or both"—are required to register through completion of a form so that the safety-related aspects of the laser environment can be reviewed and eye examinations can be scheduled. The Los Alamos National Laboratory requires that the eye examination protocol for laser personnel using any pulsed laser of any intensity or any cw laser with available power densities more than 50 mW/cm^2 and emitting wavelengths in the ocular focus region include examination of the ocular fundi by an ophthalmologist. Laser personnel employed in all other laser environments need only a measure of visual acuity and gross examination of the eyes [106].

Protective goggles are designed not only for broad-spectrum use but also for specific lasers: ultraviolet, neon-nitrogen, argon, helium-neon, ruby, gallium arsenide, and neodymium. Most filtration lenses can be had in plano, single-vision, or bifocal spectacles and with side shields. Also, goggles can be used that have a plate-holder that will accept a variety of protective plastic plates and will fit over prescription glasses.

All eyewear intended for use with lasers should carry not only the manufacturer's identification and model number or type, but also the optical density values and wavelengths for which protection is afforded and, if the wavelength range is stated, the minimum optical density in that range [107].

CONTACT LENSES

In spite of repeated publication of a policy regarding the use of contact lenses in work settings, inquiries to professional journals continue over the years in regard to the feasibility of such wear. The National Society to Prevent Blindness (NSPB) designated a special task force headed by Joseph F. Novak, M.D., an eminent ophthalmologic consultant to industry, to study the problem. A position statement that provides guidelines on the wearing of contact lenses in the industrial environment has been issued by the society [108] and follows in its entirety:

Contact lenses may be worn in many occupations. Contact lenses provide an adequate means of visual rehabilitation for employees who have had a cataract removed from one or both eyes; who are highly nearsighted; or who have irregular astigmatism from corneal scars or keratoconus. However, when the work environment entails exposure to chemical fumes, vapor, or splashes, intense heat, molten metals, or highly particulate atmosphere, contact lens use should be restricted. Certain federal or state regulations may also limit their use.*

Contact lenses, of themselves, do not provide eye protection in the industrial sense. For occupational use, contact lenses should be worn only in conjunction with appropriate industrial eye protection.†

The employer should ensure the identification of the contact lens wearer for appropriate emergency care and for protection in work areas hazardous to the eyes.

This statement supersedes those previously issued by NSPB.

It is estimated that close to two million individuals in the U.S. are fitted with contact lenses each year, and between 12 and 15 million Americans already wear them. Many of these are employed in industry.

Internationally recognized as an authority on sight conservation, NSPB in its eye safety program offers a wide range of educational materials related to eye safety on the job, in the home, in schools and on the farm. It also provides consultation service on eye safety programs.

Clarification of the position is given by the Committee on Occupational Medical Practice of the AOMA [109]:

[As is known,] there are two basic types of contact lenses, both of which are corneal; these may be either hard or soft lenses. Scleral lenses are rarely found in current use.

Hard lenses are made from an impervious plastic, and risk may result from: (1) foreign bodies, such as small metal fragments, shavings, or rust that can become entrapped beneath the lens; since the lens floats on the cornea, rather than being in a fixed position, there may be an abrading action between the lens, foreign body and cornea; or (2) chemical splashes that can be trapped beneath the lens and held in place against the cornea. The material may remain for a prolonged period or at least until the lens can be removed, thus increasing the damage from the chemical action.

The soft lens is based upon a type of plastic polymer which contains approximately 80% to 85% water. Some persons feel that the soft lens, because it adheres more tightly to the cornea and does not have as much fluid motion as the hard lens, offers some protection against corneal foreign bodies. It is still possible, however, for foreign bodies to become trapped beneath the lens. The major risk, however, is from chemical splashes and hot environments. Because of the high water content of the soft lens, caustics or materials toxic to the cornea are quickly conducted through the lens to the cornea and thus are held in place against the cornea by the proximity of the lens itself. Again, this prolongs possible damage to the cornea from accidental spills.

*Wearing of contact lenses by workers using respirators in contaminated environments shall not be allowed (*Federal Register,* Vol. 36, No. 105, Part II #1910, 134 [e][5][ii]).

†To be of industrial quality, safety eyewear devices must meet or exceed all the requirements of the "American National Standard Practice for Occupational and Educational Eye and Face Protection, Z87.1, 1979" or later revisions thereof, as published by the American National Standards Institute, Inc.

Many authorities in the field offer this advice: (1) a company policy on contact lenses should state that the wearing of contact lenses is to be prohibited where occupational safety glasses are required unless there are substantial medical reasons supported by recommendations from a physician for wearing them and then only if worn in conjunction with occupational safety glasses having sideshields or with overall goggles; and (2) there should be rigid enforcement of the NIOSH mandate (Pub. #78-210) that states that "contact lenses should not be worn when working with this (these) chemical(s)" and of the OSHA prohibition on wearing contact lenses "when a respirator is being used in a contaminated atmosphere."

Although no consensus opinion exists concerning the utilization of contact lenses in the industrial environment, some authorities believe that industrial programs can be implemented that promote eye safety requirements without placing undue constraints on those workers whose sight is best managed by contact lenses, i.e., keratoconus. In general, the wearing of hard lenses would be contraindicated in dirty, dusty environments that contain small particulates. The soft lens wearer should be prohibited in chemical areas, especially those with water-soluble materials, or in hot, low-humidity conditions that could dry the lens. Moreover, users of both types of contact lenses require protection from ultraviolet and infrared radiation. Most contact lens materials transmit wavelengths greater than 245 nanometers, offering no protection from arc-eye. Both lens types absorb infrared, thus generating heat. This effect is potentially more harmful to the soft lens wearer as it could upset the aqueous balance. Obviously, each case needs individual evaluation and under no circumstance should one believe that either type contact lens of itself provides adequate eye protection. Appropriate protective eyewear needs to be worn in conjunction with the contact lens. Backup corrective spectacles should be available for the contact user in the event that a condition exists, such as an eye infection, that might negate proper utilization of the contact lens.

In substance, apart from the rare employee with keratoconus, contact lenses should be prohibited in the worksite where eye hazards of the type indicated exist.

Although alluded to previously, mention is made again of the X-Chrom contact lens. This lens improves the individual's ability to discriminate between colors and to perceive objects blending in with their background. The lens, usually worn over the nondominant eye, is tinted a specific red. Although the uncovered eye sees some colors correctly, others are confused. This confusion is recognized by the brain, and a shift is made to the eye wearing the X-Chrom lens. Persons fitted with this lens have experienced a general improvement of color vision [110], although they may require extended wearing for optimum color vision enhancement. To date, the lens has not been approved for general or commercial aviation [111,112].

EMERGENCY CARE

Apart from the emergency care provided as part of the treatment program of employees who have sustained eye injuries,* the OHS staff should be knowledgeable regarding the type, placement, and use of emergency eyewash fountains, although their procurement and supervision are functions of operational supervisors. Such facilities are needed in work areas where chemicals are in use and the employee is exposed to potential splash hazards with the possibility of severe eye injury, if not permanent loss of sight. The presence of acids, caustic solutions, and cryogenic fluids is the primary indication for immediate access to a source of water for flushing the endangered eye or diluting the splashed eye contactant.

Weaver [113] has summarized well the OSHA standards that call for suitable facilities for the flushing of the eyes near open surface tanks containing corrosive materials; bubblers in case of caustic soda burns in pulp, paper, and paperboard mills; copious supply of fresh, clean water in textile plants where acids or caustics are used; eye-flushing capability in telecommunications utilizing storage batteries, unless the latter are of the enclosed type and equipped with explosion-proof vents; and facilities for quick drenching of the eyes in construction, within 25 feet of the work area.

In 1981, the ANSI Z358.1, "American National Standard for Emergency Eyewash and Shower Equipment" was published, and as presented in brief by Weaver [113], the types of eyewash equipment defined by the standard are as follows:

Plumbed and self-contained eyewash—one that is permanently connected to a source of potable water; a self-contained eyewash is a unit that is not permanently installed (that is, portable) and that must be refilled or replaced after use.

Personal eyewash—a supplementary eyewash that supports a plumbed unit or a self-contained unit, or both, that delivers water for immediate flushing, with less than a 15-minute supply.

Eye/face wash—a device that flushes both the eyes and the face.

Hand-held drench hoses—flexible hoses connected to a water source for the flushing of the eyes, face, and body.

*An excellent reference is *Ophthalmology for the Emergency Room Staff,* a slide-script program, produced in 1980 and available from the American Academy of Ophthalmology, 1833 Fillmore Street, P.O. Box 7424, San Francisco, CA 94120.

Combination unit—a combined emergency shower and eyewash or eye/face wash, or with a drench hose in a common assembly.

As the first few seconds following contamination are of critical importance, the eyewash unit should be as close to the hazard site as possible, preferably in the usual traffic pattern and accessible within 10 seconds and not over 25 feet from the hazardous source. No equipment or supplies should be stored in front of the fountain or in any way block the activating mechanism. Drains must be provided so there can be—without hesitation—a weekly flushing of the lines and verification of operating capability. All personnel subject to potential eye injury must be trained in the use of the unit [113]. The optimum temperature for irrigation water after chemical exposure is room temperature and certainly no warmer than body temperature [114].

Certain self-contained eyewash units available commercially are provided with an irrigating solution whose composition is isotonic (comparable to human tears) and contains a bacteriostatic agent. Refill cartridges are maintained in a standby rack, each offering 4 minutes of flushing.

Most eyewash fountains feature dual wash heads (bubblers) and are operated manually by means of a large push-plate or foot-treadle. They can be wall-mounted or pedestal-mounted. Units for external location are so devised as to operate under freezing conditions. Irrespective of the type installed, the units must be well-marked and readily identifiable. Two-color signs reading "FIRST AID—EYEWASH" or "EYEWASH STATION," or merely a large eye, with internationally recognized graphic symbols, about 8 × 18 in. can be purchased. The symbolic pictures should meet polylingual needs. As indicated before, full-flow testing and training are obligatory. The personal eyewash units—usually sealed plastic containers—are not recommended, for they may escape notice, be removed, or become contaminated. A fixed wash facility is preferred. Additional recommendations and criteria regarding emergency facilities for washing of the eyes have been provided by the National Safety Council [115].

WISE OWL CLUB

Beginning in 1948, following a suggestion of an employee in the St. Louis foundry of ACF Industries, the National Society to Prevent Blindness (NSPB) has sponsored the Wise Owl Club, an effective incentive plan to reduce costly eye injuries and visual loss through the encouragement of use of protective eyewear [116].

If it is believed necessary that a Wise Owl Chapter be established in a company, a charter application can be completed and forwarded to the NSPB* without cost to the employer. Any employee who saves the sight of one or both eyes through the use of eye protection, *either* on or off the job, is eligible for membership. The employer—through a committee of three Wise Owl Club members or an official—can authenticate the accident situation in which eye injury was averted by means of protective eyewear. A membership fee of $5.00 for lifetime enrollment to defray costs is paid by the company. The member receives a gold-filled lapel pin (a bespectacled owl), a hard hat decal, and a certificate.

The value of the club is derived from the publicity given each new member as his or her photograph appears in the company's house organ, with the cracked or broken glasses in place. A board placed at a prominent site—in the corridor of the OHS or by the ophthalmic dispensing unit—bearing the photographs of the members and the actual glasses worn can relate the effectiveness of protective eyewear usage. The fact that the workers are known to their peers carries much greater impact than were the photographs of personnel at other plants. A little ceremony in the shop for presentation of the pin and certificate will further underscore the merit of the safety effort.

Special awards are available for workers who have saved their sight on two or more occasions. The establishment of a chapter with assiduous governance by a company official is greatly encouraged, for nearly 80,000 eyes have been saved through the use of protective eyewear.

EQUIPMENT FOR THE VISUALLY IMPAIRED

While only tangentially related to vision conservation, discussion is merited regarding the placement of visually impaired persons. The ophthalmic dispensing unit personnel should be informed of the devices currently available to persons who are either blind or have low vision so that knowledgeable counsel can be provided. Also, if an employee is experiencing progressive deterioration of visual skills, as in diabetic retinopathy, assistance can be given as the job is converted, allowing the incumbent to be retained, with new equipment and new skills.

*Located at 500 E. Remington Road, Schaumberg, IL 60173.

The blind stenographer can use a portable print-reading machine,* which will verify typed copy. Printed images observed by the retina of a camera are reproduced in enlarged, raised, vibrating form by 144 individually controlled pins. Placement of the volar aspects of the distal phalanges on the vibrating letters allows the individual to "read" the printed or typed material. The author had a totally blind stenographer who transcribed all notes for entry in clinical records and typed with extreme accuracy letters that were sent to correspondents around the world. A postscript to the effect that the letter was produced by a blind typist led to comments from the recipients that they surpassed the products of their own, full-sighted secretaries.

Systems are available that allow information processing for blind persons that comprise a word processor, computer terminal, read/write notetaker, and printer driver. The system may be freestanding or interface with home computers, microcomputers, printers, or word processors. The device allows conversion of Braille input material to ink-print text and vice versa.† Equipment is available also that will display written or typed text through closed circuit television magnifiers so that the low-vision writer can see what has been written or printed.† Talking calculators are available, and a device is at hand, used for word processing, data management, programming, medical transcription, and legal research, that converts textual material to a spoken output by means of a synthetic voice.† As Stetten [117] has pointed out, however, there are hazards. Tables of data, graphs, and photographs do not, in the main, present recognizable letters, so that the output is likely to be gibberish.

There are various nonoptical low-vision aids that allow persons with diminished visual skills to continue at work, and some optical devices such as telescopic lenses are available.‡

*The Optacon (Reading Machine), manufactured by Telesensory Systems Inc., 455 North Bernardo Avenue, Mountain View, CA 94043. Other electronic visual aids are available from Kurzweil Computer Products, 185 Albany Street, Cambridge, MA 02139, and Visualtek, 1610 26th Street, Santa Monica, CA 90404.

†Manufactured also by Telesensory Systems, Inc., under the names of VersaBraille and Viewscan and Viewscan Text Systems, Apollo Products, and Vert Speech Products.

‡Information regarding these aids and others is available from the National Association for the Visually Handicapped, 305 East 24th Street, New York, NY 10010; the New York Lighthouse Optical Aids Service, 36-02 Northern Boulevard, Long Island City, NY 11101; The New York Association for the Blind, 111 East 59th Street, New York, NY 10023; and the American Federation for the Blind, 15 West 16th Street, New York, NY 10011.

PORTABLE DISPENSING CART

The Safety Division of Caterpillar Tractor Company has developed a rolling stainless-steel cart for ophthalmic service at job sites, including adjustment, repair, and replacement of protective eyewear. Trips are made regularly through the shops on all shifts to encourage the use of safety glasses. The cart measures nearly 4 feet in length, 3 feet 6 inches in height, and about 22 inches in width. The cart is compartmentalized to hold needed supplies, has large rubber-tired wheels and low guard rails on all sides, with handles at one end to facilitate mobility [118].

THE EXTREME MYOPE

In an early OHS affiliation of the author, one of the scientists scheduled to work on a particular day crushed his glasses on arising, as he had placed them alongside his bed the night before. With an extreme minus correction and without a reserve pair, he was virtually blind. As there was no taxi service in that particular situation, the employee was sent for in a company car. All persons with comparable visual needs must be encouraged to keep at home *and* on the job secondary spectacles in the event of loss or breakage so that regular functions can continue.

CLINICAL PHOTOGRAPHY

Although the point has been made previously, it must be emphasized that clinical photographs should be made of any gross eye abnormality—at the time of hire, at the time of treatment of an injury, at the time of discharge following healing—of any scarring around the lids, an ectroprion, burns, or even a strabismus. A claim can be made that a congenital deformity, old post-traumatic residual, or even post-inflammatory states resulted from a recent injury. The photographs can provide accurate documentation in refutation.

COSMETIC REHABILITATION

As certain disorders of the eye can preclude promotional opportunities, such as strabismus, corneal scarring, and the like, workers displaying these changes should be encouraged to seek professional repair. Personality changes will be noted, with a more positive person and possibly greater productivity.

TRAINING AIDS

As vision conservation can be included in an in-plant health education program, there may be need of audiovisual materials. Films, periodicals, and posters can be obtained from the NSPB, a slide-cassette program from the American Society of Safety Engineers,* and a film from Pyramid Film-Video,† among, unquestionably, many other sources. A cartoon-illustrated, 8-page brochure in color for distribution to employees—*A Guide to Eye Safety*—is available from Krames Communications.‡

OCCUPATIONAL HEALTH NURSING

Although composing the greatest number of health care professionals serving employed groups, occupational health nurses (OHNs) have undergone the same striving for recognition and growth as have their counterparts in the more traditional nursing modes. In the past three decades, the voices of the profession have become louder as its members have upgraded standards of practice, the academic programs of preparation, and qualifications for certification in the newer classifications. Breaking away from the deeply imbedded image of the bedside helper has not been easy. Aided, however, in this climb upward has been the creation of positions requiring lower levels of skill in which tasks are performed that once were the sole function of the professional nurse.

Licensed vocational nurses (LVNs) and nurses aides have assumed many of the roles formerly held by registered professional nurses (RNs), while the latter have prepared themselves through additional education for posts as nurse practitioners and clinical nurse specialists. Upward mobility in an area dominated by a strong male constituency—physicians—is undertaken only with difficulty. The rise of feminism as an issue of civil rights has given added impetus to the move of the female nurse away from the role of paraprofessional to one of strong contemporary identity, representative of a co-partnership in the provision of health care.

The OHN has been part of this change, and currently there are positions of corporate OHNs, many OHSs are headed by nurses as the only skilled professionals on a full-time duty basis, and a good number of the specialty are nurse practitioners. The struggle continues, and while the 1980s still are witness to change, it is entirely conceivable that, in the near future, nursing and medicine will share directorates in the occupational health arena.

*Located at 850 Busse Highway, Park Ridge, IL 60068.
†Box 1048, Santa Monica, CA 90406-1048.
‡Located at 312 90th Street, Daly City, CA 94015.

NUMERICAL NEEDS

While occupational health nursing and the occupational nurse were defined earlier, it would be helpful to cite the need for nurses by size of the employed group.

The American Association of Occupational Health Nurses (AAOHN) has pointed out that the number of nurses required for a comprehensive OHN program is determined by (1) the size of the company, (2) the number and health characteristics of the employees, (3) the variety of industrial processes or services, and (4) the potential health and safety hazards [119]. The AAOHN's current staffing recommendations are as follows [119]:

One RN for up to 300 employees in an industrial setting, or up to 750 employees in a nonindustrial environment
Two or more RNs for up to 600 industrial employees
Three or more RNs for up to 1,000 employees in an industrial setting
One RN for each additional 1,000 employees up to 5,000 in either setting

The larger the organization, the greater the number of shifts worked, or the more hazardous the work climate or mission, the greater will be the need for additional nursing staff. Understood, of course, is the fact that the presence of other personnel will be dictated by the same unique features of the enterprise.

FUNCTIONS OF THE OCCUPATIONAL NURSE

Much of the literature relating to the role of the nurse who works with employed groups seems to duplicate the functions expected of the occupational physician. This delineation in parallel is neither a statement of careless duplication nor the declaration of an overly ambitious professional segment. It is factual that many of the tasks performed by physicians are also carried out by nurses and often in tandem. This mutual capability is needed and desirable, for it is not possible for the physician to meet personally all employee needs. Nor is it correct that the nurse care for all patients in solo style without seeking consultative assistance when it is indicated.

The OHN, then, can perform in the following functions in toto, under medical directives, in consultation with an on-site physician, or in cooperation with the worker's personal practitioner. The functions are presented in the same framework as offered previously and are the ones expected of the staff nurse. While they are applicable to nurses in supervisory positions as well, there will be additional or other duties of persons filling the roles of OHN director, supervising nurse, or shift supervisor.

NURSING SERVICES TO THE JOB APPLICANT

Development, conjointly with work candidates, of both medical and occupational histories, and the provision of needed detail in clarification of significant historic events.

Conduct of the preplacement examination, including instrumental testing if not performed by technicians, in keeping with practitioner capability and OHS policy, and with follow-up referral to a physician when pathologic changes require confirmation, definition, or specific diagnosis.

Classification of the applicants in keeping with systems indicated in Chapter 5, Program Activities Relating to Prospective Employees, including work restrictions when needed.

Forwarding of nondiagnostic placement recommendations to the personnel authority so that the employment process can be completed.

Clarification of work restrictions—if delineated—with new employees so that they will work without jeopardy to themselves or fellow workers.

Explanation of medical surveillance requirements, as determined by knowledge of the physical and environmental demands of the position to be filled or by the physical or emotional impairments encountered during the examination.

Identification of, and counsel regarding, personal or family health problems discovered during the placement review.

Referral for issue of pertinent personal protective devices, including corrective/protective eyewear if prescription glasses are worn or plano lenses if protection only is needed.

Initiation of tetanus toxoid immunization, if previous series is outdated, and the administration of other immunizing injections as determined by job locale, travel needs, exposure to biohazards, or the history of communicable disease.

Tentative scheduling of second appointment if needed for clarification or verification of abnormal laboratory test results.

NURSING SERVICES TO THE WELL EMPLOYEE

Updating of medical and occupational histories in preparation for periodic examination or medical surveillance procedures.

Conduct of periodic examination, with explanation of, and guidance regarding, positive findings.

Forwarding of recommendations concerning continued placement in current position or reclassification and placement in other position if warranted by physiologic, functional, or anatomic change not consonant with present classification.

Conduct of health education programs including new or repetitive information in keeping with "right-to-know" legislation or material relating to personal health, physical fitness, cardiovascular risk factors, reproductive risk exposures, or stress management.

Administration, if needed, of booster immunizing injections.

Initiation of corrective action or change if malfunction of sanitation facilities is reported.

Review of periods of illness absence with emphasis on future avoidance procedures.

NURSING SERVICES TO THE ILL OR INJURED EMPLOYEE

Provision of emergency health care to employees sustaining occupationally incurred injury or illness.

Provision of limited emergency health care to employees sustaining nonoccupationally incurred injury or illness, including injuries sustained in company-sponsored sports activities.

Referral of injured or ill employee to private physician or health care facility for definitive treatment if beyond in-house medical or nursing capability or if hospitalization is needed.

Limited counseling or crisis intervention, or referral, if the stress manifested by a troubled employee exceeds the in-house staff capability of amelioration or reversal.

Referral to industrial hygienist of information indicating environmental evaluation if baseline bioassay levels are exceeded and verified or if untoward exposures require identification and correction of cause.

Transmittal to safety director of information indicating evaluation of physical and environmental factors causative of injury.

Maintenance of liaison with insurance carriers, community health agencies, the organization's workers' compensation authority, retirement board personnel, first-line supervisors, and managers as needed for purposes of illness and injury prevention or loss control.

Conduct, as indicated by reported injuries or illnesses, of physical-plant evaluations, if professional industrial hygiene personnel are not on staff, or with such personnel when needed for programs in prevention or for greater understanding of environmental health hazards.

OTHER SERVICES

Assistance with field placement of students.
Assistance with research projects.
Attendance at safety committee meetings or managerial staff meetings.
Maintenance of clinical records in keeping with standard practice and in compliance with legislative mandates.
Maintenance of supply inventories including requisition, receipt, and storage of expendable supplies.
Maintenance of capital equipment inventory.
Maintenance of special controlled-substances inventory and dispensing voucher file.
Continuation of professional growth through attendance at OHN conferences and participation in seminars and university course offerings.

PROFESSIONAL OBJECTIVES

The performance of the functions given above is aimed toward the achievement of certain objectives, and these goals have been articulated well by Gray [120] and are offered with some modification:

Utilization of the nursing process to support, modify, and promote adaptation to achieve optimal health in employed individuals and groups.
Interdigitation of theoretic and empiric knowledge derived from the natural and behavioral sciences and the humanities with nursing theory to establish a base for professional nursing practice.
Use of relevant nursing theory in the analysis of employees' levels of functioning and decision-making required in nursing practice.
Utilization of data collected in the practice of occupational health nursing to improve decision-making relative to that practice.
Participation with other personnel in the identification of group health needs and the effecting of change needed to improve the provision and quality of health care and nursing practice.
Assumption of individual responsibility and accountability for decisions, actions, and outcomes resulting from one's nursing practice.
Utilization of leadership skills in the identification and meeting of the health care needs of employed groups and in the achieving of occupational health nursing goals.
Functioning independently when appropriate, and interdependently with employees and the health team in a collaborative manner to provide, facilitate, and coordinate optimal health care.
Evaluation of research findings to determine their relevance and applicability to professional occupational health nursing practice.
Acceptance of responsibility for learning as a lifelong process to promote personal and professional growth and to meet the changing health needs of both employees and society in general.

STANDARDS OF PRACTICE

The AAOHN [121] has published a set of standards for the practice of occupational health nursing, guidelines for the protection of the public and the profession itself. The five standards, which are delineated in detail, can serve not only as yardsticks of quality in practice, but also as bases for determining managerial and professional responsibilities and for evaluating the services being provided.

Each standard provides not only a definitive statement of action but also an interpretation and the criteria needed to flesh out the standard. For example, standard I relates to *policy* and points up the need for a declared philosophy and its associated goals and objectives. The *interpretation* clarifies the roles of involved personnel, and the *criteria* concern the content of a policy manual that relates the operational components of the program and the procedures needed to implement the programmatic elements.

The *standards* as given [121], concern: I. Policy; II. Staff; III. Resources; IV. Nursing Practice; and V. Evaluation. It is suggested that use be made of *Standards of Occupational Health Nursing Practice* not only by OHNs long accustomed to practice in the work setting, but also by nurses new to an organization, and particularly in an organization embarking seminally on an occupational health program.

An opinion has been rendered by the Office of the General Counsel of the AMA [122] that where a clinic, hospital, or health maintenance organization or *other medical establishment* (emphasis added) may choose to provide care through the services of a physician, or through the services of a nurse practitioner or physician's assistant, the patient is entitled to the standard of care required of physicians. Even with the law's recognition of overlapping functions, a patient treated in a medical establishment *supervised* by physicians is entitled still to the standard of care required of physicians.

Where the health care service is provided by an independent practitioner or physician's assistant not under the immediate supervision of a physician, the patient is entitled to the same protection. Those persons holding themselves out as "having or profess to have the same expertise as doctors of medicine in performing medical tasks should be accountable for the same standard of care" [122].

CODE OF ETHICS

As most professional organizations have articulated an ethical stance in their journals, usually determined by a board of directors, so has the AAOHN. The AAOHN Code of Ethics is reproduced in its entirety below:

The Code of Ethics has been developed as a guide for registered professional nurses to maintain ethical conduct in providing occupational health services.

Occupational health nurses should:

1. conserve, protect and promote the health and safety of the employee in the workplace.
2. provide health care in the work environment with respect for human dignity, unrestricted by considerations of social or economic status, national origin, race, religion, sex or the nature of health problems.
3. safeguard the employee's right to privacy by protecting confidential information and releasing information only upon written consent of the employee or as required by law.
4. maintain individual competence in occupational health nursing practice, recognizing and accepting responsibility for individual actions and judgments.
5. participate in activities (such as research and case-finding) that contribute to the ongoing development of the profession's body of knowledge when assured that the employee's and the employer's rights are protected.
6. contribute to the ongoing efforts of the profession to define and upgrade standards for occupational health nursing practice and education.
7. incorporate standards of practice into the occupational health nursing service by using them as criteria to assure quality of care.
8. collaborate with other health professions and community health agencies to promote efforts to meet the health needs of America's workers.

Emphasis must be given item 3 in the code, for the occupational health nurse frequently is placed in the same position as the physician in industry who is requested—frequently badgered—to provide confidential diagnostic information obtained in the course of history acquisition or in the process of physical examination. The pressure can be extreme, and the less stalwart individual may concede to such demands. But, as indicated previously, almost to the point of tedium, one's moral responsibility is to adhere scrupulously to the code that permits transfer of information only by legislative mandate or with the employee's permission.

If this ethic is bypassed once, future demands will be made unhesitatingly because the concession was made in one case in response to the managerial request and thus a behavioral pattern was established. *No* confidential information is needed by supervisors to effect personnel action. Recommendations can and must be made that will aid in the administration or disposition of employees, but these recommendations must be free of data likely to prove embarrassing, upsetting, degrading, or denigrating, as judged by society's norms.

To comply with such requests will only change the perception of the professional person in the eyes of the individual asking for restricted medical information. Future interrelationships will be difficult, and no longer will the OHN be viewed as a responsible member of either the profession or management. These team ploys will neither advance a program nor gain any additional managerial support. One must adhere at all times to the principle of safeguarding personal medical information, for if knowledge of an infraction of this ethical fundamental spreads to plant personnel, one's program will suffer, for no worker will ever trust the OHS in any future interaction.

PROTOCOLS FOR NURSING PRACTICE

The occupational health nurse practices the specialty in a unique manner, different from almost any other professional nurse with the possible exception of the public health nurse. As noted previously, many occupational health nurses are the sole practitioners at the worksite and are not effecting care side-by-side with a physician and in numerous situations are isolated from peer support. This situation has been met in the past by the creation of what originally were termed standing orders, step-by-step directions for the treatment of specific medical or surgical disorders. These listings were compiled into a document that required the signature of a physician who might have been in a private office in the neighborhood of the plant, the company's medical consultant who visited a few hours weekly, or the full-time medical director.

With time, the "standing orders" became "medical directives" but still served the same purpose. In California, joint statements were prepared by the medical association and the nurses' association that outlined the services that could be provided by the nurse [123]. With the revision of the Nurse Practice Act in that state, the joint statements became obsolete, and the development of a protocol guide was required under which the OHN could function independently. In keeping with the desiderata of a hospital-medical-nursing Task Force on the Development of Guidelines for Standardized Procedures, a set of protocols was developed [124] to be used as suggested guidelines by occupational health nurses. The protocols "shall be carried out by a registered occupational health nurse specialist whose skills and knowledge have been evaluated by a company approved physician" [124].

The protocols cover treatment of a variety of disorders and the conduct of several preventive procedures. The topics that are covered could serve as the basis for a guide to be developed for a new OHS. The protocol subjects follow:

Treatment of anaphylaxis
Treatment of chemical burns
Evaluation and treatment of occupational dermatoses
Treatment of injuries to the eye (chemical burns, arc-welders' flash, foreign bodies, contusions)
Treatment of minor head injuries
Conducting a hearing conservation program
Treatment of lacerations and abrasions
Treatment of acute lumbosacral strain
Preplacement health-screening examination
Treatment of otitis
Treatment of sinusitis
Treatment of sprains and strains of extremities
Tetanus prophylaxis
Treatment of acute upper respiratory infections
Venipuncture

Each protocol follows a standard outline that provides continuity to the guides and completeness in the instruction. The outline comprises the following sections:

Policy format
Protocol format
- Definition
- Etiology
- Findings (subjective, objective)
- Treatment plan
- Consultation-referral
- Follow-up

In certain of the protocols, additional sections have been added, such as diagnostic studies, record-keeping requirements, counseling of employees, and differential diagnosis. Of special worth in guidance are the sections headed "Consultation-Referral," wherein are listed the indications for physician consultation.

The proliferation of the so-called physician extenders, or nonphysician health care providers, has beclouded the issue somewhat. In addition to the registered or professional nurse, there is the nurse practitioner, the physician's assistant, the emergency medical technician, the paramedic, and possibly others. In response to a query to the AOMA's Committee on Occupational Medical Practice concerning medical directives [125], it was pointed out that such directives or protocols must take into account such factors as (1) the functional relationship of the physician to the nonphysician health care provider, (2) the type of industry being served, (3) the availability of emergency and standard medical care and facilities, and (4) the skill and training level of the nonphysical health care provider. Emphasized was good communication—the nurses should be able to call on the physicians whenever indicated, and the physicians, in turn, should be free to provide new and updated guides to the nurses at regular intervals.

There are differences among the statutes of the states, for some jurisdictions have embraced the concept of expanded health care delivery more so than others, and in some instances, there have been changes made in existing codes to facilitate this type of practice [125]. One issue of particular significance is the provision or administration of medication by the nurse. A special committee of the AOMA studied the various regulations of the state boards of pharmacy and learned that the pharmacy regulations in all states, exclusive of Virginia [126], contain restrictive provisions regarding the nurse's ability to administer medications in the absence of the physician to the extent that the conduct of occupational health programs can be impeded under certain important circumstances, such as the drug management of life-threatening emergencies and the administration of controlled medications when and where pharmacies are not readily available [126]. It was found that most of the regulations made no reference to occupational health programs but rather stipulate that controlled substances must be procured, maintained, and managed only in the pharmacy setting. In the strict sense, any OHS is in violation of the law through storage of such medications in emergency cabinets or bags. The study was summarized with the recommendation that each state board of pharmacy and state nursing board be consulted regarding local sanctions [126].*

*A distinction must be made among certain terms. *Dispense* means to furnish medication pursuant to the lawful order of a practitioner beyond the patient's immediate needs, a quantity to "take home." *Administer* means to furnish medication for the patient's immediate needs, usually representative of the length of time before the patient could reasonably secure the medication from a phar-

In essence, any OHN currently engaged should be practicing under protocols either prepared through joint nursing-medicine consultation or by a physician consultant to or with the organization.

NURSE PRACTITIONER

Meriting particular attention has been the addition of the OHN practitioner (OHNP) to the health care team in industry. Although the nurse practitioner (NP) concept in other areas, primary care and pediatrics particularly, antedated the appearance of the specially trained nurse at the worksite, opinions have shifted somewhat over the years so that presently there are disagreements as to the value of the co-practitioner and particularly as to the infringement of the newcomer on the medical turf.

A recent summary by Spitzer [127] indicates that there has been universal and unequivocal satisfaction with the NP, and the paucity of legal claims bespeaks no evidence of substandard practice or public disaffection. There have been problems though—nonrecognition by third-party insurers, lack of legal status, inability to prescribe medication, and insufficient access to medical support or referral coverage. Initially promised was a lowering of medical care costs through use of the NP, but the nurse practitioners' push for remuneration equal to that of physicians nullifies the argument. Further, the statements of the 1970s that assured better access to care by the disadvantaged have not been substantiated [127]. It is Spitzer's feeling that the prognosis for the long-term viability of the NP concept is poor and that issues of turf, status, role, and the type of degrees needed for safety and effectiveness must be resolved.*

In Idaho, after considerable debate and many hearings, the *1980 Guidelines for Nurse Practitioners* evolved, which gave definitions and guidelines [128]. The NP was authorized to (1) perform a complete history and physical examination; (2) diagnose and manage minor illness or conditions; (3) manage the health of the stable, chronically ill patient after a medical regimen has been established by the physician supervisor; and (4) after consultation, perform repair of minor lacerations. Laboratory and radiographic privileges were allowed, but only after consultation with the supervising physician and then only if related to the diagnosis and management of a minor illness. In addition, a brief formulary of medications was drawn up that would facilitate management of patients with minor illnesses. To have this prescription privilege, though, the NP must be completely reviewed regarding pharmacologic background. There are no potentially dangerous items or controlled substances in the permitted list of drugs.

In Canada, there has been underutilization of the NP, particularly in institutional settings, which traditionally have employed the greatest number of nurses [129], and current programs hope to train NPs for practice in remote areas. At the University of Alberta program [130], the NP has been defined as a registered nurse who has received training in the medical examination of adults and children and has become familiar with common diseases and with methods of coping with medical, surgical, and dental emergencies.

But how does this discussion relate to care in industry? At one time, 222 member nurses of the AAOHN were NPs [131]. While it is not known how many of the group were actually employed in industry or commerce, there has been sufficient personal experience with a select number to substantiate the worth of such a role in an OHS. In early trials of role expansion of the OHN, particularly in the telecommunications industry, initial health reviews (preplacement health examinations) were conducted by

macy. *Furnish* means to supply by any means, by sale or otherwise, and usually implies the giving of an unbroken package or bottle of a drug, bearing no prescription legend, but carrying directions for use and the name and address of the manufacturer, essentially an "over-the-counter" medication.

If the OHS has a pharmacy, the dispensed container must be correctly labeled with the following information: (1) trade name of the drug, or the generic name, and name of the manufacturer; (2) directions for use; (3) name of patient; (4) name of prescriber; (5) date of issue; (6) name, address, and prescription number of furnisher; (7) strength of drug prescribed; and (8) quantity of drug prescribed. If the expiration date of effectiveness of the medication is required on the original label of the manufacturer, the prescription label must bear that date. State pharmacy laws must be reviewed regarding repackaging from original large-quantity containers.

*Spitzer's forecast of gloom met with rebutting letters to the editor. Molde and Diers (Nurse practitioners. *N Engl J Med* 311:535, 1984) countered with the comment that the NPs can compete effectively on their own terms; Pearson, in the same citation, pointed out that certain underwriting programs have mandated third-party reimbursement for NPs, that only six states statutorily prohibit diagnosis and treatment by nurses, that physician opposition has been strong, and that the NP movement is "very much alive." Goldberg (*N Engl J Med* 311:536, 1984), the one responding physician's voice, points out that the NP can fill in the gaps left by physicians in the areas of patient instruction, explanation, teaching, and demonstration, in addition to the provision of direct medical care.

OHNs at first on female employment applicants and later on both men and women. The new delegation of responsibility saved one company $30,000 per year and released 1,500 hours of physician time for services unique to the traditional practitioner [132].

At about the same time, 1971, "nurse clinicians" in another company, after a course in physical diagnosis, carried out physical examinations, differentiated normal from abnormal or suspicious findings, and were able to separate employee-patients or work applicants with normal findings from those individuals with physical variants [133]. It was concluded that such a move away from the orthodox mode served to upgrade the quality of medical care that the physicians provided their patients, for the physician who has responsibility for oversight of growing professionals will become more competent. Physicians relieved of repetitive, undemanding tasks would become more interested in their work and perform better [134]. Finally, in another setting, nurses' and physicians' findings were compared, and in 10.3 percent of 16,000 independent variables selected for evaluation from the examination by both nurses and physicians of 1,000 presumed well individuals, there was positive concurrence of findings. Both the physician and nurse agreed that there was no finding in 70.3 percent of the variables. The physician found a sign or symptom undiscovered by the nurse in 5 percent of the variables, and in the remaining 14.4 percent of the variables, the nurse disclosed signs not found by the physician. In short, few serious differences between the two groups of examiners were found [135].

In the experience of the writer, where NPs obtained histories from and examined both applicants for employment and incumbent workers, it was found that the nurses obtained more detailed histories than the physicians, who probably had a certain amount of burnout in the performance of repetitive procedures in an unchanging workload—one that comprised examinations solely, without dilution by patients in need of care or counseling. The rapport established with the examinees was excellent, and the interaction was heightened by the worker's being intrigued by the change in examiners.

In contemporary times, such programs continue. At the IBM Corporation, in 1980, nurses performed nearly four times as many examinations (40,427) as did physicians (10,708). The change in procedure has seen professional revitalization of the nurses, sparing them from technical obsolescence. They have felt more independent, worthy, recognized, and professional [136].

The movement continues, for the number of NPs will unquestionably increase as nursing professionals "become less acquiescent in clinical decision making and more assertive in demonstrating their autonomy" [137]. If one compares an OHS, in the institutional sense, with a hospital, where members of a full-time staff are salaried, there is little evidence of rivalry for fee-paying patients. In the open marketplace there has been acrimony where some NPs have been viewed as highly aspiring competitors. It is hoped that more NPs will become members of the occupational health team so that physicians can spend additional time with employee-patients who present with alleged adverse health effects, or frank occupational disease secondary to contact with hazardous substances, or with more complex medical or counseling problems. The skills of the OHNP are needed at the worksite and will improve the service provided in both the one-nurse unit and the fully complemented OHS.

As pointed out by Mechanic and Aiken [138] in their review of the interface between medicine and nursing, there must be more effective collaboration in the future for the benefit of the patient who is in need of the skills of both disciplines. Only with close academic ties between the educators of physicians and nurses will a better, more trusting partnership result. Occupational health could benefit from a closer involvement of the two at the professional school or preparatory level. Given further substance to the need for closer cooperation was the concluding objective of the AMA's position statement of over a decade ago—"Medicine and Nursing in the 1970's"—constructive collaboration of medicine with the various elements of the nursing profession is essential to attain optimal utilization of physician and nursing talent [139].

LEGAL ASPECTS OF OCCUPATIONAL HEALTH NURSING

As the skills exercised by today's nurse have so broadened and as the technology of medical and nursing practice has so changed the pattern of care, the professional nurse, irrespective of the specialty selected for career development, has become more vulnerable legally than ever before. The nurse is carrying out procedures previously considered the sole operational area of the physician, and the many new classifications of professional nurses, particularly in the hospital setting, point to both the expansion of practice and the particularizing of a skill (for example, the "IV nurse").

This growth has given the nurse the same potential exposure for suit in a litigious society as the physician. The situation is compounded by the great variation in definitions as provided by the Nursing Practice Acts of the various states, many of which are much more generic than specific in their mandates. Because of the dynamic nature of the profession today, the tenets offered by the AMA still hold [140]: The limitations on the procedures that a nurse may properly perform are governed by (1) the nature of the relationship between the medical and nursing professions in the community; (2) the scope of training offered in recognized nurses' curricula; and (3) the training, experience, and proficiency of the individual nurse. It was put well by Murchison [141], who commented that the nurse is becoming increasingly independent in a practice that is growing steadily more complex and that medical direction, while still there, is becoming more distant. Because of these changes, it is incumbent on the nurse to know the law, particularly as it applies to the jurisdiction in which he or she is practicing, so that the nurse will know when and how to take risks and when to set limits. She adds that knowledge of the law adds confidence to professional practice, whereas a superficial overview of the law merely generates fear and a lack of confidence in making decisions.

While the Good Samaritan Act of most of the states protects the person providing care and covers situations usually unrelated to the care needs in industry, the nurse does well to know the "do's" and "don't's" of emergency care as given by a seasoned defense attorney for nurses. Horsley [142] has listed the following:

The "Do's"

Use good nursing judgment in assisting an ill or injured person in an emergency.
Avoid attempts at diagnosis and attend only to the emergency needs of the patient.
Try only to contain shock, control bleeding, promote breathing and circulation, and provide ordinary first aid.
Get medical assistance and more experienced help if available.
Call for an ambulance or rescue squad that's emergency-trained and equipped.
Turn over diagnosis and treatment to competent medical personnel when available.
Continue to assist and provide nursing care at one's level of expertise until the emergency is over or care is taken over by equally competent personnel.

The "Don't's"

Don't announce one's professional qualifications as if in charge and by ordering bystanders around. Let them know one is a nurse and do ask for assistance. But—they have no obligation to help.
Don't get in over one's head, by attempting treatment that one is neither qualified for nor skilled at performing.
Don't act the part of a physician; stay within one's professional limits.
Don't make diagnoses of a medical nature or attempt to give medical treatment. In an emergency situation, a nurse does not have the same legal obligation as a physician. The nurse's duty is to stabilize the victim until medical help is available.
Don't just walk away from an emergency, for one could end up charged with negligence, even though it is the physician's, not the nurse's, duty to provide medical treatment. The law is fluid and in a case may decide that the nurse's skilled assistance was vital to the victim.
Don't abandon a victim one has begun to care for until medical help arrives.

The matter of consent has been discussed earlier, and the OHN must follow the same caveats indicated there, when appropriate. If a patient, frequently the "belligerent" or "impatient patient," refuses treatment when a particular disorder logically requires therapy and wishes to leave the OHS against medical advice, the OHN should explain the consequences of such action and have the patient sign a form releasing the OHS staff and the company from liability for nontreatment. If such a request is refused, all the circumstances should be documented in the patient's health record, and the entry should be read and signed by another staff member, as a witness [143].

As more and more OHNs are performing examinations, preplacement or periodic, they have the same responsibility as physicians of informing applicants or incumbents of abnormal findings, even though the job candidate may not be employed. Even if there is no so-termed nurse-patient relationship, such information is considered part of reasonable care. If this duty is performed negligently, the employer who required or requested the examination, as well as the examiner, may be held liable for any untoward effect [144].

Another case has highlighted the need for a nurse to relay all of the history obtained from a patient in an emergency situation to a physician to whom the patient is referred for treatment. The case cited by George [145] was one of misdiagnosed Rocky Mountain spotted fever presenting as the initial rash in two brothers. The emergency service nurse was told of the removal of ticks from the boys, but the treating physician who inquired regarding ticks was not given the positive tick history by either the parents or the nurse. Treatment continued for measles, and one boy died. A negligence suit was filed, and the hospital was held liable for the nurse's failure to relay the important item in the history.

Under Canadian law, the Emergency Medical Aid Act, and as cited by Inions [146], a nurse is legally justified in providing care in an emergency without obtaining prior consent provided certain conditions are met, that is, the patient is an adult, is in need of treatment in the written opinion of two physicians, is incapable of consenting, and has not previously withheld consent, and the treatment is reasonably necessary in the best interests of the individual. Were these requirements to be met in the United States, most likely the OHN in a comparable situation would not be liable for adverse action.

In connection with professional liability insurance, it has been expressed [147] that an OHN should have this coverage if in a position of responsibility such as director of a nursing service, if there is considerable independence in practice such as in a single-nurse unit, or if the OHN is concerned or worried about having this type of policy. As the cost is not excessive, this insurance is recommended. In most instances, however, a company will provide professional liability insurance that will cover the nurse and the employer if a malpractice claim is made against the OHN. Usually, all that is required is the attachment of a rider clause to a standard policy carried by the company [148] wherein the nurse is specifically designated by name. However, Gallagher [149] has advised that even though the employer provides coverage for on-the-job negligence or malpractice, the OHN should carry individual insurance as well in case the misfortune arises of having to defend a suit if the employer opts to sue the nurse. Such insurance will not offer protection (1) if there has been a violation of the medical practice act of the state; (2) if the nurse is practicing without a license; (3) for professional acts performed in addition to the nursing functions for the employer, when coverage is provided by the company; and (4) against an illegal act.

Lastly, in an interpretation by the Judicial Council of the AMA [150], it was stated that, in the performance of reasonable care, a nurse may be justified in acting contrary to a physician's standing orders for the safety of the patient. The ethical physician should neither expect nor insist that a nurse comply with orders contrary to standards of good medical and nursing practice. Such an act should not be deemed a breakdown in professional relations.

THE OCCUPATIONAL HEALTH NURSE AS MANAGER

In most large OHSs there is a hierarchy in the nursing staff that requires certain supervisory positions. Many nurses coming into occupational health nursing as a first experience or after a period of hospital service will be ill-prepared, as are many physicians, to serve as a leader of a shift or a group. Professional education offers little in the area of people governance, and nurses appointed to superordinate positions are frequently so designated because of certain technical skills or because of seniority rights. Rarely considered is the individual's ability to motivate a group of workers or to build an esprit that will conjointly lead to effective health care and obviate professional burnout. Often persons given supervisory assignments have personality or behavioral deficits that will emerge under the stress of new responsibilities and alienate the group rather than bringing out their productive or practice potential.

The point to be made is that skills in administration are behaviorally determined, and a nurse headed for a managerial role must be prepared through appropriate education at a graduate level or through continuing educational opportunities. If there have been difficulties in interpersonal relations, the self-reflection provided by counseling or therapy will remedy the problem. Too often problems carried over from childhood or teenage youth manifest themselves in the work setting and lead to troublesome mishandling of contributing personnel. Only through adequate preparation can one become a good manager—a person with "people" skills in addition to possession of a body of professional nursing knowledge.

THE ROLE IN SAFETY OF THE OCCUPATIONAL HEALTH NURSE

Frequently, in a smaller organization, the OHN is asked to supervise its occupational safety activities in addition to undertaking occupational health nursing duties. Haag [151] has outlined well these additional functions, as follows:

INJURY STATISTICS AND EPIDEMIOLOGY

Prepares monthly and quarterly reports for management, noting injury statistics and explanatory tables.

From these statistics, determines high hazard areas or groups; notifies appropriate supervisors.

Remains alert for possible connection between apparently unrelated accidents or illness.

Keeps accident and injury statistics.

HAZARDOUS SUBSTANCES

Is aware of new processes in plant and the hazards involved.

Keeps up-to-date on hazardous substances, appropriate MSDSs, and notification of employees.

JOB REQUIREMENTS

Does preplacement physical assessment and recommends job assignment on the basis of the physical examination findings.

Consults with safety officer in evaluation of preplacement physical examination to ensure safe job placement.

Is aware of the type and amount of work each job requires.

Evaluates ability of absentees to return safely to work.

CONSULTANT-LIAISON

Answers questions from safety officer regarding what happened in an accident and whether the description of the accident and type of injury are compatible.

Mediates between employee and safety officer by gently obtaining requested information without scolding or reprimand.

Consults and collaborates with a large variety of people—safety, personnel, union, management—to provide a safer working environment.

Notifies safety officer of suspicious injuries that may need investigation.

Receives complaints from employees, acts on them, and/or refers them to the safety committee and/or safety officer.

COUNSELING-EDUCATION

Participates in employee's safety orientation classes by lecturing, demonstrating, and reinforcing safety rules and regulations.

Publishes articles for the company newsletter.

Plans general safety courses and special programs for high-risk areas.

Encourages display of safety posters and other safety information.

Offers safety counseling to employees on a one-to-one basis.

SAFETY COMMITTEE

Serves as a member of the safety committee.

Reviews accident reports; establishes causes.

Tours plant to identify hazards and violations.

May initiate action to resolve hazards.

Monitors progress of action taken on the committee's recommendations.

May initiate a committee if plant does not have one or revamp the committee if one exists and change is needed.

ACCIDENT INVESTIGATION

Initiates accident report; may include employee's description of accident and description of injury.

Notifies supervisor of probable cause and encourages him to talk to employee.

Interviewing and investigation with or without line foreman or supervisor.

SAFETY EQUIPMENT

Is aware of protective clothing necessary for all areas.

Remains up-to-date on new and available safety equipment.

Orders and distributes safety equipment; fits equipment as necessary.

ERGONOMICS

Works with safety engineer in locating areas where there is an ergonomics problem and in designing a solution by using knowledge of human anatomy and physiology.

MISCELLANEOUS

Encourages development of safety manual if one does not exist. Assists in revision of preexisting manual.

DRESS CODE

Times and customs change. With the assumption and exercise of new skills previously in the practice of the physician, there has been an associated move away from the traditional white garb to street clothing. Many nurses have adopted the white laboratory coat of the physician and, with a stethoscope slewed around the neck in the contemporary mode, are indistinguishable from a physician, or, in fact, from any of the many related health specialists.

In a recent changeover in one large medical center, it was claimed that white or pastel uniforms were "not associated with the wearer being intelligent or powerful," the uniforms relegating nurses to second-class citizenship in medicine by fostering a "handmaiden image" [152]. This struggle for professional power has not been manifested so strongly outside the large teaching institutions, and nurses in sizable metropolitan hospitals are still in traditional white, either in dresses or pants. What previously had been seen as pride in the wearing of caps from eminent schools is no longer visible among the many nurses who have foregone this portion of attire.

The writer, perhaps temporarily slack in some of his beliefs, feels that the uniform worn traditionally but in contemporary styling appeals to employee-patients and gives an immediate signal as to who is who and who does what. The symbols of a trade or profession are meaningful and should give some clue as to the nature of the bearer. On one occasion when visiting a large teaching center, a custodian dressed in work gray was seen moving an active floor polisher down a corridor, with a stethoscope slung around his neck. Such ambiguity is not needed in an institution where the mores are strange at best to the bewildered patient.

In essence, it has not been this author's experience in several settings that the uniform is, in any way, demeaning or detracting from the skills of the person wearing it. The attire is neat, demands an appearance of cleanliness, and is professional. With the assumption of white dress by technicians, receptionists, records clerks, and the like, there can be confusion as all wish to identify with the medical image. It is hoped that one day the striving for a higher professional status can be separated from the movement for feminism and that equality will arise from merit and not from superficial trappings. Although these statements may seem superficially as misogynic, they are not intended so, for there is no place where respect for the nurse is greater than in a well-run OHS.

RESEARCH

As nursing practice has broadened in scope, the speciality has seen undertakings in research. While much of the investigative effort has stemmed from academic centers, practitioners could, and should, explore the potential at their various OHS settings. Rogers and Spencer [153] have indicated that nursing has been a late bloomer in research, and although research activities in occupational health nursing have been slower to develop, there have been substantial gains in this segment of the specialization area [154].

The potential research problems are legion, and university personnel would be pleased either to assist in the development of the design or to work conjointly. OHNs can make a considerable contribution to the current body of knowledge in occupational health, for they have good rapport with sizable employed groups and can be more effective in carrying out investigative projects than outsiders unknown to the workers. Every OHN should explore this relatively untouched portion of occupational health nursing practice.

THE FUTURE

The declaration of a stance is never accepted readily in an area of controversy. It is believed that in the near future there will be equity in the directorates of occupational medicine and occupational health nursing. A few health services in industry are providing full care to workers and their families, where nursing diagnoses, nursing care plans, and expanded nursing practice will be not only necessary but also mandatory. In the main, employee education in health matters has not been undertaken with any enthusiasm by physicians for whatever reason—disinclination, disinterest, or inarticulateness. Clarification of existing clinical disorders in understandable layese is usually accomplished more readily by the OHN, who somehow seems to identify more closely with the patient's need to know.

Physicians are not taught nursing procedures, and where most care plans for ill or injured employees seen in an OHS are based on nursing principles, it seems logical that that element of the therapy be under the direction of the nursing group. Cross consultation can be a reality and is envisioned, as indicated previously, as a more functional mode of occupational health practice.

That the OHN has moved to the corporate level has been given testimony by Scharon and Bernacki [155], who point out that Tenneco, Inc., based in Houston, has expanded its occupational health program to include primary care and disease prevention services for its 3,500 employees at corporate headquarters. While Dr. Bernacki is Vice President of Tenneco Corporate Medical Services, Scharon (an occupational health nurse practitioner) is Manager of Health Services. In another example, a nurse, Charlene M. Mosckau, R.N., B.S., C.O.H.N., serves as Employee Services Manager in charge of health, safety, and security for the Ordinance Division of FMC Corporation in Minneapolis, having moved up from the full-time position of shift nurse occupied initially in 1969. She oversees 54 employees and works smoothly with the part-time medical director [156]. With continuing preparation for activities beyond the basic skills of occupational health nursing, the movement will continue.

The future of occupational health nursing was expressed well by Babbitz [157], who stated that OHNs were going to

> continue to maintain and improve their professional competence;
> continue to expand their role as independent health managers, change agents, and worker advocates;
> be responsible and accountable as professionals for the quality of health care provided, and equally important, for health care not provided;
> develop efficient, cost-effective health programs responsive to the health needs of workers and the management needs of employers; and
> remember that the overall goal of OH nursing is a safe and healthful workplace and a safe and healthy worker.

The firmness of the resolve is given further testimony in another statement of Babbitz [158] when she declared, "For years, nursing has been a passive profession and we're not willing to be that any more. We're assertive and we're going to become more assertive. We feel that we're well educated, competent professionals. We provide excellent, much-needed services for the nation's workers in a cost-effective manner. And that's what we will continue to do."

As the number of single-nurse units remains high, with the likelihood of increasing, and with many of today's newly trained occupational physicians opting for consultant careers rather than positions in plants, the role of the nurse will attain greater significance in the future. To reach the equity mentioned earlier, there will have to be more curricula available in occupational health nursing so that the new OHNs will be prepared not only for certification but more knowledgeably for their roles as codirectors of health programs in industry.

A message was directed to nurse educators by the 12 NIOSH educational nursing program resource centers, together with 12 other educators preparing nurses for specialty areas of practice, that indicates the needs in the teaching/learning arena. It follows [159]:

As occupational health nurse educators we believe that:

All workers in all settings have a right to a healthful and safe work environment.
A dynamic interaction exists between worker and environment.

Therefore, we believe:

Occupational health nursing practice is based on a holistic approach to worker health and the individual ability to adapt to a changing environment.
Occupational health nursing practice is based on the knowledge and skills of the nurse and is responsive to the needs of the worker population, policies of management and the existing state of technology. It is also influenced by the present state of the art of nursing, available resources, the political, economic and social climate, and current laws and regulations.
Occupational health nursing is based on a body of knowledge and theory that is communicated in practice and research.
Occupational health nurses have a responsibility to develop quality occupational health programs to meet the needs of the working population.
The primary focus of occupational health nursing practice is to promote and maintain the health of working populations.
Occupational health nursing practice contributes to the continuity of health care for working populations.
Occupational health nurses are health advocates.
The occupational health nurse works cooperatively with management toward meeting management goals of productivity through insuring worker health and quality of the work environment.
Occupational health nurses are responsible for their own professional growth and development.
Occupational health nurses have the opportunity to impact upon quality nursing practice through role modeling.

Therefore we believe that the preparation of the occupational health nurse specialist should reflect these beliefs and include:

Specialized knowledge and skills beyond basic nursing education.
Learning that is interdisciplinary.
Educationally sound programs which include well defined goals, objectives and expectations.
Incorporation of public health concepts, management and organization theories and the nurse's use of power and influence to promote the health of the worker community.
Research, with application and communication of research findings, because practice and teaching incorporate as well as nurture research.
Specialization as nurse practitioners, clinical specialists, educators, consultants, administrators and researchers in master's level programs.

SUCCINCT SUMMARY

Often one must turn to our British confreres for enablement of our language. Over three decades ago, when Spickett [160], the Chief Medical Officer for an English firm, was asked what is occupational health nursing, he replied in the terminology of the day, "An industrial nurse is an active member of a team employed in maintaining health in industry, in the prevention of ill-health, in the treatment of disease, in the encouragement of a healthy interest in the work of the employee and in *soothing out the wrinkles of unrest.*" How better could the role be described than in that last phrase?

REFERENCES

1. Industrial hygiene: Definition, scope, function and organization. *Am Ind Hyg Assoc J* 20:428, 1959.
2. Hendricks, N. V. Industrial hygiene today. *Med Bull* (Standard Oil Company, New Jersey) 11:496, 1951.
3. Hendricks, N. V. The industrial hygiene engineer's role in an integrated occupational health program. *Med Bull* (Standard Oil Company, New Jersey) 25:107, 1965.
4. King, E. Occupational hygiene: 1. The hygienist. *Trans Soc Occup Med* 16:45, 1965.
5. Talty, J. T., and Konzen, R. B. Occupational health engineering control technology: Report on a workshop. *Am Ind Hyg Assoc J* 42:157, 1981.
6. Fernandez, L. Senior manager's view of industrial hygiene. *Am Ind Hyg Assoc J* 41:A-57, 1980.

7. Bardsley, C. A., Lichtenstein, M. E., and Nusbaum, V. A. Industrial hygiene career planning. *Am Ind Hyg Assoc J* 44:229, 1983.
8. Anderson, W. M. Managing occupational health performance: A view from the corporation. *Am Ind Hyg Assoc J* 41:A-53, 1980.
9. Smith, R. G. What the young industrial hygienist needs to know to advance. *Am Ind Hyg Assoc J* 41:A-61, 1980.
10. Schulte, H. F. The industrial hygienist as a social scientist. *Am Ind Hyg Assoc J* 33:360, 1972.
11. Sheriff, R. E. [Letter in the Forum . . .]. *Am Ind Hyg Assoc J* 41:A-36, 1980.
12. Keane, W. T. More about malpractice. *Am Ind Hyg Assoc J* 39:313, 1978.
13. First, M. W. Obituary: In memoriam, Leslie Silverman, D.Sc.—April 27, 1914–March 4, 1966. *Health Physics* 12:988, 1966.
14. Booth, R. Safety: Too important a matter to be kept to the engineers. *Occup Health* 31:228, 1979.
15. Kilian, D. J. The Relationship Between Safety Management and Occupational Health Programs. In H. H. Fawcett and W. S. Wood (Eds.), *Safety and Accident Prevention in Chemical Operations* (2nd ed.). New York: Wiley, 1982. Pp. 173–174.
16. Premature mortality—United States, 1982. *MMWR* 33:13, 1984.
17. Wetzler, H. P. Loss of working years in accidents. *N Engl J Med* 294:1348, 1976.
18. Occupational injuries and illnesses in 1982. *News*—United States Department of Labor. USDL—83-471.
19. Occupational injury surveillance—United States. *MMWR* 30:578, 1981.
20. Baker, S. P., Samkoff, J. S., Fisher, R. S., et al. Fatal occupational injuries. *JAMA* 248:692, 1982.
21. Kraus, J. F. Homicide while at work: Persons, industries, and occupations at high risk. *Am J Public Health* 77:1285, 1987.
22. Speca, J. M., and Cowell, H. R. Minibike and motorcycle accidents in adolescents: A new epidemic. *JAMA* 232:55, 1975.
23. Cycling accidents in the United States. *Stat Bull Metrapol Life Insur Co* 62:4, Oct–Dec 1981.
24. Krissof, W. B., and Eiseman, B. Injuries associated with hang gliding. *JAMA* 233:158, 1975.
25. Flying in balloons, blimps, gliders, and kites. *Stat Bull Metrapol Life Insur Co* 56:5, Sept 1975.
26. Selected outpatient morbidity rates reported to NEPMU #5 from sentinel ships during month of February. *Prev Med Notes* (Navy Environmental and Preventive Medicine Unit No. 5, San Diego), March 1982. P. 3.
27. Waller, J. A. Chronic medical conditions and traffic safety: Review of the California experience. *N Engl J Med* 273:1413, 1965.
28. Waller, J. A. Traffic accidents: Chronic medical conditions as a cause. *Calif Med* 105:197, 1966.
29. Waller, J. A. Cardiovascular disease, aging, and traffic accidents. *J Chronic Dis* 20:615, 1967.
30. Waller, J. A. Medical conditions: What role in crashes? *N Engl J Med* 283:430, 1970.
31. Baker, S. P., and Fisher, R. S. Alcohol and motorcycle fatalities. *Am J Public Health* 67:246, 1977.
32. Motorcycles not authorized for state errands. *Am J Public Health* 66:476, 1976.
33. Suskind, F. Another look at the link between work injuries and job experience. *Month Labor Rev* 105:38, Feb 1982.
34. Council on Scientific Affairs, American Medical Association. Automobile-related injuries: Components, trends, prevention. *JAMA* 249:3216, 1983.
35. Boylston, R. P. Managing loss control. *Occup Health Saf* 50:206, Nov 1981.
36. *Guidelines for Setting Up Job Safety and Health Programs.* Washington, D.C.: U.S. Department of Labor, Occupational Safety and Health Administration, Oct 1972.
37. Abercrombie, S. A. (Ed.). *Dictionary of Terms Used in the Safety Profession* (2nd ed.). Park Ridge, IL: American Society of Safety Engineers, 1981.
38. American National Standard ANSI Z 16.4-1977. *Uniform Recordkeeping for Occupational Inquiries and Illnesses.* New York: American National Standards Institute, 1977.
39. *Scope and Functions of the Professional Safety Position.* Park Ridge, IL: American Society of Safety Engineers, 1982.
40. Directory of [Safety] Products. *Occup Haz* 46:123, Jan 1984.
41. Dunbar, F. *Psychosomatic Diagnosis.* New York: Hoeber, 1943.
42. Dunbar, F. Susceptibility to accidents. *Med Clin North Am* 28:653, 1944.
43. Carroll, R. E., and Haddon, W., Jr. Pitfalls in the use of "accident" victims as comparison groups. *J Chronic Dis* 18:601, 1965.
44. Hirschfeld, A. H., and Behan, R. C. The accident process: I. Etiological considerations of industrial injuries. *JAMA* 186:300, 1963.
45. Behan, R. C., and Hirschfeld, A. H. The accident process: II. Toward more rational treatment of industrial injuries. *JAMA* 197:85, 1966.
46. Hirschfeld, A. H., and Behan, R. C. The accident process: III. Disability—acceptable and unacceptable. *JAMA* 197:85, 1966.
47. Enelow, A. J. Industrial injuries: Prediction and prevention of psychological complications. *J Occup Med* 10:683, 1968.
48. Public Law 91-596, Occupational Safety and Health Act of 1970, Sec. (2)(b)(5).
49. Public Law 91-596, Occupational Safety and Health Act of 1970, Sec. 20(a)(4).
50. Cohen, A., Smith, M., Kroes, W., et al. NIOSH Behavioral Research in Industrial Safety. Unpublished typescript. Cincinnati, OH: NIOSH, [n.d.].
51. Cohen, A., Colligan, M. J., and Berger, P. Psychology in health risk messages for workers. *J Occup Med* 27:543, 1985.
52. Margolis, B. L., and Kroes, W. H. (Eds.). *The Human Side of Accident Prevention.* Springfield, IL: Thomas, 1975.
53. *NIOSH Certified Equipment List as of October 1,*

1985. Atlanta, U.S. Department of Health and Human Services, Public Health Service, Centers for Disease Control, National Institute for Occupational Safety and Health, Oct 1985. P. 1.
54. Occupational Safety and Health Administration. *General Industry Safety and Health Regulations*. Part 1910.134.
55. Skretvedt, O. T. and Loschiavo, J. G. Effect of facial hair on the face seal of negative-pressure respirators. *Am Ind Hyg Assoc J* 45:63, 1984.
56. No facial hair for safe respirator use. *CAL/OSHA News* 8:7, Feb 1984.
57. Johanson, R. E., and Morgan, M. S. Some observations of frequency of respirator fit tests. *Am Ind Hyg Assoc J* 45:134, 1984.
58. Facial hair ban upheld by court. *Occup Health Saf* 53:21, Sept 1984.
59. Holt, G. L. Employee facial hair versus employer respirator policies. *Appl Ind Hyg* 2:200, 1987.
60. Endorsement. ACHIG *Billboard* 28:1, June 1983.
61. Culver, J. C. Noise control: A congressional view. *ASHA* 21:897, 1979.
62. Ramazzini, B. *Diseases of Workers*. The Latin text of 1713 translated by W. C. Wright. New York: Hafner, 1964. Pp. 437, 439.
63. Steinberg, J. C., Montgomery, H. C., and Gardner, M. B. Results of the World's Fair hearing tests. *Bell System Tech J* 19:533, 1940.
64. Meyer, A. F. The United States Noise Control Act: Comprehensive Noise Control Legislation. An unpublished working document prepared for the Sixth Meeting of the Urban Environment Sector Group, held in Paris, April 22–24, 1974. P. 1.
65. Rules and Regulations, Occupational Safety and Health Administration. Occupational Noise Exposure, Hearing Conservation Amendment. *Fed Reg* 46:4078, Jan 16, 1981—29 CFR 1910.
66. Rules and Regulations, Occupational Safety and Health Administration. Occupational Noise Exposure; Hearing Conservation Amendment. *Fed Reg* 46:42622, Aug. 21, 1981—29 CFR 1910 and as amended by *Fed Reg* 48:9776, March 8, 1983.
67. Lancianese, F. W. Legal battle over OSHA's Hearing Conservation Amendment continues. *Occup Haz* 47:53, March 1985.
68. Lancianese, F. W. Appeals court puts Hearing Conservation Amendment on hold. *Ind Saf Hyg News* 19:13, Jan 1985.
69. Federal court to rule on OSHA's Hearing Conservation Amendment. *Occup Haz* 47:57, July 1985.
70. *Hearing Conservation,* OSHA 3074, pamphlet published by the U.S. Department of Labor, Occupational Safety and Health Administration, 1983.
71. Burchett, C. At last: The Hearing Conservation Standard. *Occup Health Saf* 52:45, Apr 1983.
72. Committee on Noise and Hearing Conservation of the American Occupational Medical Association. Guidelines for conduct of an occupational hearing conservation program. *J Occup Med* 23:56, 1981.
73. Selecting noise measurement and hearing protection equipment. *Ind Hyg News* 4:46, July 1981.
74. Mellard, T. J., and Geier, S. R. Personal Hearing Protection and Employee Education Programs. In M. H. Miller and C. A. Silverman (Eds.), *Occupational Hearing Conservation*. Englewood Cliffs, NJ: Prentice-Hall, 1984. Pp. 182–203.
75. Berger, E. H. Laboratory attenuation of earmuffs and earplugs both singly and in combination. *Am Ind Hyg Assoc J* 44:321, 1983.
76. Riko, K., and Alberti, P. W. Hearing protectors: A review of recent observations. *J Occup Med* 25:523, 1983.
77. Singer, E. E. Physical Environment for the Performance of Basic and Follow-up Audiometric Studies. In M. H. Miller and C. A. Silverman (Eds.), *Occupational Hearing Conservation*. Englewood Cliffs, NJ: Prentice-Hall, 1984. Pp. 62–74.
78. Miller, M. H. *Manual for Training Occupational hearing Conservationists* (2nd ed.). Cherry Hill, NJ: Council for Accreditation in Occupational Hearing Conservation, 1981.
79. Selection charts: Medical screening instruments—audiometers. *Ind Hyg News* 7:48, March 1984.
80. Computers can monitor hearing conservation. *Natl Saf News* 195:36, April 1984.
81. Cook, G., and Creech, H. Reliability and validity of computer hearing tests. *Hearing Instruments* 34:10, July 1983.
82. Morrell, J. C., and Sterrett, M. L. Quality controls for audiometric testing. *Occup Health Inf* 50:26, Aug 1981.
83. Final Rule. Occupational Safety and Health Administration. Occupational Noise Exposure; Hearing Conservation Amendment. *Fed Reg* 48:9739, March 8, 1983—29 CFR 1910.
84. Olishifski, J. B. Subjective Aspects of Sound. In J. B. Olishifski and E. R. Harford (Eds.), *Industrial Noise and Hearing Conservation*. Chicago: National Safety Council, 1975. P. 77.
85. Sataloff, J., Sataloff, R. T., and Vassallo, L. A. *Hearing Loss* (2nd ed.). Philadelphia: Lippincott, 1980. P. 43.
86. *Control of Noise Exposure*. California Administrative Code, Title 8 General Industry Safety Orders, Group 15 Occupational Noise, Article 105 Control of Noise Exposure, Aug 1982, Sec. 5099 Training Program.
87. Pell, S. An evaluation of a hearing conservation program. *Am Ind Hyg Assoc J* 33:60, 1972.
88. Pell, S. An evaluation of a hearing conservation program: A five-year longitudinal study. *Am Ind Hyg Assoc J* 34:82, 1973.
89. Pell, S., Dear, T. A., and Karrh, B. W. The Long-Term Affectiveness of a Hearing Conservation Programme Based upon Personal Hearing Protection. In P. W. Alberti (Ed.), *Personal Hearing Protection in Industry*. New York: Raven, 1982. Pp. 541–557.
90. Royster, L. H., and Royster,J. D. Methods of Evaluating Hearing Conservation (Ed.), *Personal Hearing Protection in Industry*. New York: Raven, 1982. Audiometric Data Bases. In P. W. Alberti. Pp. 511–539.

91. Ear, Nose, Throat and Related Structures. In *Guides to the Evaluation of Permanent Impairment* (2nd ed.). Chicago: American Medical Association, 1984.
92. *Background for Loss of Hearing Claims* (2nd ed.). Technical Guide No. 9. Chicago: Alliance of American Insurers, 1981. P. 3.
93. *HCI, Inc. Phase and Hearing Test Management System.* Part I-Basic Information. Rockford,IL: HCI, Inc., 1984.
94. Glorig, A. Hearing conservation or compliance. *Sound and Vibration* 16:5, Jan 1982.
95. Billings, B.L. Personal communication, August 10, 1977.
96. Cited in G. M. Price, *The Modern Factory.* New York: Wiley, 1914. P. 153.
97. Kuhn, H. S. Industrial Ophthalmology. In M. Wilner (Ed.), *Ophthalmology in the War Years.* Chicago: Year Book, 1946. P. 438.
98. Cited in *A Systems Approach to Eye Protection.* Rochester, NY: Bausch & Lomb, [n.d.]. P. 5.
99. Turnbull, V. H. A new eye chart in mass pre-employment vision testing. *Trans Soc Occup Med* 19:64, 1969.
100. *Glaucoma Control: A Report on the Second National Conference on Glaucoma Detection and Treatment.* Amelia Island, Florida, March 1981. New York: National Society to Prevent Blindness, [n.d.].
101. Rushmore, C. H. Personal communication, Feb 16, 1981.
102. *A Guide for Controlling Eye Injuries in Industry.* New York: National Society to Prevent Blindness, 1982.
103. *Occupational and Environmental Health—Occupational Vision.* Technical Bulletin 506. Washington, DC: Headquarters, Department of the Army, Dec 15, 1981.
104. Occupational Safety and Health Standards, Section 1910, 133, Eye and Face Protection. *Fed Reg,* Oct 18, 1972, Part II.
105. Sliney, D. H. Biohazards of ultraviolet, visible and infrared radiation. *J Occup Med* 25:203, 1983.
106. Winburn, D. C. Guideline protects laser users. *Natl Saf News* 129:51, May 1984.
107. Envall, K. R., and Murray, R., Jr. *Evaluation of Commercially Available Laser Protective Eyewear.* Rockville, MD: U.S. Department of Health, Education, and Welfare, Public Health Service, Food and Drug Administration, Bureau of Radiological Health, May 1979.
108. Reproduced with the permission of the National Society to Prevent Blindness. *NSPB Cautions against Use of Contact Lenses in Industry.* New York [n.d.—circa 1981].
109. Committee on Occupational Medical Practice, American Occupational Medical Association. Use of contact lenses in industry. *J Occup Med* 26:330, 1984.
110. Committee on Occupational Medical Practice, American Occupational Medical Association. Clinical occupational health inquiry [X-Chrom Hard Contact Lens]. *J Occup Med* 23:593, 1981.
111. Welsh, K. W., Vaughan,J. A., and Rasmussen, P. G. *Aeromedical Implications of the X-Chrom Lens for Improving Color Vision Deficiencies.* Washington, DC: U.S. Department of Transportation, Federal Aviation Administration, Office of Aviation Medicine, Apr 1978.
112. Welsh, K. W. A red-tinted contact lens for color blindness. *JAMA* 244:2457, 1980.
113. Weaver, L. A., III. Eyewashes and showers: Ensuring effectiveness. *Occup Health Saf* 52:13, Aug 1983.
114. Faye, E. E. Water temperature at eye wash stations. *J Occup Med* 14:638, 1972.
115. National Safety Council. *Natl Saf News* Emergency shower/eyewash recommendations. 131:49, Apr 1985.
116. *The Wise Owl Club of America.* New York: National Society to Prevent Blindness, Nov 1980.
117. Stetten, D. W., Jr. Coping with blindness. *N Engl J Med* 305:458, 1981.
118. Information courtesy of Gerald W. Grawey, M.D., Corporate Medical Director.
119. *Occupational Health Nurses: The Answer to Health Care Cost Containment.* Atlanta, GA: American Association of Occupational health Nurses, Inc., [n.d.].
120. Gray, A. J. Personal communication, 1984.
121. *Standards of Occupational Health Nursing Practice* (revd.). Atlanta, GA: American Association of Occupational Health Nurses, 1983.
122. Devlin, M. M. Nurse practitioners and physician's assistants: Standard of care. *JAMA* 249:652, 1983.
123. Joint Statement on the Role of the Registered Nurse in a Hearing Conservation Program—California Nurses' Association—California Medical Association, Jan 1973.
124. Stockman, J. F. (Ed.). *Protocol Guide for Occupational Health Nursing Specialists.* California State Occupational Health Nurses Association, [n.d.].
125. Medical directives for the non-physician provider. *J Occup Med* 25:263, 1983.
126. *Regulations of the Board of Pharmacy.* Richmond, VA: Commonwealth of Virginia, Department of Health Regulatory Boards, 1980. Regulation 27, Drugs in Industrial Infirmaries/First Aid Rooms, PC-1.
127. Spitzer, W. O. The nurse practitioner revisited: Slow death of a good idea. *N Engl J Med* 310:1049, 1984.
128. Sorenson, D. E. Nurse practitioners: The Idaho experience. *Private Practice* 12:59, May 1980.
129. Draye, M. A., and Pesznecker, B. L. Where are the nurse practitioners? Some insights of utilization. *Nurs Admin Q* 4:55, 1980.
130. Herbert, F. A., and Little, C. Nurse practitioner program: University of Alberta. *Can Med Assoc J* 128:1311, 1983.
131. Babbitz, M. A. Personal communication, July 10, 1984.

132. Bews, D. C. Personal communication, Feb 23, 1971.
133. Cipolla, J. A., and Collings, G. H., Jr. Nurse clinicians in industry. *Am J Nurs 71:1530, 1971.*
134. Plotz, C. M., Weiner, M., Collings, G. H., Jr., et al. The training of nurse-clinicians. *J Occup Med* 13:515, 1971.
135. Kaku, K., Gilbert, F. E., Jr., and Sachs, R. R. Comparison of health appraisals by nurses and physicians. *Public Health Rep* 85:1042, 1970.
136. Hannigan, L. J. Nurse health assessment: The new "physical" in American industry. *Occup Health Nurs* 30:30, Aug 1982.
137. Steel, J. E. Cited in Nursing practice increases scope: "Physicians will need to adjust." *Intern Med News* 17:11, Feb 1–14, 1984.
138. Mechanic, P., and Aiken, L. H. A cooperative agenda for medicine and nursing. *N Engl J Med* 307:747, 1982.
139. Committee on Nursing [of the AMA]. Medicine and nursing in the 1970s: A position statement. *JAMA* 213:1881, 1970.
140. The legal scope of industrial nursing practice. *JAMA* 169:1072, 1959.
141. Murchison, J. A. Law: An element of quality control in occupational health nursing practice. *Occup Health Nurs* 22:9, Nov 1974.
142. Horsley, J. E. How to avoid the "Good Samaritan" trap. *RN* 42:97, Feb 1979. Copyright © 1979 Medical Economics Inc., Oradell, N.J. Reprinted by permission.
143. George, J. E. (Ed.). Law and the emergency nurse: Consent problems. *J Emerg Nurs* 5:46, Sept–Oct 1979.
144. Bowyer, E. A. Occupational health nurses face growing number of lawsuits. *Occup Health Saf* 53:48, Apr 1984.
145. George, J. E. (Ed.). Law and the emergency nurse: Failure to relay history. *J Emerg Nurs* 5:38, Jan–Feb, 1979.
146. Inions, N. The Law and the lamp: The emergency doctrine. *Alberta Assoc Reg Nurs Newsletter* 38:6, May 1982.
147. Anderson, R. D. Personal communication, Oct 9, 1981.
148. Lee, J. A. *Community Health Nursing for Working People.* Cincinnati, OH: U.S. Department of Health, Education, and Welfare, Public Health Service, National Institute for Occupational Safety and Health, 1970. P. 20.
149. Gallagher, P. M. Occupational health nursing: Autonomy and interdependence. *Occup Health Saf* 50:43, Feb 1981.
150. Recent opinions of the judicial council of the American Medical Association. *JAMA* 251:2078, 1984.
151. Haag, A. B. The Occupational Health Nurse: The Answer to Health Care Cost Containment. Typescript, [n.d.]. Pp. 3–4.
152. Abrams, G. UCLA nurses nix whites for civvies. *Los Angeles Times,* July 23, 1982. P. W8.
153. Rogers, B., and Spencer, G. A. Nursing research in occupational health. *Occup Health Nurs* 32:552, 1984.
154. McKecknie, M., and Rogers, B. Developing research skills in occupational health nursing: Where to begin? *Occup Health Nurs* 33:515, 1985.
155. Scharon, B. M., and Bernacki, E. J. A corporate role for nurse practitioners. *Business Health* 1:26, Sept 1984.
156. Palisano, P. Nurse moves up the management ladder. *Occup Haz* 47:53, Nov 1985.
157. Babbitz, M. A. The practice of occupational health nursing in the United States. *Occup Health Nurs* 31:33, June 1983.
158. Nurses' changing role. *Occup Haz* 46:66, Apr 1984.
159. Prosser, L. E., and Richard, E. Statement of beliefs about occupational health nursing. *Am Ind Hyg Assoc J* 41:A-24, 1980.
160. Spickett, J . S. The nurse in industry. *Nursing Times* 50:58, 1954.

APPENDIX 15-1 POTENTIAL PROTOCOLS FOR AN OCCUPATIONAL HEALTH NURSING SERVICE

The listing below represents a number of titles of possible protocols that can be developed for an occupational health nursing service. Other subjects can be added, or some of the headings can be deleted, depending on local needs.

- Abdominal injuries
- Amputations
- Anaphylaxis
  - Emergency procedure
  - Supplies
- Asphyxiation
- Asthma
- Back injuries
- Bites, animal and human
- Blisters
- Burns
  - Thermal
  - Chemical of the eye
  - Chemical of the skin
  - Electric
  - Radiation
- Cardiac emergencies
- Cerebrovascular accidents
- Chest wall injuries
- Common cold
- Communicable disease
- Contusions
- Convulsive disorders
- Cough
- Critical illness or death
- Dermatitis
- Diabetes, emergencies
  - Insulin reaction
  - Diabetic coma
- Diarrhea
- Dysmenorrhea
- Earache
- Ear injuries
- Electric shock
- Eye injuries and other emergencies
  - Use of contact lenses
  - Basic principles
  - Basic supplies
  - Drugs and solutions
  - Foreign bodies
  - Protruding foreign bodies
  - Perforating or intraocular foreign bodies
  - Burns of the eye
  - Contusions of the eye
  - Laceration of the eyelid
- Fainting
- Fractures and dislocations
- Gastrointestinal complaints
- Headache
- Head injuries
- Heat stress emergencies
  - Heat exhaustion
  - Heat stroke
  - Heat cramps
- Hernia emergencies
- Nosebleed
- Respiratory irritation
- Resuscitation
- Shock
- Sore throat
- Splinters
- Sprains and strains
- Toothache
- Wounds
  - Severe or moderately severe
  - Abrasions
  - Lacerations
  - Puncture wounds
  - Infected wounds
  - Tetanus immunization status
    - No previous immunization
    - Previous immunization

16. OCCUPATIONAL HEALTH PROGRAMS IN VARIED SETTINGS

No pleasure endures unseasoned by variety—Maxim 406.
It is a bad plan that admits of no modification—Maxim 469.

Publilius Syrus

A discussion of occupational health programs (OHPs) usually calls to mind a medical activity within the heart of an industrial undertaking, most likely fixed but subject to the changes demanded by the progress of the enterprise. Not every occupational health service (OHS) is so located, for the populations may shift, or the mission may present challenges in extraordinary physical settings or provide hazardous exposures rarely matched elsewhere.

Industry, in its genericness, fails to connote the worldwide facilities of a multinational company, the admixture of workers and activities on a large university campus, the unique demands of a military installation, or the intermittent presence of a maritime workforce. The labor-intensive but relatively short-duration construction projects, the world-touring theatrical and musical groups, and the mixed permanent/transient population of an airport present problems in administration greatly different from the needs of either a fixed health service or a fixed personnel.

While it is not feasible to review the variety of solutions applied to this mix of work settings, certain features pertinent to some of these operations will be discussed. Bodies of employees on the move—a circus, a ballet company, a symphony orchestra—may, but rarely, include health care professionals in the entourage. The usual custom is to make contact in the locality of the moment with physicians who have worked with opera singers, dancers, or actors and are cognizant of the urgency of fitness for performance. Nothing is more disturbing to an eager audience than the last-minute announcement of a substitution for the lead of a show. Certain physicians have made regular calls to New York theaters to meet the needs of stage personnel. Most hotels provide the names of physicians who will provide care for guests and who are accustomed to seeing patients who are strangers to the city.

As the military bodies have been altered by the newer technologies of warfare, the armed services have become accustomed to the need for occupational health facilities in their repair installations, ports of embarkation, and air bases. Today's equipment provides exposures and stressors new to the traditional between-wars ethos. Because of legislative mandates, university campuses have had to establish environmental health offices to ensure meeting the demands of standards and clinical surveillance. The energy crisis of the early 1970s accelerated oil-exploratory efforts in the jungles and offshore, offering new and hazardous work locations and conditions.

A standard OHP conceived in a comfortable corporate headquarters will not suffice in many instances, and medical directors of multinational companies frequently fly to corporate outposts to resolve problems among their expatriate employees.* Arctic and Antarctic research and fixed installations in northernmost Alaska, carry the stressors of general isolation, infrequent communication, and the closeness of community living. Some of the issues of occupational health inherent in these situations will be considered.

MILITARY OCCUPATIONAL HEALTH

As implied previously, both the technology of preparedness and warfare and the legal requirement of

*One corporate medical director had to visit an installation abroad because the company's workers far afield felt that American physicians were the only qualified practitioners to whom they would go for care. Any accent—including British—was immediately viewed as negative. So, the medical director had to visit the worker enclave and explain the care with which physicians were selected and the qualifications that were demanded.

compliance with occupational safety and health standards are relatively new and constantly changing. At no time in the future is the United States likely to return to the relaxed kind of service duty encountered between earlier conflicts. With mobile units on the ready, with the constant threat of peace disruption, and with the enhancement of a defense capability, workers continue to face both long-known and new job-related potential health hazards.

A difficulty that is constantly present is the distance between policy-making offices and sites of operation. Frequent exchange visits by both personnel groups to the offices of either the headquarters or the field activities aid in breaching the experiential gaps. While civilian employees of the armed services have seen concerned on-site health care as an effort secondary to care for military careerists, the demands of the Occupational Safety and Health Act of 1970 have required the same compliance of federal installations as private-sector industry. Medical personnel, primarily physicians, have been sent for specialized training in occupational medicine so that Navy, Army, and Air Force programs in occupational health are, more and more, seeing knowledgeable practitioners as medical officers in charge of the occupational health efforts. The extension of occupational health surveillance to uniformed personnel has broadened the total OHP at military bases. The undertaking by the armed services is part of the overall requirement that all federal agencies provide OHPs for governmental employees.*

The programs at various bases have included the usual components: examination of applicants and employees; selective placement; hearing and vision conservation programs; industrial hygiene; counseling or employee assistance programs; emergency health care; surveillance of workers exposed to potential heath hazards; referral of seriously injured or ill personnel to outside treatment sources; immunization programs; health education concerning both work contactants and nonoccupational health behavior; special efforts in absenteeism control; fitness and disability evaluation; computerization of records; development of reports; where feasible, research or epidemiologic study of workers; and cooperation with managers in the resolution of problems involving health-related issues.

Some of the exposures encountered have included a broad variety of chemicals (metals, solvents, carcinogens [asbestos], fuels, acids, mutagens, and teratogens among others), ionizing and nonionizing radiation, lasers, abnormalities of temperature, humidity, pressure, and illumination, noise, vibration, and microbiologic hazards. In addition, there are responsibilities in environmental health, previously subsumed under the general heading of sanitation, that may or may not be included in the occupational medical officer's portfolio. In the Air Force and Navy, the effort in aviation medicine may likewise be combined with the activity in occupational medicine or may be a separate aspect of preventive medicine.

Needless to add, the selection of astronauts at the beginning of the ventures into space required intensive physical and psychological evaluation of crews for space vehicles, as did the introduction of the nuclear reactor into submarines.

MARITIME MEDICINE

Care for the seafarer has a long history, coursing back to vessels propelled by wind and sail, through ships of steam and diesel engines, to undersea craft with nuclear power plants. Responsibility for the health of the crew in early days was assigned to the captain and later to the contemporary equivalents of today's emergency medical technicians. Eventually, physicians came aboard, and probably the largest medical facilities afloat now are the medical staffs and hospitals on the heaviest of the aircraft carriers.

But maritime medicine has not been the exclusive territory of the uniformed service. Cruise ships carry physicians, and the tanker fleets of the world's petroleum companies have provided problems to corpo-

*The OHP for the U.S. Army is described in a series of manuals: *Occupational Health Surveillance Manual,* with changes, DOD 6055.5-M. Washington, DC: Department of Defense, Assistant Secretary of Defense (Manpower, Reserve Affairs, and Logistics (July 26) 1982; *Hearing Conservation.* TB MED 501. Washington, DC: Headquarters, Department of the Army, (March) 1980; *Occupational and Environmental Health—Respiratory Protection Program.* TB MED 502, DLAM 1000.2. Washington, DC: Headquarters, Department of the Army and Defense Logistics Agency, Feb 15, 1982; *Occupational and Environmental Health—The Army Industrial Hygiene Program.* TB MED 503. Washington, DC: Headquarters, Department of the Army, Feb 1985; *Occupational and Environmental Health—Occupational Vision.* TB MED 506. Headquarters, Department of the Army Dec 1981.

The directives for the OHP for the U.S. Navy are to be found in OPNAV Instruction 5100.23B, *Navy Occupational Safety and Health (NAVOSH) Program Manual.* Washington, DC: Department of the Navy, Office of the Chief of Naval Operations, Aug 31, 1983, with Change 1, dated Oct 23, 1984.

Occupational Health in the U.S. Air Force is outlined in *Occupational Health—Standardized Occupational Health Program.* AFOSH Standard 161-17. Washington, DC: Headquarters U.S. Air Force, June 25, 1982.

rate medical departments. Of concern in recent years, though, has been the health care—selection and emergent attention—of workers on offshore drilling rigs, where personnel may remain on assignment days at a time or be subject to disastrous accidents at sea through mishap to the platform or tower. Governmental regulations also apply to the merchant marine in the examination and provision of care for its members. Freight-carrying vessels in commerce usually have no health personnel aboard, but today's communication systems do allow contact with shore-based medical facilities, so guidance can be obtained. Efforts have been made in the United Kingdom to establish an umbrella area of interest termed Medical Services in Transport, including occupational health practice for all forms of transportation—surface, sea, and air—but no such focusing of effort has been attempted in the United States.

MERCHANT MARINE

Lindsay [1] has pointed out that while most seamen serve in cargo ships—vessels of up to some 13,000 tons—there are, however, a number of other types of craft where working and living conditions are varied and where different standards of fitness may be required: large passenger ships, bulk carriers, oil tankers, cross-channel steamers, fishing vessels, and oddments such as offshore supply rigs.

The physical demands are greatest of deck ratings, who must be able to climb up masts and rope ladders, climb down vertical ladders into holds,and climb back out again. They handle heavy ship's gear and mooring ropes and must be able to row ship lifeboats. Deck officers or mates start as midshipmen, but when certified, leave the tasks of the ratings. They are concerned with navigation at sea and supervision of cargo when in port, which involves multiple trips in and out of the hatches to ensure stability of the vessel with the loading. After 10 to 15 years, they advance to captain or master. This position is primarily administrative, and they are more often "office-bound." Although less demanding, the position requires daily inspection of the ship and carries responsibility for the safety of the ship, the cargo, the crew, and the passengers. In persistent fog, there are long periods of watch on the bridge, and in long river estuaries duty may be for hours in the dark.

There is the problem of loneliness during long voyages, and the captain cannot fraternize excessively with junior officers, occasioning much time by himself. It is not possible to "pass the buck" at sea. Engine-room personnel work in noisy, limited, malodorous space with steep ladders for ingress and egress.

Other positions at sea match their counterparts ashore—catering officers, lounge stewards, bedroom stewards, hairdressers, musicians, radio operators, and the like. Lindsay [1] indicates that the entry examination must be a searching one, for certain medical conditions can be troublesome at sea when no medical attendant is available. Separation from home can exacerbate previous mental or emotional difficulties, and some skin diseases worsen in hot climates. Otitis externa and media can return in tropical areas, and an individual with recurrent peptic ulceration should not be accepted, as hemorrhage or perforation in mid-ocean, without a physician, could be fatal. Good hearing is mandatory for men on watch, particularly for audibility of orders and ships' whistles in fog. A history of renal calculus questions the wisdom of employment away from a source of care [1].

Blais [2] has indicated that even though the numbers of jobs in the deep-sea maritime industry are the lowest in over half a century,* the mean age of mariners on United States ocean-going vessels is 53+ years. There are twice as many reported illnesses and injuries and four times as many reported illness-related deaths in the over-40 age group. Problems at sea include an unstable platform for both work environment and home, which speeds through all kinds of seas and weather. As noted by Lindsay, no physician is available, and the master or chief mate may not have adequate knowledge for emergent care. Means for evacuation of a patient may be either nonexistent or delayed, and even when a port is reached, there is a lack of quality assurance in the care received—care given by persons unknowing of the demands of life at sea. Problems exist in learning the names or dosage of nongeneric medications used in port. Repatriation of ill seamen is costly, let alone the high charges involved in diversion† of the vessel and users' fees for boats or helicopters employed in medevacuation.

Fitness of seamen is mandatory, for any ship that puts to sea with infirm or physically unfit personnel is at risk [2]. In an emergency, the safety of an entire

*Low employment has resulted from there being fewer ships under the American flag, increased automation, less manpower needed per ship, and an increase in the skills and knowledge required. In 1951, there were 86,000 seamen's jobs, but this number dropped to 13,154 in 1985, as reported to the Marine Index Bureau in New York City. (Statistical Analysis No. 93, July 23, 1986.)

†Anderson [3] has provided numbers. The cost of operating a 31,000-ton tanker is about $1,000 per ton per day. In the case of a patient bleeding from esophageal varices who required ship diversion, the fuel cost exceeded $10,000, and the loss of steaming time and other expenses exceeded $100,000.

crew can be jeopardized by the inability of a few to complete their regularly assigned duties.

Currently concerned groups are working on both the improvement of maritime medical care and the development of fitness standards. In addition, a familiarization program is underway so that examiners become knowledgeable of the work demands at sea and the hazards involved. In addition, there will be upgrading of both the medical equipment and stores used at sea and the instructions concerning their employment. In substance, efforts are being directed toward developing all aspects of a full OHP for use with seafarers—examination, knowledge of the work environment, provision of good care by trained paramedical personnel, and a central depository for medical records.

A separate statute governs personal injuries sustained by maritime personnel. In 1920, the Jones Act was passed, which gave to seamen an effective personal injury and wrongful death remedy. The Sieracki decision of the Supreme Court in 1946 gave to longshoremen the important right of seaworthiness. Affected by the decision were not only longshoremen, but passengers, visitors, and repairmen of all types. While originally a seaman was defined as a person who could hand, reef, and steer, case law has come to include such diverse persons as radio operators, stewardesses, ferry hands, musicians, clerks, barbers, bartenders, divers, pursers, wreckers, and laundresses, among others [4]. For practitioners specializing in maritime medicine in the larger port cities, the potential clientele can extend far beyond the usual understanding of the master, the officers, and the crew. Usually these questions are asked to reach a definition of "seaman:" (1) Is the vessel in navigation? (2) Is there a more or less permanent connection with the vessel, as distinguished from a visitor or passenger? and (3) Are the services rendered maritime in character? The Jones Act and the decisions reached under its coverage without question allow liberal interpretations [5].

A serious change occurred in relation to the health of merchant mariners when, in late 1981, all U.S. public health service (USPHS) hospitals and clinics were closed, and U.S. seamen were disentitled for care.* Historically, the USPHS has provided a system across the nation that coordinated occupational health care delivery to a highly mobile patient population with special needs in health care [6]. To fill the gap, in part, that was created by these closures, a health care system was devised, not only to meet recognized needs but also to improve on the design of the USPHS. Serving over 600 commercial vessels and offshore oil rigs, a workforce approximating 40,000 persons, is the Medical Telecommunications Response Center (MTRC).* Hall and his coworkers [6] relate a 20-month experience with the MTRC, to which more recently had been added the Pharmaceutical Inventory Control Program and the Seafarers' Health History Program. Previous efforts at therapeutic intervention were inadequate because of delays in communication. As an example, a Coast Guard study covering the period 1972 to 1977 demonstrated a 93-percent mortality rate for patients sustaining a "heart attack" while at sea [3].

The MTRC is staffed around the clock by a physician and a communications coordinator. A physician's assistant may be added during peak shifts. About 10 percent of United States vessels are equipped for direct contact by telephone or telex, using the International Maritime Satellite System (INMARSAT). Voice communication, even at great distances, is of near-perfect clarity, and the satellite permits the sending of telex messages with delay by a high-seas operator relay. Printed instructions can be sent, backing up voiced recommendations. Special formats for sea-to-land and land-to-sea messages have been designed, as has a medical protocol manual for reference use by the ship's captain. While the communications equipment on-board ship and connect-time charges are high, INMARSAT has been used in 19 percent of the situations requiring consultation.

The MTRC has, in addition, a single-side band radio station that provides communication over a radius of 3,000 to 5,000 miles, operating over 15 separate frequencies. Through bilateral use of a medical protocol manual—prepared in language clear to a ship's master—the patient can be stabilized, and then a decision can be reached regarding evacuation. The average case has seen two to three follow-up contacts and 48 minutes of total communicating time.

The Pharmaceuticals Inventory Control Program provides a standardized medicine chest for all vessels. There are periodic reviews and updating of the items included. Included under each medication are synonyms of its designation, its category, use, usual dosage, and special notes, if needed. The Seafarers' Health History Program allows storage of baseline

*As the USPHS hospitals were in place, no workers' compensation scheme was ever initiated for the merchant mariners. The hospital closure created considerable chaos as plans for in-patient care particularly began to be formulated.

*Medical Telecommunications Response Center, Medical Advisory Systems, Inc., Box 193, Chaneyville Road, Owings, MD 20736, (301) 855-8070. The European Office is located at Golden Lane, Western Street, Brighton BN1 2Q6, United Kingdom 44-273-202141.

medical information of a seaman in the MTRC data bank. Newly occurring events at sea are added to the records, and with the patient's authorization, the information can be relayed to a facility when land-based care is sought.

A Responder Training Course, designed specifically for ships' medical officers, has been initiated that focuses on physical examination of the patient and radio communication of this medical information to the MTRC [7]. In addition, a Health History Storage and Retrieval System has been established at the MTRC, allowing rapid access by the medical staff to baseline history and physical examination information while communication is in progress [7]. Another system that has been created is an organized network of independent medical clinics in the major port cities of the United States, allowing a systematic determination of duty status, the uniform application of entry and retention physical standards, and organized routing of medical records for centralized storage at the MTRC [7].

Currently, as pointed out by Hall and his colleagues [6], the Seafarers' Health Improvement Program (SHIP)* has working groups from all areas of the maritime community addressing such issues as entry and retention physical standards, access to land-based care, seagoing care and services, shipboard occupational and environmental health monitoring, and medical records storage. Health care for merchant seamen was provided by industry during the 17th and 18th centuries,† subsequently by the federal government from 1790 through 1981, and is again the responsibility of the employer [6]. The training segment of ships' masters has been undertaken by the Maritime Institute of Technology and Graduate Studies (MITAGS).* Training in shipboard medicine has been available also through the Center for Advanced Maritime Studies sponsored by the Maine Maritime Academy† and the Staff Officers' Association of America [10].

The standard source book is still a USPHS publication that has undergone several revisions. *The Ship's Medicine Chest and Medical Aid at Sea* [1] (first published in 1881) provides not only material on the human body and medical care but the suggested instruments, supplies, and equipment for the sickbay and a complete list of recommended pharmaceuticals. Further, a full list of drug products by generic names with corresponding brand or proprietary names is given, along with the names of their manufacturers. The list of pharmaceuticals is offered also by Urner [10] with some additions suggested by the Lykes Lines. While the drugs are suggested, their availability or stocking is not mandatory. Forms are shown for use in the inventory of controlled substances, which are equally applicable to use in shore installations. A comparmentalized freestanding ship's locker has been designed by Urner and associates [12] that serves as a medical dispensing system and is commercially available.‡

One additional group in need of care warrants discussion. About 300,000 new divers are trained each year in the United States [13], and currently it is estimated that there may be nearly 3 million active sport SCUBA (self-contained underwater breathing apparatus) divers who undertake an undetermined number of dives each year. According to clinicians operating Duke University's Divers Alert Network in Durham, NC, about 500 such divers may encounter problems.

To meet this need—caring for persons with specialized injuries—the Duke team maintains a 24-hour emergency hotline that accepts collect calls concerning diving accidents. The telephone is (919) 684-8111. Medical questions of a nonemergent nature relating to diving may be placed through a second line—(919) 684-2948—Monday through Friday, 9A.M. to 5 P.M. EST. The officials may be

*Seafarers' Health Improvement Program, 17 Battery Place, Suite 2233, New York, NY, 10004-1283, (212) 269-1200. The SHIP adopted "Reference Guide—Physical Examination Standards for Original Entry into the U.S. Merchant Marine" in 1982 (latest edition, 1984) and "Guidelines for Physical Examination for Retention of Seafarers in the U.S. Merchant Marine" in 1985. See also C. J. Urner, Ship: The Seafarers Health Improvement Program *J Occup Med* 29:531, 1987.

†Although he was British, not American, one can recall the surgeon aboard the *HMS Bounty*. "Our sawbone's name was Thomas Huggan . . . but he was known as Old Bacchus. . . . This normal state was what sailors call 'in the wind' or 'shaking a cloth,' and the signal that he had passed his normal state earned him the name by which all hands on the *Bounty* knew him. . . . He had been afloat so long that he could scarcely recollect the days when he had lived ashore, and viewed with apprehension the prospect of retirement. He preferred salt beef to the finest steak . . . to be obtained ashore, and confided . . . that it was almost impossible for him to sleep in a bed." [8].

*MITAGS, 5700 Hammonds Ferry Road, Linthicum Heights, MD 21090, (301) 859-5700. This organization is the training arm of the International Organization of Masters, Mates, and Pilots, and the courses developed to assist the masters and deck officers on American flag merchant ships in responding to shipboard emergencies have included Hazardous Materials and Shipboard Medical Care and others [9].

†Maine Maritime Academy, Castine, ME 04421.

‡Available from Delta Export Pharmacy, Inc., 4714 Earhart Boulevard, New Orleans, LA 70125.

reached care of Box 3823, Duke University Medical Center, Durham, NC 27710. The network is supported by memberships ($10), which include a newsletter, *Alert Diver,* and a manual.*

Fitness for Duty

Probably most irksome in the entire area of marine medicine has been the irresponsible declaration of fitness for duty of many examinees whose health status would certainly dictate unseaworthiness. Physicians close to the problem have cited negligence in the medical recommendations submitted following physical examinations to determine fitness for duty at sea, particularly on deep-water ships. Recommendations have followed review of applicants not only for service on ocean-going vessels, but also on "lakers," fishing vessels, and barges. Urner [10] has related some of the results of impaired physician judgment:

> Modern ships are being built larger and the crews tend to get smaller. When a seaman is ill or injured there is no replacement. To send a man to sea who has to stand lookout duty, or go aloft, or over the side of a vessel, or work with fast-moving machinery when his diagnosis is "controlled epilepsy" puts this individual and his working community at risk. Yet this has been done. Men have been sent to work with known psychotic conditions, suicidal tendencies, and some have died as a result. Men have been found fit for duty with acute liver failure; following a cardiac bypass and while taking anticoagulants; while receiving long-term steroid medication; and even with multiple sclerosis since "there is an elevator aboard." Men have been injured because of unstable backs or knees which did not allow them to respond properly to a sudden motion of the vessel, e.g., permanent leg brace (this person lasted two hours) or a lower-limb prosthesis (one seaman fell and broke his sound leg).

Anderson [3] has voiced similar frustration when noting the approval for duty of maritime personnel who had chronic alcoholism—some of whom were on dry ships and became psychotic—or were suicidal, who had type II diabetes out of control when injured, who incarcerated or strangulated hernias, or who developed severe asthma, acute glaucoma, or urinary tract obstruction. And now that seamen are seapersons, the pregnancy rate has been found to be high, and vaginal bleeding from miscarriage and ruptured tubal pregnancies have been encountered. Added to these pathologic states has been drug abuse.

As most deep-water ships today are crewed by third-world-nation seamen, tropical medicine has become a significant segment of marine medicine. They have presented with infestations unknown among American mariners, complicated by language difficulties* and frequent self-medication.

Offered as absolute contraindications to duty on deep-water ships are the following clinical conditions [14]:

- Contact lenses (corneal irritation from hard lenses; discoloration of soft lenses on fume contact)
- Glaucoma
- Tympanic membrane perforations (preclude gas mask use on parcel tankers or oil rigs)
- Asthma, when constant medication is required (hazard of status asthmaticus)
- Emphysema, advanced
- Hypertension, when multiple medications are required
- Pulmonary blebs (potential spontaneous pneumothorax)
- Coronary artery disease (when symptomatic and requiring vasodilators)
- Post–coronary bypass status (unless with evidence of post-surgical exercise test clearance and no need of medication)
- Thrombophlebitis, symptomatic
- Peripheral vascular disease
- Peptic ulceration
- Panceratitis (even on history exclusively)
- Cirrhosis, particularly with esophageal varices
- Prostatic hypertrophy, symptomatic, with frequency and nocturia
- Renal calculi
- Pregnancy
- Pelvic inflammatory disease
- Diabetes, type II
- Inguinal hernia
- Lumbar disc disease
- Spondylolisthesis
- Epilepsy
- Psychiatric states, including schizophrenia, depression, and severe anxiety ("Seamanship is voluntary servitude," and mental disorders worsen at sea.)
- Alcoholism, alcoholic psychosis
- Drug abuse

*Mebane, G. Y., and Dick, A. P. *Underwater Diving Accident Manual.* Durham, NC: Duke University, 1982. Among the topics discussed in the 24-page publication are such entities as air embolism, decompression sickness, nitrogen narcosis, mediastinal emphysema, and motion sickness. Each clinical disorder is discussed from the aspects of cause, symptoms, signs, prevention, and treatment.

*Anderson [14] related the problem of obtaining adequate histories when Asians use dictionary language. As an example, a Korean handed him a note printed in English reading, "Love hot when rain—medicine no do rain clear." The diagnosis was gonorrhea—penicillin resistant.

Any condition requiring regular use of corticosteroids (Addison's disease, nephrotic syndrome)
Any condition requiring anticoagulants

Urner [15] has produced excellent guidelines for examiners that include job descriptions of marine personnel. Urner adds these states as contraindicating sea duty:

Any communicable disease, including carrier stage
Any known disorder likely to need treatment for acute manifestations (malignancies; heart disease functional class III, IV; hemophilia)
Severe speech impediment (inability to transmit orders)
Any condition that seriously limits balance
Permanent tracheostomy
Senility
Mental deficiency
Parkinsonism
Chorea
Neurosyphilis
Extreme obesity (limits ordinary activity)
Back surgery, with patient's remaining symptomatic following surgery, or more than one surgical procedure on the back
Repetitive repatriation—more than twice—or inability to complete several voyages because of health reasons

While medical standards have been drawn up in the United States by working groups representing all concerned parties—employers, unions, physicians—no action has been taken because of the current administration's desire to refrain from imposing regulations of any sort. This inaction, plus the shutoff of care for merchant seamen, has left maritime occupational medicine in a state of suspension, if not total inconclusivity. In Great Britain, however, medical standards were revised in 1984 by a Working Party from the Faculty of Occupational Medicine at the London Royal College of Physicians [16] and have been issued by the Department of Transport as a formal Merchant Shipping Notice [17].

In the notice, examinations are called for on a regular basis:

All seafarers below the age of 18 shall have a yearly medical examination.
Seafarers between the ages of 18 and 40 shall be examined at intervals not exceeding 5 years.
Seafarers aged 40 years and over shall be examined at intervals not exceeding 2 years.
Seafarers serving on bulk chemical carriers shall be subject to annual examinations and blood tests at yearly or more frequent intervals, according to the nature of the cargo.

The problem of physical health maintenance of merchant mariners has not been resolved because of the inequality of medical care in various ports, language problems, the unwarranted approval of unfit personnel for sea duty, and the lack of formalized medical standards in many, if not most, countries.

Emotional Health

The British notice recognizes the demands on a seafarer's emotional economy with these comments [17]:

> . . . [A] ship is not only a place of work requiring attention throughout the day and night but also a temporary home in which the crew must eat, sleep and find recreation. Most important of all is the need to adjust to each other, often for long periods, during a voyage.
>
> Much is done to ameliorate living and working conditions but certain inherent characteristics remain. A crew is a closed community living in a ship that is seldom quiet or still. Individual eating habits and tastes cannot be met; facilities for physical exercise are limited; forced ventilation systems are used; the tedium of routine can easily become oppressive in the absence of normal diversion enjoyed by those ashore. An inability to fit in, or unwillingness to take responsibility, or to accept a reasonable measure of necessary discipline, could impair the safe and efficient working of the ship.

The appearance of supertankers—ships designed to carry liquid cargo in bulk—in the fleets of the world's petroleum companies was not occasioned by the simple desire to create a larger mode of transport. Changes in tanker fleets came about as a result of several actions, as indicated by Gerst [18]: political, in the closing of the Suez Canal; technical, in the increased installation of advanced automation in ships; and economic, in that studies and their application have demonstrated that increasing the tonnage reduced the cost of transportation per ton of cargo. In 1950, the tanker fleet of the world was limited to ships under 25,000 tons. Over the years, larger and larger tankers were built so that today's supertankers, the largest ships afloat, carry more than 500,000 tons deadweight. The only obstacles to increasing the size even further are the lack of shore facilities to handle such huge carriers and the objections by conservationists because of biodamage from large spillages.*

With the enlargement of the sea carriers, the amenities for the crew have increased. There are fewer per-

*The mid-1980s drop in oil prices has been paralleled by a lessened use of the large tankers, some being released or scrapped.

sons aboard, and each person has an individual cabin with adjoining toilet facilities. The fare served is sumptuous, and there is no question whatsoever regarding water quality. For leisure hours there are miniature amphitheaters for motion pictures, television, card tables, pinball games, a fully equipped gymnasium, a hobby shop, a library, an indoor pool, and finally, a complete sound system in every cabin, with a radio, turntable, tape recorder, and speakers—all of these benefits for 30 men and an apprentice.

The pay scale is excellent and competitive. Yet, the members of the crew seek a return to the "classical" tankers. There has been a general psychological discomfort, which Gerst [18] believes results from the reluctance to accept these plush assignments and is "the cause of true neurosis."

There is almost too much room aboard; the seamen are isolated from the rest of the world for 4 months; there are no ports of call; and "life on board orders and determines everything, it becomes the only universe" [18]. Thirty men break into subgroups that are too small for a coherency in social living. Separate mess rooms by rank, some clique-formation by service, work by watches, and shift schedules fragment further the homogeneity of the subgroups. Members facing stressors seek isolation, and there are no shore-type duties to consume the 18 hours off duty. There is even no travel time required to get to work.

Resulting from these factors is the use of free time only in a passive manner—film and television viewing. In the facilities provided for active participation, the groups are too small for true social gatherings with their lack of admiring onlookers and social rewards. The men remain in their cabins, awaiting the end of the voyage.

As remedies, Gerst suggests shorter crew service periods and teaching men to live in groups and to occupy their leisure time. Efforts to raise the cultural level so that more effective use could be made of free time are unrealistic. A motivator is needed, preferably from the junior officer group, so that the crews could become involved and compelled to revive themselves by having returned to them their original feeling of team spirit.

Some time ago, commensurate with exploration on the North Slope of Alaska, an Arctic test voyage of a tanker was reported by Clark and Montgomery [19]. The ship was refitted as an icebreaker and made the run to the Canadian Arctic through the fabled "northwest passage." The trip was made from Chester, Pennsylvania, to Prudhoe Bay and return. An enlarged crew of 60 was on board, in addition to many observers and scientific personnel, and the ship carried a physician for the initial run. Modest use was made of the medical facility, there being 272 visits in the 45-day period.

It was determined that a physician would not be needed on future trips, for it was in only four presenting conditions that a nonphysician might have requested assistance. Interestingly, the movies were fairly well attended, but the exercise and game facilities were rarely used. It was felt that presail dental prophylaxes for the crew would be extremely worthwhile and that there be some selection of the crew. The writers concluded that tanker crews seem to comprise middle-aged, self-selected, self-sufficient men who are not prone to accidental injury and that the captain of such a vessel should have training in contemporary first aid. A last recommendation pointed to the helpfulness of medicine in prepackaged containers of individual-dose size.

OFFSHORE DRILLING

Initially with oil exploration in remote parts of the world, the petroleum companies provided those medical facilities that would offer adequate care for the employees and their dependents. Usually such care was obtained in a small clinic or major hospital, the program representing ordinarily a general practice of a slightly special type, together with the basic tenets of occupational medicine as applicable to the petroleum industry [20].

With the beginning of drilling offshore, new challenges arose in health care. The practitioners were separated from their patients by both time and distance, which made even minor disorders of significance. The disaster potential on a drilling platform was ever present, and the biotechnology of work underwater offered new questions for resolution. As the offshore communities grew, there were the difficulties of overcrowding, lengthy work shifts, and separation from families. These challenges were seen in both the southern segment of the North Sea and the deep-water, hostile, remote environment of the upper sector of the North Sea [20].

The same needs will, indue course, appear off the waters of Eastern Canada, where fog and icebergs abound, to the project in the Beaufort Sea, and eventually in the southern oceans and the Antarctica land mass [20]. The North Sea challenge had the problem of the involvement of multiple companies and many countries. Most offshore personnel are trained in first aid, and as a second care source there has been developed the life support escort who not only is trained in first aid but also is intelligent and interested in the health arena and is further trained to escort the seriously ill or injured patient from the offshore facility to the hospital. The escort is able to support the airways, measure blood pressure, care for intravenous infusions, and communicate medical information [20]. The presence of several such persons obviates the need for a so-called rig medic, who is usually a specially trained nurse.

The third person to provide aid is the diving paramedic, who is versed in the treatment of diving casualties and is knowledgeable in relation to both diving and intercurrent illness in saturation systems [20]. All report to the company's medical director.

With good communications systems to shore bases, the level of emergency is determined; specialists can be called on, such as those physicians willing to go offshore, mobile specialist teams, diving medicine experts; and facilities such as hyperbaric chambers can be readied. As Norman [20] has expressed it, the training of both medical and paramedical personnel has been developed to an advanced stage, but if "high standards of nursing and medical care are to be maintained within an acceptable career structure . . . the work has to be undertaken in more and more difficult circumstances and involve more and more people"—meaning that it must be married to academic research and teaching so that progress will continue "for tomorrow when the exploratory activities penetrate the much more difficult areas" now being entered. All activities, because of the multinational and multicontractor involvement, must be pooled so that training, public health policy offshore, equipment evaluation and research, and physical fitness determination can be coordinated.

Cox, who published previously on the subject of medical service to offshore facilities [21], has included most currently available knowledge in his monograph, *Offshore Medicine: Medical Care of Employees in the Offshore Oil Industry* [22] which covers in detail such topics as preplacement and periodic medical examinations, provision of back-up services, special problems (for example, hydrogen sulfide, methanol, obesity, noise, scabies, and diving. Appendices offer complete lists of drugs and dressings for offshore installation sickbays (both types of items are given, those required by law and those recommended), the same materials for merchant shipping, medical supplies to be kept at diving sites, medical equipment for offshore emergencies, contents of a medical chest for use in offshore disasters, extra medical equipment to be kept on rigs for use in major disasters, and major items of furniture and medical equipment for offshore installations.* For definitive treatment of any of these areas, *Offshore Medicine* is the reference to be sought.

The contraindications to platform employment are stringent and match fairly well the standards given for merchant marine activity listed earlier in this chapter. Such terms as "absolute contraindication," "bar to offshore work," "not suitable," "should not be allowed offshore until . . . repaired," "cause for rejection," and "should not be accepted" bespeak the need for rigorous prehire physical review because of the absence of definitive care in that work setting. Confidentiality is stressed in all recordkeeping, and Cox [22] indicates that a clinical condition found on examination may not affect current employment but may bear an influence on the individual's future career. He advises that the personal file be endorsed, "Not to be promoted or transferred without reference to [the] Medical [Department]"* [22].

CIRCUMPOLAR HEALTH

With the development of the oil fields on the North Slope in Alaska, special medical difficulties were anticipated with the transfer of personnel to that region from less challenging climates. However, Stallard [23] has expressed it well in that "Alaska is no longer a frontier in the sense that health problems are not understood. The usual problems of cyclic work patterns, remoteness, and behavioral abnormalities, including substance abuse, are all common to medical practice everywhere, although the percentages or the emphasis may differ in Alaska."

An American Society for Circumpolar Health was established in 1980, and state and international congresses have been held. There have been discussions of such topics as cross-cultural treatment, alcoholism and drug abuse, cold exposure, primary hepatocellular carcinoma and other malignancies in Alaskan natives, stress in the Arctic, traditional health practices, health care in the Alaskan bush, occupational health programs in the Alaskan seafood processing industry, the woman in the Arctic, and Arctic industrialization, among others. Crippen and Davis, around 1970, produced a valuable booklet for the American Petroleum Institute, *Staying Alive in the Arctic* [24], which deals with self-preservation in a survival situation, including the prevention of losing one's way and frostbite or other injury. More re-

*Infrequently British terminology may seem puzzling, but American-English equivalents can be determined readily, although there are differences in the designation of pharmaceuticals.

*Often there are unpredictable stress responses. An engineer from one of the country's largest petroleum companies was sent to Oak Ridge for training in nuclear engineering. As he was required to read reports, it was learned that he claimed that all the documents in the technical library were radioactive and he was being contaminated. He had to be returned to his parent company with appropriate recommendations.

cently, the American Public Health Association published a booklet, *The National Arctic Health Science Policy* [25]. While not dealing with occupational health directly, the policy outlined was designed, in part, to protect and promote the health of persons living and working in circumarctic lands.

COLLEGES AND UNIVERSITIES

It has been customary practice to have student health services (SHS) on nearly all college campuses because of the special needs of students, particularly young persons living away from home. The occupational health of students has been given little thought, and most SHSs have been reluctant to add a capability in occupational health for university faculty and nonacademic employees.* Safety offices are found commonly, and even environmental health services, but no clinical activities—emergency care, periodic examinations, hearing conservation, and the like—have been established except on certain large campuses. At one eminent institution where there were separate SHSs for the undergraduate students, the law school, the medical school, and possibly others, there was an OHS for the employed personnel. The consortium of services was headed by a psychiatrist, which may imply a sharpened insight into needs.

Because of the multiplicity and complexity of university activities—administration; teaching at all levels; research in hundreds of scholarly and professional disciplines; maintenance of the physical plant; hosting of cultural, educational, and athletic events and conferences; evening extension classes; state psychiatric hospital care; demonstrations in gardening and farming; food service; museum and art gallery preparation; animal husbandry and dairying; and the provision of consultation to industry and government in the United States and abroad, among other undertakings—a campus frequently is a broader section of industry than industry itself. The problems of hazards exposures, safety violations, traffic mishaps, substance abuse, assaultive behavior, and psychotic breaks are as ubiquitous as in any manufacturing plant.

HAZARDS ON CAMPUS

The environmental health problems in institutions of higher learning have been addressed by Tabershaw and Fuenning [26]. Although underplaying some of the realities, they describe a few of the elements of academe:

> The campus population is composed of highly intelligent and *usually* [emphasis added] socially cooperative individuals. The physical activity is normally sedentary and the pace leisurely. Work connected injuries are relatively infrequent because responsible work habits overcome many physical conditions which in any other setting would be disastrous. Cerebration is pervasive and mental trauma may be rampant, but untoward effects of these activities are not highly visible and work-induced mental and emotional illness is not easily recognized nor often admitted. Since the finished products, the graduating student and scholarly and research publications, cannot be subjected to quality control and because accounting practices are difficult, the efficiency of a university cannot be evaluated.

The range of health problems includes water, air, and solid pollution; hazards of physical safety—fire, traffic, explosion, and athletics; sanitation—housing, food services, swimming pools; and the potential environmental hazards in lighting, ventilation, and noise. These conceivable endangerments are in addition to the usual trilogy of risks: biologic, physical, and chemical sources of health jeopardy. While there are experts in all fields, it is with difficulty that the theoretician can be brought face-to-face with the practical.* Otherwise the sources of consultative help on a large campus would be legion.

Over the years, various occupational health hazards have been rated by on-site observers. Michaelsen [27] recalls these exposures, since corrected, at the University of Minnesota, a campus where occupational health considerations were given a position of primacy:

A sergeant in charge of the armory rifle range became ill with lead poisoning.
Lead and solvent hazards in the print shop.
Welding fume in the maintenance shops.
Carbon monoxide in underground garages.
Excessive noise in the wind tunnel, in jet engine testing, and in jet fuel combustion research.
Mercury in scores of laboratories.
Potential dangers in the handling of organic, phosphate-type insecticides in the laboratory, the greenhouse, and the field.

*The author has had consultative opportunities to study occupational health needs on various campuses, and in most settings, including statewide multicampus systems, there has been extreme hesitancy (frank negativity) on the part of administrators to initiate this kind of activity and of SHS directors to broaden the scope of their programs.

*An example of this disparity was experienced once when discussing cartography with a geography professor at UCLA. He informed the author that if he wanted a map of the interior of Burma or Mongolia it could be supplied, but he did not have a map of Los Angeles.

The issue of ionizing radiation has been discussed by Prince [28], and the occupational allergy to laboratory animals has been noted [29]. Mercurialism was diagnosed in a university chemical laboratory assistant [30]. Edmonds [31], in commenting on the British scene, pointed to the use on campus of epoxy resins, epoxypropane, osmium tetroxide, phosphorus pentoxide, and benzene. Microbiologic hazards, lead, solvents, chromic acid, organophosphate pesticides, hydrofluoric acid, and both ionizing and non-ionizing radiation were found on a large campus.

But more telling than an inventory of potential health hazards are the comments of Edmonds [31] regarding the work environment itself. The outstanding features, he relates, are the multiplicity of small pockets of men exposed to risk and the varied nature of the occupational tasks. There may be, he continues, as many as 70 or 80 different departments all separated topographically and administratively in which almost every activity covered by factory legislation is being pursued.

He quotes a vice-chancellor as illustrative of the antediluvian attitude toward health concerns as late as 1972: "The University does not exist to ensure adequate physical training or health; it exists primarily for the purpose—call it medieval if you like—of training the intellect in the pathway of truth. Everything else is subordinate."

The issue of biohazards has been faced by Dreesen [32], who offers the definition as developed on the University of Georgia campus. These hazards are defined as biologic agents that are capable of reproduction and that could be detrimental to various forms of life if they escaped from laboratory situations into the environment. The six types of biohazards in keeping with that university's standards are the following:

Type I	In vitro construction and/or propagation of rDNA molecules
Type II	Organisms of demonstrated human pathogenicity
Type III	Oncogenic animal viruses
Type IV	The laboratory culture of animal cells
Type V	Venomous vertebrates and invertebrates
Type VI	The movement into the state of Pathogens that adversely affect plants or animals Any non-indigenous species of plants or animals Any indigenous species of plants or animals infected with pathogenic organisms outside the state

Dreesen [32] emphasized the need in a litigious society for university administrators and researchers to comply with governmental regulations as well as the basic concepts of biologic containment. "Individuals in communities contiguous with research centers are no longer complacent to unrestrictive research and are not hesitant to speak out when they feel threatened" [32].

AMERICAN COLLEGE HEALTH ASSOCIATION RECOMMENDATIONS

Singularly significant has been the inclusion in the Recommended Standards and Practices for a College Health Program of a section devoted to occupational health [33]. The fact is addressed that faculty, staff, and students are the college's most important assets and that an occupational health program is a part of any comprehensive and effective plan designed to protect these assets. The recommended program elements in an occupational health effort include

- Preplacement health evaluations
- Assistance in the development of written physical and emotional demands of positions within the college or university.
- Periodic health evaluations
- Coordination and arrangement of medical care and rehabilitation of workers sustaining job-related illnesses or injuries.
- Immunizations
- Control of chemical, physical, and biologic hazards in the environment
- Educational program concerning the identification and control of environmental stressors, personal health maintenance, and motivation of faculty and staff to participate actively in the development of an environment for healthful living
- Retention (or release) of medical records in keeping with legislative mandates and practice of confidentiality
- Psychiatric consultation for emotional problems*

Responsibility for the occupational health segment should be vested in one coordinator who reports to the director of the overall health program.

ONE UNIVERSITY EXAMPLE

As an example of occupational health programming on a large university campus, the staffing at Ohio State University is cited. The division of Environmental and Occupational Health and Safety (EOHS) is one segment of the university health service, and the chief is an occupational physician. In addition, there is a doctoral-level bio-safety officer, a master's level

*Inexplicably, this component, which appeared in the 1977 *Recommended Standards and Practices*, 3rd edition, was omitted in the current edition.

industrial hygienist, one occupational health nurse, one safety engineer at the master's level, five research assistants who are cross-trained in industrial hygiene, bio-safety, and industrial safety who serve as extenders of the health and safety professionals, a part-time nurse epidemiologist, and two clerical support persons, for a total staff of 13 [34].

The EOHS division provides the following program services:

Occupational medicine and nursing
Safety in educational, research, and service areas
Identification and analysis of environmental problems
Compliance with federal, state, and local environmental regulations and health and safety codes or statutes
Control of physical, chemical, and biologic hazards in the work place
Employee occupational health and safety education

In addition, there are these specific activities:

Hazardous waste pickup, transport, and storage
Biologic and chemical hood surveillance
Broad-scope occupational medicine and nursing services
Industrial hygiene evaluation and consultation
Bio-safety evaluation and consultation
Occupational accident investigation, training, and preventive services

Educational presentations are made to various university departments, and EOHS staff members serve on several departmental and college safety committees. A management training series for health and safety staff was conducted by the health educator, including university credit for those persons enrolled, with the objective of developing new insights into their current administrative procedures and of establishing a common basis for the team effort deemed so necessary in occupational health and safety [35].

ADVANTAGES OF A CAMPUS PROGRAM

As no survey has been conducted recently, it is not possible to determine the scope of OHSS in our colleges and universities. It is hoped that new understandings will develop concerning the actual hazards to health existing or potential in university laboratories, shops, superannuated* buildings, residence halls, athletic facilities, and health science centers. In essence, a university-based program in occupational health could

Conserve manpower
Protect the health of the university
Increase actual work time
Minimize the frequency and severity of job-incurred injuries
Lower absenteeism alleged to be due to illness
Increase work-effectiveness through a counseling program
Serve as a fringe benefit to attract and retain employees
Provide medical surveillance of employees exposed to hazardous substances
Integrate environmental control and clinical observations
Serve as a base for health-educational activities
Serve as an adjuvant agent in the health-and-accident benefit or major medical insurance programs
Build health precautions into new construction at the planning stage

Chalfen [37] summarized the effort at the Massachusetts Institute of Technology well when he wrote, "The approach at MIT is to foster the work of a collegial and consultative group of experienced environmental, medical, veterinarian, and safety personnel in an interdisciplinary manner."

AIRPORT MEDICINE

While some discussion was given previously of airport* facilities, no comments were directed to the airport as the site for OHPs. An airport hosts a melange of populations—airline flight personnel; airline ground and maintenance workers; municipal officials and employees (law enforcement, airport department); concessionaires (restaurants, gift shops, auto rental firms, ground transportation companies, foreign exchange branches, in-flight caterers); passengers; airline reservation and counter staffs; state employees (highway patrol, police); federal employees (Federal Aviation Administration [FAA], PHS, Department of Transportation [DOT], postal service, weather bureau, Department of Justice, Department of Agriculture, Immigration and Customs Service); volunteers (Travelers' Aid); vendors and delivery per-

*Not all facilities presenting hazards need be old. On several college campuses demolition of asbestos insulation has been undertaken in dormitories or classrooms when free fibers became airborne because of deterioration of the ceiling, wall, or pipe-wrap materials. The buildings, in some instances, were less than a decade in age [36].

*Larsen [38] has defined an airport simply as a facility that consists of an aggregation of industrial, business, and commercial establishments, governmental as well as private, collectively engaged in the air transportation of people and goods.

sonnel; noncommercial airmen; visitors, including primary school students; relatives; extramural transport personnel (cab, hotel van, shuttle, and municipal bus drivers); and construction workers. Some of these groups have access to OHSs external to the airport, but all are subject to emergent needs while at work, visiting, or travelling. A bomb explosion can involve any number of these disparate individuals, giving an immediate sense of commonality to all persons who are injured. The crash of an airliner on takeoff or landing can fuse many of these diverse employees into a single, helping force.

The medical facility in an airport, therefore, serves a variety of clients and does perform many OHP functions.

AIRPORT HAZARDS

In 1974, a questionnaire prepared by the National Institute for Occupational Safety and Health (NIOSH) was completed, during interview, by the managers of five major airports, and a preliminary industrial hygiene survey with a walk-through was conducted by an experienced industrial hygienist.

Of some 40 potential exposures to toxic materials in various airport facilities, the following were mentioned: noise, paint mist, welding gases, ultraviolet radiation, cleaning solvents or degreasing compounds, metal fume, carbon monoxide, dust, jet exhaust gases, lead, ammonia, ionizing radiation, and microwave radiation. Paint stripping, electroplating, metalizing, use of epoxy resins, battery charging, filling of mercury manometers, nondestructive testing, magnetic particle inspection, and fuel-tank cleaning were some of the operations observed.

MEDICAL SERVICES

In most instances, the airport medical facility is located within the main building or as close to the center of passenger traffic as possible. Usually, these units are freestanding, are physician-owned, and are not company functions of any of the airlines or the municipalities controlling the airports.* Port authorities represent a variant. These offices may provide service to airline personnel, but in those cities where the company has its headquarters and primary maintenance shops, there will most often be an OHS that is part of the headquarters installation.

A unit of this type is prepared to render emergent care and also to conduct such health evaluations of food-service personnel, or others, as are mandated by federal or local code. The following represent the program elements that an airport medical service should be prepared to deliver.

Examinations

- Preplacement evaluations of ground personnel
- Periodic examinations of
  - Airline flight personnel FAA class I
  - Commercial flight personnel FAA class II
  - Private flight personnel FAA class III
  - Air traffic controllers FAA class III
  - Aviation industry employees
  - Aviation industry managers
  - Federal, state, municipal employees
  - Motor vehicle operators
  - Contractor/concessionaire employees
- Disability evaluation of
  - Employees returning to work after injury
  - Employees returning to work after illness
- Termination examinations for
  - Transfer
  - Retirement
  - Disability retirement
- Physical fitness examinations
- Medical surveillance examinations of
  - Workers exposed to potential occupational health hazards such as
    - Asbestos or other fibrogenic dusts
    - Solvent vapor
    - Lead
    - Other substances
  - Workers subject to sensory organ change
    - Auditory skills determination
    - Visual skills determination
- Food-handler examinations (if required at time of hire or subsequently)

Emergency Health Care

- Aircraft crew
- Enplaning passengers
- Deplaning passengers
- In-transit passengers
- Airport employees (airlines, concessionaires, and so on)
- In-transit employees (bus drivers, vendors)
- Visitors
- Persons manifesting acute psychiatric disorders
- Visitors or passengers with problems of acute alcohol or drug intoxication
- Pregnant women in labor

Immunizations

- In keeping with requirements of country of destination

*The organizational patterns for an airport medical service may be any one of the following: a cooperative scheme initiated and administered by airport tenants, a private group equivalent to a concession, a facility operated by physicians employed by the airport authority, or provision of services by physicians and nurses of a group under contract with the airport authority [39].

Tetanus toxoid immunization of airport personnel
In keeping with disease prevalence in countries of stopover for airline personnel

Consultative Participation
Airport planning regarding environmental, industrial, and passenger safety
Airport planning regarding access for the physically limited, aged, or obese passenger or visitor
Assistance to the public health authority regarding airport sanitation (food service, washing facilities, drinking water, waste disposal, rodent and insect control)
Assistance to the public health authority regarding industrial hygiene problems, their evaluation and control
Training in first aid of ground or flight personnel

Disaster Preparedness
Established plan in event of major disaster (earthquake, flood, tornado, fire, explosion, terrorist attack) to include health care person in charge
Established plan in event of aircraft crash at airport or within adjacent perimeter of airport
- Availability of mobile equipment and supplies and professional personnel
- Medical examination of survivors, casualty collection at predetermined area, triage, and evacuation to hospitals
- Skilled on-the-scene care for special injuries—burns, smoke inhalation, hemorrhage, shock
- Crowd and traffic control
- Communications system from site of disaster to site of emergency care and for medical communication with hospitals, relatives, and the news media

AIRPORT DISASTER PLAN

At the least, any handling of casualties in an airport disaster will be difficult because there is always a time delay in deploying health care personnel. The situation is fraught with extreme tension because of the injuries sustained and the deaths. The news media representatives crowd the scene, relatives may still be in the airport, and crowd control may take a while to effect. The airline involved must mobilize its staff to provide assistance and support. The weather most likely is bad, and other departing or arriving planes are held pending clearance of the scene. Federal inspectors must begin their investigation. In essence, few medical facilities, including community hospitals, are ready for mass casualties because no matter how smoothly a disaster drill may proceed, nothing matches the real event for confusion, delay in coordination of effort, anxiety, fright, and the press of curious onlookers.

Klinghoffer [40] has described the plan developed at one time at O'Hare International Airport. The problems at an airport of that size are similar to difficulties that would arise in any densely populated industrial area: the type and site of the accident, extrication and identification of the victims, traffic, inclement weather, and *immediate* lifesaving care for the casualties. The echelons of pretriage care are (1) emergency care at the site, continuous care during extrication, and care enroute to second echelon; (2) further pretriage care and stabilization (at O'Hare the main fire department is used); and (3) transportation to neighboring hospital [40].

To succeed, the program requires (1) highly mobile equipment for sustaining life and personnel employed in the area trained in the basics of life support; (2) a "backup" supply of equipment for further patient care set up in a predetermined area, established after consideration of accessibility, temperature, and lighting; and (3) preplanned modes of transport from the second echelon to neighboring hospitals, with patients always accompanied by emergency-trained personnel. Klinghoffer [40] indicates further that the mobile phase of pretriage involves the use of 15 medical bags stored in a secure area in the main fire department. In an adjacent locked vault there are 15 cartons, each with a supply of injectable narcotics, one carton to accompany each bag. The contents of the disaster bags, the inventories for the backup supplies and equipment, and the triage table boxes may be found in the original writing [40].

The sterile state of the equipment is maintained for several years through appropriate sealing. When the bag is put into use, a 6 × 6 ft plastic sheet and four spikes are immediately available to allow fixation in snow, mud, or ice, thus providing a site that is reasonably clean and dry. The bags weigh 23 pounds and are readily portable.

Backup supplies, located and inventoried by row and column, are stored in the basement of the fire station. Persons trained for emergent action include freight handlers, ticket agents, administrative personnel, mechanics, pilots, post office employees, and restaurant workers. In addition, at O'Hare, paramedics on 24-hour duty can head up the emergency teams until physicians are available. Comparable personnel who happen to be in the terminal can be called by the public address system.

If needed, 19 "pagers" can be activated from any O'Hare telephone, signaling all pretriage personnel to report to "Crash 1" Fire Station. After dividing into two groups, one group with the 15 bags is taken to the accident site, and the remaining group moves the backup equipment to the firemen's bunk room where they establish Echelon Two. When emergent care is concluded at the crash scene, the first group returns to the fire station for assignment in the stabilization of the casualties.

Eight folding, aluminum pretriage tables are used, measuring 3 × 6 ft when open. The divisions of the table top accommodate resuscitation equipment, fracture supplies, dressings, IV supplies, and records. A morgue, *separate* from the treatment area, must be established nearby.

The disasters at O'Hare and San Diego in late 1978 warrant the kind of preparation described by Klinghoffer [40].

An example of prompt reaction to a catastrophic situation has been given by George Bergot, M.D., Director of the Paris Airports Medical Department [41]. On July 15, 1983 at 2:12 P.M., a powerful bomb exploded in front of the check-in counter of the Turkish Airlines, in the South Terminal of the Orly Airport. Airport emergency planning was activated immediately to face on-site 3 persons killed, 21 severely injured (5 to die in the hours or days following), and about 40 individuals "slightly injured." With the exception of two persons taken in an "uncontrolled way" by some witnesses to the nearest hospital, which was not prepared to render care to severely burned patients, all involved individuals had been checked within 2 hours and given care on site before transport to hospitals by ambulances or helicopters. In exactly 2½ hours after the explosion, the area was cleared, and cleaning had begun.

Bergot, in another working paper for a workshop held in Dakar,* "Medical Aspect[s] of . . . Airport Emergency Planning in the Case of Holding of Hostages" (January 1984), points up the differences between an aviation accident and such a situation. When hostages are taken, there generally is time to react. The number of victims needing care is not known and will change unexpectedly with the negotiations. With the passage of time it becomes more difficult to maintain substantial and high-quality medical facilities on site, as the service may be required elsewhere at the same time. When word is received that a hijacked plane is due to land, the airport medical staff is alerted, and reinforcements (hospital emergency teams, Civil Defense, Red Cross teams, and so on) are warned to stand by. At the Orly and Paris Charles De Gaulle Airports, the green alert is initiated.

Automatically, medical aid adequate for fewer than 10 persons injured in an aircraft accident is placed on the ready—"local red alert." In the event of piracy with maximum risk, it is estimated that 50 percent of the passengers will be injured, 10 percent seriously. Additional preparations are then made in anticipation of the worst. A medical command post is established, and teams are readied for response as soon as intervention is authorized.

Certain potential risks must be appreciated—such as the use of gas by police, boobytrapping of the aircraft—and the medical personnel must be equipped appropriately: gas masks, bulletproof jackets, and respiratory protection for both the staff and the injured. With the passage of time, vigilance may diminish and must be reinforced constantly.

The physically uninjured will require care, for the passengers will have suffered psychic trauma. Certain chronic disease states—heart difficulties, diabetes—will not have been treated during the crisis. A psychiatrist and a cardiologist are considered necessary members of the medical team.

Bergot advises strongly that the white coat be worn solely by medical personnel and no one else. Were the garment to be worn by others the terrorists would become suspicious and no longer permit physicians to intervene in the aircraft. There is the fear also that the physician will be taken hostage. From the point of boarding, the triage and evacuation proceed as they do following an aviation accident.

COMMENT

Casual users of airports may not be aware of the medical needs of various transient population groups, but some years ago data were gathered by Bergot [42]. A survey was conducted of 10 million outbound passengers, 10 million inbound passengers, and slightly over 10 million visitors. Three types of situations encountered were recorded as follows:

Among enplaning passengers	2 deaths (or 0.2 per million) 9 heart attacks (or 0.9 per million)
Among deplaning passengers	22 deaths (or 2.2 per million) 38 heart attacks (or 3.8 per million)
Among visitors	3 deaths (or 0.26 per million) 7 heart attacks (or 0.6 per million)

*Other working papers prepared by Bergot for the same conference include such titles as "Importance of the Medical Part in . . . Airport Emergency Planning"; "Casualty Distribution"; "Emergency Medical Facilities to be Provided at an Airport in Case of an On-Airport Aircraft Accident"; and "Practical Procedures." All are dated January 1984, and copies may be obtained from Dr. Bergot at the Medical Department, Aeroports de Paris, Orly Sud 103, 94396 Orly Aerogare Cedex.

The role of anxiety and tension in-flight becomes apparent with such data. The figures give substance to the declared need for an airport medical service and particularly one that is open around the clock.

As late as mid-1983, the issue arose at the Los Angeles International Airport when a lengthy article appeared in the *Los Angeles Times* [43] under the six-column headline of "Lack of Medical Facilities at L.A. Airport Poses Serious Problem." The question was raised by adjacent fire department installations that rolled 6,000 times to the airport within 3 years in response to emergency calls. The majority did not require an ambulance and could have been cared for on site were a facility present. The population base cited was 47,000 employees, over 53,000 passengers, and unknown thousands of visitors. The O'Hare system was cited as exemplary—a physician on duty from 8:00 A.M. until 11:00 P.M. with nurse or paramedic coverage during the remaining 9 hours. The lack of action seemed to be based on cost.*

Boston's Logan Airport OHP is actually a branch of the Massachusetts General Hospital, with three physicians, one nurse practitioner, and one health center assistant in attendance. Initially, when there was but one nurse (circa 1962), closed-circuit television to the hospital made physician viewing of the patient and subsequent diagnosis possible.

Another problem reviewed by some writers concerns psychiatric behavior disorders at airports. Miller and Zarcone [44] comment on some 49 persons brought by police for psychiatric observation from the San Francisco International Airport to a county hospital, during a 7-year period. Statistically this number represented about one "suspected mental case" per million airport passengers and visitors. Most of the disorders presented were schizophrenia, primarily of the paranoid type. Of the group, 35 displayed bizarre behavior, 9 were disoriented, and 6 were aggressive and threatening. In all cases where such judgment was possible, it was clear that the illness preceded the trip and that the travel was an expression of the illness rather than a causative factor. The authors felt that most of the persons seen could be expected to be out in open society again, and in light of their acting-out of the psychotic disorders and an apparent tendency to be drawn back to the airport and air flight, an important public health problem is posed. This difficulty appears in a world where "technological competence is greatly increasing the dependence of each individual's safety upon the sane and appropriate behavior of the next" [44]. Recommended was training of contact persons at the airport in detection and management.

*By late 1986, a multistoried medical facility was completed at the perimeter of the airport. It is an extension of a local hospital.

In another report involving persons brought in from Kennedy International Airport in a 5-year span, Shapiro [45] indicated that of some 21,000 psychiatric emergency service patients, 359 were referred from the airport, of whom 79 percent were from the New York City area. Again, most (74 percent) manifested symptoms of schizophrenia, and 82 percent had neither been on a plane nor were in transit during the psychotic episode. Involved also was considerable wandering about the airport, some persons living in the area for 6 to 7 days. There would be a return to the airport during subsequent episodes of decompensation. Shapiro concluded that the psychosis occurred in relation to the family, and the facility was a symbolic representation of connection with the family, rather than being an independent event or pertinent to travel.

In a later article, Shapiro [46] discussed aimless airport wandering as a psychotic symptom and emphasized once more a causal relationship between the attraction to the airport setting and ideas relating to abandonment and reunion with family.

All types of medical problems can and do arise at a metropolitan airport, from birth to death, and from exultation to disaster; an on-site health care facility should be available to meet the multiple human needs. The needs will persist, for there is neither a pretravel selection of passengers and visitors nor a healthy-worker effect. The airport medical arm represents a crossover or combination of the skills of both occupational and aerospace medicine, operating at a distance from nearly all community centers. There should be greater awareness of the potential contribution of such a facility.

THE OFFICE

When Morris [47] published his article on "Dermatoses among Office Workers" in 1953, it was a rare reporting of afflictions endured by a group of employees believed to be free of job-associated illness or injury. But with "stress" being given recognition by retirement authorities as a legitimate reason for declared disability and with the persisting claims of adverse health effects from working with video display terminals (VDTs), white-collar workers have brought new concerns to the OHS.

VDTs are now ubiquitous, and soon every manager and clerical person will face a small screen much of the workday. With the advent of air conditioning and the concomitant "sealing" of buildings, attention has been drawn to office health hazards and the tight-building syndrome, and new battlefields have appeared for the contests between smokers and nonusers of tobacco. The problems of indoor office air have been voiced in both the professional and lay presses, yet little preventive or corrective momentum has been seen, and medical verification of these many ills is still in the wings.

Much that is disputatious in the office setting has related to changes in work modes, impaired supervisor-employee relations, monotony, fractionated job assignments, and repetitive, unstimulating tasks. Complaints of ill health are the end product, and the physical plant frequently is scapegoated as the cause. Are there any merited findings?

THE CLOSED BUILDING

In a review emanating from the University of Washington [48], the freshet of symptoms, either single or in combination, in closed buildings is acknowledged and associated with the move toward "energy conservation." Complaints vary, including headache, nausea, eye and upper respiratory tract irritation, vertigo, pruritus or frank dermatitis, dyspnea, and "sinus congestion." Buildings are being tightened with little attention directed to untoward effects on the occupants. More of the office air is being recirculated, often with less than 25-percent outside air. During periods of nonuse, contaminants build up and are not diluted. Temperatures climb, and air velocities and humidities drop because of inadequate ventilation.

Most office occupants can attest to the economies sought through less and poorer building maintenance with the resultant accumulation of dust. Added to these environmental circumstances are crowding, noise, inadequate illumination, poor seating, and the release of nuisance vapors or ozone from office machines and their needed liquid accessories.

Studies conducted by NIOSH have been inconclusive as to single-source etiologies for symptoms indicated by affected workers. All air contaminants were measured at levels below the permissible exposure limits. Poor ventilation and excessive indoor temperatures were noted, and trace amounts of formaldehyde were found to which some workers were probably sensitized [48].

In studies conducted by the University of Washington, certain conclusions were reached. Because contaminant levels rarely are in excess of federal or state occupational health standards, enforcement under current Occupational Safety and Health Administration (OSHA) regulations is not possible. Companies that complain seldom own the buildings they occupy, and the actual owners do not wish to expend money for "comfort" reasons only, which further complicates the issue of control.

The chronic discomfiture resulting will eventually impair productivity and most likely lead to feelings of stress. If the goal of energy conservation is still ahead in building construction and maintenance, then potentially health-damaging materials must be used sparingly in tight buildings [48]. Examples follow:

Furniture, partitions, subflooring of particle board (formaldehyde)
Asbestos-containing materials
Natural-mineral building materials (radon)
Carpets and carpet adhesives (organic compounds such as styrene)
Cigarette smoke (particulates, carbon monoxide, and so on)
Carpet cleaners (perchloroethylene)
Pesticides (chlorinated compounds, organic phosphates, and so on)
Air-conditioning systems (*Legionella,* molds, and so on)
Urea formaldehyde foam insulation (formaldehyde)
Carbonless copying paper (possible formaldehyde)
Blueprint machines (ammonia)
Ditto machines (methyl alcohol)
Photocopiers (ozone)

The contemporary low-partitioned, open office mode is the design most likely to develop indoor air problems. Current distribution systems do not deliver the quantities of air needed in habitable areas but stratify over the dividers. Improvement could be seen through use of linear diffusers [48].

Arndt and Chapman [49,50], authors of a report prepared for the Congressional Office of Technology Assessment (OTA), noted that although indoor air pollution, stress, and low-level radiation from VDTs are neither life-threatening nor life-shortening, they may prove disabling, causing unnecessary discomfort, and can be costly because of lost workdays. However, it was conceded that the effects of long-term, low-level exposures are in many cases unknown. While reactions to work with VDTs were mixed, some operators have mentioned monitoring, piecework, and quotas as stress productive. Other negative elements included low pay, monotonous, repetitive work, and lack of worker participation and control. There is no evidence to associate visual or reproductive problems with work involving VDTs.

The matter of tight buildings arose in California in connection with a 2½-year-old building in the state capital. The building was presumably energy-efficient, utilizing solar energy for heating and cooling.

Shortly after occupancy, the physical complaints began to surface, and there were illnesses over and above the number expected. Air sampling revealed no contaminants, but it was found that the ventilation system and the air flow at the diffusers failed to meet design specifications, resulting in inadequate air circulation. With balancing of the system, the symptoms cleared. Also advised was improved illumination.

However, it was recommended that a "building close-out procedure" be developed and used for all newly constructed or substantially renovated buildings. The building is to be tested well before occupancy, it is to be "baked out" at maximum system temperatures, and furniture should be "aged" before placement. It is anticipated that this protocol will prepare newly completed work structures for healthful human habitation [51].

A survey of working women that produced 1,300 responses [52] indicated that problems with office air quality were noted most frequently, along with job stress. Over 80 percent reported temperature extremes; more than 70 percent stated that the supply of fresh air in their offices was inadequate or nonexistent; 40 percent claimed that there was "no fresh air at all"; two-thirds of the respondents mentioned that the air was either stale, stagnant, or drafty; and 25 percent reported irritating fumes*—cigarette smoke; from photocopying, duplicating, and other printing equipment; laboratory or industrial fumes; car exhaust, and from chemically treated paper. One-fifth had lost time from work because of job-related health problems. The bases for the difficulties, as pointed out by Gregory [52], lie in energy conservation; "fume"-emitting new building and furniture materials; sealed "weatherless" office, computer-controlled; faulty ventilation and humidifying systems with recycling of contaminants; overcrowding because of cost of premium space; or old rental buildings with inadequate maintenance or sealed antiquated ventilation systems.

Strange office illnesses have appeared with no identifiable cause. The Centers for Disease Control (CDC) has reported two outbreaks of respiratory illness among employees in large metropolitan office buildings [53]. In one instance, symptoms appeared with the start-up of a heating–ventilation–air-conditioning system that was contaminated with bacteria, fungi, protozoa, nematodes, and mites. No single agent could be assigned responsibility for the outbreak. In the second building, a flooding-contaminated water-drainage system presumably caused the illness. With refurbishing, there was no recurrence, even though no specific relationship, apart from epidemiologic evidence, could connect etiologically the isolated organisms to the disease pattern.

*Used in the lay sense of a generic designation for vapors, fumes, dusts, aerosols, gases, and particulates.

VISUAL DISPLAY TERMINALS

Given considerable publicity in recent years has been the anxiety created among operators of VDTs.† The use of these devices has occasioned much comment concerning possible adverse health effects among their operators. The designation VDT is usually limited to a self-contained unit that generates an alphanumeric or graphic display on a cathode ray tube (CRT) [54]. In many situations the unit interacts with a computer through a keyboard and thus becomes a true visual display *terminal.*

The main components include a keyboard, a display screen, an electronics circuit pack, and a power supply. These parts are encased in a housing of metal, fibrous glass, or plastic and are cooled by a motor-driven fan [54]. Certain potential health and safety hazards have been studied because of operator complaints in a telecommunications organization. In an investigation of directory assistance operators—"Information" to the caller—with one group using a VDT screen and the controls referring to printed-paper records, a variety of discomforts was indicated [55]. Complaints included headache; difficulties in seeing; burning, tearing, soreness, or itching of the eyes; afterimages; discomfort in the neck, shoulders, and upper and lower back; nausea or abdominal cramps; and discomfort in the buttocks or "bottom of thighs." The only issue that was of statistically significant difference at the 0.5 level was discomfort in the neck of the VDT operators versus that of the paper readers.

Job satisfaction was studied also, and no difference was found between the study group and the controls. Starr [55] did believe, though, that there was a factual basis for some of the complaints reported anecdotally. Persons wearing bifocal spectacles can experience some unique problems, as indicated earlier.

The issue of radiation has presented itself, and measurements have been made. Several investigators [54,56–59] have concluded that the amount of radiation—actual and potential—presents no hazards to health. There is no evidence that work with VDTs has caused miscarriages or birth defects. Air sampling has shown no hazardous exposure to chemicals including carbon monoxide, formaldehyde, hydrocarbons, acetic acid, and ozone [58]. The levels of illumination were generally acceptable, but glare was

*Also known as visual display units.

a problem at many of the work stations. Most of the complaints offered by operators could be traced to the physical dimensions encountered, such as excessive height of the keyboard or of the VDT screen.

Because of continuing concern, the American Academy of Ophthalmology published a brief position paper, "Video Display Terminals (VDTs) and the Eye" [60], in which it was concluded that such devices are safe for normal use and present no hazard to the eye. Further, there is no evidence, experimental or epidemiologic, that exposure to VDTs produces cataracts or any other organic damage to the eye.

Ergonomics Recommendations

Recommendations have been made to reverse the physiologic or health-related difficulties experienced by operators of VDTs [54,57–59,61–63].

Desk or Table Top. The top should be 24 to 26 inches high and no thicker than 1 inch. Space under the table should be at least 27 inches wide and 27 inches deep. Recessed areas for the keyboard are not recommended.

Keyboard Height. The space from the top of the table to the top surface of the space bar and the bottom row of keys should be 2½ inches. (These dimensions allow the elbows to be flexed at 90 degrees in the working position, with arms hanging comfortably at the operator's sides.

Screen Height. The screen should be detached, and the top of the screen should not be higher than eye level so as to minimize oculomotion, and the center of the screen should be 15 to 20 degrees below eye level.

Viewing Distance. The screen should be 18 inches from the eyes of the operator, but adjustable between 15 and 32 inches.

Viewing Angle of Screen. The face of the screen should be tilted back 10 to 20 degrees for easier viewing, provided screen glare is not increased. The screen should be tiltable from about 5 degrees forward to 15 degrees backward, and the bottom of the screen should be no lower than 40 degrees below eye level.

Chair. The seat should be adjustable for height between 14 and 20 inches above the floor and at least 16 inches in width. The angle between the seat surface and seat back should be 100 to 120 degrees. Support for lumbar back should be centered 9 to 10 inches above the lowest point on the seat. There should be no pressure on the thighs from the leading edge of the seat.

Illumination. The walls of the surrounding area should be of a matte finish to diminish the amount of reflected light. Lighting needs are lower than the levels required in the average office, which reduces the amount of contrast between the illuminated screen and the general work area. About 500 to 700 lux (46–65 foot-candles) is advised, with a room-light to screen-light ratio of 5:1 to 7:1. If the operator of the VDT works concomitantly with other materials, properly placed supplemental lighting may be needed. Work requiring greater illumination should not be placed in juxtaposition to the VDT.

Supplemental Illumination. To reduce glare, the screen should be placed perpendicular to the windows, not in front of or opposite them. Recessed overhead and downward lighting is best. To direct light downward, fluorescent fixtures can be baffled or have special louvers attached. To reduce glare further, drapes or blinds placed over adjacent windows, a hood over the screen, or tilting or rotating the screen will be effective.

Keyboard. The keyboard should be detachable, be as thin as feasible, and have a nonskid base. The keyboard angle should be between 5 and 15 degrees, and the surfaces of the keys should be concave and the tops in matte finish.

Screen Characters. Operator should be able to adjust for brightness, flicker, contrast, and sharpness. The font selected should maximize legibility. The smallest acceptable dot matrix size is 5 × 7, which is adequate for capitals and numerals but there is the bare minimum for combined upper- and lowercase letters.

Accessories. A wrist rest can be helpful, and a foot rest should be available for short operators if the table and chair cannot be adjusted for height. An adjustable document holder should be available for tasks involving data entry and dialog.

Rest Breaks. With most VDT operation, a 15-minute break is advised for every 2-hour work span, or a break each hour for operators on extremely tedious tasks such as data entry. Alternating work away from the terminal may reduce the stress resulting from the continuum of intense work "while providing the operator with other more fulfilling roles in the workplace" [57].

Eye Precautions. VDT operation is visually fatiguing because of rapid changes in accommodation and fixation. To minimize visual problems for the wearer of bifocal lenses, the recommended corrective lenses, in order of preference, are monofocal, full-width (straight-line) bifocal ("executive" bifocal), flat-top bifocal, and progressive addition lens. The round segment or crescent segment is not advised. The usual bifocals may not meet VDT operating needs if frequent neck flexion is experienced. Special occupational eyewear may be required to handle the viewing distance inherent in work with the terminal. Contact lenses may be worn if a single-vision lens offers adequate correction. They are not suitable if a bifocal or trifocal correction is needed, unless spectacles are worn in addition to the contact lenses.

Other Environmental Factors. Ambient temperature, humidity, and ventilation should allow for comfort.

Medical Procedures

Preplacement examinations of applicants for positions involving VDT operation should include the following [59]: (1) complete ophthalmologic history and examination, including refraction testing for accommodation, and the instrumental visual screening procedures indicated earlier; (2) examination of the cornea, lens opacity, and retina; and (3) prescription for or referral for prescription of corrective occupational lenses, if needed.

Recommended for the periodic examination is an annual review of the protocol given above in addition to other diagnostic procedures as indicated by the medical history, intercurrent injury or illness, or aging.

Comment

That there is continuing controversy concerning health effects from work with VDTs is seen in the consideration by several state legislatures of bills to regulate, in some way, the use of such equipment. The proposed legislation points to more frequent rest breaks and eye examinations, the prevention of glare, and the option of alternative work for pregnant operators. The bills are supported strongly by organized labor and are opposed by airlines, banks, newspapers, and business and computer equipment manufacturers [64]. The National Association for Working Women had established a VDT "hotline," and the calls confirmed the fact "that health complaints of VDT operators are widespread and serious." A questionnaire study with 873 returns revealed "a personal health profile for the VDT operator which is truly frightening." Whether the investigation utilized rigorous epidemiologic principles is not determined [64].

In an investigation conducted by Frank [65] and by the Newspaper Guild, AFL-CIO, the findings showed that the workers suffered more somatic symptoms than did the nonusers. In addition, they reported being more irritable, having greater difficulty sleeping and waking up, and feeling overworked. The VDT operators were absent one-half day more than the nonusers during the study period. It was pointed out that male operators, although in the minority, reported more birth defects among their newborns than did the women workers.

Because of the anxiety created among pregnant operators, some of the women have taken to the wearing of lead aprons while using the equipment [66]. Such additional devices could increase the potential for postural problems by forcing the operator to carry extra weight across the front of the body, displacing forward the center of gravity.

The Council on Scientific Affairs of the American Medical Association (AMA) published a definitive article [67] of the research and state-of-the-art papers on the health effects of work with VDTs. The conclusions were reached that there was no association found between radiation emissions from the devices and reported spontaneous abortions, birth defects, cataracts, or other injuries. Monitoring of representative equipment for all forms of electromagnetic and other emissions showed that the levels have been well below presently accepted standards of exposure. Confirming what has been mentioned in this chapter, health complaints, both perceived and real, were most likely related to stressors peculiar to the work or its environment. Corporate management was encouraged to be more cognizant of the operator-machine interface and to stimulate more effective communication between the system planners and the users.

While no permanent adverse health effects have been demonstrated, the population involved is large and is concerned. Education of the workers is needed, and their participation in altering the equipment-operator interface should be helpful in eliminating many of the ergonomic errors currently productive of the spectrum of musculoskeletal symptoms. Support furniture is commercially available for the automation office that is "ergonomically designed [and which will] improve the working relationship between people and machines so each work station is more comfortable and productive," reads the catalog. And now "Videoterminal Glasses" are being manufactured for use with different-colored displays. Perhaps the prophecy of Emerson* will see fruition in this age of information processing.

CONSTRUCTION INDUSTRY

The building of new structures for man's housing, commerce, transport, power and water supplies, research, and space-vehicle launch sites has seen the replacement of old methods in construction by gigantic time- and labor-saving apparatus. Also, there has

*"If a man . . . can make better chairs or knives, crucibles or church organs than anybody else, you will find a broad hard-beaten road to his house, though it be in the woods." Ralph Waldo Emerson, *Journal*, Feb 1855.

been the addition of new materials, introduced to recapture trades lost to automation or electronic controls or to provide more appealing, useful, and enduring structural surfaces. With these changes, though, new occupational health hazards have appeared to make the construction industry even more dangerous than it traditionally has been.*

Even though the erection of single-family dwellings has slowed considerably for a variety of fiscal reasons, the construction of hotels, office buildings, condominiums, and shopping malls has persisted at an unabated rate. In much of today's building, prefabricated sections are brought to the site, having been assembled in specialty shops dedicated to a particular structural part. Contemporary construction methods employ huge cranes—which topple occasionally with lethal results—the lifting into place of complete floor slabs, the elevation of entire walls, and the inclusion of large precast, prestressed concrete elements. With these changes have come the pneumatic application of plasters, the use of expanded aggregates, the necessity of grinding irregularities from concrete surfaces, the increased use of solvents, and airless spray painting. Huge sections of heavy building exteriors are lifted into place by cranes at street level in situations where hand signals can readily be misread in the murk of inclement weather.

Construction is not limited to the continental United States. Worldwide builders undertake projects at remote sites where the type of medical care or facility varies. One such engineering-construction organization, although based on the West Coast, has had as many as 120 major projects in some 25 different countries. These undertakings have involved 35,000 permanent employees, of whom 4,000 were overseas, and anywhere from 75,000 to 100,000 temporary workers, mainly abroad [68]. Employees are examined before departure and are immunized.

*Perhaps even riskier than construction is the removal of buildings, wherein injuries have been great in number and workers have been exposed to asbestos dust or residual radioactive contamination. It is of interest that as labor costs have exceeded the salvage value in old buildings, the swinging iron ball has come into full pendulum, making this form of methodical destruction safer than ever. Paralleling this change has been the alteration of the industrial tag. One large firm whose advertising content previously read "house wreckers" now utilizes the designation "demolition engineers."

Evidence of change in building materials is seen in the shift of end products at the once largest marble company in the world. The plant in Vermont that previously supplied the beautiful marble exteriors to such structures as the U.S. Supreme Court now grinds the marble it quarries for sale throughout the world merely as calcium carbonate.

The medical facilities provided at the construction area will vary with the remoteness of the jobsite, the type of camp (single status or family), the emergency evacuation capability, the time and distance factors in the access to quality medical care, the project population growth curve, the availability of medical equipment and supplies and their maintenance potential in the host country, and the availability of a medical import license. The level of employer involvement in the provision of facilities and staffing will vary: (1) use of local medical care after evacuation, approval, and recommendation by company medical authority, such as in London, Paris, and so on; (2) participation in expansion, upgrading, or both of existing medical care resources, such as in Taiwan, South Korea, and so on; (3) provision of all new facilities and staff as a company unit, such as in Sumatra, New Guinea, and so on; and (4) subcontracting of care to providers, such as in Riijadh and Jubail, Saudi Arabia [68].

While the above comments only cover the provision of care superficially, there is commonality in the hazardous exposures to which construction workers are subject, irrespective of the location of the worksite.

HEALTH HAZARDS

The concept that construction work is fraught with considerable risk is given substance by some data. In 1982, 2,100 construction workers lost their lives on the job, while thousands were seriously injured. As such workers are employed on the average of 1,500 hours per year—about 187 days only—it means that 1.4 workers are killed each hour [69]. In Finland, during 1979, 14,640 accidents resulted in at least a 3-day absence from work in construction[70].

Several factors characterize the industry that make for the high morbidity and mortality among its members. Turnover of employees is common, which renders difficult the maintenance of records, particularly of short-term workers. Seasonal unemployment is rampant, and with a high level of worker mobility, it is merely impossible to generate, maintain, or forward individual exposure records. The constraints of the weather force construction personnel to seek jobs where work outdoors can proceed. The labor force in various building trades is highly transient, many workers are unskilled or semiskilled, and language difficulties with migrant workers preclude fairly basic comprehension of, or instruction in, safe or healthful work practices [71].

The mix of trades within a single construction area leads to multiple exposures, many not usually associated with the craft of the incumbent. The situation is comparable to the work done in the spaces below deck of a vessel undergoing overhaul. In a small compartment, riggers, welders, pipefitters, painters, and electricians can be working simultaneously, all sharing a common exposure that normally may not be considered a concomitant of that trade's activities.

As much work is performed outdoors, wind and temperature changes are frequent, materials normally solid or viscid can volatilize, and particulates can be given greater excursion with resulting inhalation. As tunnels are advanced and excavations are developed for high-rise buildings, toxic materials are released for which the workers may not have been prepared or that, may compromise further already impaired pulmonary tissue in unexamined personnel. The salvage or reuse of old buildings—part of the conservancy effort of historical societies* and the need to contain new construction costs—offers, as noted before, exposure to asbestos, noise, and other fibrogenic dusts. In summary, the industry has been characterized by greatly increased mechanization (noise, whole-body vibration, and static physical work), prefabrication (new materials), computerization (alteration of working patterns with some effect on safety, both positive and negative), and energy conservation (greater attention to insulating materials) [71].

Because of the costs of new construction, many homeowners are attempting, through remodeling, to bring their dwellings into conformance with current codes, which means exposure to both old and new hazardous materials. The "do-it-yourself" movement of a few decades ago is undergoing rebirth, and knowledge of the exposures incurred may be extremely limited. The constant in construction is change, which makes lifelong recordkeeping nearly impossible.

The physical hazards are numerous—noise from both stationary and mobile heavy equipment, blasting, impact pneumatic tools, and gasoline- or electrically-powered hand-held tools; exposure to whole-body vibration; excessive solar radiation; cold (Raynaud's phenomenon, frostbite); and lasers, as examples. Ergonomic problems are universal because of the nonphysiologic positions required in the completion of many tasks within the constraints of strange structural configurations. Weight-lifting limits may not be adhered to, available chainfalls or hoist systems will not be used, or certain space limitations will preclude load transport and placement by materials handling equipment.

*Outstanding is the conversion of the old textile mills of New England into condominiums, high-technology work areas, and shopping malls; Ghiradelli Square in San Francisco; and Cannery Row in Monterey.

Dermatogenic agents, both allergenic and irritant, are in use everywhere—cement, concrete, brick, plaster, rubber, epoxy fixatives, and degreasing chemicals, for example. Exotic woods, polyurethane materials, formaldehyde, and phthalic acid, among others, are troublesome contactants.

Lead is still present, and welding produces zinc, chromate, or nickel fume, in addition to ozone and nitrogen oxides. Pyrolysis of chlorinated organic compounds can produce highly toxic gaseous products (carbonyl chloride).

Substitutes for asbestos are being used—zeolite and wollastonite. The former has been found to be carcinogenic, while the second natural fiber requires further study of its health effects [71]. The inhalation of fibrogenic dust from the grinding, finishing, and resurfacing of cement surfaces, granite, marble, or other quartz-containing stone is ever a possibility. Potential malignant responses lie in contact with synthetic resins, lacquers, paints, plastics, rubber, and wood-treatment chemicals.

Superimposed on all of these physical, chemical, and biologic stressors (organic materials encountered in tunneling) are the psychosocial factors seen in work-pacing; unchecked individual fitness; aging; assimilation, acceptance, or rejection of immigrants by indigenous workers; and work in isolated regions—the arctic, deserts, the continental shelf—or in highly restricted enclaves in vastly different cultures. Added to these expatriate problems is the hesitance of certain illegal aliens to report work-related illness for fear of deportation.

HEALTH SERVICES

For all the reasons presented, the provision of health services at construction sites has been inconsistent. Skilled nurses have cared for iron workers on the skeletons of new high-rise structures, first-aid personnel have been provided on site in certain projects, and completely equipped trailers staffed with physicians and nurses have been installed near long-term undertakings such as in dam construction. Adjacency to the so-called industrial clinics has allowed care for physical injury.

But lacking in this entire industry are systematized methods of job placement, environmental evaluation, medical surveillance, and recordkeeping. Little research has been devoted to the building trades, although some data have been collected by the occupational health and safety specialists employed by certain of the trade unions at their national headquarters. Some studies of specific craft workers have been conducted, and cancer surveillance data banks have been searched for work-disease associations.

But because of the mix of financiers, designers, engineers, builders, construction and transport unions, and a mobile labor force, little has been seen in the true occupational health programming for this population at high risk. The care for traumatic injury is insufficient. The hope seen currently is that hospitals with OHSs will offer outreach capabilities to construction firms so that services in both the care-for-injury and preventive medicine arenas will be available. Education of workers must be undertaken in both safe *and* healthful work practices, in the use of labor-relieving devices, and in the elimination, as much as possible, of the machismo ethos that is productive of not only illness, but also injury and death.

While the International Labor Organization (ILO) and the World Health Organization (WHO) have been able to make some progress in the developing countries, the presumably civilized and cultured world is yet to see a construction industry that is free from accruing harm to its members.

HEALTH CARE FACILITIES

One of the last bastions to accept a formal OHS is the hospital, with its multiple inpatient and outpatient services. For reasons enumerated previously [72], this facility, central to the provision of definitive care in any scheme of regionalization or echelons of treatment, has been backward in the development of employees health services. Where practitioners of all stripes are present throughout the day, the seeking of a diagnosis and treatment by a lesion-laden staff member has been conducted informally, frequently "on the run."

Lacking has been an established OHS, appropriately sited, staffed, and equipped, separate from the institution's emergency service. While a certain number of large metropolitan hospitals have created such units for their employees, most hospitals have failed to develop an occupational health activity headed by a physician and chartered to deliver the program long familiar to industry.

Over the years hospitals were viewed as charitable organizations and were in no way competitive in the labor market. Benefits were few and turnover high. Employees, in many instances, were itinerants using the institution as a stopgap in career advancement and having little intention of remaining permanently. The creation of the health maintenance organizations (HMOs), the development of the large national hospital chains, and the growth of health service employees unions have altered the eleemosynary tradition of the care facilities. In spite of these moves into modernity, the OHS has not become a universal segment of the hospital structure. The Joint Commission on Accreditation of Hospitals (JCAH) has not asked that a hospital have an employee health service as one of the desiderata for approval.

ARE HOSPITALS AN INDUSTRY?

In 1982, hospitals* had 3,959,000 full-time employees [73], or about 3.5 percent of the total labor force. Nursing homes add another 798,000 workers.† All employed persons in 1983 in selected health occupations numbered 5,576,000, of whom 76.5 percent were female [73]. Total expenditures for health care in 1983 came to $355,400,000,000, or nearly 10.8 percent of the gross national product ;[73]. Expenses in 1982 for all hospitals reached $123,200,000,000 [73].

Conant and Stent [74] a decade-and-a half ago viewed the large general hospital as an industrial complex that had failed to provide adequate health services for its employees and asked that the mantle of "benign neglect" be removed. Shortly thereafter Conant [75] pointed up the growth in health care, the rapid sophistication of services, and the need for better trained personnel. The hospital, as he described it, was not only a hotel caring for sick guests, but also an assembly line of sick persons being transformed into well beings, a production line of newborn and of prosthetic replacements for injured extremities, a laundry, a college, a restaurant, "a radioisotope laboratory and a bacterial zoological garden." The traumatic injuries and the dermatoses sustained by hospital employees do not differ from the disorders seen in manufacturing industry. Superimposed on these untoward work effects are the infections, the ubiquitous needle-puncture wounds, and the reagent exposures unique to the hospital operation.

In essence, the health care institution is an industrial operation, simulating other organizations in many ways, but characteristically different. What business is comparable in the use of its facilities by daily visitors—private physicians—who are neither employees nor stockholders of the establishment yet dictate policy formally or informally? How many companies offer the amount of education obtainable in a hospital to both insiders and outsiders? And what institutions have as a final product the strange

*Includes general, psychiatric, chronic disease, tuberculosis, and federal hospitals.
†1980 data.

dichotomous choice of wellness or death and the relationship to human beings from prebirth to termination? And, apart from the aerospace industry, in how many enterprises must the product be protected against the worker?

THE BACKDROP

Concerned interest has been manifested for many years in the lack of health services for hospital personnel. As early as 1945, Geiger [76] wrote of this "neglected branch of industrial medicine." Feeling the need for recognition, a Joint Committee on Health Program for Hospitals Personnel for the AMA and the American Hospital Association (AHA) met in 1957 and produced "Guiding Principles for an Occupational Health Program in a Hospital Employee Group" [77]. Apart from material added in 1964 and 1965 regarding immunization programs, the statement has held firmly over the years subsequent to publication.

In 1964, Mammen [78] surveyed the hospital environment and concluded that today's institution presented many physical hazards to its workers. Corrective educational goals could be reached by "an enlightened management which would insist upon procuring for its employees the benefits to be derived from good occupational medicine, industrial hygiene engineering, and a safety program." A full-time personnel physician was required. The need for a hospital-employee OHS was given further support by *JAMA* in an editorial comment [79].

Kagey [80] gave additional emphasis to the need for an OHS, stating that while most attention had been given the *patient's* safety, solid application of basic environmental safety standards to *all* hospital areas would enhance patient safety and care. In the intervening years, though, some definitive studies had been conducted, and some new guidelines were produced. The USPHS promulgated the booklet, *An Occupational Health Program for Hospital Employees* [81], and the Wisconsin State Board of Health published in 1964 the first edition of *A General Guide for an Occupational Health Program for Hospital Employees* [82]. Ultimately, NIOSH conducted the definitive study of the OHS in hospitals, and a seven-volume report resulted* [83]. From this query of nearly 4,000 general hospitals, certain principles and guidelines were evolved, which will be referred to later in this chapter.

As the JCAH requires on a broad sense (1) that hospitals maintain records of examinations conducted on employees at the time of hire and of care given them subsequently and (2) that workers are free from communicable disease and are physically able to carry out their assigned duties, a review was indicated of the content of "effective" programs. As OSHA general industry standards and state equivalents offer no protection to the hospitalized patient, many states adopted supplementary codes [84]. To determine the status of such codes, the Committee on Medical Center Employee Occupational Health Services of the American Occupational Medical Association (AOMA) conducted a national survey, the results of which were reported by Lewy [84]. Of responses from 49 states, 26 (55 percent) indicated no regulations concerning occupational health in hospitals. In 21 states, preemployment and periodic examinations were mandated. The content of such examinations, or the actual conduct of these required reviews, remained vague. Previous studies showed an inadequate immunization of hospital personnel—workers at great risk in the acquisition and transmission of infectious disease. Lewy [84] concluded, "Hospitals are responsible and socially conscious institutions, but without the specific regulatory authority of state health codes, cost-containment pressure may impede the implementation of rational employee-screening policies." The committee produced some program guidelines, which will be cited later.

The absence of occupational health care for 800,000 persons in Britain's National Health Service and 200,000 individuals in general medical and dental practices, community and school-health services, and the private sector has been comparably lamented by Blackadder [85].

Guidelines were prepared in late 1983 by the AOMA committee referred to previously [84] for employee health services in hospitals, clinics, and medical research institutions, which, it is hoped, may serve as incentive for the initiation of appropriate and effective programs [86]. That the problem is still unsettled and evolving was given evidence by Messite [87] in late 1984 when she indicated that 53.1 percent (17 of 32) of hospitals inspected on request had health hazards. In 1983, there were 126,000 injuries and 2,900 work-related illnesses in that industry, coursing from exposure to solvents and pesticides in the maintenance worker to burnout in the nurse overloaded with emotional stress response. Recommended was a program to monitor all chemical, physical, and biologic hazards and preventive maintenance of all equipment and facilities.

*In April 1976, NIOSH published a summarizing brochure, *Highlights of the NIOSH Hospital Occupational Health Services Study* (20 pages).

HOSPITAL HAZARDS

A hospital presents, as mentioned earlier, most of the hazards familiar to industry and many, in addition, qualitatively and quantitatively unique to its many operations. The hazards are physical, chemical, microbiologic, and psychosocial, and some examples of all of these kinds of exposures have been recorded for decades in the professional literature [88,89].

In the beginning of the present century, when many disease entities went unabated because of the absence of appropriate therapy, health care personnel manifested high levels of morbidity and mortality. Laboratory infections were common, primary care physicians and psychiatrists were attacked with deadly weapons, and there were few, if any, staff members assigned the tasks of accident prevention or epidemiologic study as they related to nosocomial infections.

The Occupational Safety and Health Act of 1970 has applied to hospitals as well as general industry, and the sensitivity to work-associated hazards has been sharpened. There still remain, however, the ubiquitous high-risk tasks of lifting and transferring impaired or unconscious patients, facing terminally ill adults, and even more emotionally searing, working with children destined for early demise. The demands of crash-team activity, of emergency-service duty, and of the always unexpected community disasters—airplane crashes, earthquakes, riots, floods, multiple highway accidents—remain as the ultimate evocation of psychic energy. Few occupations, including the media, the performing arts, politics, or professional athletics, drain the participants as does medical care.

It is not unusual, then, for the physical injuries, the chemical intoxications, the microbiologic invasions, and the burnouts to be incurred. Are there preventive measures possible in the hospital worksites?

THE HOSPITAL OCCUPATIONAL HEALTH FACILITY

As mentioned, the OHS of the hospital is still to come of age. In those institutions where such employee health care centers have been established, the path of creation and acceptance has not always been clear. Why is the obvious so unheeded? Medical leaders have had little exposure to occupational health principles or modes of practice in the medical school curricula of recent decades and cannot then extrapolate an unknown to their work environment. Further, in an institution staffed by health care professionals, it may seem superfluous, even unnecessary, to establish a unit that appears duplicative of all the natural talent present in the ubiquitous full-time and attending staffs. But none of the available skill is organized or dedicated solely to the health of the workers. In these days of strikes, high health care costs, and unionization of workers—including house staff members—it is unconscionable to administer a hazard-laden enterprise without protection of exposed employees.

About 15 years ago, a New York City group known as the Greater Metropolitan Hospital Health Services Directors and Associates was meeting informally for discussion of recurring health center problems, such as hepatitis B and "the general lack of awareness for the need to implement effective employee health programs [90]. In an effort to find national representation, the group met with the AOMA and shortly thereafter became a formal committee associated with the parent organization. The group, comprising physician and nurse representatives of some 14 medical institutions in 14 states, met and developed "guidelines for Employee Health Services in Hospitals, Clinics and Medical Research Institutions" [86,91]. The guidelines, as stated by the Committee on Medical Center Employee Occupational Health Services, set forth only minimum recommendations. They are subject to strengthening or change as determined by the institution's geographic location, employee turnover rate, and local or state regulations, among other considerations.

The essence of the guidelines follows [86]:

Every prospective employee should undergo a job-specific health evaluation. Each institution should develop a list of job categories that requires periodic evaluation.

Hospital employee health services should establish a close working relationship with the infection control staff and develop a method for recording annually the interim health history of employees involved in the care of patients having infectious diseases.

Annual tuberculin skin testing should be carried out on all employees except those workers known to be tuberculin positive. For positive reactors, initial chest x-rays should be taken.

All employees, especially those persons in obstetric services, should have their immune status for rubella evaluated and be vaccinated if found not to be immune. Each hospital should develop a policy for counseling pregnant workers for specific hazards.

Employees whose work assignments place them at high risk of hepatitis B should be tested for hepatitis B antibody at time of employment.

A program aimed at reduction of risk and injury should be developed. The program should include preventive education, early treatment, full rehabilitation, and return to work at the earliest date compatible with satisfactory convalescence.

Stress-prevention programs should be developed for supervisory personnel.

Except where required by law, or for the protection of others, employee medical information must be kept in strict confidence.

Employee-health personnel should cooperate freely with employees' personal physicians, specifically in the matter of referral for the care of illness, reports on progress, imposition of work restrictions, and return-to-work evaluations.

In 1986, because of advances in occupational medicine, the committee updated and expanded the guidelines published previously but still indicated that they set forth minimal recommendations only [92]. Recognizing hazards specific to the health care setting, the suggested program was brought more in line with the elements encountered in most of the occupational health efforts seen in industry.

The more detailed program comprised these services [92]:

- Preplacement and periodic health assessment
  - Determination of health status, including evaluation of physical and emotional health and presence of or susceptibility to communicable disease
  - Informing employee of results and, when required, recommendation of follow-up care
  - Job placement, with restrictions, if indicated
  - Periodic review of health status as determined by age, nature and duration of job assignment, and degree of exposure to risk
- Infection control
  - Prevention of nosocomial infections in both personnel and patients through:
    - Close working relationship with the infection control staff
    - Preplacement and periodic health evaluations
    - Immunization programs
    - Care of personnel for work-related exposures and illnesses
    - Monitoring of exposures to infectious disease
    - Establishment of guidelines for work restriction because of communicable disease
    - Provision of appropriate health education, stressing personal hygiene
    - Maintenance of employee health records
- Control of specific infections
  - Minimization of risk of exposure to parenteral or mucosal contact with potentially infectious material from patients with *AIDS* or suspected *AIDS*
  - Immunization against *diphtheria, polio, tetanus, measles,* and *mumps,* with appropriate subsequent booster inoculations
  - *Enteric pathogens*–cultures and examination for ova and parasites at time of hire of dietary personnel and required reporting to the employee health service (EHS) of significant gastrointestinal illnesses
  - *Hepatitis B*—preexposure and postexposure prophylaxis, as indicated, and counseling of carriers
  - *Influenza*—immunization in the fall of each year of employees with patient contact
  - *Special health risks in international travel*—predeparture evaluation and education
  - *Pneumonias*—pneumococcal vaccination as determined by age, health, and other risks
  - *Rubella*—immune status affirmed through statement of vaccination from authoritative health care source or documentation of protective titer, vaccination at time of hire except during pregnancy
  - *Tuberculosis*—screening by Mantoux skin testing, chest radiography of positive reactors, testing postexposure, and INH prophylaxis when indicated
  - *Varicella*—documentation of immune status and work restrictions as needed
- Diagnosis and treatment of occupational injuries and illnesses
  - Diagnosis, treatment, reporting, and rehabilitation
  - Knowledge of and safe work practices concerning chemical hazards:
    - Anesthetic gases
    - Asbestos
    - Chemotherapeutic agents
    - Ethylene oxide
    - Formaldehyde
    - Mercury
  - Knowledge of and safe work practices concerning physical hazards:
    - Electrical hazards
    - Slippery floors
    - Heat
    - Poor lighting
    - Inadequate ventilation
    - Work with lasers and radiation sources
    - Needle puncture wounds
    - Back injuries sustained in the lifting and transfer of patients

Environmental control and surveillance
Health education—counseling concerning reproductive hazards
Substance abuse—evaluation, referral for treatment, and return-to-work clearance
Stress management
Maintenance of complete health and safety records
  Confidentiality
  Retention
Cooperation with private physicians
Periodic evaluation of the OHS

It is presumed, of course, that these functions are conducted in a formalized OHS,* and not elsewhere in the institution. Some elaboration of the guidelines may be helpful.

HEALTH EVALUATIONS

Health examinations should be conducted at time of hire and periodically thereafter as determined by the exposure and level of risk inherent in the position, as delineated in the job description. House staff physicians should be included in the protocol, for they are, at least, at risk equivalent to that of other personnel. Lewy [94], of the EHS of Columbia-Presbyterian Medical Center in New York, believes that the preplacement examination serves these purposes: (1) It identifies illness or disability that might prevent performance of an assigned job function; (2) it provides baseline medical information to be used as a standard if subsequent injury or illness were to develop; and (3) it identifies for the examine previously unrecognized or inadequately managed health problems. Special attention must be directed to the presence of or susceptibility to communicable diseases. Protection against attendant-borne infectious disease is needed by hospitalized patients, particularly individuals who are immunosuppressed. The hospital worker also must be shielded from the acquisition of such disease. That the prospective health care employee was either susceptible to infectious disease or potentially capable of transmitting it was given testimony by the study of Schneider and Dykan [95] conducted at New York's Montefiore Hospital and Medical Center. Of 2,866 applicants examined, the following were the observations made with greatest frequency:

Problem Noted	*No. of Individuals (of 2,866 Total)*
Inadequate diphtheria immunization	1,872
Susceptibility to rubella	274
Tuberculin-positive by skin test	194
Tuberculin-positive by history	293
Intestinal parasites	19
Positive HBsAg	14

Other conditions found included 93 with hypertension, 67 with anemia, and 26 with urinary tract infections.

The presence of 52 percent of applicants who had not been immunized against diphtheria in the preceding 10 years was astonishing in light of contemporary medical practice and the decennial requirement for such protection in hospital workers.

Lewy's protocol [94] for incoming house staff members included not only the history and examination, but a complete blood count, a 20-channel biochemical profile, a urinalysis, a serodiagnostic test for syphilis, determination of the presence of HBsAg and antibody by radioimmunoassay, a hemagglutination inhibition test for rubella antibody, a posteroanterior chest radiograph, and an intradermal skin test using 0.1 ml of PPD containing 5 TU in applicants whose tuberculin status is unknown or normal.

It is a prudent idea that physicians early in their careers be given a sense of preventive medicine in the form of periodic health evaluations and protective immunization. Although it has been some centuries since Luke cautioned practitioners, "Physician, heal thyself" [96], there has been little spontaneous effort to maintain health-affording practices. As examples of the disinclination to follow advised protocols, in a voluntary mass immunization program involving hospital personnel after an outbreak of rubella, participation of physicians was the lowest at 19 percent in a group of nearly 2,000 who received the injections* [97].

In a medical center serosurvey of about 2,500 high-risk employees, 345 were shown to be susceptible to rubella [99]. Of the group, 53.3 percent were vaccinated; only 1 of 11 known susceptible obstetrician-gynecologists received the immunization, and physicians, as a whole, totaled only 21.9 percent participation. This negative behavior among better-knowing professionals was explained by Barrett-Connor [101] as relating to a "lack of perceived vul-

*The term *employee health service* (EHS), in contradistinction to *occupational health service,* seems to be preferred by the committee for use in the hospital setting. It is conceivable that volunteers, private duty nurses, student nurses, blood donors, visitors, and even attending staff, on occasion, might receive care in the facility [93].

*Physicians can be motivated. In commenting on an article concerning the health screening of physicians, Babb [98] sent the editor of the journal this succinct message: "[T]he Palo Alto Medical Clinic requires its physicians to have annual physical examinations. Enforcement of this rule is simple and effective: if you don't do it, you don't get paid."

nerability and the press of other priorities." Strickler [102] has noted the same lack of response by health care professionals to offered preventive measures, but with more direct comments. When personnel of a general hospital were offered hepatitis B vaccine, but 37 percent of some 700 persons at risk indicated that they wanted the immunization, Strickler commented, ". . . Much of the resistance is irrational and emotional, and therefore difficult to overcome even with education and the best available information." He did not feel that "sensible behavior" correlates particularly well with the advantages of being either educated or informed.

Clever and Arsham [103] reviewed physicians' health practices and observed that although life-span statistics were encouraging, they do work more hours *and* more years, which results in shorter periods of retirement: 3.1 years versus 7.8 years for the general population. Suicides have been high, and substance abuse has directed attention to "the impaired physician."* But physicians have ceased smoking at a greater rate than any other professional group. Pressures of modern practice have increased—malpractice action, peer review, threat of physical harm, decreased autonomy, increased regulation, increased competition, decreased financial rewards, and emergence of greater roles for other health professionals [103].

Clever and Arsham [103] laid out these health recommendations for physicians:

Determine your current health status and the positive and negative factors involved.
Equate your health practice with your own values, personality, and life—pleasure versus risk.
Provide yourself incentives for, and remove barriers to, the change of destructive health behavior.
Document the changes.
Get help when needed.
Stop smoking.
Get immunized against hepatitis B virus (if in contact with blood or blood-contaminated patient products), tetanus, and rubella.
Drink alcohol in moderation only.
Avoid recreational drugs.
Undertake an enjoyable form of aerobic exercise.
Decrease dietary cholesterol.
Develop interests outside of medicine [emphasis added].
Plan for retirement.

*One preventive program has been initiated at UCLA—a Mental Health Program for Physicians in Training. Physician volunteers provide free psychiatric evaluation and short-term psychotherapy to medical students and house officers. The ultimate goal was conceived as promoting "a respect for the inner life among those who labor under the delusion that they have no time for such self-indulgence" [100].

INFECTION CONTROL

Tuberculosis

Tuberculosis has not been eradicated, and in areas of high southeast Asian immigration, the disease rate has attained new heights. Tuberculin skin testing should be conducted annually on hospital personnel, except on those individuals known to be tuberculin positive. On positive reactors, baseline chest radiographs should be obtained. The rate of repetition of x-ray studies should be determined after consideration of the extent and intensity of exposure. As advised [86], more frequent radiographs should be obtained in personnel working in newborn nurseries and other services where there is contact with immunosuppressed patients. If not specifically contraindicated, INH prophylaxis should be considered for use with converters of any age and with all newly determined reactors under 35 years of age.

While concern was high in the early pre– and post–World War II years regarding tuberculosis in student nurses and medical students, interest flagged as disease-specific medications appeared that put an end to lengthy hospitalizations. In recent years, however, interest has been redirected to the problem of tuberculous infection among health care personnel [101,104–111]. Two questions arise in this renewed attention. The first relates to the frequency of post-employment chest radiography. Some states have changed their requirements regarding repetitive chest films. In Oregon [110], for example, it is now asked that hospital personnel with significant tuberculin reactions have only one chest film on entry into employment if their tuberculin reactivity has been documented for 3 or more years. If such is not the case, and chemoprophylaxis is either contraindicated or refused, then three negative consecutive yearly chest radiographs are required. However, those individuals with significant reactions and high-risk factors who have not completed 1 year of INH therapy must have annual chest films for the duration of their employment. The risk factors include (1) inadequately treated past tuberculosis, (2) close exposure to communicable pulmonary tuberculosis in the past 2 years, (3) a negative tuberculin reaction in the last 2 years, (4) immunologic deficiencies and immunosuppressive therapy, (5) diabetes, (6) silicosis, (7) alcoholism, and (8) a previous gastrectomy. In these groups, the tuberculin test is of little value as a survey method in detecting bacteriologically positive tuberculosis in populations at high risk. Further, radiographic chest surveys of these high-risk groups are useful in detecting new cases and in identifying reactivated tuberculosis in longitudinal studies.

The second issue concerns the use of the controversial BCG vaccine [112,113]. Barrett-Connor [101] indicates that the use of BCG is an alternative to the employment of INH prophylaxis. It is purported to be safe and effective in young adults and is inexpensive. As she points out, the historic argument against the vaccine's use has been the fact that the BCG-induced tuberculin conversion limits the value of skin-testing as an epidemiologic and diagnostic tool. In the U.S. medical student, though, the value of preserving the tuberculin test may not be relevant when two-thirds of negative-reactor physicians fail to monitor themselves for possible recent infection.

The AHA has recommended that BCG be given whenever the infection rate of tuberculosis exceeds 1 percent per year and other disease-control measures cannot be implemented. These criteria have been met in the physician population Barrett-Connor [101] reviewed but may not apply to other health care workers more compliant with both annual tuberculin-testing activities and chemoprophylaxis. Before beginning a BCG program, the actual in-hospital risk should be evaluated in addition to the potential risk present in the community in which the employees live.

The protocol suggested in part by both the AHA [107] and the USPHS [108] consists of new personnel having both a standard chest radiograph and a tuberculin skin test at time of hire, using 5 TU PPD. Tuberculin-negative individuals are then given BCG vaccine,* to be followed by annual chest radiographs, or more often if clinically indicated. It is suggested that skin testing be repeated to determine if conversion did take place. If the test result remains negative, it is not necessary to reimmunize. Prior to the initiation of a BCG program, the AHA advises that each hospital assess the tuberculosis risk among its workers. In addition to the hospital exposure risk, there is the hazard of contact within the community of residence.

While the surveillance program recommended by the USPHS [108] parallels the suggestions of the AHA as to skin testing, it provides additional detail. If the first test results in 0 to 9 mm of induration, a second test should be given at least 1 week and not later than 3 weeks after the first test. The result of the second test is to be used as the baseline in determining treatment and follow-up. A history of BCG vaccination does not preclude initial screening, and a reaction of 10 mm or more should be managed as a tuberculous infection. Employees with a significant reaction to the skin test or who have symptoms compatible with pulmonary tuberculosis are to be given a chest radiograph to determine the presence of current disease. The use of BCG vaccine is *not* recommended by the USPHS.

The policies for skin-test repetition after the initial examination should be established by the risk of acquiring a new disease. Somewhat similar to AHA guidelines, the following factors are to be considered in the determination of risk:

The number and location of tuberculous patients admitted to the hospital—the issue of employee exposure.
The number and location of tuberculosis patients in the community
The number of employees already infected
The number of employees who become infected
The flow of air throughout the hospital—for the possibility of airborne transmission

If the risk of exposure to tuberculosis is small or infrequent, it is not necessary to repeat skin testing on a regular basis.

If there are certain hospital areas or categories of workers with greater exposure to diagnosed and undiagnosed cases or with a higher rate of new infections, the skin testing may be repeated every 3 to 6 months, until the exposure risk is reduced. Preventive treatment is advised as is contact investigation when there has been exposure to a "potential transmitter."

After the first evaluation of individuals with significant tuberculin reactions, repeated chest radiographs are not advised. "They are not a substitute for preventive therapy" [108]. Those workers who have completed an adequate course of treatment or preventive treatment should be exempt from further screening unless they become symptomatic.

The records advised by the USPHS include the following:

1. Date of each tuberculin test with method and antigen used
2. Measurement in millimeters of skin-test reaction
3. Date of any known exposure to infectious tuberculosis
4. Date and result of chest radiographic examination of significant skin-test reactors
5. Dates of initiation and completion of preventive treatment
6. Dates of diagnosis, if disease occurs, and initiation and completion of treatment

*Available from Eli Lilly and Co., Indianapolis, IN, and Research Foundation, Chicago, IL.

Rubella
Although discussed earlier, it should be emphasized that all workers, particularly in hospitals with obstetric services, should have their status of immunity from rubella determined and be vaccinated if found to be susceptible. Rubella vaccine should not be given during pregnancy, and instructions should be given regarding the avoidance of conception immediately after the immunization [114–116].

Varicella
Workers in contact with children and immunosuppressed patients should have their level of immunity from varicella evaluated. The EHS should be notified if there is contact with a varicella patient either at work or in the community [86].

Enteric Disease
While the conduct of repeated stool examinations in food handlers is not productive, such examinations for the presence of ova and parasites should be completed on employment, at the time of *significant* gastroenteric disease prevalence, and on return to work subsequent to such illness.

Diphtheria, Polio, Tetanus, Measles, Mumps
An immunization record should be initiated at the time of hire that will show past protective inoculations and all injections given during the period of employment. Many individuals well immunized during youth fail to maintain an adequate immune status. Fresh series or vaccinations should be carried out to protect the worker, and a recall schedule for subsequent stimulating injections should be established.

Hepatitis B
While discussed earlier, attention must be given those employees at greatest risk of acquiring hepatitis B. Employees new to the hospital setting and headed for placement in high-risk positions* should be tested for hepatitis B antibody (anti-HB_s). Because of the cost of hepatitis B vaccine, there has been considerable review of the indications and cost-effectiveness of its use and of the indications for preimmunization serotesting [117–126].

The vaccine has been used extensively in spite of cost. Kreider and Lange [127] indicated that in a single program year the incidence of clinically evident hepatitis B in employees decreased 80 percent. Its successful use has been reported by Szmuness and coworkers [128], who noted that even in the first 75 days following the first injection, there was a lower incidence of hepatitis B among the actively immunized group. In 30 healthy adults, Beasley and Hwang [129] demonstrated antibody (anti-HBs) response in 40 percent following the first dose and in 90 percent 1 month subsequent to the second dose. From another view, in a retrospective study by Lohiya and associates [130], no excess morbidity due to hepatitis B was noted among 2,000 employees in a 10-year period, and it was felt that in an institution for the mentally retarded, hepatitis B vaccine was neither warranted nor at that time (early 1984) cost-effective for most client-care personnel.

The safety of hepatitis B vaccine has been assured by joint conclusions of the Inter-Agency Group to Monitor Vaccine Development, Production and Usage the CDC, the Food and Drug Administration (FDA), and the National Institutes of Health (NIH) [131–133]. The findings are that (1) immediate side effects are minimal after receipt of hepatitis B virus, (2) no long-term reactions have been reported, (3) the purification and inactivation process is known to inactivate representatives of all known groups of animal viruses, (4) each lot is safety tested in primates, (5) no known cases of hepatitis B or non-A, non-B hepatitis have been transmitted by the vaccine, and (6) *no known occurrence of AIDS has been associated with the vaccine.*

Some additional observations regarding hepatitis B vaccine are in order. While immune globulin (HBIG) has been advised as protection against hepatitis of a viral origin [134], prophylactic treatment after accidental percutaneous exposure to HB_sAg-positive blood should be considered, using a combination of hepatitis B vaccine and HBIG. Concurrent administration of HBIG does not impair the response to hepatitis B vaccine. The combination of the vaccine and one dose of HBIG produces immediate and sustained high levels of protective antibody to hepatitis B surface antigen (HBsAg) [135]. The joint use will provide prolonged immunity to subsequent exposures and may also heighten the efficacy in preventing hepatitis B in postexposure situations. The dosage recommended is HBIG, 0.06 ml/kg or 5.0 ml for adults, given as soon as possible after exposure, preferably within 24 hours. The hepatitis B vaccine, 1 ml (20 μg), should be injected intramuscularly at a separate site as soon as possible and certainly within 7 days. The second and third doses should be given 1 and 6 months after the first injection. If HBIG is unavaila-

*Personnel at risk in the hospital include medical technologists, operating room staff, phlebotomists, pathologists, oncologists, dialysis staff members, and oral surgeons. Dental personnel, staff of institutions for the mentally impaired, morticians, and any other health workers based outside of hospitals who have frequent contact with blood or blood products are comparably at risk [117].

ble, IG (formerly gamma globulin) may be used in equivalent dosage—5.0 ml for adults or 0.06 ml/kg. If the affected individual has received two doses of hepatitis B vaccine prior to exposure, no treatment is needed if serotesting slows adequate levels of anti-HB_s, that is, greater than 10 S/N (sample-negative ratio) by radioimmunoassay [135].

It has been observed by London [136] that, from evidence accumulated in the 1970s, hepatitis B virus may be the principal, if not the only, etiologic agent of primary hepatocellular carcinoma. In a chronic carrier, the lifetime risk of developing the malignancy is about 40 percent. It is hypothesized that such disease might be prevented through the administration of hepatitis B vaccine, which gives two valid reasons for its use.

Proposed by Mostow [137] has been the concept that physicians should be actively immunized against hepatitis B, not only to prevent their acquiring the disease, but also to protect themselves from litigation resulting from their spreading the virus to their patients. Cases are presently being evaluated for possible court action.

Lastly, the formulation of a hepatitis B vaccine from HBsAg produced by a recombinant strain of the yeast *Saccharomyces cerevisiae* has been announced [138], and its use recommended [139]. The vaccine currently in use is hepatitis B vaccine utilizing HBsAg purified from the plasma of human carriers of hepatitis B virus infection. The supply, therefore, is potentially limited by the availability of adequate sources. The problem is constantly present of ensuring, through appropriate inactivation, that none of the major groups of animal viruses survives the purification process. The use of recombinant DNA technology could avert such a hazard. This human immunogenicity-safety trial of the yeast recombinant hepatitis B vaccine is the first time that such a vaccine has been used in humans.

The definitive recommendations concerning use of hepatitis B vaccine have been published by the CDC [139] and in part by the U.S. Preventive Services Task Force [140]. Revaccination may be necessary after 3 years [141].

ACCIDENT PREVENTION/EMPLOYEE EDUCATION

Needless to say, complete records must be maintained of injuries accidentally sustained by hospital workers, including work-associated illnesses. The records should be reviewed by a health and safety committee. The advisory or governance group is usually designated as a safety committee, but the causative episodes and the resultant adverse effects frequently are closely related. Conrad [142] gave as an example of the interrelatedness of health and safety the avoidance of contact with antineoplastic drugs. Good needle disposal practices are essential and diminish as well the number of needle puncture wounds. Also, good chemical storage and transfer procedures help avert toxic exposures as well as slippery spills.

In employee educational efforts, as well as in committee reviews, both subjects should be included in the instructional effort. Brown [143] has reported an educational program regarding hospital hazards that was conducted through the union. It was believed that working with the organized employee group would be more effective, in light of their greater power in bringing about health and safety improvements in the workplace by virtue of established grievance procedures and negotiated contract agreements.

Teaching aids are available for use in such programs. For example, St. Elizabeth Hospital of Cleveland* has produced on videocassette "The Choice is Yours . . . A Total Hospital Risk Management Program," which covers personal safety, body mechanics, radiation, and gases, infectious diseases, complex equipment, and toxic substances. A second production entitled "Kitchen Safety" explores injuries encountered in the hospital's dietary department—falls, back strains, lacerations, burns. The American Hospital Association has publications that can be used as support materials in an educational program.†

A special course was developed in biohazards and laboratory safety at the Sloan-Kettering Institute, which is mandatory for all institute personnel who work with radioisotopes, carcinogens, or cells in tissue culture. The course is given annually, with "special topics" throughout the year [144]. The topics covered included general laboratory safety, physical and chemical safety, radiation protection, personnel practices, barrier systems, emergency procedures, basic principles of contamination control, biocontamination dissemination, chemical containments

*St. Elizabeth Hospital, c/o Care Video Productions, P.O. Box 45132, Cleveland, OH 44145.

†For example: *Fire Safety Training in Health Care Institutions,* 60-page book published in 1975; *Safety Guide for Health Care Institutions,* 160-page book published jointly with the National Safety Council in 1983; *Fire Emergency in a Patient Care Facility: Rehearsal for Survival,* a packaged program comprising 80 slides, a 30-minute audiotape, a 30-minute videotape, a 32-page instructor's manual, and ten 32-page staff manuals; *Flashover—Point of No Return,* a 9-minute videocassette (Beta-Matic or VHS) made in 1980; and *Nuclear Waste Disposal and Radiation Accident Planning,* a 3-part audiotape made in 1981. Available from the American Hospital Association, 840 North Lake Shore Drive, Chicago, IL 60611.

and toxic agents, chemical carcinogens, risk assessment, and hazards associated with research animals [145].

STRESS MANAGEMENT

While there are admittedly a greater number of stressors in the hospital work setting than in other occupational arenas where emergent situations involving "life-and-death" challenges do not arise, the mode of managing the resultant stress does not differ. There must be a trained person or facility available to provide counseling. Most hospitals have social workers, and while their primary functions relate to patients, they could be asked or directed to provide assistance to troubled hospital employees.

In various consultative reviews with hospital authorities, the problems of alcoholism, absenteeism, drug abuse, and obesity have been indicated as nearly ubiquitous in large urban health care settings. It seems strange that in a social institution possessive of all the disciplines needed for patient care that the full-time staff is not given the advantage of nutritional counseling, brief psychotherapy, or its own inhouse Alcoholics Anonymous group. But then that is the theme of this section—hospital workers are not, in the main, afforded these employment perquisites common to most industrial enterprises. Companies of a size smaller than many large-city hospitals provide these facilities, for it means lower overhead costs; hospitals have yet to appreciate the dividends from a broad-based EHS.

CONFIDENTIALITY

As medical care protocols are commonplace in the hospital and patients' records are constantly being scanned and used by greater numbers of staff personnel, a sense of openness of records can pervade the care of all patients. Because of this frequent slippage in privilege, hospital employees can rightly suspect the lack of confidentiality in the maintenance of their records. Without being repetitious of the caveats presented previously in the discussion of medical records and documentation, one can only say that these clinical records are completely privileged and *at no time* are to be included in the patients' files maintained by the central medical records authority. Only with this kind of protection can the confidence of the employees be developed and have it endure.

COMMUNITY RELATIONS

As noted previously [86], one of the AOMA's desiderata concerning the EHS of hospitals was the free professional cooperation with the workers' private physicians. As in any business or industrial establishment, employee-patients are referred to their own practitioners for care of illness, the placement of work restrictions when indicated, and return-to-work recommendations.

Another relationship with the community might be the creation of a hospital-based OHS that would provide service to local industry. Such a service has been described knowledgeably by McCunney [146,147], and it could be offered in conjunction with the EHS of the hospital. Such a facility would be highly advantageous to neighborhood enterprises because of the total health care capability of the hospital, but, as outlined by McCunney, the program should provide all of the program elements encountered in any in-plant OHS.

Since worker turnover in hospitals is high and employees tend to seek comparable work in other institutions, Hamory [148] has suggested that a standard health record be developed by the AHA, similar to the International Certificate of Vaccination issued to travelers by the CDC and the WHO. Such a record would document the results of screening of hemodialysis workers for antibody to hepatitis, the vaccination for hepatitis B and cytomegalovirus, tuberculin skin testing, and other antibody levels. When a worker moves from one hospital to another, the record would be forwarded, and much needless test duplication would be avoided. As many institutions demonstrate 40-percent turnover per year, or higher, much time and money could be saved, and the worker could be spared unnecessary exposure and anxiety [148].

DAY-CARE CENTERS

In some hospitals, centers for the day care of employees' children have been established as an answer to aid recruiting in light of the shortage of nurses and the high percentage of young women in both nursing and other areas in health care. It is estimated that nearly half of the 415 employer-sponsored child care programs in the United States are operated by hospitals [149]. Since 1947, there has been a fourfold increase in the number of working mothers with children under 6 years of age—from 12 percent to 47 percent. Of this group, 54 percent of women with children between ages 3 and 5 and 42 percent of women with children less than 3 years are in the labor force [150,151].

The rationale for the growth of these hospital-centered facilities has been the attraction and retention of highly trained staff and the difficulty in shift scheduling. On-site care has improved worker productivity and has decreased turnover and absenteeism [152]. This activity is mentioned because in some institutions the day-care center has been a responsibility of the OHS, and there have been problems of a health nature. In California, the state administrative code mandates licensure of such facilities when nonresidential care is provided for more than 10 children, or fewer if the facility is institutional.

Various infectious disease outbreaks have been associated with day-care centers. The presence of *Giardia, Shigella, Campylobacter,* and hepatitis A—agents transmitted by the fecal-oral route—have been reported [153] in children, staff, and contacts of persons in day-care centers. In addition, there have been respiratory tract–generated disease outbreaks of measles, scarlet fever, and bacterial meningitis. Pediculosis and scabies have also been noted. Holmes [154] has advocated the use of prophylactic immunoglobulin in the reduction of center-related episodes of hepatitis A.

While the day-care center may not be related organizationally to the EHS, the idea may arise that there should be a central facility responsible for the care of all nonpatient, full-time residents of the hospital. If the concept is carried out, all public health intelligence should be brought to bear by the medical director.

Further, because of the low hospital census occasioned by the use of diagnosis-related groups (DRGs) in cost-containment, unused hospital facilities may be the site of choice by industry for its day-care centers in the near future. It is viewed as the location of preference over creation of new facilities at the worksite.

DISASTER PLANNING

The hospital will become the focus of care in the event of a disaster, which may be internal—bomb threats, fire, strikes, natural phenomena, and utility failure, including telephone service—or external in the form of civil disorder, earthquakes, airplane crashes, warfare, floods, tornadoes, multiple or chain-reaction highway accidents, and the like. Whatever the role of the EHS proves to be, the plan should be documented, and staff members of the EHS should know and check their assigned duty stations. As indicated in Chapter 9, Emergency Medical Care, an overall company or institutional plan is needed. The same concept is applied to a hospital, and a checklist is provided in an AHA publication, *Safety Guide for Health Care Institutions* [155].

INFECTIOUS WASTES

While ordinarily the responsibility of county health authorities, the EHS of the hospital may become involved with the supervision of the proper disposal of infectious waste materials, as part of its responsibility in environmental control.

A classification of infectious wastes (unless autoclaved), has been developed as they are encountered in acute-care hospitals. The categorization follows [156,157].

Infectious Wastes Classification

Microbiology laboratory: blood; tissue cultures; stool specimens; microbiologic cultures; viral cultures; urine and excreta specimens; all pathologic waste and specimens; secretions (sputum) and needle and syringes handled separately.

Hemodialysis (all double red-bagged): used tubing from dialysis machines, used kidneys (artificial); equipment contaminated with blood; all patient equipment (disposable) and needles and syringes handled separately.

All trash from patients in strict wound, skin, enteric, and blood isolation, including dressings (placed in impervious bags prior to being placed in trash); diet trays, respiratory equipment (disposable), used items (such as urinary bags and tubing, IV tubings), and needles and syringes handled separately.

Operating room: patient-contaminated disposable articles (double red-bagged and picked up by housekeeping) and all pathologic waste and specimens.

Pathology: pathologic waste (such as organs, tissues, and limbs).

Research laboratories: specimens (all red-bagged); tissue specimens; animal cultures; blood; excreta and secretions.

Emergency room (communicable-disease room): all trash to be red-bagged; specimens (sent to laboratory); drainage (such as pus); dressings, disposable equipment and isolation garb (caps, gowns, masks, and gloves).

Outpatient department: drainage and dressings from contaminated wounds.

Neonatal intensive care: all trash from patients in isolation (all red-bagged).

The following items from physicians' offices are classified as infectious waste:

Laboratory wastes, particularly cultures of etiologic agents.*

Pathologic specimens, including human tissues, blood elements, excreta, equipment, disposable materials and secretions that contain etiologic agents.

*As used in the above categories, *etiologic agent* means a type of microorganism, or virus that causes, or significantly contributes to the cause of, increased morbidity or mortality of human beings.

Any other material that, in the determination of the physician, presents a significant danger of infection because it is contaminated with, or may reasonably be expected to be contaminated with, etiologic agents.

Recommended Methods for the Handling and Processing of Infectious Waste

Infectious waste generated from physicians' offices should be placed in disposable plastic bags and stored separately from the office's solid waste. The infectious waste should then be disposed of by one of the following methods:

The infectious waste may be autoclaved at the physicians' offices so as to render the waste noninfectious and subsequently discarded with the office's solid waste. If an autoclave is not available in the physician's office, then arrangements may be made elsewhere to autoclave the infectious waste.

Physicians' offices in the immediate vicinity of an acute-care hospital may, if agreed on by the hospital, utilize the hospital's disposal system for infectious waste.

Infectious waste in the liquid form (such as excreta, blood) may be discarded into the sewer followed by adequate flushing.

Physicians, or groups of physicians, may contract with an approved off-site infectious waste processor to have the waste picked up for off-site treatment.

RISK MANAGEMENT

As it has been done in certain companies, the concept of risk management has been proposed for the hospital setting. Brown [158] notes that the terms *loss prevention* and *liability* might be used synonymously and that the objective is the elimination of problems that may result in harm to the organization, its staff, and most importantly, to the public. He delineates the objectives further: (1) the avoidance of the causes of loss, (2) the lessening of the operational and financial effects created by losses that are unavoidable, and (3) the provision for inevitable losses at the lowest practical cost. Involved are the identification, measurement, and control of the hospital's basic risks.

The functional elements subsumed under risk management may include any or all of the following:

Infection control
Security
Safety
Incident/accident reporting
Drug management
Noise control
Smoking
Traffic control
Patient transfer and transportation
Environmental control
Material to and from hospital premises
Occupational injury and illness
Employee health
Employee deaths
Employee education

Other proposed functions, such as personnel selection and employee evaluation, are obvious activities of the industrial relations or human resources area, as employee health and occupational illness are within the purview of an EHS. This organizational scheme is mentioned because it may be found in some large facilities. Loss prevention, as a unit, in a few companies is usually assigned workers' compensation administration and small OHSs staffed by occupational health nurses solely. It may or may not include safety.

There is no knowledge of research conducted to determine the advantage of this larger functional umbrella. If hospital unions strengthen further and if malpractice suits against organizations or their officers increase, risk management may demand greater cognizance.

LEGAL IMPLICATIONS

That the hospital may be not only an unsafe place to work, but also an unsafe place to be treated has been observed by Manes [159], who cites specific cases. In *Guy et al.* v. *Arthur H. Thomas et al.*, the Ohio Supreme Court ruled that when a hospital is in a dual-capacity position, that is, a capacity created by being not only the employer of an injured worker but also the treating medical facility for that worker, that hospital can be held accountable in medical negligence for treatment rendered at the facility, even though the employee is receiving workers' compensation benefits for the work-related injury. The plaintiff developed symptoms of mercurialism as a hospital laboratory technician operating a Thomas–Van Slyke Magnamatic Blood Gas Apparatus. In essence, the diagnosis was missed, the symptoms usually being attributed to "nerves."

Action was initiated against both the hospital employer and the manufacturer, the issues being product liability, negligence in warning, and strict liability. The employer argued that a separate cause of action was barred, as the injury was covered under the state workers' compensation law. After ruling in favor of the hospital, the case went to the Supreme Court. The ruling there, and in other cited cases, stated in essence that the cause of the action set forth in the claim was entirely independent and distinct from the claim from which the plaintiff recovered compensation. The mercurialism arose from negligence and not out of and in the course of employment.

Actually, there was total naivete, if not ignorance, in the handling of an exposure to mercury. The point made in the several cases was that medical facilities, administrators, and other employees should be knowledgeable not only in the dangers and symptoms of hazardous exposure, but also in the application of the dual-capacity doctrine.

ACQUIRED IMMUNE DEFICIENCY SYNDROME (AIDS) AND THE HEALTH CARE WORKER

Because of the continued appearance of AIDS in selective elements of the population, workers in various health facilities have been apprehensive about contact with patients and the possible acquisition of the disease. The epidemiologic findings unquestionably point to transmission by intimate sexual contact, by percutaneous inoculation of blood or blood components, or perinatally from the mother to the neonate, but only blood, semen, vaginal secretions, and possibly breast milk have been implicated in the transmission [160].

As of June 12, 1987 (date of source publication), six persons who provided health care to patients with HIV infection and who denied other risk factors were reported to have HIV infection [161]. Four of the cases resulted from needle-stick exposures to blood from patients infected with HIV, while two additional cases involved individuals providing nursing care to persons with HIV infection. The latter pair had not sustained any needle-stick injuries but did have extensive contact with blood or body fluids of the infected patient, neither one having observed the regularly recommended barrier precautions.

Three more cases, not involving needle sticks, have been reported in health care workers—while assisting with an unsuccessful effort at arterial catheterization, while phlebotomizing (with a 10-ml vacuum blood collection tube) a patient with suspected HIV infection, and while manipulating an apheresis machine (a device separating blood components). Although such events are rare, they underscore the need for rigorous adherence to infection-control procedures that minimize the worker's exposure to the patient's blood and body fluids.

Because of the increasing morbidity and mortality of HIV infection, the precautions concerning health care workers have been strengthened in that blood and body-fluid precautions should be used consistently with *all* patients—termed "universal blood and body-fluid precautions" or "universal precautions." Particular care is to be exercised in emergency-care settings where exposure to blood is greater. The essence of the "universal precautions" follows:

1. Use gloves in all procedures involving contact with blood, body fluids, mucous membranes, and nonintact skin of *all* patients. Masks and protective eyewear are to be added if droplets of blood or other body fluids are likely to be generated. If splashes of fluid are anticipated, gowns are to be worn.
2. Wash hands or other skin surfaces immediately and thoroughly if contaminated and after glove removal.
3. Avoid injury by needles and sharp instruments. Do not bend or break needles, but place used syringes and needles in puncture-resistant containers.
4. In areas where resuscitation may be indicated, have ventilation devices available.
5. Health care workers with exudative lesions or weeping dermatitis should refrain from patient care.
6. Particular precautions must be taken by pregnant workers to avoid possible perinatal transmission of HIV infection development during the pregnancy.

Special precautions are advised in dentistry, for autopsies or morticians' services, in dialysis, and in laboratories, and reference should be made to the most recent CDC recommendations [160].*

Employers of health care workers should ensure that policies exist for

1. Education and training of all health care workers on the epidemiology, modes of transmission, and prevention of HIV and other blood-borne infections and the need for consistent use of the universal precautions for *all* patients.
2. Provision of equipment and supplies needed to minimize the risk of infection with HIV and other blood-borne pathogens.
3. Monitoring adherence to recommended measures, with counseling, education, retraining, or disciplinary action as indicated by infractions.

*Available from the Centers for Disease Control in Atlanta, Georgia 30333.

The matter of testing health care workers has arisen, and although transmission of HIV from health care workers to patients has not been reported, the possibility remains during the conduct of invasive procedures. The transfer of hepatitis B virus—a blood-borne agent with much greater potential for nosocomial spread—from health care workers to patients has been noted. When such transmission did occur, the concentration of virus particles in the blood was much higher than is found in HIV infection. In keeping with the views of CDC [160], the usefulness of regular testing of health care workers cannot be assessed. If such a program for workers engaged in invasive procedures is considered, the issues of frequency of testing, consent, confidentiality, and the consequences of the test results must be addressed.

In substance, the precautions advised follow the hepatitis B model of transmission. The recommendations given to prevent the spread of hepatitis B will also prevent the transmission of AIDS. Studies of exposed groups have been reported and are ongoing, and the body of literature continues to grow [162–167]. Encouraging, though, is the approval of an HIV vaccine for clinical trials (Vax Syn HIV.1), with others in various stages of development [168].

SUMMARY: PRINCIPLES AND GUIDELINES FOR HOSPITAL OCCUPATIONAL HEALTH AND SAFETY PROGRAMS

The OHP in a hospital is not greatly different from an in-plant medical activity in any other organization. Particular employee exposures need to be known and environmental, surveillance, and immunizing precautions taken.

On the completion of the NIOSH Hospital Occupational Health Services Study, certain principles and guidelines wee developed [169]. They follow, with some modification.

PREPLACEMENT MEDICAL EXAMINATIONS

Preplacement medical examinations should be performed on all new employees by a health care professional to include

- History, including family, past medical, and occupational histories, review of systems, and details of present complaints, if any
- Physical examination, including
  - Height, weight, temperature, pulse, and blood pressure measurements
  - Vision and hearing tests
  - Examination of skin, eyes, ears, nose, teeth, mouth, heart, lungs, breasts, lymph nodes, peripheral blood vessels, abdomen, inguinal regions, genitalia, rectum, spine, and extremities
  - Assessment of obvious emotional and mental status
- Additional procedures
  - Blood tests:
    - Hemoglobin or hematocrit determination
    - Total and differential leukocyte counts
    - Serologic test for syphilis
    - Blood chemistry determinations as deemed necessary by examiner
    - Urinalysis, including microscopic examination
    - Chest radiograph
    - Tuberculin skin test, unless known to be positive
    - Cervical cytology (for women aged 18 or older, unless performed within past year)
    - Cervical culture for *Neisseria gonorrhoeae*
    - Electrocardiogram
- Other procedures and consultations as indicated by history, physical findings or *special job requirements*

PERIODIC HEALTH MAINTENANCE PROCEDURES

- General examination, as outlined above, repeated triennially to age 30, biennially to age 40, annually thereafter, and under certain circumstances, on retirement.
- In intervals between, cervical cytology with culture for *Neisseria gonorrhoeae* annually and tuberculin skin test unless known positive.
- Periodic health appraisals to be conducted at intervals consonant with job assignment and potentially hazardous exposures, or with federal or state mandates.
- Special health appraisals to be conducted after 3- to 5-day periods of illness absence. Records to be reviewed on interservice or interdepartmental transfer to determine if incumbent physically or emotionally fit to undertake new assignment.

HEALTH AND SAFETY EDUCATION

An ongoing program should include job orientation, safe work practices, relevant health information, and use of EHS for reporting injury and illness. It should include discussion of known and potential work-related hazards affecting conception and pregnancy. The educational program should be a joint effort of the occupational health physician, the occupational health nurse, and the industrial hygienist.

IMMUNIZATION PRACTICES

Diphtheria-tetanus immunization initially, if needed, and booster injection decennially.

Oral polio immunization.

Special screening and immunizations, as indicated by patient or laboratory contacts.

Establish a recall system to maintain currency of immune status, in keeping with CDC recommendations.

CARE OF ILLNESS AND INJURY AT WORK

Arrangements should be provided to give occupational medical, surgical, psychological, and rehabilitative services to all employees.

A specific, identified site should be designated for this purpose.

A panel of medical and surgical consultants either from the hospital staff or the larger medical community should be available.

A formalized procedure should be developed for liaison with employees' physicians or clinics.

Establish procedures to ensure continuity of care for all employees.

Treatment and reporting of occupational injuries and illnesses should conform to state workers compensation laws and OSHA standards.

PERSONAL HEALTH COUNSELING

A counseling program should provide assistance for employees having problems with weight control or chemical substance abuse (drugs, alcohol, tobacco) or for pregnancy, family problems, or retirement.

A referral system should be developed for employees in need of more definitive intervention by mental health care specialists.

ENVIRONMENTAL CONTROL AND SURVEILLANCE

Service should be headed by a specialist knowledgeable regarding hospital work environments, particularly as they affect women of child-bearing age.

A competent person should be responsible for radiation safety, and the services of a consulting health-physicist should be obtained as needed.

Compliance with regulations pertinent to radiation hazards must be maintained.

HEALTH AND SAFETY RECORDS SYSTEM

A health record must be maintained on each employee to include all material relating to health and all environmental data collected at the employee's worksite.

Records must be prepared monthly and annually showing illness and injury rates and all environmental measurements made in accordance with OSHA standards.

Records must be maintained with full confidentiality and are to be made available only to appropriate medical personnel unless signed authorization of the employee has been secured for transmittal to other individuals or institutions.

COORDINATED PLANNING WITH OTHER HOSPITAL DEPARTMENTS AND SERVICES

A committee should be available to consult on employee health policies as they pertain to various hospital departments, services, and unions.

Specialized committees, such as health and safety and infection control, should consider the health of all hospital employees in their planning.

A representative of the EHS should be on the committees indicated and other appropriate hospital committees.

CLOSURE

While most health care professionals take for granted the employees of a hospital and the completion of their duties, one practitioner gained insight into the energy demands of such employment. Rosner [170], a physician, reported his personal participation as a covering volunteer during a New York City hospital workers' strike, under the telling title "A Humbling Experience." Departmental heads undertook the tasks of admitting clerk, food service worker, and the like. His assignment was that of hospital messenger, and during his shift he had walked, run, jogged, skipped, hopped, lunged, and otherwise locomoted over 9 miles. At shift's end, he was totally exhausted, but better able to "appreciate the indispensable tasks performed by the ancillary and support staffs of a hospital."

In light of their contribution, is not an EHS the least that can be offered? Let not today's hospital workers go the way of Ignaz Philipp Semmelweis (1818–1865), who died from the disease to the prevention of which his entire professional life had been devoted [171].

REFERENCES

1. Lindsay, G. G. General Principles in the Assessment of Fitness for Work in the Merchant Navy. Presented

to the Society of Occupational Medicine, Oct 29, 1971.
2. Blais, B. R. Delivery Patterns of Medical Care to Seafarers: Medical Care at Sea. Presented to the American Occupational Health Conference, Apr 1982.
3. Anderson, W. R. Medical Care at Sea. Presented to the American Occupational Health Conference, Apr 1982.
4. Norris, M. J. *The Law of Maritime Personal Injuries Affecting Harbor Workers Passengers and Visitors.* Mount Kisco, NY: Baker, Voorhis, 1959. P. v.
5. Norris, M. J. *The Law of Seamen* (2nd ed.). Mount Kisco, NY: Baker, Voorhis, 1962. Vol. 1, pp. 1–7.
6. Hall, T. M., Herring, S. A., and Jozwiak, T. J. Basic elements of maritime health care. *J Occup Med* 26:202, 1984.
7. Hall, T. M. Personal communication, Feb 22, 1985.
8. Nordhoff, C., and Hall, J. N. *Mutiny on the Bounty.* New York: Pocket Books, 1943. Pp. 32–33.
9. Bobb, J. K. Shipboard Emergency Preparedness. Deliveries Before the American Occupational Health Conference, Kansas City, MO, Apr 18, 1985. P. 3.
10. Urner, C. J. Occupational medicine at sea: The seafarer as a patient. *J Occup Med* 24:917, 1982.
11. Duffy, J. C. (Ed.). *The Ship's Medicine Chest and Medical Aid at Sea* (revd.). Rockville, MD: U.S. Department of Health, Education, and Welfare, Public Health Services, Health Services Administration, Bureau of Medical Services, 1984.
12. Urner, C. J. Campbell, R. S., Stanton, A. B., et al. *The Ship's Medicine Chest at Sea.* New Orleans, LA: Delta Export Pharmacy, Inc., [n.d.].
13. Gunby, P. Medicine at a glance [divers alert network]. *JAMA* 258:623, 1985.
14. Anderson, W. R. Problems of Treatment of Merchant Seamen. Presented to American Industrial Health Conference, Atlanta, GA, Apr 29, 1981.
15. Urner, C. J. *Physical Examination Guide Lines; Basic Duties of Ship Board Personnel* (revd.). New Orleans, LA: Lykes Bros. Steamship Co., 1980.
16. Dean, D. Personal communication, Jan 7, 1985.
17. The Merchant Shipping (Medical Examination) Regulations 1983, SI 1983, No. 808. Notice to Shipowners, Agents, Master, Seafarers, Approved Medical Practitioners and Approved Medical Referees. Department of Transport, Merchant Shipping Notice No. M1144. London: Department of Transport, Marine Directorate, Aug 1984.
18. Gerst, D. A review of psycho-sociological problems in crews on board supertankers. *Med Bull* (Standard Oil Co. of New Jersey) 32:164, 1972.
19. Clark, W. R., Jr., and Montgomery, C. H. Arctic tanker medicine. *Ind Med* 39:37, Mar 1970.
20. Norman, J. N. Medical Support Offshore. In *Health & Hazards in a Changing Oil Scene.* Proceedings of the Institute of Petroleum 1982 Annual Conference, London, UK. Chichester: Wiley, 1983. Pp. 105–111.
21. Cox, R. A. F. Medical services to offshore drilling. *Injury* 1:217, 1970.
22. Cox, R. A. F. *Offshore Medicine: Medical Care of Employees in the Offshore Oil Industry* (2nd ed.). New York: Springer-Verlag, 1987.
23. Stallard, C. W., Jr. Personal communication, March 21, 1985.
24. Crippen, E. F., and Davis, K. *Staying Alive in the Arctic.* Washington, DC: American Petroleum Institute, [n.d.].
25. American Public Health Association Task Force. *National Arctic Health Science Policy.* Washington, DC: The Association, [n.d.].
26. Tabershaw, I. R., and Fuenning, S. I. Environmental health problems in institutions of higher education. *J Occup Med* 10:663, 1968.
27. Michaelsen, G. S. Occupational health at a university. *Public Health Rep* 73:941, 1958.
28. Prince, J. R. Radiation safety in a university. *Health-Physics* 9:347, 1963.
29. Rutsky, I. I., Kalbfleisch, J. H., and Fink, J. N. Occupational allergy to laboratory animals: Employer practices. *J Occup Med* 25:372, 1983.
30. Goldwater, L. J., Kleinfeld, M., and Berger, A. R. Mercury exposure in a university laboratory. *Monthly Rev* (New York State Department of Labor, Division of Industrial Hygiene) 35:13, 1956.
31. Edmonds, O. P. Health hazards on the campus. *Occup Health* 24:435, 1972.
32. Dreesen, D. W. Identifying biohazards in university research. *Am J Public Health* 70:1108, 1980.
33. Recommended standards and practices for a college health program. *J Am Coll Health Assoc* 32:20, 1984.
34. Garner, W. R. Personal communication, Aug 6, 1981.
35. Garner, W. R. Personal communication, Mar 1, 1981.
36. Sawyer, R. N. Asbestos exposure in a Yale building. *Environ Res* 13:146, 1977.
37. Chalfen, M. G. Old and new environmental issues for college and university health services. *J Am Coll Health Assoc* 4:175, 1982.
38. Larsen, L. B. *An Occupational Health Survey of Selected Airports.* Salt Lake City, UT: U.S. Department of Health, Education, and Welfare, Public Health Service Center for Disease Control, National Institute for Occupational Safety and Health, Division of Technical Services, 1974.
39. Guide to organization and operation of airport medical services. *JAMA* 182:957, 1962.
40. Klinghoffer, M. A pre-triage plan for mass casualty care. *Occup Health Saf* 47:32, Nov/Dec 1978.
41. Bergot, T. P. Airport Emergency Planning and Criminal Attacks. Typescript, May 1984. P. 1.
42. Bergot, G. P. Airport Medical Problems. Presented as part of Seminar on Airport Planning Operations and Mangement, June 2–4, 1971.
43. Klatt, J. R. Lack of medical facilities at L.A. airport poses serious problem. *Los Angeles Time* VII:1,19, June 19, 1983.
44. Miller, W. B., and Zarcone, V. Psychiatric behavior

disorders at an international airport. *Arch Environ Health* 17:360, 1968.
45. Shapiro, S. A study of psychiatric syndromes manifested at an international airport. *Comp Psychiatr* 17:453, 1976.
46. Shapiro, S. Airport wandering as a psychotic symptom. *Psychiatr Clin* (Basel), 15:173, 1982.
47. Morris, G. E. Dermatoses among Office Workers. *JAMA* 152:1218, 1953.
48. Indoor air problems—The office environment—A national epidemic. *Environ Health Saf News* 30/31:1, 1981–82.
49. Office health hazards may be costly. *Occup Haz* 46:33, 1984.
50. Environmental, organizational, psychosocial factors in office may pose health hazard. *Int Med News* 17:28, Nov 15–30, 1984.
51. Building close-out procedure to prevent "tight building syndrome." *CAL/OSHA News* 8:1, Nov 1984.
52. Gregory, J. Office Air Quality, "Tight Buildings," and Job Stress: The Impact on Women Office Workers' Occupational Health. *Transactions of 1981 American Conference of Governmental Industrial Hygienists*. Cincinnati, OH: ACGIH, 1982. Pp. 36–46.
53. Outbreaks of respiratory illness among employees in large office buildings—Tennessee, District of Columbia. *MMWR* 33:506, 1984.
54. McGrath, J. G. Health safety and ergonomic aspects of visual display units. *Med Bull* (Exxon) 41:79, 1981.
55. Starr, S. J. A study of video display terminal workers. *J Occup Med* 25:95, 1983.
56. Weiss, M. M. The video display terminals: Is there a radiation hazard? *J Occup Med* 25:98, 1983.
57. American Council on Science and Health. *Health and Safety Aspects of Video Display Terminals* (2nd ed.). New York: The Council, Jan 1985.
58. Murray, W. E., Moss, C. E., Parr, W. H., et al. *Potential Health Hazards of Video Display Terminals*. NIOSH Publication No. 81-129, 1981.
59. Video Display Terminals. In *Navy Environmental Health Bulletin*. NAVMED P-5112. Norfolk, VA: Navy Environmental Health Center, [n.d.]. Pp. 1–7.
60. Video Display Terminals (VDTs) and the Eye. In *Information about Eye Care*. San Francisco: American Academy of Ophthalmology, 1984.
61. Vortouni, L. Tips on proper use of VDTs. *Saf Loss Control Bull*, No. 3, Apr 1984. Pp. 1, 4–5.
62. *Video Display Terminals . . . The Human Factor*. Chicago, IL: National Safety Council, 1982.
63. AT&T Bell Laboratories (Short Hill, NJ). *VDTs: Preliminary Guidelines for Selection, Installation and Use*. Cited in VDT guidelines made available. *Occup Health Saf* 53:17, Apr 1984.
64. Nine states now considering VDT safety bills. *Occup Health Saf Letter* 14:4, March 22, 1984.
65. Returns in on VDT study. *Occup Haz* 46:34, 1984.
66. Lead aprons for VDT users? Unnecessary—CCOHS. *At the Centre* 7:9, June 1984.
67. Council on Scientific Affairs (American Medical Association). Health effects of video display terminals. *JAMA* 257:1508, 1987.
68. Allbaugh, R. D. Personal communication, Jan 22, 1981.
69. Stafford, E. Cooperative programs cutting costs, accidents in construction. *Occup Health Saf* 54:40, Jan 1985.
70. Niskanen, T. Construction accidents and their prevention. *Saf Practitioner* 1:30, Apr 1983.
71. Grandjean, P. *Occupational Health Aspects of Construction Work*. Copenhagen: World Health Organization Regional Office for Europe, 1983. P. 2.
72. Felton, J. S. Hospital employees: Corridor consultations or health maintenance? *JAMA* 168:1854, 1958.
73. *Statistical Abstract of the United States, 1985* (105th ed.). Washington, DC: U.S. Department of Commerce, Bureau of the Census, 1984.
74. Conant, R. G., and Stent, P. A. The large general hospital, an industrial medical complex. *J Occup Med* 12:364, 1970.
75. Conant, R. G. The hospital as an industry. *J Occup Med* 13:561, 1971.
76. Geiger, A. J. A neglected branch of industrial medicine. *Yale J Biol Med* 17:483, 1945.
77. Guiding principles for an occupational health program in a hospital employee group. *JAMA* 166:777, 1958.
78. Mammen, H. W. The need for employees' health services in hospitals. *Arch Environ Health* 9:750, 1964.
79. Health services for hospital employees. *JAMA* 191:163, 1965.
80. Kagey, K. S. Hospital employee safety. *JAMA* 220:728, 1972.
81. *An Occupational Health Program for Hospital Employees*. USPHS Publication No. 725. Washington, DC: U.S. Department of Health, Education, and Welfare, Public Health Service, 1959.
82. *A General Guide for an Occupational Health Program for Hospital Employees* (1st ed.). Madison, WI: Wisconsin State Board of Health, Occupational Health Division, 1964.
83. *Hospital Occupational Health Services Study*. Cincinnati, OH: U.S. Department of Health, Education, and Welfare, Public Health Service, Center for Disease Control, National Institute for Occupational Safety and Health, Division of Technical Services, 1975. Vol. I, Environmental Health and Safety Education; Vol. II, Employee Health and Safety Statistics and Records; Vol. III, Organization and Administration of Hospital Employee Health Services; Vol. IV, Staffing of the Hospital Occupatinal Health Unit; Vol. V, Occupational Health Services for Hospital Employees; Vol. VI, Special Information; and Vol. VII, Summary and Conclusions.
84. Lewy, R. The regulatory status of hospital occupational medicine: A need for change. *J Occup Med* 24:133, 1982.

85. Blackadder, E. S. Occupational health services for NHS staff: Health and safety at work for the health-care industry. *R Soc Health J* 99:137, 1979.
86. Brown, T. C., Kreider, S. D., and Lange, W. R. Committee on Medical Center Employee Occupational Health Services of the American Occupational Medical Association. Guidelines for employee health services in hospitals, clinics and medical research institutions. *J Occup Med* 25:771, 1983.
87. Messite, J. Cited in P. C. Smith, Hospitals may be hazardous to workers' health: NIOSH. *Med Trib* 25:72, Dec 26, 1984.
88. Lohman, J. Hospital safety strategies. *Occup Health Saf* 51:46, Dec 1982.
89. Pines, A., Skulkeo, K., Pollak, E., et al. Rates of sickness absenteeism among employees of a modern hospital: The role of demographic and occupational factors. *Br J Ind Med* 42:326, 1985.
90. AOMA approves set of guidelines keyed to medical workers. *Occup Health Saf* 52:10a, Nov/Dec 1983.
91. AOMA issues guidelines for employee health services in medical institutions. *AOMA Rep,* July/Aug 1983. P. 1.
92. AOMA Committee on Medical Center Employee Occupational Health. Guidelines for employee health services in health care institutions. *J Occup Med* 28:518, 1986.
93. Hospital obligation to nonemployee personnel. *JAMA* 224:1329, 1973.
94. Lewy, R. M. Occupational health programs for house staff physicians. *JAMA* 246:1432, 1981.
95. Schneider, W. J., and Dykan, M. The preplacement medical evaluation of hospital personnel. *J Occup Med* 20:741, 1978.
96. Luke 4:23.
97. Polk, B. F., White, J. A., De Girolami, P. C., et al. An outbreak of rubella among hospital personnel. *N Engl J Med* 303:541, 1980.
98. Babb, R. R. Physical examinations for physicians. *West J Med* 142:698, 1985.
99. Orenstein, W. A., Heseltine, P. N. R., Le Gagnoux, S. J., et al. Rubella vaccine and susceptible hospital employees: Poor physician participation. *JAMA* 145:711, 1981.
100. Borenstein, D. B., and Cook, K. Impairment prevention in the training years: A new mental health program at UCLA. *JAMA* 247:2700, 1982.
101. Barrett-Connor, E. The epidemiology of tuberculosis in physicians. *JAMA* 241:33, 1979.
102. Strickler, A. C. Hepatitis B Vaccine: Implications for Hospitals. Presented at the American Occupational Health Conference, April 1955, Kansas City, KA. Typescript P. 6; personal communication, May 30, 1985.
103. Clever, L. H., and Arsham, G. M. Physicians' own health: Some advice for the advisors. *West J Med* 141:846, 1984.
104. Gaeuman, J. V. Tuberculosis surveillance of hospital personnel. *J Occup Med* 23:695, 1981.
105. Berman, J., Levin, M. L., Orr, S. T., et al. Tuberculosis risk for hospital employees: Analysis of a five-year tuberculin skin testing program. *Am J Public Health* 71:1200, 1981.
106. Testing medical students for TB is recommended. *Intern Med News* 16:42, Jan 1–14, 1983.
107. *Infection Control in the Hospital* (4th ed.). Chicago, IL: American Hospital Association, 1979. Immunization of Personnel, pp. 32–35; Appendix E, Guidelines on Tuberculosis Control Programs for Hospital Employees, pp. 207–216.
108. *Guidelines for the Prevention of TB Transmission in Hospitals,* (revd.). Atlanta, GA: U.S. Department of Health and Human Services, Public Health Service, Centers for Disease Control, Center for Prevention Services, Tuberculosis Control Division, Oct 1983. Pp. 12–14.
109. Barclay, W. R. Annual tuberculosis screening for hospital employees. *JAMA* 246:1838, 1981.
110. Cope, R., and Hartstein, A. I. The annual chest roentgenogram for the control of tuberculosis in hospital employees: Recent changes and their implications. *Am Rev Respir Dis* 125:106, 1982.
111. Committee on Occupational Medical Practice, AOMA. Tuberculosis screening in the hospital setting. *J Occup Med* 25:174, 1983.
112. Clemens, J. D., Chuong, J. J. H., and Feinstein, A. R. The BCG controversy: A methodological and statistical appraisal. *JAMA* 249:2362, 1983.
113. Barclay, W. R. BCG: An effective immunizing agent. *JAMA* 249:2376, 1983.
114. Rubella outbreaks in Los Angeles County: The need for a hospital screening program. *Public Health Letter* (Los Angeles County Department of Health Services) 4:5, 1982.
115. Preblud, S. R., and Hinman, A. R. Rubella vaccination of hospital employees. *JAMA* 145:726, 1981.
116. Wakefield, M., and Alexander, W. J. Screening for rubella susceptibility. *JAMA* 247:2500, 1982.
117. Golenda, F. G. Hepatitis B vaccine: An overview. *Sex Med Today* 7:30, June 1983.
118. Krugman, S. The newly licensed hepatitis B vaccine: Characteristics and indications for use. *JAMA* 247:2012, 1982.
119. Mulley, A. G., Silverstein, M. D., and Dienstag, J. L. Indications for use of hepatitis B vaccine, based on cost-effectiveness analysis. *N Engl J Med* 307:644, 1982.
120. Costs and benefits of hepatitis B vaccination. *Lancet* 2:1195, 1982.
121. Hashimoto, F. Cost effectiveness of serotesting before hepatitis vaccination. *N Engl J Med* 307:503, 1982.
122. Seligman, S. J. Cost effectiveness of hepatitis B vaccine. *N Engl J Med* 308:104, 1983.
123. Papaevangelou, G., Roumeliotou-Karayannis, A., Tassopoulos, N., et al. Hepatitis B vaccination policy. *Lancet* 1:533, 1983.
124. Francis, D. B. Hepatitis B virus vaccine: An opportunity for control. *JAMA* 250:1891, 1983.
125. Hamilton, J. D. Hepatitis B virus vaccine: An anal-

ysis of its potential use in medical workers. *JAMA* 250:2145, 1983.
126. Egilman, D., and Lichty, P. Costs and benefits of hepatitis prophylaxis. *JAMA* 251:2794, 1984.
127. Kreider, S. D., and Lange, W. R. Hepatitis B vaccine. *N Engl J Med* 310:466, 1984.
128. Szmuness, W., Stevens, C. E., Harley, D. J., et al. Hepatitis B vaccine: demonstration of efficacy in a controlled clinical trial in a high-risk population in the United States. *N Engl J Med* 303:833, 1980.
129. Beasley, R. P., and Hwang, L.-Y. Immunogenicity of hepatitis B virus vaccine (hepatavax-B): Response of healthy adults. *West J Med* 140:731, 1984.
130. Lohiya, G., Lohiya, S., Caires, S., et al. Occupational exposure to hepatitis B virus: Analysis of indications for hepatitis B vaccine. *J Occup Med* 26:189, 1984.
131. Hepatitis B virus vaccine safety: Report of an interagency group. *MMWR* 31:465, 1982.
132. Geretz, R. J., and Tabor, E. Newly licensed hepatitis B vaccine: Known safety and unknown risks. *JAMA* 249:745, 1983.
133. Trends: Safety of hepatitis B virus vaccine. *MMWR* 32:134, 1983.
134. Immune globulins for protection against viral hepatitis: Recommendation of the Immunization Practices Advisory Committee (ACIP). *MMWR* 30:423, 1981.
135. Postexposure prophylaxis of hepatitis B: Recommendations of the Immunization Practices Advisory Committee (ACIP). *MMWR* 33:285, 1984.
136. London, W. T. Cited in B. Merz, Antiviral vaccines/ cancer prophylactics? *JAMA* 250:15, 1983.
137. Mostow, S. R. Cited in Hepatitis vaccine may prevent lawsuit as well as illness. *Int Med News* 17:3, May 1–14, 1984.
138. Scolnick, E. M., McLean, A. A., West, D. J., et al. Clinical evaluation in healthy adults of a hepatitis B vaccine made by recombinant DNA. *JAMA* 251:2812, 1984.
139. Recommendations of the Immunization Practices Advisory Committee Update on Hepatitis B Prevention. *MMWR* 36:353, 1987.
140. U.S. Preventive Services Task Force. Immunizations, immunoprophylaxis, and chemoprophylaxis to prevent selected infections. *JAMA* 257:2464, 1987.
141. Horowitz, M. M. Cited in hepatitis B vaccine protection lessens with time. *Int Med News* 20:12, Aug 1–14, 1987.
142. Conrad, F. Hospital safety committees. *Occup Health Saf* 52:50, Feb 1983.
143. Brown, M. P. Hazards in the hospital: Educating the workforce through its union. *Am J Public Health* 69:1040, 1979.
144. Biohazards and laboratory safety lectures. *Clin Bull* 10:39, 1980.
145. *Sloan-Kettering Institute Course in Biohazards and Laboratory Safety.* New York: The Institute, 1976.
146. McCunney, R. J. A hospital-based occupational health service. *J Occup Med* 26:375, 1984.
147. American Occupational Medical Association Committee on Occupational Medical Practice. Hospital cooperation with local business. *J Occup Med* 25:501, 1983.
148. Hamory, B. H. Health records for hospital employees. *N Engl J Med* 304:56, 1981.
149. Reece, C. A hospital day care center. *Human Dev News,* Aug-Sept 1983. Pp. 6–7.
150. Employed parents. *Human Dev News,* Aug-Sept 1983. P. 7.
151. Friedman, D. E. The employer response to child care. *Human Dev News,* Oct 1982. P. 5.
152. Ricks, A. E., and Ricks, S. Hospitals should provide day-care for children of employees. *JAMA* 249:2090, 1983.
153. Infectious diseases and day care centers. *Public Health Letter* (Los Angeles County Department of Health Services) 5:1, Aug 1983.
154. Holmes, A. W. Prevention of hepatitis in day-care centers. *JAMA* 250:1841, 1983.
155. *Safety Guide for Health Care Institutions* (3rd ed.). Chicago, IL: American Hospital Association, 1983. Fig. 28, Disaster Preparedness Plan Checklist. Pp. 114–120.
156. Infectious wastes. *Physician's Bull* (Orange County [California] Health Care Agency, Public Health and Medical Services) 32:1, Apr/May 1982.
157. Infectious wastes update. *Physician's Bull* (Orange County [California] Health Care Agency, Public Health and Medical Services) 33:1, Feb 1983.
158. Brown, B. L. *Risk Management for Hospitals: A Practical Approach.* Germantown, MD: Aspen Systems, 1979. Chaps. 1 and 3, pp. 1–8, 49–77.
159. Manes, M. P. The dual capacity doctrine of treating hospital employees. *Occup Health Saf* 50:46, Jan 1981.
160. Recommmendation for prevention of HIV transmission in health-care settings. *MMWR* 36(Suppl. 28):18-18s.
161. Update: Human immunodeficiency virus infections in health-care workers exposed to blood of infected patients. *MMWR* 36:285, 1987.
162. *Surgeon General's Report on Acquired Immune Deficiency Syndrome.* U.S. Department of Health and Human Services, 1987.
163. Revision of the CDC surveillance care definition for acquired immunodeficiency syndrome. *MMWR* 36(Suppl. 18 S):38.
164. Francis, D. P., and Chin, J. The prevention of acquired immunodeficiency syndrome in the United States: An objective strategy for medicine, public health, business, and the community. *JAMA* 257:1357, 1987.
165. Public Health Service guidelines for counseling and antibody testing to prevent HIV infection and AIDS. *MMWR* 36:509, 1987.
166. Kuhls, T.L., Viker, S., Parris, N. B., et al. Occupational risk of HIV, HBV and HSV-2 infections in health care personnel caring for AIDS patients. *Am J Public Health* 77:1306, 1987.

167. Vlahor, D., and Polk, B. F. Transmission of human immunodeficiency virus within the health care setting. *State Art Rev—Occup Med* 3:539, 1987.
168. Kirn, T. F. HIV vaccine approved for clinical trials. *JAMA* 258:1433, 1987.
169. *Highlights of the NIOSH Hospital Occupational Health Services Study.* Cincinnati, OH: U.S. Department of Health, Education, and Welfare, Public Health Service, Center for Disease Control, National Institute for Occupational Safety and Health, 1976. Pp. 15–20.
170. Rosner, F. A humbling experience. *JAMA* 253:199, 1985.
171. Sinclair, W. J. Death of Semmelweis. In E. F. Griffith, *Doctors by Themselves.* London: Cassell, 1951. Pp. 187–188.

549409

17. OCCUPATIONAL HEALTH AND SPECIFIC WORK GROUPS

Si jeunesse savait, se vieillesse peuvait.
(If youth but knew, if old age but could.)

Henri Estienne

Your huddled masses yearning to breathe free,
The wretched refuse of your teeming shore.
Send these, the homeless, tempest-tost to me . . .

Emma Lazarus

Each time there has been a drive by women for equal status with men there have been attempts to ridicule, to become outraged at the new demands that are raised, but each time these demands have been satisfied, there has been a step forward not only for women but for men and therefore for all members of society.

Leonard C. Frank, M.D.

The move of the world's disabled people forward from primitive times was due to improved social attitudes as well as improved technology and the economy of nations. They moved first to the right to survival, then to the right to dependency, and finally to the right to independency. But the transitional stages have been terribly slow and are still not complete in even the wealthiest and most advanced nations. Social attitudes revert at times to even primitive levels as expressed in the treatment accorded disabled individuals.

George Nelson Wright, Ph.D.

YOUTH IN THE WORKPLACE

Changes in society, economic waves and troughs, and altered technologies affect the constituency of any employed group. Certain segments of a plant population will increase in number or diminish as a company prospers, declines, or ages or as certain groups become heard in their demands for greater representation in the labor market. While it was traditional in earlier years for high school graduates not proceeding into higher education to seek employment in industry, the turmoil of the late 1960s and early 1970s saw youth turning angrily against the so-called establishment and rejecting the opportunities for beginning-career training. Only 4 of 10 students queried then felt that "hard work will always pay off" [1]. The press, comprising both slick and thoughtful publications, documented the national and analytic concerns arising from the destructive rebellion to which the country was bearing witness [1–5].

Somers [6] indicated that in 1973, 18,032 young Americans between 15 and 24 years of age died in motor vehicle accidents,* 5,182 were murdered, and 4,098 committed suicide—leading to a death rate that was 19 percent higher in 1973–1974 than it had been in 1960–1961. In addition to this wasting of life, the war in Vietnam was scattering youth to other countries, and business was reluctant to hire young people. As voiced by Hodgson, then Secretary of Labor, "For some strange reason, except for a few large companies, industry has remained strangely apathetic to the problems of the [vocational] schools" [8]. Further emphasis was given by the Assistant Secretary of Labor, who observed that "American big business is anti-youth employment without a conscious policy" [9].

With the changing years, though, the attitude of America's young has changed, and the strident vocalists of the 1970s have become today's parents, seeking work and, in the main, remaining in jobs. Those persons wishing better preparation have gone on to college for further study.† Through apprentice-training programs, skills have been acquired, and many of the former critics of both academe and industry have become either journeymen in their crafts or teachers of the next generation.

*This age group was still high in 1983—20,040 were killed in motor vehicle accidents [7].

†As of early 1984, more than twice as many persons (45.2 percent) had completed 4 years of high school as had finished fewer than the 4 years (21.6 percent). Individuals completing 1 to 3 years of college composed 26.4 percent, while 6.74 percent had finished 4 years or more of college [10].

Today, youth is seen in all positions—clerical, law enforcement, manufacturing, computer science, service, and the distributive trades. Men are in jobs formerly held solely by women, and female youth is seen in the crafts and in heavy work, previously thought inappropriate for the less-muscled gender. But certain problems remain to be addressed.

EXPOSURE

Ely [11] voiced it well when he pointed out that the various quantitative guidelines in the form of standards and regulations that have been developed for the control of physical and chemical hazards were designed for adults and that uniform application to younger humans would be incorrect. He asked that occupational health personnel advise line managers with young workers in their groups that when effecting controls of hazardous operations, they should consider age, the magnitude and duration of the potential exposure, the ease of controlling the level, the adult makeup of the group assigned to the task, and what is known of sensitivity versus age. The counsel of occupational or industrial health specialists should be sought, as some noxious agents are more toxic to younger persons than adults. Other materials, conversely, are less hazardous to youth. In many instances, the vulnerability of the one exposed is unknown, but caution would suggest that the younger worker would be more sensitive. Ely indicates that control would take the form of reducing the level of the offending agent, limiting the duration of exposure, or a combination of the two. While his comments then (1976) were directed to the age group of "conception to, classically, age 18 years," much work has been done subsequently on hazards to the reproductive system in both working women and men.

But in light of continued summer employment opportunities, the lightening of controls on the working minor, and the eagerness of many youths to drop out of school and take any kind of job, occupational health specialists should carry on the educational effort suggested by Ely.

HEALTH EVALUATION

Legislators in England historically have been much more concerned about working youth than have the lawmakers in the United States because of the traditional use of child labor and the young age of the "school leavers." While their system of the examination of youngsters by certifying surgeons dates to the Factories Act of 1844, the contemporary use of appointed factory doctors (AFD) had its birth in 1948 [12]. The designation of a practitioner as an AFD required that certain functions be carried out: medical examination of all young persons under 18 when they enter work and change employment and at annual intervals; medical examination of all persons required by special regulations to have periodic assessment; and the investigation and reporting of injuries or deaths caused by noxious exposures or cases of occupationally related poisoning specifically prescribed by regulation.

In the course of such examinations the defects found have been analyzed, and while the major defects were relatively few—those findings affecting employment working capacity—minor defects, however, were encountered in 34 percent of some 863 examinations of boys and over 44 percent of 566 examinations of girls* [13]. Highest among the conditions uncovered were visual defects and dental caries. Orthopedic defects were exhibited in 74 of the youngsters, and 59 demonstrated ear, nose, or throat deficits.

The content of the examination differs in no way from the components of the health assessment of older workers. In physically hazardous job sites, such as mines, where the stronger, younger men might be called on to participate in rescue operations, it must be determined that they are sufficiently fit to handle the extra demands of such arduous tasks [14]. It must be remembered that in many school systems physical education is no longer mandated, so that not every graduate, or school dropout, is necessarily in peak physical condition to undertake energy-demanding tasks.

The preplacement examination does allow counseling that, when related to the beginning of employment, is more readily accepted than from parents, the ministry, or social agencies. Problems such as persisting adolescent acne, substance abuse, overweight, or malnutrition can be reviewed, as can unclear issues in human sexuality. The young person entering the blue-collar world is quickly subjected to the pressure of the work group and readily adopts the mores of his peers where "machismo" is king and anything less is to be shunned.

SELF-DESTRUCTIVE BEHAVIOR

Young workers are risk-takers, and any occupational health specialist who provides emergency care to a

*The examinations conducted were the evaluations at time of "entry," "change of employment," or "recheck."

large workforce will begin to see repeatedly many of the same young workers who accept the concepts of safe work practices extremely slowly.* To demonstrate muscular strength, some young laborers will vie with each other in unapproved and even prohibited contests while at work to show physical superiority.

Many of the youth group drive motorcycles to work, as can be judged by a scan of company parking lots. Often they are involved in accidents and, if near the plant, will be brought into the occupational health service (OHS) for care. In spite of educational efforts by manufacturers and more mature motorcycle enthusiasts, the collisions, spills, and rear-endings continue. Particularly vulnerable are the riders who scoff at the use of protective helmets, clothing, and shoes. In the California beach cities on weekends, it is a common experience to see the youthful riders of the heavy cycles and their passengers wearing sandals only, being subject to crushing injuries, denudation of a foot, and friction burns, if not deep lacerations and fractures.

When engaged in athletic events, particularly in team activities that are company-sponsored, younger workers, not always adequately conditioned, will be injured. These amateur contests rarely are accompanied by the sage counsel of trainers, and the coaches are usually equally unprepared fellow employees. In these instances of sustained trauma, there is time lost from work, and the injured persons are given care through the workers' compensation system,† which may be both protracted and costly. These injuries need not be limited to after-hours play, for noontime horseshoes can be equally damaging if there is no supervision of the activity.

*Recalled is one young man who worked with heavy steel plating. A piece of steel one-half inch thick and about 3 × 6 feet in dimension had to be lifted from a metal table. A manual hoist, complete with chainfall, was immediately above the table, but this young man attempted to lift the part with his ungloved hands. Two fingers were caught with slippage of the piece, causing compound fractures. The response on querying: "I know I should have used the lift."

†There is considerable case law to substantiate the rule that workers injured in employer-sponsored events (office parties, picnics, or touch football) are covered through workers' compensation insurance.

As an additional example of foolhardy participation by inadequately conditioned players, although not deemed old, the author recalls the preparation in the Philippine islands of an army unit for the invasion of Japan. To while away some of the time, a pickup baseball team was formed, comprising eminent medical specialists from a cardiac surgeon to a psychiatrist to an internist, which proceeded to play several innings of hard ball. Most of the officers were unable to walk comfortably for a full week.

Forssman and Coppee [14] discuss risk-taking among adolescents—who in some classifications are extended to age 25 years—and point out that this characteristic is bound up with their need to express and to surpass themselves. One is cautioned, though, not to condemn the action, necessarily. Nor should one exercise multiple, repeated prohibitions. Such action would only produce behavior antithetic to the one being sought. That youth can be cautious is seen in the strict discipline employed in practicing such hazardous sports as scuba diving, parachuting, or mountain climbing [14].

The injury repeaters should be identified early and counseled, for a serious injury with residua that will limit work performance can affect a much longer potential work life than the same injury sustained by an older employee awaiting retirement. Ideally, the best instruction takes place informally when seasoned craftsmen can serve as role models. The veterans have developed the techniques in working that allow them to continue their duties beyond an otherwise controlling chronologic age. The work patterns of a respected senior can and will be emulated when the role of the elder is avuncular rather than paternal.

WORK ATTENDANCE

In some ethnic groups, work newly acquired in the larger community is an undertaking that may be derogated by fellow gang members or other peers, and continuance may be difficult. Every support at the worksite must be exercised so that the simplest of work habits can be encouraged and nurtured—coming to work each day and reporting and leaving on time. In some areas, work may be viewed as a mechanism productive of a paycheck, which implies absenting oneself until the money is spent and then returning to acquire another payment. Not every youth may understand that work is carried on daily and that one's absence may either slow or halt an operation or bring down the wrath of fellow workers who have to cover for the absentee.

Young women, not removed much in time from the menarche, may find the energy-intensive tasks of nontraditional jobs upsetting to cycles that are yet to establish themselves in a regularly recurring mode. They may assume that remaining home from work may be done with the same ease as their previously absenting themselves from school. Industry is not that understanding, and counsel, redirection, or even referral by wise occupational health nurses may help develop a greater capacity of the young woman to cope with unsettling menstrual difficulties.

SMOKING

Workers in plants smoke, many heavily. The freely influenced youngster recently come to the job may believe that this behavior characterizes a good, skilled mechanic and will adopt the habit. Again, appropriate educational effort by the OHS may thwart the adoption of a health-hazardous lifestyle. At one time, when the epidemiologic findings regarding the association of smoking and cardiopulmonary disease were still to become firm, a health professional in industry might have shown some trepidation in delivering the message to hardy, toughened workers. But, today, with nonsmokers demanding recognition of their rights, with the conclusiveness of the data concerning the smoking-disease relationship, and with the passage of local ordinances limiting smoking, one can assume an extremely strong stance and press the facts home concerning the hazard of cigarette use. This action *must* be taken in a company where the pulmonary tree is challenged daily by materials toxic to respiratory tissue. The young worker, particularly, must be assisted in this and other areas of substance abuse.

THE YOUTH AND THE PARENT

An issue somewhat tangential to a consideration of youth in the workplace is a view of youth at school, when a particular youngster's parent is an employee of the company offering an OHS. It has been the author's experience that working with school counselors has been productive of insights into the problems of parents who happen to be employees. In a community of 30,000 persons where there was essentially a single industry, apart from supporting services and shopping facilities, all professionals concerned with mental health cooperated closely. The head of school counseling would determine, when a student was doing poorly, if the parent(s) was an employee of the plant in which the author served in the OHS. If this were the case, the counselor would apprise the author of the child's difficulties, and we would seek out the parent and initiate some assistance. With counseling being given to both child and parent, a family could be directed toward a restyling in relationships.

The opposite also would be effective. If an employee were receiving counseling at work, inquiry would be made as to the children's progress in school. If there were deficits, then, again, bilateral intervention would help both the parent and the children. Occupational health need not be practiced in a vacuum.

AGING IN THE WORKPLACE

LEGISLATIVE BACKGROUND

Several enactments by the Congress have pointed to a new concern relating to the great increase in the population of the aging and the aged. A White House Conference on Aging held in 1961 recommended federal legislation to help states initiate or expand state and community programs for older persons. Two years later, President Kennedy recommended an expanded program to include research, demonstration, and training projects in aging. In 1965, the Older Americans Act was passed, and in succeeding years various amendments enriched the original law, giving emphasis to advocacy for the elderly within all levels of government* [15].

Further, in 1978, by passage of the Civil Rights Commission Act of 1978,† the words *age* and *handicap* had been inserted in the original civil rights legislation, so that the Civil Rights Act of 1957 would not tolerate discrimination or denials of equal protection of the laws under the Constitution because of race, color, religion, sex, age, handicap, or national origin [15]. More pertinent to occupational health, though, was the action of Congress in passing the Age Discrimination in Employment Act of 1967,‡ which aimed at promoting the employment of older persons based on their ability rather than age, prohibiting arbitrary age discrimination in employment, and helping employers and workers find ways of meeting problems arising from the impact of age on employment [16]. Particularly underscored was the protection of persons aged 40 to 65 years from age discrimination in employment in such matters as hiring, discharge, leave, compensation, and promotions, among other areas of employment [17].

That the legislation is binding is seen as recently as early 1985, when a 69-year-old employee of a telecommunications company filed suit against the company in 1980 because he was passed over for promotion despite high performance ratings. He was awarded, in Massachusetts, $425,215, representing

*Public Law 89-73 (July 14, 1965), as amended, particularly by Public Law 95-478 (October 18, 1978).
†Public Law 95-444 (October 10, 1978).
‡Public Law 90-202 (December 15, 1967).

$122,574 for financial losses, $150,000 for emotional distress, and $152,641 in interest [18].

NUMBERS

That the age group 25 to 64 years will increase in number in the years ahead is well-known. As pointed out in a statistical review [19], Americans in that age segment make many personal decisions that affect society as a whole: choice of career, marriage, family formation, housing, insurance portfolio, financial plan, health behavior, medical care utilization, and participation in elections. Their demographic extrapolations are important, for this group is the workforce age, and these kinds of decisions allow for either stability or disruption of workers' lifestyle and the need for supportive assistance by a concerned OHS.

By the year 2000, this productive age group will increase by one-fourth—from 114,387,000 to over 141,000,000 [19]. The growth will continue and will peak at 153,700,000 in 2020. Following a dip, the increase will reappear and reach 151,600,000 by 2050. In the study of three age divisions—25 to 34, 35 to 44, and 45 to 64—the most rapid rise will be in the third segment. The number of men will increase 75 percent between 1983 and 2050—from 21,195,000 to 36,709,000 [19]. The number of women will increase 60 percent, to reach a total of 37,612,000. By century's end, the number of men will exceed slightly the number of women, the ratio being 99 females for 100 males. Of significance in this discussion is the aging of the workforce. Whereas in 1980 the 45- to 64-year age group made up more than 40 percent of the total age bracket, by the year 2050 it will represent half.

Other numbers are important. Ninety percent of the men of the entire group are in the labor force, with the great majority gainfully employed. In early 1970, less than half of the 25- to 64-year-old women were working or seeking employment; in 1985 this group reached over 60 percent, and even of the women aged 45 to 64, over half were in the labor force [19]. A further change will be noted in that the younger workers have had more education than today's 45- to 64-year group, so that there may be a different health behavior pattern and change in morbidity with aging.

The mortality rates among both men and women are declining [20] so that a more active post-retirement life can be anticipated, which implies better preparation for the separation from work period. Further, if certain individuals remain at work until age 70, then the task of the OHS is increased in the screening for chronic disease and the matching of older workers against the demands of the job.*

WORK CAPACITY

That the older worker cannot sustain the load undertaken at career's beginning is uncontested. Gage [21] has pointed out that the worker is treated as a highly flexible commodity who can be fitted in almost as an afterthought to operate equipment that is becoming increasingly complex and costly. Some jobs are age-specific, and some are performed well by virtue of the experience and judgment developed over the years. In the completion of light to moderate work, there is little age dependence up to age 65 [21]. However, as indicated by Gage, the capacity to carry out heavy, exhausting physical work is strictly related to age. Yet there are many workers in the crafts or laborers who, because of limited education or mental capacity, do not rise to less demanding jobs and who are still expected to produce in the same capacity they manifested when they entered the labor force. Ten percent of strength is lost by age 40, 15 percent by age 50, and 20 percent is gone on reaching 60 [21]. What happens, as Gage indicates, is that an older person cannot maintain high maximum oxygen consumption levels and high cardiac output for as long as one could earlier in life. If the task required 50 percent of the man's capacity at age 25, he will be able still to perform the task when older, but then it will consume as much as 75 percent of his maximal capacity. To continue at such a pace, more frequent rest breaks and a slower rate may be necessary.

Other changes take place. With aging, there is a loss of ability to accommodate visually; the sensitiv-

*In this connection, the age group classifications offered by Walter B. Pitkin (*The Consumer, His Nature and His Changing Habits*. New York: McGraw-Hill, 1932. P. 421) are of interest: infancy, up to the third year; childhood, ages 3 to 6; prepuberty, ages 6 to 12; adolescence, ages 12 to 17; pre-adulthood, ages 19 to 22; adulthood, 22 to 45; middle age, ages 45 to 65; presenility, ages 67 to 70; and senility, after age 70. Points of view have changed in the subsequent five plus decades.

Braceland (*Int Med News* 12:5, Jan 1, 1979) has suggested the replacement of the term *senility* by the nonpejorative word *senescence*—a gentler designation and more descriptive of the normal process of aging.

In his usual inimitable style, Ogden Nash, in "Crossing the Border," wrote, "Senescence begins/And middle age ends/The day your descendants/Outnumber your friends." (*Verses from 1929 On*. Boston: Little, Brown, 1959. P. 522.)

ity to glare increases; there is some loss of hearing (presbycusis) in the upper frequencies*; some workers experience difficulty in adjusting to widely differing levels of temperature,† humidity, and rate of air circulation; physical work stress, in the form of vibration, acceleration, and fatigue, is less well tolerated by the older worker; body agility drops; there is a loss of stature‡; short-term memory deteriorates; and performance slows [21]. A long-experienced and respected design engineer put it well when he commented just before retirement, "I'm just not so sharp as I used to be." Not every aging worker will concede this change.

All of these alterations in function must be considered in the placement of the aging worker, possibly less at time of hire, but more importantly at time of job transfer or move to a new process or line of operation.

The Administration on Aging has prepared a fact sheet that lists a series of myths concerning older workers. The following are the **myths** that, in keeping with the definition, **are all untrue** [24]:

- Older workers are less productive than the average worker.
- It costs more to prepare the older worker for the job than it does to prepare other workers.
- The costs of employee benefits outweigh any possible gain from hiring older workers.
- Older workers do not get along well with others.
- Older people want to retire as soon as they can and remain in retirement.
- Older workers are too frequently absent because of age-related infirmities and above-average rates of sickness.
- Older workers have an unacceptably high rate of accidents at work.
- Older people are well provided for by their retirement income.
- Older people do not want to work because they lose Social Security benefits.
- Older people are unwilling to learn new jobs and are inflexible about the hours they will work.
- Older people who want to find jobs and cannot just do not have the experience or qualifications.

*Glorig [22] has used the term *socioacusis*.

†In a packing plant once visited by the author in Oklahoma, workers coursed between an outside temperature of 107 degrees F and that of walk-in freezers. The extent of physiologic shock was not determined.

‡In a study by Bert Hanman [23], the maximum loss in height of men was 5 inches.

ROLE OF THE OCCUPATIONAL HEALTH SERVICE

HEALTH MAINTENANCE

The OHS must maintain its health vigilance over the older segment of the plant workforce. Not only should periodic examinations be conducted in keeping with the age increment but in parallel with mandates concerning surveillance of workers exposed to hazardous materials and as continuing review of certain chronic health deficits. The employee with coronary artery disease, discomforting osteoarthritis, hypertension, chronic bowel disorder, post-traumatic residua, or dermatologic dysfunction should be followed through recurring functional assessment, supportive counseling, and referral. Of essence is the review with the individual of the regimen advised by the private practitioner to determine that the recommendations made, the medication prescribed, and the dietary precautions offered are completely understood and followed. The function of interpretation is one of the most important contributions of occupational health nurses, and it is they who can give emphasis to the need for the continuing of a care plan. Employee-patients do not always understand a physician's message or it may not be clear, and the patient is hesitant to ask for clarification. It is important that the OHS staff member providing the counsel ensure the worker that knowledge of various chronic disorders will not jeopardize employment. Often workers will fail to disclose certain chronic health states, as they fear that such information will be used in adverse personnel actions. The confidentiality of the interchange must be emphasized and preserved.*

PRE-RETIREMENT COUNSELING

If such pre-retirement counseling programs are not undertaken by the industrial relations authority of the organization, they should be initiated by the OHS. Often this kind of group counseling effort is offered by the personnel department, and the OHS is asked to participate. Preparation for job discontinuance—the move from employment to a nonwork status—is of extreme importance. Many individuals fail to do any planning at all for such separation or begin their planning late in their careers. Much of the fan-

*It would be desirable for OHS personnel, in their preventive and counseling efforts, to recall constantly the observation of Williams and Hadler (*N Engl J Med* 308:1357, 1983) that even though chronic conditions are incurable, the discomfort or disability may be substantially modified, and it is the intervening in the illness that constitutes healing.

tasy connected with retirement activity is totally unrealistic because of current and future health status, because of unanticipated disappointment with long dreamed-of undertakings—fishing or golf every day begins to pall—or because the chore of redoing a home is completed more quickly than expected.

In a study of attitudes toward retirement [25], it was shown that the experience of retirees indicates that pre-retirement planning is critical to a secure retirement. Retirees who had planned inadequately for their change in status were considerably more likely than others to have an inadequate amount of retirement income. Among persons who felt they had done enough planning, 10 percent claimed their income was less than adequate. The same claim was made by 56 percent of the retirees who said they had done far too little or no planning at all. Thirty percent of the then current employees had done no planning at all for their retirement, as had 20 percent of persons between the ages of 50 and 64. Of employees between 50 and 64 years, 48 percent (and 58 percent of all employees) had given no thought to the amount of money needed for retirement. Interestingly, more than one in five of these older workers intended to retire without a pension [25].

Most pre-retirement programs will involve consideration of the following topics:

- Home retention or relocation
- Money management
- Activities: exercise, reading, church, travel, study, voluntarism
- Clubs or other organizations
- Second careers
- Legal matters—wills
- Health

Having an employee's spouse attend the sessions will frequently produce more significant questions and discussion than were the worker only to attend.

In a discussion of preparation for retirement from a health point of view, the following subjects should be discussed:

- Outlook toward retirement
  - Anxiety
  - Pleasure
  - End of boredom
  - Separation from stress
  - Self-actualization
  - Fear
- Turning point for all people
  - For well people
  - For successful and still capable people
  - For deadwood people
  - For sick people
- One retires the way one lives and works—productively or in idleness.
- Physical health
  - Care of the skin
  - Heart—exercise testing and prescription for activity and fitness
  - Arthritis
  - Diet—obesity, eating habits, and mythology of "health foods"
  - Chest diseases and smoking
  - Vision—presbyopia, cataracts, preparation of the person with complications of diabetes, glaucoma, corrective lenses
  - Hearing aids
  - Dentition
  - Bowel habit
  - Prostatism
  - Accidents—driving patterns, injury control
  - Personal hygiene—bathing, grooming
  - Sleep
  - Corrective or elective surgery (to be accomplished while still on maximum income, with insurance coverage and sick leave)
  - Medications and their safe use
  - Alcohol use and abuse
  - Smoking cessation
  - Sexual activity
  - Preventive medical reviews
- Mental health
  - Undertake several activities.
  - Refrain from boring discussions of health or deadly reminiscences; live in the present.
  - Develop rewarding friendships.
  - Exercise emotional control.
  - Avoid involvement in family turmoil.
  - Have an amount of privacy.
  - Nurture a good husband-wife relationship.
  - Understand and do not deprecate (too loudly) contemporary ways, language, arts, and change.
  - Be interested in others.
  - Help with youngsters.
  - Exercise hobbies.
  - Try new things—cooking, gardening, painting.*
  - Do not rot or ossify by the tube.

*"To die with one's boots on is the keynote of the mental hygiene of old age. Never to know that one is through, never to feel superfluous, never to lack significance, never to be without use, never to be without an outlet for the creative urge, never to be without a word in the affairs of men—these are the other notes" [26].

It has been the author's experience that a frank discussion of health issues will provoke a freshet of questions, most of which have been occasioned by a medical experience or a disorder needing care that was never adequately explained by the treating physician. If the material was not understood at the time of consultation, there were few requests for clarification—"My doctor is a busy man, you know." Preretirement discussion of these various health areas will help direct the employees to timely understanding, action, and care.

DISABILITY RETIREMENT

In many organizations the OHS is asked to perform medical evaluations on employees seeking to retire because of disability. While some of the applicants for this form of work severance are truly incapable of continuing in the jobs they hold, many persons seek this more remunerative method of ending a career. The protocol involves the completion of an application by the prospective retiree indicating the medical rationale for the separation, the obtaining of a medical history, and the conduct of a complete health examination with such adjuvant laboratory procedures as are indicated by the bodily organ system presumably affected. For the individual with a severe cardiac disorder, post-trauma residua, or a debilitating cerebrovascular accident, there is usually little question that continuing at work would be hazardous, possibly nonproductive, and even costly.

But there are many workers who cannot adjust to changes undertaken by the company such as a redirection in mission, the computerization or robotization of a former hand or mechanical operation, the introduction of a new pacing or different objectives, or the placement of bright young supervisors over the "old hands." In one situation where disability retirement applications were reviewed by the author because of their increasing number—and there were no health-hazardous exposures—certain operative words were found throughout the documents: strain, stress, and pressure. The applicants were unable to cope with the change, whatever it might have been in their particular cases, and here was a way out from an untenable or unacceptable work situation.

In an earlier study [27], comparable feelings were expressed more openly with such reasons as "Fed up with bosses," "Unhappy with the company," "Didn't enjoy my work," and "Earned right to retire." Of 742 persons seeking *early* retirement, but 103, or 13.9 percent, indicated that they were too ill to work.

In some instances, it was possible to retire through this avenue before the regular service retirement age, thus allowing an earlier escape. Myers [28] has indicated that, in addition to the reasons given, the closing of a facility, a transfer of functions to a new locality, or reduction in force actions will frequently trigger a number of disability retirement applications. While some of the requests are "legitimate," some will require careful scrutiny.

Brodsky [29] has been concerned about retirement and has pointed up three categories of employees who retire early because of a disability for which they can claim compensation: (1) "worn out" workers with no special plans, (2) persons who have hobbies that they intend to pursue actively, and (3) workers who want to engage in a different occupation after retirement. He shows that extensive testing reveals no physical basis for the disability, and treatment does not alter its course. Both the patient and the physician are involved in this transition from occupational function to subjective nonfunction. Brodsky feels that unless the circumstances are recognized, rehabilitation workers and vocational counselors are led to futile activity. Although these individuals may be happy in their retirement, this fulfillment of their wishes is costly to society in time, money, and frustration. Brodsky advises retraining of certain motivated persons into new occupations before the disability becomes fixed. Such action would be particularly applicable to incumbents in jobs requiring great physical stamina and agility in which the workers wear out early.

Wherein lies the solution to the retention of personnel to the point of the less costly years-of-service retirement? Some of these efforts may be made by the OHS directly or in cooperation with top managers:

Initiation early of rehabilitative or counseling measures at the first indication of alleged or real disability.

Training of supervisors to identify, early, disaffection, impaired job performance, or changes in mood, affect, or cooperative work pattern and seek counsel through referral to the OHS.

Prepare or retrain aging workers in physical labor–intensive jobs for assignment in less demanding positions or lateral transfer.

Modify the current set of tasks.

Develop a part-time workforce for these individuals.

Allow employees to prepare for a second career while still at full-time or part-time work.

Recognize early through periodic evaluation signs of potentially disabling chronic disease, refer for definitive care, and *follow-up* supportively the prescribed regimen.

The last of the suggested actions is given emphasis because chronic disorders can appear early and can be detected during employment. Early identification will allow gainful employment when those persons with pending limitation are given prudent guidance. As has been observed by Portnoi [30], there is no scientific evidence to support the concept of "natural" death in the aged. Rarely encountered on autopsy are cases of elderly subjects without pathologic findings. Aging per se is not an illness, and that percept is rejected by gerontologists [30]. Chronic disease is rising, and the OHS must share the responsibility with managers of forestalling early departure of both the disaffected and the pending impaired through sagacious counseling and creative health surveillance.

VISUAL NEEDS

The older employee presents certain needs in vision that can be met readily, particularly if the OHS has the capability of an ophthalmic dispensing service. Certain procedures must be followed to allow the aging eye to function in the work setting:

1. Obtain an accurate measurement of the normal work distance.
2. Correct for that distance through appropriate lenses.
3. Determine secondary work distances, if any.
4. Correct for that distance, if such correction is desired.
5. Conduct or have the worker obtain an accurate and comfortable fitting of the corrective device.

Each point is of equal importance in allowing older workers to carry out their tasks as they had done prior to presbyopic change.

As the work distance may vary considerably from job to job and individual to individual, an accurate measurement should be made for that person while at his or her own job site. This step is of extreme importance, since nearly all of these individuals require considerable lens power to correct their vision for near work, and the depth of focus of these lenses is shallow. For example, a given correction may provide clear vision for its wearer from a work distance of 12 inches at a minimum to 15 inches at a maximum. One can see readily that if the correction were based on a work distance of 13.5 inches, that correction would be useless at a distance of 19 or 20 inches.

The matter of adequate correction for that distance is within the province of the vision specialist. If given accurate information regarding the work distance, the correction will be appropriate.

The spectacles must fit—that is, they must be optically correct and fit the face comfortably without being skewed or in need of constant repositioning by the wearer.

An ideal solution for many workers—and they include professional persons as well—is to have prescribed trifocal lenses, which would provide intermediate power through the additional segment, a power between the two extremes of the distance and near powers. Such a triple correction, for instance, would allow a machinist to read a micrometer or lay out work, run a lathe, and see across the shop or drive an automobile. Such corrections provide essentially an unbroken depth of focus from the near point to infinity and clear, comfortable vision at all distances. It is suggested by the vision specialist that any correction that calls for an ADD of +1.75D or more for near correction is best utilized in the trifocal, rather than the bifocal mode. With that much ADD there is so great a difference between the distance and near corrections in a bifocal that there is a point at about arm's length where neither correction will be adequate—one is too weak, the other too strong. While there may be some slight difficulty in adjusting to three areas of lens correction, the wearer will soon be unaware of the differences and will become totally accustomed to their use at work and at home.

Some variants have been indicated by Hodgson [31] in connection with vision and the use of video display terminals (VDTs). Whether a company furnishes glasses up to a certain price, or gratis, or requires employees to provide their own, certain thorny problems must be addressed.

Bifocals and varifocal or trifocal lenses are not ideal for VDT operation. There are ergonomic difficulties with current equipment such as the lack of flexibility of work stations and the position of the head when using the reading component of the spectacles. Optical specialists are willing, it seems, to prescribe a specific pair of "dedicated" full-field spectacles for operators, which will include the enhanced reading distance up to 39.25 inches (1 meter) that may be required at a VDT station.

A number of older workers—aged 50 or more—may find screens blurred at 19 to 20 inches (50 cm), for reading glasses have been prescribed for 12-inch (30 cm) distance. The problem is compounded in that the reading material may not be on a lectern but flat on the desk at about 12 inches (30 cm), thereby involving considerable accommodation—effort between the screen and the material and vice versa, resulting in "eyestrain."

Both groups should have prescribed a pair of intermediate-distance reading glasses that will include the VDT reading distance of between 15 and 31 inches (40 to 80 cm). It may be necessary for companies to consider furnishing "dedicated" spectacles to these operators, as are some other work glasses.

IMMIGRATION AND HEALTH

The move of people to the United States has been characterized by successive waves since the early 17th century. The sites of indigenous oppression, hardship, or starvation have varied, but the goal was to reach America, where freedom was extant, where no class system persisted, and where personal ambition could carry one to almost any height. Most of those persons emigrating to this country became the source of labor for growing industry and established fairly discrete enclaves of foreign stock. Morin, Pickle, and Mason [32] have developed maps of ethnic concentration for use in the study of disease patterns. In many areas, specific national groups have populated certain industries, while in others there have appeared a greater number of individual entrepreneurs.

While the great surge of immigrants reaching these shores between the 1850s and the 1920s desired acceptance, and assimilation was the ethos of the day—Americanization—more recent bodies of people have wanted to retain their identifiable ethnicity. That large movements of various populations affect the patterning of health is given evidence in almost any study of troop movements, of the Holocaust, or of evacuees. As early as 1847, "the Irish immigrants' fever" was reported from Canada [33], and all of the new arrivals processed through either Castle Garden or Ellis Island were examined by medical officers, some individuals with disease being refused entry.

In more recent years, however, great numbers of immigrants from Southeast Asia, the Pacific Basin, Mexico, and Western Europe have arrived, only to introduce new or exacerbate old disease states. Most noteworthy has been the recrudescence of tuberculosis, a disease that in 1959 at the Arden House Conference stocktaking was believed due for eradication through drug therapy and the destruction of all remaining reservoirs of tubercle bacilli [34]. The goal was not reached, and the prediction now, according to Lillington [35], is that eradication is possible by the end of the next century. He feels that until the 25,000,000 positive tuberculin skin test reactors die off in perhaps 50 to 75 years, active disease will continue.

In 1983, about 22,300 cases of tuberculosis were reported to the Centers for Disease Control (CDC), representing a 6.7-percent decrease from the 1982 total. In 1968 to 1978, the average annual decrease in U.S. cases was 5.8 percent. However, the period 1979–1982 saw a large influx of Indochinese refugees, and the annual decline was only 1.4 percent. The estimated deaths from tuberculosis in 1982 came to 1,807, a decrease of 6.7 percent from the number reported for 1981 [35]. The control of tuberculosis has been limited by several factors, precluding the elimination of the disease prior to the year 2100. Each year over 20,000 new cases and 1,800 deaths still occur. The elements hampering control are the following: (1) Many public and private-sector health care providers do not believe that a problem exists, the viewpoint being reinforced by sanatorium closures and the initiating of outpatient treatment programs; (2) noncompliance with prescribed treatment; (3) the emergence of tuberculosis organisms resistant to commonly used drugs such as isoniazid and streptomycin, more commonly encountered among the foreign-born; and (4) the limitations of the currently available technology in prevention—in persons over age 35 years, preventive therapy is not recommended because of the risk of isoniazid toxicity outweighing the benefits of treatment [36].

The reason for concern in connection with the reintroduction of the disease is that many older individuals who were previously infected have apparently outlived their initial infecting organism, as indicated by a negative tuberculin test, and are subject, on contact, to a second primary infection [37]. Also, most adults in the United States today were not infected as children and are vulnerable. As Davidson expressed it, there are no grounds for complacency about this still-menacing disease [37]. The numbers among the foreign-born have been high. It was reported in 1982 that the tuberculosis rate among Latinos in the United States was double that of the nation as a whole and among Southeast Asians was 40 times greater than for the general population [38].

Beginning with the 1985–1986 school year, it has been mandatory that all kindergarten through twelfth-grade students entering a California school for the first time have a tuberculin skin test (5TU) by the Mantoux method. Those students with a significant reaction—10 mm of induration or greater—are required to have a chest radiograph as well. All schools are included—public, private, and parochial. As it is believed that the infection rate in Los Angeles is higher than the 1 percent or less throughout much of the United States, this program will provide a measure of the prevalence of infection among the selected group [39].

In addition to the concern with tuberculosis among Indochinese refugees [40–42], there are additional disease states being presented: parasitism [43–47], hepatitis B antigenemia [46–49], other infectious diseases including gonococcal infection, measles, abnormal VDRL results, and epidemic conjuctivitis [46,49–52], anemia and hemoglobin disorders [48,53], and dermatologic conditions [53]. The

Southeast Asian immigrants have manifested also differences in pregnancy outcome, such as lower birth weight and pregnancy complications [54], and there has been recorded the unexplained nocturnal phenomenon, predominantly in males, of sudden death [55–57].

More recently Chagas' disease has been reported among immigrants from Latin America [58] and cysticercosis has been encountered primarily among Hispanics from Mexico, the increase in cases coinciding with the introduction of computed tomography [59].

Identification of the various disease states is important as refugees move into the American labor force. While many open their own businesses and engage in other entrepreneurial activities, some of the professional groups will enter industry. It has been indicated in cited writings that no public health problem exists but that the recorded disease entities do represent personal health difficulties. With the persisting elevated rates of tuberculosis and parasitic disease, care must be exercised in early detection and referral for treatment. Jones and his coworkers [44] have recommended certain health screening procedures for Indochinese refugees requiring medical care. The same protocol could, and most likely should, be used at the time of the prehire evaluation. The recommendations, with additions, follow:

A general physical examination, including dental and nutritional status evaluation.

Tuberculin skin testing: All persons reacting positively should have chest radiography.* Local or state health departments should be notified of persons found to have tuberculosis so that therapy can be initiated or continued. The CDC further advises bacteriologic examination with smear culture and susceptibility studies for suspected or follow-up cases. Multidrug regimens for active cases are advised and have been delineated because of the significant possibility of isoniazid-resistant organisms.

Serodiagnostic test for syphilis.

Serologic test for hepatitis, with results to be entered in both medical and dental records.

Stool examination for intestinal parasites.

Thick and thin blood films for malaria on all individuals with fever.*

Persons manifesting falciparum malaria should be referred immediately for, as Jones and coworkers have indicated [44], the disease is a medical emergency because of the overwhelming parasitism that may occur. As malaria will persist for months or years without becoming clinically apparent, continued follow-up is recommended if the applicant is employed. Because of the adequacy of most sewerage systems in the United States, intestinal parasitism is not considered an important public health hazard. In areas of poor sanitation—and such arenas might be the early living sites after resettlement—*Ascaris* and hookworm may be transmitted. *Giardia, Entamoeba histolytica,* and hepatitis B are public health hazards in comparable areas or when encountered in food handlers [44].

Efforts have been made to bring greater understanding of the Vietnamese culture to American practitioners who treat refugees. Medical directors facing the issue of examination and emergency care of these groups are advised to consult a recent writing of Nguyen [61].

Other migrant groups have been reviewed from the perspective of health care, some presenting problems unique to the culture from which they have come. Puerto Ricans have been studied for parasitism [62], and the health of Pilipinos† coming to the United States has been reviewed [63]. The values retained by immigrant Japanese have been presented [64], and observers have described issues in the health care of Middle Eastern migrants [65] and Soviet Jewish emigres [66].

The "importation" of Hansen's disease has attracted comment with the new waves of immigration [67–69], and the illnesses of incoming Cubans has been discussed [70,71]. The Haitians have come under scrutiny [72,73], and migrants from the Pacific Basin have presented distinct needs [74,75]. Because of their number in Southwestern United States, the Hispanics have been the subject of medical survey [76,77], as have the Chinese [78–80].

Irrespective of the cultural group represented in a plant population, it is desirable that an opinion-maker or informal leader be identified. Working closely with such a person will aid in establishing the

*While annual chest radiography on employed groups has been considered unproductive, the World Health Organization (WHO) has indicated that there are "exceptions to this statement in countries or areas where there is a high prevalence of tuberculosis and similar infections" [60]. It is from such countries that many immigrants arrive, not only in the United States, but also in Canada and the United Kingdom.

*Vital signs are frequently not taken during a preplacement medical examination. These measures should be added in evaluating refugees.

†A preferred term because of the absence of the letter "f" in the national language of the Philippines.

best possible relationship with employees frequently hesitant in seeking medical care.

EMPLOYMENT OF WOMEN IN COMMERCE AND INDUSTRY

Characterizing a portion of the tumult of the early 1970s was the move for the liberation of women. Ever increasing in number in the workforce since World War II, in 1980, 51.2 percent of all women were working, representing about 42 percent of the labor force and about 43 million women, increasing to 43.7 percent of the labor force in 1984 [81]. Extrapolation of current data puts the participation in the work market for 1990 at nearly 46 percent [82]. This growth, in addition to the entry of women into blue-collar jobs, speaks for unprecedented changes in the concept of the American family: a decline in the single-income, male-breadwinner role and alteration of the traditional homemaker/rearer-of-children functions of the wife/mother. By 1990, 70 percent of two-parent families will have both mother and father working [82].

In contrast to the "auxiliary" status of uniformed women early in World War II, there were, in March 1985, 77,617 women on active duty in the U.S. Army [83], 67,034 in the U.S. Air Force [83], and 49,856 in the U.S. Navy [83].

The placement of female personnel in industrial and military white- and blue-collar positions has evoked both operational and research interest in reproductive system hazards occasioned by exposure of the unborn child to known or unidentified toxic materials. That this interest is warranted is seen in the data descriptive of working mothers, as released by the U.S. Department of Labor for mid-1984 [84]:

> About six out of every 10 mothers with pre-school or school-age children were in the labor force in March 1984. A record 19.5 million women with children under the age of 18—including 8.0 million whose youngest children were under 6—were working or looking for work. In 1970, just four out of 10 mothers (12.1 million) were in the labor force.
>
> Mothers of infants and toddlers under age three were a substantial part of the increase. By March 1984, nearly half of these women were labor-force participants compared with about 30 percent in 1970. As in the past, divorced women continued to have the highest labor force participation rates of any marital status group, especially when they were rearing school-age children.
>
> These data are compiled from supplementary questions to the March Current Population Survey. Other highlights from the March 1984 survey:
>
> Regardless of their marital or child status, most employed women work at full-time jobs (35 hours or more per week). About 73 percent of all employed mothers of school-age children and 67 percent of the mothers of pre-schoolers worked full time. Divorced mothers were the most likely to work full time.
>
> About 32.7 million children—well over half of all children under age 18—had a mother in the labor force in March 1984. More than nine million of these children were under six, and 14.7 million were six to 13, age groups requiring either full-day care or after-school care. Whatever their ages, a smaller proportion of white than black children in married-couple families had working mothers. In families maintained by women, the opposite prevailed.
>
> About 27 percent of all children were in families in which the father was either absent (10.9 million), unemployed (2.7 million), or not in the labor force (2.2 million). More than half of all black children and nearly one-fifth of all white children were living in one of these situations.
>
> Of the 24.4 million married-couple families with children under age 18, 14.9 million—61 percent—were families where both parents were earners at some time during the year. In about four out of 10 such families, both parents worked full time for 40 weeks or more.
>
> Over 12 million families were maintained by persons living without a spouse—10.3 million by women and 2.1 million by men. Families maintained by women were more likely than those maintained by men to have children in the home and were less likely to contain an earner. About 71 percent of the families maintained by women with children contained an earner, compared with 89 percent of those maintained by men.

HISTORY

When Edith Abbott [85] was writing from Hull House in 1916, she indicated that most men were employed in agriculture, and industry, such as it was in the early years of this century, was primarily in the hands of women and girls. With the establishment of the factory system in the United States, it was believed that his new kind of work was identical with the work that women had long been doing in their home. Hamilton, along with other early statesmen, felt that the great advantage of the establishment of manufacturers was "the employment of persons who would otherwise be idle" and that "women and children are rendered more useful by [factories] than they otherwise would be" [85].

World War I saw a huge influx of women into production plants both in Great Britain and the United States, and in England, the protective mandates of the Factory Acts were put aside, and women frequently worked 12 hours plus overtime, lacked seating, eating facilities, and proper toilets, and had to travel long distances over inadequate roads leading to the newly built munitions plants [86]. The health risks were many, including exposure to TNT and metals and pinpricks while making uniforms, in addition to the constant presence of explosives.

At war's end, Andrews [87] pointed out that, in a New Hampshire study, 1.8 percent of some 79 stillbirths occurred among mothers gainfully employed at home, while 7.5 percent, more than fourfold, were encountered among mothers working away from home. By the time of the second great war, of 54 plants visited by Sappington [88] to determine what was the "woman problem" under wartime conditions, there were 131,000 women among 452,000 workers, or 29 percent. In some plants there were as high as 52-percent and 77-percent female employees. In nearly all installations visited, the illness-absence and work-related injury rates were equal to or lower than those levels for men. The primary deficit encountered was inadequate or inappropriate shoes for the work being conducted, and little consideration had been given the need for sanitary facilities. Advised, though, was an initial hiring of a few women to form a group that could be built upon rather than beginning with a large group before working conditions could be matched to the replacement personnel.

By 1967, sex discrimination in the federal government was prohibited by an executive order [89], and in 1972 the Equal Employment Opportunity Commission ruled that to deny a woman a job because of pregnancy was in violation of the Civil Rights Act of 1964 [90]. The following year, 52 job titles considered sex-stereotyped in the Census Bureau's Occupational Classifications System were changed—for example, airline stewardesses became flight attendants, firemen were changed to firefighters, and not for the sake of brevity, foremen were to be known as blue-collar worker supervisors [91].

In the 1980s, women were found in an extensive variety of positions that were formerly the exclusive domain of men. Women in 1981 accounted for 6 percent of craft workers. They have become miners [92], workers on offshore drilling platforms [93], craft personnel in shipyards [94], roustabouts in the oil fields [95], and construction workers [96], as examples of the changes in the workforce. These kinds of job assignments and current data [97] negate longstanding **myths** concerning the employment of women [98,99].

A woman's place is in the home.
Women are not seriously attached to the labor force; they work only for extra pocket money.
Women are out ill more than male workers; they cost the company more.
Women do not work so long or so regularly as their male coworkers; their training is costly and largely wasted.
Married women take jobs away from men; in fact, they ought to quit those jobs they now hold.
Women should stick to "women's jobs" and should not compete for "men's jobs."
Women do not want responsibility on the job; they do not want promotions or job changes that add to their load.
The employment of women leads to juvenile delinquency.
Men do not like to work for women supervisors.

The reality of work situations has given the lie to all of the myths delineated above. Women are as dedicated as men, are as desirous of upward mobility and increased responsibility as their male counterparts, and have proved themselves in all areas—as workers, as first-line supervisors, as managers, and as executive/owners. Yet, unfounded beliefs endure, as given evidence by the response encountered in a study involving both physicians and employers [100]. A physician indicated his bewilderment regarding the patient's work: "How the ___[sic] do I know what she does when she tells me she has to 'surge a shell on the monorail every six seconds'?" And from employer/supervisor interviews one heard these comments: "Women are more emotional when they are pregnant. No matter where I put them, it's wrong, and they gripe and won't work up to par," or "No, you'll never see any women around this place. They sure can't handle the big jobs here—just too heavy for women. Geez, all I'd need was one of 'em here and pregnant, too.'"

Such concepts disappear slowly, and possibly, only with persisting demonstration of capability and skills of women workers, and the retirement of older supervisors who grew up in another era, will acceptance become universal. Inequity remains, however, in wage and salary scales, but the issue of comparable worth has already come into the courts. A recent decision involved the city of Los Angeles, which, in a settlement reached with employees, agreed to increase the pay of 3,900 women, underscoring the dimension of the problem [101]. The state of Washington would have been liable for billions of dollars to female employees as a result of a ruling in which the court concluded that women were being discriminated against because the wages paid in predominantly female occupations were less than in predominantly male occupations of "comparable worth," that is, in occupations requiring "similar skills" [102]. In late 1985, the Ninth Circuit Court of Appeals reversed the lower court decision. However, the state has moved ahead with a comparable worth plan, its outcome pending legal action.

HEALTH ISSUES

Several health-related entities present themselves for consideration in the employment of women. Of primary concern has been the exposure to the industrial environment, with both its known and unknown work materials, of the unborn child. Numerous conferences have addressed the issue,* and various organizations have endeavored to establish medical guidelines. More important, however, is the pertinent supportive legislation concerning women in the workplace.

The summary prepared by Stellman [103] includes the various federal acts germane to the rights of working women (Table 17-1).

Under *Title VII of the 1964 Civil Rights Act,* there can be no discrimination in employment, in this issue, based on sex. The various elements in employment that are pertinent are hiring and firing; wages; fringe benefits; classifying, referring, assigning or promoting employees; extending or assigning facilities; training, retraining, or apprenticeship; or any other terms, conditions, or privileges of employment. The groups subsumed under the employer rubric include companies of 15 or more employees, employment agencies, labor organizations with 15 or more members, and labor-management apprenticeship programs. The guidelines have been issued by the Equal Employment Opportunity Commission, and they bar hiring based on stereotyped characterizations of the sexes, classification or labeling of "men's jobs" and "women's jobs," advertising under male and female headings, or preference in the content of the advertising based on sex [104].

The Pregnancy Disability Act of 1978 was an amendment to Title VII† and became effective May 1, 1979. Under its mandates, employers cannot discriminate against pregnant workers in any area of employment or in any benefit program. Pregnancy and childbirth are to be considered the same as any other health problem that interferes with a worker's ability to perform an assigned task. Employers are prohibited from requiring a medical statement in writing concerning the disability of pregnancy unless a similar document is required for all disability claims.

Similarly, the employer cannot require that a worker remains on leave until after delivery, even though she has been absent from work because of the pregnancy and then recovers. The job previously held by a pregnant worker on leave cannot be eliminated unless the employee has notified the employer that she does not plan to return to work after delivery. If a job applicant is pregnant and can perform the major tasks required of the job, she cannot be rejected merely because of the pregnancy. Special waiting periods of eligibility for pregnancy benefits cannot be required if not required for other disabilities. The employer can refuse benefits if a pregnant woman was hired and if medical and hospital coverage for employees with other preexisting conditions are also denied. Lastly, hospital and medical benefits for an abortion not performed to save the woman's life need not be provided by the employer, but there must be granted sick leave or disability benefits for abortions undertaken voluntarily. Most recently, it was ruled by the Supreme Court that pregnant employees had the right to a 4-month leave to have a child and a guarantee that they would have their jobs back on completion of the leave.

Executive Order No. 11375 prohibited discrimination against women by federal contractors and, in addition, mandated affirmative action, measures enforced through the Office of Federal Contract Compliance.

The OHS may be consulted regarding certain personnel actions by the industrial relations authority. Before any counsel can be given, it must be determined that the pregnancy has been made known. If communication is needed for administrative purposes, signed authorization for the transfer of information is mandatory [105].

Within the constraints of this varied legislation, what are the health issues? Messite [106] has indicated that approximately 5,700 mutagens, teratogens, or other substances that affect the reproductive system are listed in the NIOSH registry of toxic effects of chemical substances *(RTECS)* [107], and a significant number of such materials "could affect the reproductive health of workers." The effects comprise menstrual disorders, changes in sexual behavior such as decreased libido or impaired ability to engage in sex, and reduced fertility or sterility resulting from diminished sperm production or production of defective gametes.

*For example, "Reproductive Health Hazards in the Workplace," held September 29–30, 1980 in Washington, DC; "Reproduction—The New Frontier in Occupational and Environmental Health Research," sponsored by the University of Utah and the National Institute for Occupational Safety and Health (NIOSH), held April 5–8, 1983 in Park City, Utah; and "Reproductive Hazards in the Workplace," held under the aegis of the Harvard School of Public Health, Boston, MA, on November 2–4, 1984.

†Public Law 95-555, Oct 31, 1978.

TABLE 17-1. *Legislation Affecting the Rights of Women Workers*

U.S. constitutional amendments	*Legislation*	*Administering agency*
Article XIV: Section 1: "All persons born or naturalized in the United States and subject to the jurisdiction thereof, are citizens of the United States and of the State wherein they reside. No State shall make or enforce any law which shall abridge the privilege or immunities of citizens of the United States; nor shall any State deprive any person of life, liberty or property without the due process of law; nor deny to any person within its jurisdiction the equal protection of the laws." (The Fifth Amendment provides the same protections as regards the federal government.)	Civil Rights Act of 1964, Title VII: guarantees the rights to employment without sex, race, color, creed, religion, or national origin discrimination	Equal Employment Opportunity Commission
	Equal Employment Opportunity Act of 1972: amends and broadens Title VII	
	Pregnancy Disability Act of 1978: requires employers to treat pregnancy-related absences like absences for other disabilities	
	Fair Labor Standards Act of 1938: establishes minimum wage, overtime, etc.	Wage and Hour Division, Department of Labor
	Equal Pay Act of 1963; most recent amendment to the Fair Labor Standards Act	Occupational Safety and Health Administration
	Occupational Safety and Health Act of 1970; guarantees a safe and healthful workplace to all workers	Department of Labor
	State Fair Employment Practices Statutes	Appropriate state agency

Source: From *Women's Work, Women's Health: Myths and Realities,* by Jeanne Mager Stellman. Copyright © 1977 by Jeanne Mager Stellman. Reprinted by permission of Pantheon Books, a division of Random House, Inc.

Further, other potential undesirable reproductive effects include genetic damage and chromosomal aberrations in both ova and sperm, which can lead to spontaneous abortion or stillbirth, premature delivery, and birth defects, which might be structural, behavioral, or functional [106]. While no occupationally related cases of transplacental carcinogenesis have been reported, the history of diethylstilbestrol (DES), as it was prescribed to prevent miscarriage, must be remembered.

Messite [106] noted also that contamination of the maternal breast milk may affect a newborn's health, and contaminating materials brought home on workers' clothing can have deleterious effects on the health of the employee's spouse and children. Specific examples of toxins that have been known to alter reproductive function or outcome have included carbon disulfide, which may cause menstrual disturbances in women and loss of libido and impotence in men; chloroprene exposure in the rubber industry, which has resulted in decreased motility and numbers of sperm in male workers and an elevated incidence of miscarriage among their wives; and Kepone (dibromochloropropane [DBCP]) exposure, which has led to marked changes in spermatogenesis. In lead exposure, decreased sperm counts, teratospermia, and diminished libido have been recorded; menorrhagia and intermenstrual bleeding have been seen in women working in the manufacture of synthetic estrogens, while the male workers have manifested gynecomastia, altered libido, infertility, and feminization; and the wives of employees exposed to vinyl chloride have shown adverse pregnancy outcome and fetal loss. Personnel working at high altitudes and those individuals such as bakers and glassblowers who are subjected to high temperatures have experienced adverse effects on spermatogenesis, and lastly, in ionizing radiation workers, impaired spermatogenesis and reproductive capability have been documented [106]. These instances of unfavorable health effects are some that have withstood critical review. Many other chemical substances have the potential, but possibly there has been insufficient epidemiologic scrutiny to date to document direct cause-effect relationships.

This knowledge warrants control problems, particularly as women in the labor force increase their numbers and are brought into contact with a broader variety of deleterious agents. While efforts have been made to exclude women from jeopardizing work exposures [108], little has been done to preclude contact among male employees, an action or inaction that has led to further implications of discrimination. The policy to be followed is that of decreasing exposure levels to those limits that are safe for all men, women, and the developing fetus]108].

Le Clercq [109] has outlined a program specifically targeted toward this area of protection. The corporate guidelines offered are the following:

Review workplace exposures to identify potential reproductive hazards.
Inform exposed employees of potential hazards.
Control exposures to acceptable levels for *all* [emphasis added] employees.
Implement protective work assignment practices where necessary for particularly susceptible employees.
Provide continuing research on potential reproductive hazards.
Terminate manufacture or use of any substance if unacceptable risks cannot be prevented.

Underscored is the caveat that selective work restriction of high-risk employees may be used, but only as a last resort. Le Clercq [109] has provided some elaboration of the guidelines. To identify the reproductive hazards, an inventory of all chemicals used by the company must be developed and maintained through constant updating, including feedstocks, intermediates, and end products. As discussed in chapter 12, under Medical Records and Documentation, this information is readily coupled with the records of environmental measurement, clinical evaluation findings, and personnel data in the data bank. Once listed, the substances are compared with currently available information on known or suspected mutagens and teratogens to establish which materials are significant as reproductive hazards. Subsequently, more extensive risk analyses can be formulated by toxicologists and industrial hygienists. Then, a pinpointed number of chemicals can undergo more extensive testing, increased engineering control, and consideration for reassessment of the allowable workplace exposure levels [109].

The educational effort is part of the right-to-know activity, and both managers and workers are informed of the potential reproductive hazards extant in their work areas, and the use of personal protective equipment and the adherence to safe work practices are emphasized. The training program is a combined activity of occupational physicians, industrial hygienists, and occupational health nurses. A discussion concerning reproductive capacity may prove embarrassing or offensive to some older workers, so the subject matter should be treated openly, with complete professionalism, and without causing undue anxiety.* The point must be made that the responsibilities of safety and health preservation are shared jointly by *both* managers and workers.

In the control of exposure, acceptable levels are obtained through a combination of (1) process or equipment engineering design, (2) work practice arrangements, including shortened exposure times when necessary, and (3) the use of personal protective equipment. When a potential reproductive hazard has been identified, yet there is insufficient information to establish a definitive exposure level, an interim standard with an appropriate safety factor should be designated, and then substantive data should be gathered so that a permanent standard can be developed. With a standard, the traditional industrial hygiene control technology will bring exposures within acceptable levels [109]. If it is felt that total restriction from exposure is necessary—which is rare—such prescription should be instituted only with a sound scientific rationale and only after all control measures have been exhausted [109].

The need for new information remains, and it is imperative to obtain continuously data concerning potential reproductive toxicity relating to the company's activities. Such research must be coordinated with studies being undertaken by trade associations, independent laboratories, governmental agencies, and university investigators. Caution is suggested in the immediate extrapolation of laboratory findings to human workers as they relate to reproductive toxicology. As Le Clercq [109] points out, new short-term predictive toxicologic tests in animals, as well as noninvasive diagnostic tests in humans, such as serum hormone determinations and cytogenetic tests, need development and validation before insertion into worker surveillance programs. The program's future lies in good epidemiologic study, and as many of the large chemical manufacturers have epidemiologists in their medical activities, the future will see the use of validated questionnaires, scientifically based medical surveillance programs, the creation of data banks, and the ability to identify quickly reproductive hazards at the workplace [109].

By way of summary, an American Medical Association (AMA) Council of Scientific Affairs report [110] updated information concerning the effects of

*There are geographic differences found in worker populations that reflect varying attitudes toward discussions of "personal" issues. While the author was medical director of an OHS in the South, it had been the custom to have job applicants and employees collect urine specimens in the appropriate restrooms and then return the opaque container cartons to the clinical laboratory. A worker found this procedure offensive—it was a brief walk of possibly 15 feet in a side corridor—so the system was changed. Collecting points were established in the restrooms.

physical forces on the reproductive cycle. The conclusions reached include the following:

At levels above 3,636 meters (12,000 ft), adverse reproductive effects have been observed in men, women, the conceptus, and certain species of animals.
Hyperthermia in excess of 40°C (104°F) may affect humans and the conceptus, as well as the reproductive capacity of certain animals.
Hypothermia has been demonstrated as adverse only in animals.
Ionizing radiation can injure men, women, the conceptus, and animals, depending on the dose and duration of exposure.
Radiofrequency-microwave radiation has had no injurious effect on the human reproductive system, but the thermal effects have resulted in untoward reproductive limitations in animals.
No harmful effects have been noted from electronic and magnetic fields (although early research may indicate the opposite), gravity and acceleration, noise, optical radiation (ultraviolet, visible, infrared, and lasers), ultrasound, and vibration.

Further studies are needed. This information, combined with the data concerning exposure to chemicals, can serve as the basis for a program that will be rational in the protection of the reproductive system of the worker, at any stage.

In a second report from the AMA [111], recommendations are made concerning the continuance of work of pregnant women presenting with certain clinical disorders that are severely compromised by pregnancy and other conditions that predispose the worker to an increased likelihood of complications of the pregnancy. The disorders indicated are not in themselves disabling, nor is the pregnant woman disabled because she has one or more of them.

Workers with the following conditions must be carefully evaluated to determine whether they may continue to work during the pregnancy or whether it would be best to cease working until after the delivery:

Women who have been delivered of two premature infants weighing less than 2,000 gm
Women with an incompetent cervix and history of previous fetal loss or cervical cerclage (encirclement of an incompetent cervix)
Women with uterine anomaly who have lost a fetus
Women with cardiac status greater than class II, which affects the ability to tolerate the massive increase in cardiac output and blood volume imposed by pregnancy
Women with Marfan's syndrome
Women with hemoglobinopathy including thalassemia
Women with pulmonary hypertension or arterial hypertension
Women with retinopathy greater than stage I, renal changes with abnormal creatinine clearance, preeclampsia, or polyhydramnios
Women with herpes gestationis, if discomfort is great
Women with severe anemia—8 gm/dl of hemoglobin or less

TABLE 17-2. *Guidelines for Continuation of Various Levels of Work During Pregnancy*

Job function	*Week of gestation*
Secretarial and light clerical	40
Professional and managerial	40
Sitting with light tasks	
Prolonged (> 4 hr)	40
Intermittent	40
Standing	
Prolonged (> 4 hr)	24
Intermittent	
(> 30 min/hr)	32
(< 30 min/hr)	40
Stooping and bending below knee level	
Repetitive (> 10 times/hr)	20
Intermittent (between 2 and 10 times/hr)	28
Climbing	
Vertical ladders and poles	
Repetitive (≥ 4 times/8-hr shift)	20
Intermittent (< 4 times/8-hr shift)	28
Stairs	
Repetitive (≥ 4 times/8-hr shift)	28
Intermittent (< 4 times/8-hr shift)	40
Lifting	
Repetitive	
> 23 kg	20
Between 11 and 23 kg	24
< 11 kg	40
Intermittent	
> 23 kg	30
Between 11 and 14 kg	40
> 11 kg	40

In the same council report [111], guidelines were provided concerning the continuance of certain tasks during pregnancy, as seen in Table 17-2.

A third report, "Effects of Toxic Chemicals on the Reproductive System" [112] concluded the series prepared by the AMA Council on Scientific Affairs. Some 120 chemicals were considered for review based on an estimation of their imminent hazard, that is, widespread use, inherent toxicity, or both. Three chemicals—acrylonitrile, inorganic arsenic, and carbon disulphide—were presented in moderate detail, as models, consideration being given (1) description and uses, (2) reproductive effects, (3) human data with references, and (4) summary opinion. A glossary concerning reproductive hazards in the workplace provides definitions or discussion of 33 entities. While three substances only are given with analyses, information concerning the remaining 11 compounds is available from the AMA on request.

SAFETY

The definitive treatise on pregnancy and work is still *Guidelines on Pregnancy and Work* [113], produced by the American College of Obstetricians and Gynecologists (ACOG). Attention is directed in that book to certain ergonomic/physical energy conditions. The tolerance to strenuous exertion—lifting, pulling, pushing, or climbing—will vary widely, as determined by differences in the woman worker's physical fitness and strength, the load demands, and the environment. The pregnant woman may be small or large, strong or weak, and her strength, balance, agility, and internal burdens change month by month. The packages or loads involved in meeting work demands may vary in size, shape, and consistency, coursing from a bale of towels, to a case of food, to a patient in a nursing home. The job may or may not permit any modification in the conduct of the required physical tasks in their intensity, frequency, or pattern. Here, as in any issue of placement or possible job-associated illness, a detailed work history is necessary, so that both the private and occupational physicians can provide the most intelligent and useful guidance [113].

An alteration in the established order of work, such as extreme changes in the daily set of tasks or frequent changes in work shift, that may cause anorexia or excessive or constant fatigue is to be avoided. As many nonspecific symptoms are present during pregnancy, such as headache, backache, and nausea, inordinate changes in the work pattern are to be averted.

It is recommended in the ACOG report [113] that in the third trimester low-heeled shoes be worn to lessen the shift of the weight-bearing angle. Women unaccustomed to flat shoes may be allowed medium-height heels. Spike heels and shoes with inadequate support should not be worn because of the risk of slips and falls. Weight-lifting restrictions previously codified in most jurisdictions have been discarded, and it is believed that whatever the load that can be handled readily by the nonpregnant woman will not be stressing when she is pregnant. If the load is lifted in the front of the body, then obviously this task will be difficult in the third trimester because of the protruding abdomen.

Because of stresses on the lumbar spine during pregnancy, a load that was maximum before pregnancy should be reduced 20 to 25 percent during late pregnancy. Because of the awkwardness developing after the twentieth to twenty-fourth week of gestation, work should be avoided that demands a strained posture or a good sense of balance. Special care must be given in certain work situations. Any blow to the abdomen, even the most minor, must be avoided, and the worker must be scrupulously attentive to the avoidance of falls. She cannot climb ladders. Belts and safety harnesses may be worn if not constricting [113].

In the work setting, the backrest of the chair must be low enough to support both the lumbar and sacral spines, and the seat must be sufficiently wide to permit the worker to sit with both lower extremities in a semi-abducted and supported position. The use of a small footrest will remove pressure by the seat pan on the suprapopliteal region.

The pregnant worker may work standing or seated, and particularly in the last trimester, there should be frequent postural changes. It is suggested that a high stool matched to a fairly high workbench be used, so that the height of the work surface does not change when she alternates sitting and standing positions. In this situation, the legs must be supported by a footrest, when seated, so that the venous return from the legs is not compromised [113].

While not involving pregnancy, one study conducted by the Mine Safety and Health Administration [114] points up the differences—favorably—in the injuries sustained by male and female coal miners. Data from the period 1978–1980 were analyzed and revealed the following: Approximately 4 percent of all women coal workers were involved in a lost-time accident, as compared with 7 percent for men; female workers lost approximately 1.1 days each, in contrast to 2.4 days for men; and only 0.01 percent of the female workforce were fatally injured, as compared with 0.05 percent among the male miners. The injuries sustained by both groups consisted primarily of back sprains, the majority of others comprising sprains and fractures of joints and bones of the extremities. Women made up 4.3 percent of the coal mining workforce in 1980, and their jobs included such demanding tasks as the continuous shoveling of coal that has fallen from conveyor belts, the transport of heavy timbers to lay track for the mine's rail system, and operation of shuttle cars.

PERSONAL PROTECTIVE EQUIPMENT

In the 1970s, when women began to seek and obtain nontraditional jobs, there was little in the collection of personal protective devices that they could use. The equipment and work clothing were designed primarily to fit the average male frame, which left the women workers and the small or extra-large man without adequate protection [115].

Some manufacturers have responded to the need and have produced protective eyewear and footgear appropriately sized, in many instances designed in some simulation of current high-fashion spectacles and contemporary women's shoes. More slowly to arrive have been ear defenders, hard hats with accessories, and respirators in sizes required by women workers. It is astonishing, but not different from the retail clothing market, that comparably numbered sizes made by different manufacturers will vary in dimension. There is yet to be a standardization among producers who make gloves, respirators, or safety eyewear. As Rosenberg and Stellman [115] have indicated, much personal protective equipment is still being made as reduced versions of items made to match the male anthropometry, with the strange belief that women are miniaturized men, a fact readily refutable by the most fleeting observation.

Clothing must recognize the unique bathroom needs of women workers, irrespective of the quality of the facilities provided. A prototype of work coveralls that zip from knee to knee, precluding the need for removal, has been developed, which may see greater use [116]. The problem has been even more severe among women miners, who must wear a lamp and walk in a bent-over position or crawl. The hard hat wobbles, slides to the side, or actually falls off [117]. The need for tool redesign by the specialists in ergonomics is slowly being identified [118].

While standards finally are recognizing the need for specifically designed personal protective equipment for women, the OHS can check the work device fit at the time of placement or during visits to the health care facility. Prompt cooperative action with the safety authority may avert accidental injury and, sometimes of greater significance, disaffection toward the job.

HEALTH CARE ASPECTS OF ILLNESS

There has been some investigational activity centered around the health of women who have moved into jobs previously held by men. Would they sustain the same physiologic response to work-environmental stressors as have men? Would the usual stress-related disorders—coronary artery disease and hypertension among others—increase in female workers performing comparable tasks in the same kinds of demanding workplaces? Ibrahim [119] has noted that most studies have focused on the male candidate for coronary heart disease, and the early epidemiologic efforts were most often carried out by men and interpreted from the male point of view. "Stress and strain" are appearing between men and women, among women themselves, and within families. Women, in their new work settings, are being uniquely exposed to the pressures brought about by multiple roles and conflicting expectations. The health consequences, Ibrahim feels, are complex and relatively unknown. Studies initiated by women investigators have indicated that in opposition to a greater reporting of illnesses and disabilities by women, more visits to physicians, and higher rates of hospitalization, women do live longer than men [119]. The disorders reported by women do not seem to be major ailments—possibly a matter of perception—while there are a greater number of serious and life-threatening conditions seen among men. Proposed in explanation are such factors as more frequent contact with the health care system, allowing earlier diagnosis and treatment; an inborn sex-linked resistance to serious illnesses; or possibly a more limited exposure to damaging physical and social stressors [119].

In the summary review of relatively current studies, Ibrahim [119] stated these research conclusions:

Married employed women show fewer psychiatric symptoms than married nonemployed women.

Although elevated blood pressure is less prevalent among married, employed women, when the woman is committed excessively to the work role, the prevalence rate of hypertension rises.

Gainfully employed women were more likely to report type A behavior, daily stress, and marital dissatisfaction than were housewives.

Women in clerical positions and women who had been married and reared three or more children were at increased risk of developing coronary artery disease.

Certain factors may invalidate the results of such studies. While being married is usually associated in both men and women with a better physical health status, better mental health is not associated with women unless they are gainfully employed. Continuing research is needed to identify factors in employment that may prove to be traditionally stressful to women or elements in the job hazardous to men that may actually be health-constructive for women [119].

Among the factors predictive of coronary heart disease (CHD) in clerical workers [120] were suppressed hostility, having a nonsupportive boss, and decreased job mobility. The group at highest risk for CHD consisted of women clerical workers, with children, and married to blue-collar workers. In a subsequent study by the same investigators [121], it was demonstrated that type A men were at increased risk for CHD if their wives were highly educated or worked outside the home. The development of CHD was most marked in pairs where the husband was type A and the wife type B.

The difficulties of determing the effect of work on health were shown by Waldron and coworkers [122], who indicated that labor-force participation, "on the average," had neither harmful nor beneficial effects on the general health of middle-aged married women in the United States. On the other hand, women reporting poorer health were more likely to leave the labor force and less likely to participate.

Two other observations place the working woman advantageously in health status. In a nationwide analysis [123] that corrected for possible confounding factors, employed women showed a lower prevalence of serum cholesterol elevation than did housewives, and thus less risk for CHD. The "healthy worker effect" was not held responsible, and an explanation for the difference was not forthcoming. The second study [124] manifested other evidence of the beneficial effect of outside employment insofar as protection against CHD is concerned. While certain risk factors—total serum cholesterol, systolic and diastolic blood pressure, and obesity—were similar in both working women and homemakers, the levels of high-density lipoprotein cholesterol were significantly higher in currently employed women, a finding not readily explained. In essence, work did seem to provide a protective factor against CHD.

These studies are cited preliminarily, for personnel of an OHS who provide in-plant care should be aware of current research concerning the effects of work on women in the organization. Such knowledge will be helpful in the health counseling conducted and in the consultation offered managers who supervise female employees.

Other elements arise, though, in the interactive process of providing preventive care or definitive treatment for women workers. There has been criticism of the male-dominated specialty of obstetrics and gynecology and the surgery-mindedness of its practitioners [125]. In addition, it has been argued that while women use the health care system more than men, their symptoms are treated or viewed less seriously than the complaints presented by men [126]. It is contended that physicians and other health professionals quickly dismiss women's symptoms as trivial or psychogenic, not worthy of serious effort at diagnosis or treatment. Studies in all three bodies of writing—the lay press, medical publications, and the social science literature—support this view [126]. An investigation of the care that was provided gave strength to the notion that the male was considered "typically stoic and the female as hypochondriacal" [126]. Women patients who press practitioners for more thorough workups, Ruzek [126] indicates, or who return for repeated visits run the risk of being labeled "crocks" or "neurotic complainers." Physicians bring into practice from medical school this inculcated denigration of the complaining patient and do not seem to break out of this mold of the superior being whose skills are being trivialized by the emotionally ill patient or the individual with a submaximal organic sickness who is not presenting with an exotic disease subject to sophisticated diagnostic study and a complex mode of treatment.

This kind of stereotypical response is inappropriate in an organization where the employees return for care repeatedly to the same unit and staff. They cannot readily change health professionals. Further, it is almost axiomatic that the intelligent employee-patient who asks questions and is not immediately accepting of the response manifest by the physician or nurse is distanced even more so in the interaction, which proves to be antitherapeutic rather than helpful and supportive. A plea was made previously that complaints be listened to, the patient be "heard out," and the care given be as personal and empathic as the treating person is capable of rendering.

This level of reception and consideration is mandatory in a setting where supervisors might be over-demanding and impersonal and where deadlines are commonplace. The woman employee's complaints may be the first evidence of much more serious symptoms or illness to follow, especially if early signs are misjudged or mishandled. There is a reason for every OHS visit, particularly those calls that are self-generated and made for considerations outside the surveillance programs. An erroneous response, a deprecating attitude will alienate the worker and most likely exacerbate a difficulty that initially could be easily reversed through compassionate listening and serious concern.

SEXUAL HARASSMENT

Women employees are subject to sexual harassment, and the OHS rather than a department head may be the source for assistance used by a woman employee. Female workers in nontraditional jobs may find themselves subject to this treatment, and if the supervisor joins the "sport," there may be only the medical unit to which they can turn for aid. As Crull and Cohen [127] have pointed out, harassment by groups of men that include a supervisor creates a situation of "the old boy" network, which isolates the victim, protects the guilty, and leaves no mode of redress. In the nontraditional job, the new woman worker often faces resentment because of the entry into a previously all-male domain. This continuing badgering, overt or hidden, coupled with sexually motivated behavior in the guise of chivalry, reminds the employee blatantly that her proper place is either at home or in a stereotypical "woman's" job [127].

The OHS can be helpful in resolving the problem either through counseling or direct review with the department head of the activity involved. If the unit chief tends to downplay the harassment with a "boys-will-be-boys" approach, the consultation must take the form of confrontation for ultimate resolution.

Mendelson [128] elaborated on the subject when she cited the guidelines adopted by the Equal Employment Opportunity Commission [129]. *Sexual harassment* was defined as "unwelcome sexual advances, requests for sexual favors, and other verbal or physical conduct of a sexual nature" that takes place under any of the following circumstances:

When submission to the sexual advance is a condition of getting or keeping a job, whether expressed in explicit or implicit terms.

When a supervisor makes a personnel decision based on an employee's submission to, or rejection of, sexual advances.

When sexual conduct unreasonably interferes with a person's work performance or creates an intimidating, hostile, or offensive work environment.

Few companies have policies addressing the issue, possibly because the policy makers are too high on the managerial hierarchy to be aware of the practice, and proof is difficult to obtain and the complaints either are not taken seriously or are not believed. To reiterate, it may be the OHS that proves to be the sole supportive unit in a company where sexual harassment is encountered.

SOURCES OF INFORMATION

For some years, there has been based at Columbia University, the Women's Occupational Health Resource Center,* which has been headed by Jeanne M. Stellman, Ph.D., Executive Director, whose writings have been cited in this section.

The center has publicized hazards attendant upon female-dominated jobs and has produced fact sheets that describe modes of protection against such hazards. The organization was created in 1978 to help working women, trade unions, managers, professionals, and government policy makers become aware of women's occupational health and safety needs and the necessity for adequate programs to deal with them [129]. Available from the center are a bimonthly *Newsletter,* a quarterly *Technical Bulletin,* publication lists, and selected bibliographies, in addition to the fact sheets mentioned previously. Consultative assistance should be sought by health professionals in areas not adjacent to other occupational health resource facilities.

The Women's Bureau of the U.S. Department of Labor is placed in the Office of the Secretary and has produced over the years many publications related to the employment of women, pertinent legislation, and child care. Research has been conducted in such areas as the impact of technologic change on women's employment opportunities; the needs of immigrant, refugee, and entrant women; career transitions of women in professions; the impact of job dislocation; and the effect of military service on the postservice employment of women [130]. Information may be obtained directly from the Women's Bureau, Washington, DC 20210.

EMPLOYMENT OF THE IMPAIRED PERSON

Although the first legislative concern for the employment of the physically limited individual dates back nearly 70 years ago, certain negative philosophies regarding the vocational placement and utilization of the somatically or emotionally impaired person still persist. While the mandates provided by the Rehabilitation Act of 1973 are still in force and have not been diluted by deregulation, there are still fair numbers of rejections of so-called handicapped applicants, so that appeals to various fair employment practice commissions, or their equivalent bodies, continue to be filed.

Fears die hard, and employers' beliefs that less than physically perfect individuals will injure themselves, or will prove to be an eventual drain on what-

*Located at Columbia University, School of Public Health, 600 West 168th Street, New York, NY 10032.

ever benefit scheme is undergoing scrutiny, remain in constant need of rebuttal. Not too many corporate medical directors or their staff physicians have attempted to reverse employers' attitudes and to demonstrate the worth of hiring the impaired candidate for work. That there are companies that have undertaken such additions to their personnel has been given testimony by the organizations receiving awards from the various governors' committees and the President's Committee on Employment of the Handicapped. What the determinants of such positive policies might be or what the motivating factors are have not been subjected to much research inquiry. In some instances, involved relatives of industrial managers or their immediate family members who were born with impairments bring about attitudinal fixings rather early, and they remain to be converted into business stances later in life. Some other employers believe that commerce and industry can manifest a social conscience beyond the awarding of foundation grants, and they will hire the capable, although physically variant, applicant.

DEFINITIONS

The terms used in writings on disability seem to vary with the profession, the discipline, the agency, the retirement function, the workers' compensation authority, and the legislative bodies, among others. A consensus has not been reached so that nearly anyone who voices a point of view must lay down some basic understandings.

Physical impairment, as used here, means an anatomic or physiologic variance that might be congenital in origin, the result or residua of trauma, illness, metabolic change, or the process of aging and is an abnormality that persists after treatment.

The term *physical limitation,* again, as utilized in this writing, is considered synonymous with physical impairment. *Disability* represents the inability to execute certain tasks or functions. *Handicap,* although used in a generic sense, is employed in legislative language, by lay persons, frequently for added emotional appeal, and in such agency designations as the president's, governors', and mayors' committees on employment of the handicapped. It is not a term included in the lexicon of this monograph, except as an official label for the bodies just mentioned.

There is confusion because a person with paraplegia, with diabetes mellitus, with an amputation, or with any limiting physical condition, if employed, is not disabled. Such an individual is only disabled for the performance of certain tasks or functions and, with careful placement, is not required to complete assignments outside the demands of a particular job or beyond his or her abilities.

As pointed out by Blumenfeld and Menkes [131], there are other factors entering into an individual's ability to engage in substantial gainful activity, such as age, sex, previous training, and previous work experience. To cite the example they used, a college graduate, 30 years of age, should be able to continue working even though he or she has a below-knee amputation and would not be considered disabled under the law governing the social security disability program. However an uneducated laborer, 60 years of age, would not be expected to work were he or she to have a similar physical impairment and thus would be considered disabled.

As discussed previously, persons who have been working for years in spite of certain physical limitations may be granted disability retirements because of the entry of new influencing factors or the interpretation of the regulations of a particular retirement system.

DEMONSTRATION OF POLICY

As in other areas relating to occupational health, it is the medical directors' function to provide the employers—the chief executive officers (CEOs)—with a philosophy that they can articulate understandably to their industrial peers. Such action goes beyond having the CEO read a speech prepared by the plant physician, for no matter how skilled a reader one might be, the text will lack conviction unless the executive truly comprehends the message and believes in what is being delivered. For there to be true commitment, there must be both intellectual and emotional involvement. The CEO has credibility in the community, and a statement of belief in the worth of the employment of the impaired will go far in emphasizing that, as promulgated by others, it is good business, in light of the group's record in attendance, productivity, loyalty, and minimal injury rate.

There are two other ways in which visual evidence of faith in the job performance of the physically impaired can be demonstrated. Assigning an individual in a wheelchair or an amputee, for example, at the reception desk of an organization—the first contact point of a visitor—is the equivalent of a declaration of policy. When the author was associated early on with a research laboratory in nuclear energy, the receptionist at the front desk was an above-elbow amputee veteran of World War II, and all visitors, vendors to consultants, learned immediately of the laboratory's hiring policy.

The other mode of nonverbal communication that

will relate a belief is for the OHS itself to employ as many physically limited staff members as it can. Again, to refer to personal experience, in a large OHS that the author had the professional pleasure to develop, the following individuals were added, and they served well: an achondroplastic dwarf (occupational health technician); a man in a wheelchair, status post-polio (occupational health technician); a woman with osteoarthritis of the hip joint, with gait impairment (occupational health nurse); recovered problem drinkers (one as a counselor, one as a secretary); a hypertensive man (physician); a woman with anorexia nervosa and cerebral palsy (clerk); a woman with bronchiectasis (administrative aide); and a woman with rheumatoid arthritis (nurse/health educator). In other OHS configurations, the same principle of giving solidity to preachments was adhered to as workers with achrondroplasia, Legg-Perthes disease, recovered alcoholism, diabetes mellitus, congenital paraplegia, and compensated hearing loss were added successfully to various occupational health staffs. Outstanding was a totally blind stenographer who transcribed, *and proofread* via a special tactile device, all of the author's clinical notes at a time when a great number of patients would be seen each day. This mode of hiring not only educates skeptical managers but convinces rather tough-shelled craft foremen that (1) the handicapped employee can do a job and (2) the OHS does exactly what it expects other departments to do.

INITIAL INTERVIEW

It has long been believed that the impaired individual should be interviewed either by the OHS director or a designate skilled in meeting with job applicants who are ill at ease, primarily because of repeated rejections in the hiring process, compounded by weak rationales for the rebuffs. It is the latter that is so frustrating and disheartening to trained and experienced job candidates, for they realize that the excuse given for the declination rarely contains the truth, which is simply, "We don't want you."* A chemist who was applying for a research position told the author of his experience. He was kyphotic and scoliotic from childhood polio and had been rejected by nine possible employers, and presenting an extraordinarily thin reason for nonacceptance. His explanation was that even though he had the experience, the graduate education, and a good work record, he did not match the Hollywood prototype of the tall, handsome white-gowned researcher gazing intently at a hand-held test tube, while the colored contents of retorts boiled furiously nearby on a laboratory bench. The moment was a poignant one because no "make-over" by a skilled beautician could change his appearance. He was what he was physically, and he had a great deal to offer, but we, only, were the buyers.

A special interview will allow the applicant to decant off his or her life's experiences and, while doing so, acquire the feeling that, at long last, a caring person has been found. Such an individual, irrespective of the impairing disorder, particularly if it is a visible difference, will appreciate the opportunity to review the rebuffs, the compensatory and overcompensatory mechanisms, the altered lifestyle that have been experienced or adopted. The difficulties in transportation, ambulation, or interpersonal relationships must be teased out for a full and empathic understanding of the personality and the person inside the altered body. Recalled with considerable pathos is an interview that was being conducted before a class on a field visit to Goodwill Industries. The objective of the sessions was to demonstrate the technique of discussing impairments with the persons concerned. The worker was a 17-year-old extremely attractive Hispanic girl who, after being shot in the back, had sustained a spinal cord injury with resultant paraplegia. The conversation led to the adjustment to her job, her continuing therapy, and her living situation, but more importantly, how she was coping with the lack of dating, a burgeoning activity of all of her friends. She poured out her feelings, oblivious to the group, expressing the loneliness, the needs, the disappointment. The class sat in utter stillness, astonished that in a new situation, with a strange interviewer, these highly personal emotional responses to her situation could be verbalized. The point was made that the concern expressed with the employee would be felt and that this initial interaction would serve as a continuing bond throughout the individual's employment.

During such an interview there should be a "laying out of hands," when indicated. Healed surgical or incisional traumatic scars should be palpated. Prostheses worn on extremity amputation stumps should be removed, hefted, and checked for fit, and the healed scar on the stump palpated. The reason for this kind of supplementary examination is that the impaired person feels the bond created by the touching, as does an unimpaired person. The move

*One is reminded of the opening scenes of the excellent, insightful, and comedic film "Tootsie," in which the protagonist, following several readings for possible casting, was told he was too short, too tall, too young, too old, etc. when the real message was, "We don't want to hire you."

is not the shallow, meaningless "touchy-feely" approach of the pseudo-therapist, but one that will carry meaning that the physician or nurse wants to share in the feeling of physical difference or deficit. Many are the employees or patients who detect immediately reticence or hesitancy on the part of the professional and who will state later, "He didn't want to touch me."

It is helpful if clinical photographs are taken of old scars, amputation stumps, disfigurements, or congenital anomalies. Changes can be detected secularly, and particularly, when the beginning of a new job might be stressful for the above-knee amputee, there can be an accompanying weight gain and loss of fit of the prosthetic socket. In the event of burns sustained over a previously scarred or otherwise traumatized area, clinical photographs prior to the injury are helpful in judging the amount of change. Such documentation has special relevance in pigmented skin, when a burn may cause loss of pigment, gain of pigment, or both and a claim is filed alleging more change than was actually sustained.

All physical alterations that are subject to mensuration should have data recorded, such as length and width of scars (and height if a keloid), diameter of thighs when there is unilateral atrophy, and the like.

FOLLOW-UP

As indicated previously, it is helpful if the individual has diabetes, particularly if insulin-dependent, or has a convulsive disorder to have the employee's permission to apprise the immediate supervisor of the clinical state so that if an emergency were to arise, appropriate aid can be provided, without panicking adjacent workers. Rarely does an employee refuse permission.

The initial interview at time of hire is not the end of the interaction, for there must be follow-up visits either of the worker to the OHS or the medical director to the worksite, in addition to continuing contact with the employee's physician or referring agency (or counselor). During such contacts it can be determined if special parking facilities are needed or, in the event of fire, explosion, or other accident, if the impaired individual will be able to have ready egress from his or her customary work place. For some employees it is necessary to determine that toilet and washroom facilities are close to the work station.

If transportation and time loss are significant factors for the newly hired person, and the lack of accumulated sick leave will be a consideration, the OHS can undertake blood glucose determinations, repeated urinalyses, or whatever other laboratory test procedures might be requested by the employee's physician.

The process of employment and placement of the physically impaired worker is seen in Figure 17-1.

INDUSTRY-CREATED DISABILITY—THE RETURN TO WORK

Not all physically marginal workers come from outside the plant as job applicants in need of selective placement. Many of those persons requiring care in job assignment are the company's own personnel who have been permanently partially impaired by traffic or recreational accidents, or they are employees who have been injured at work and return following treatment and rehabilitation. It is conceivable that the injuries sustained were of sufficient severity as to preclude resumption of the former job, and a new post will have to be found in keeping with the incumbent's current physical and emotional capacities.

In some jurisdictions, rehabilitation following occupationally incurred injury has been mandated, and rehabilitation plans must be developed for every employee whose injury precludes, or is likely to preclude, the worker's engaging in his or her usual occupation or time-of-injury employment and who can be reasonably expected to benefit from such a program. Usually, a special unit in the state workers' compensation structure will review the proposed plan and will approve, disapprove, or modify the envisioned program. The "qualified rehabilitation representative" may be a vocational rehabilitation consultant employed by the state, a public or private agency, or an agent of the employer. The passage of such a law has led to the establishment of many counselors in private practice who follow the client through the entire process from initial evaluation and determination of need to return to work. The phrases *private rehabilitation* and *private-for-profit rehabilitation* are relatively new in the physical restoration vocabulary [132].

In the private sector, certain expectations are offered the employer, and ultimately the client, in the form of loss control by [133]

Management of the injured worker's treatment plan
Management of the injured worker's attitude toward recovery and return to work
Prevention of the development of the disability syndrome
Early identification of the barriers to recovery

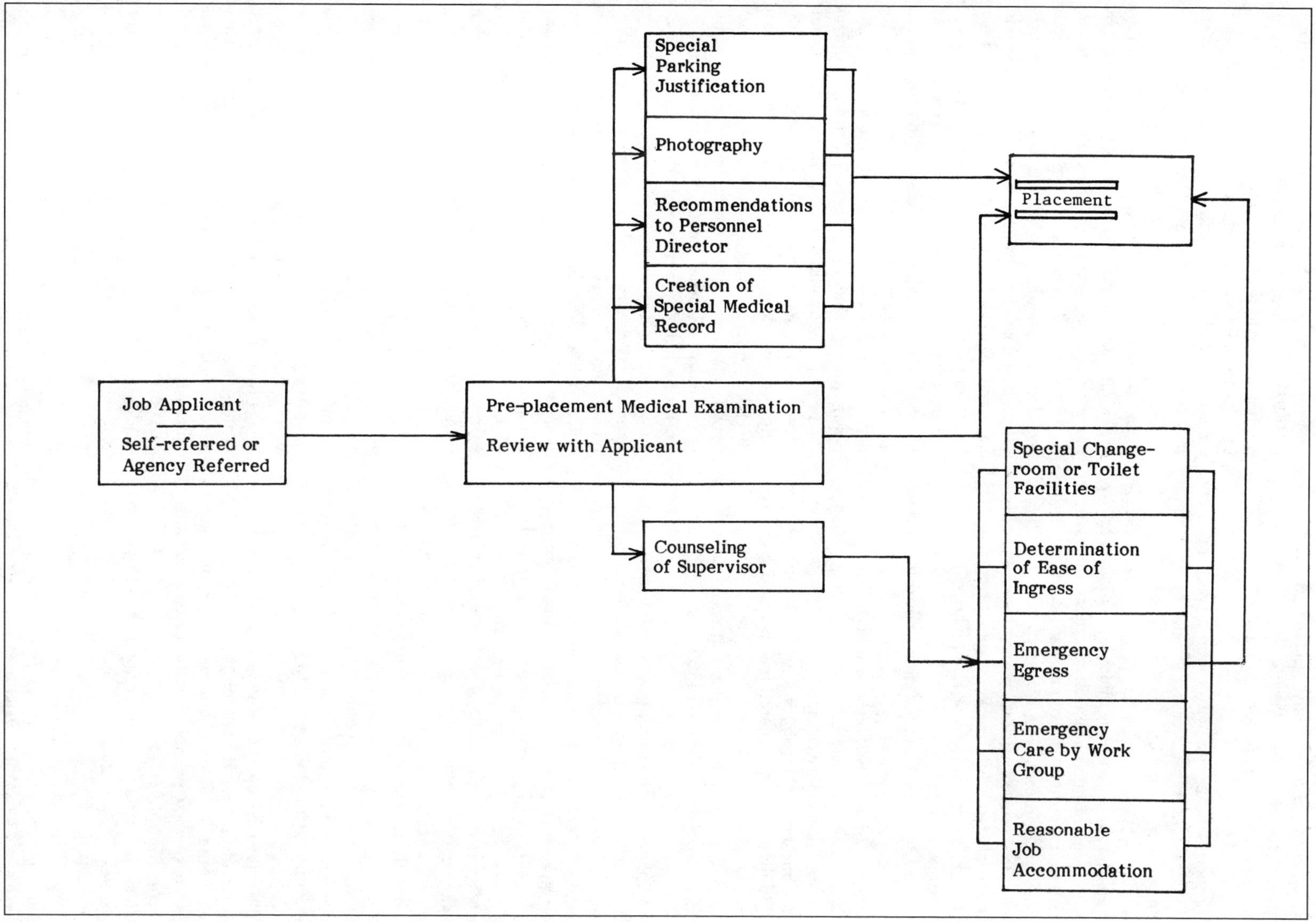

FIGURE 17-1. *Employment process of the physically impaired person.*

The provision of file visibility (enabling the early setting of accurate reserves)
The reduction of the period of disability

In the first interview with the injured client, a rehabilitation nurse, a member of the rehabilitation management team, will

Establish rapport with the injured worker and clarify confusion or misconceptions on the injured worker's part regarding either medical treatment or the insurance process.
Obtain the injured worker's perception of his or her medical status, the worker's view of current and future treatment, and a comprehensive medical history.
Obtain educational and vocational histories, including vocational skills.
Note the injured worker's current financial status and document daily activities, including pre- and postinjury activity changes.
Note the family dynamics and the attitude of the family toward the injured member and his or her recovery.
Document the injured worker's attitude, as well as any barriers toward return to work.

A report will be submitted to the carrier, and in addition to frequent oral communication, written reports will follow on a tri-weekly basis. If needed, a complete job analysis will be done for review by the treating physician. The rehabilitation nurse will work with the physician in coordinating needed medical services and in assessing the current care. When necessary, recommendations will be made regarding a change of treatment or facility, always a sensitive subject, but often indicated because of differences between the treater and the treated, because of prolonged unsupervised ineffective care in the form of physical therapy, or because of the lack of communication. In substance, it is believed that this early intervention and follow-up [133]

Allow the development of goodwill between the carrier and the injured worker.
Lessen the likelihood of attorney representation.
Ensure the best possible medical care, which aids in cost control.
Effect the earliest and most complete recovery possible.

Some large companies have created their own inhouse or rehabilitation (postinjury) programs for these reasons: (1) The rehabilitation staff is on the scene and can identify more readily employees who may require help, even if such persons have not been referred for assistance; (2) the staff's knowledge of the inner workings of the company enables them to find potential job opportunities for rehabilitated employees; and (3) the staff can provide important follow-up services to ensure that rehabilitated employees are performing useful work [134]. Return-to-work programs have been formalized in many organizations, and the objectives, as hypothesized by one writer [135], could be (1) to reduce absenteeism by 45 percent, (2) to reduce long-term disability costs by 25 percent, and (3) to reduce workers' compensation time-loss costs by 15 percent, all in year one. Such activities can be undertaken by an occupational health nurse or a rehabilitation counselor.

Such rehabilitation will include, as needed, tuition, books, training fees, tools necessary to learn or start a new job, transportation, and additional living expenses. There is no cost to the employee, and temporary total disability payments will continue during the period of rehabilitation services. Again, with reference to one state, rehabilitation is offered by the employer mandatorily after 180 days of temporary disability. Acceptance of the program may be postponed, but in any event and irrespective of the kind of settlement reached, benefits are not affected.

This program is mentioned because there have always been workers who will settle a claim and never return to work who, with some rehabilitative assistance, could resume working and not become disabled. While there has been success with the program,* industry will continue to produce its own impairments, challenging acceptance and placement. OHS personnel should encourage all injured workers to take advantage of such restorative or retraining programs when needed.

ASSISTIVE DEVICES/SENSORY AIDS

Employees who undergo degenerative organic change or sensory organ loss through the aging process or who, by virtue of a congenital defect, present at the time of job application with a deformity of an extremity or other appendage can often obtain a compensatory cosmetic or prosthetic device that either will assist in the performance of a set of tasks or will, by concealing a deformity, allow the candidate more readily to be accepted by peers. These various corrective and assistive devices can be obtained from a

*In California, 85 percent of workers undergoing rehabilitation in the 1978–1980 period returned to work; the figure dropped to 78 percent in 1982 because of economic conditions [136].

variety of vendors, but they are listed here as suggestive of the kinds of appliances available.

AMBULATORY DEVICES

Wheelchair, standard, basic
Wheelchair, special models:
- Double-rimmed wheels for one-hand propelling
- Models for persons with lower extremity amputations
- Models for persons with hemiplegia
- Models that are heavy-duty
- Special sizes for small, tall, and extra-large persons
- Battery-powered chair (wheelchair, three-wheeled scooter or cycle chair)
- Stand-up wheelchair
- Elevating wheelchair
- Wheelchair for airborne use

Wheelchair, special features:
- Detachable arms
- Desk-length arms
- Pneumatic tires
- Attachment to standard wheelchair of a power and steering unit similar to that used with the scooter-type vehicle
- A narrowing, cranking device that will allow the chair to proceed through a narrow doorway
- Hand controls for driving an automobile

Wheelchair stair-lift, fixed, for both indoor and outdoor applications
Wheelchair stair-lift, portable—utilizes rubber tracks similar to tractor tracks

WRITING AIDS

Board supports for typewriter
Devices to increase grasp of a pen or pencil by creating a wider diameter of the writing implement

TELEPHONING AIDS

Lightweight headset
Loudspeaker for incoming calls and a microphone
Extra earpiece to allow binaural hearing
Hearing-aid adapter
Card-dialer telephone, with or without braille markings
Push-button telephone in place of dial and one-touch dialing using touch-sensitive dial surface
Handset for faint-speech amplification
Large-number dial overlay
Special breath-activated telephone for persons with motion impairment (connects user to operator who dials call)
Lamp signal to flash with ringing tone or to remain lit until call is answered
Teletypewriter (TTY)
Handset for hearing amplification

SPEAKING AIDS

Spelling board
Picture chart
Lightwriter (a typewriter that produces a luminous line of capital letters on a board)
Speech-recognition keyboard, computer-compatible
Blissymbols (a symbol language)
American Sign Language (Amsalan)
Fingerspelling (a one-handed manual alphabet is used in the United States)

ELECTRONIC AIDS

Remote control of such devices as taperecorder, TV set, radio, alarm system, door-entry mechanism with intercom, curtain opener and closer, heating and lighting, and typewriter (Systems of operation may include shining of a light, minimal movement of a hand, foot, cheek, or toe, or voice activation.)
Hearing aids

SPEECH AIDS, ELECTRONIC

Transcervical electronic larynx
Transoral electronic larynx
Transoral pneumatic larynx (not powered electronically, but by stoma air)

VISION AIDS

Telescopic lenses
Tactual watches
Braille labeler
Talking paper-money identifier
Image-enlargement for visually impaired typist
Communication device for use with person who is deaf and blind and knows braille; uses pinfield
Writing guides
Reading machines that convert printed material into easily understood speech

MISCELLANEOUS AIDS

Wheelchair-accessible drinking fountains and electric water coolers

PUBLICATIONS

Several publications provide information concerning sources of assistive devices. As an example, one directory that relates the device to the job is *The International Directory of Job-Oriented Assistive Device Sources,** compiled by Marjorie Golter, M.S., C.R.C. Two examples of the ties among the device, the job, and the disability are seen in the following descriptions from the directory, reprinted with permission:

*Published in 1983 by Lifeboat, Fox Hills Garden Offices, 5855 Green Valley Circle, Culver City, CA 90230.

Job (or Function): Carpentry
Disability: Vision Impaired
Problem: Difficulty in using handsaw.
Solution: Tactile Saw Guide
How it Works: The fixed portion of the guide has raised dots on the left and right sides marked at 45 and 90 degrees. The moving portion has one raised reference dot. Settings can be established at any 15 degree point between 45 and 90 degrees through the use of the notches cut into the tool. These notches make it useful for any size handsaw for square and angled cuts, and it can be adjusted for right and left hand workers.
Contact: American Foundation for the Blind
15 West 16th Street
New York, New York 10011
(212) 620-2169

Job (or Function): Inspector
Disability: Vision Impaired
Problem: Difficulty in inspecting machine parts.
Solution: Optical Projection Equipment
How it Works: The work station aligns, inspects, gauges, fits or measures machine parts. The products of these operations were to be inspected. A screen and special projector were installed. The projector used 10×, 20×, 31.25× or 50× magnification lenses. With this system magnified images of the parts are projected on the screen which make measurement and inspection easier. The inspector can view a part without removing it from the machine. The system can be adapted to various machines, using a reversible arm support or an extension boom arm. The unit can be mounted in various relationships to the work area: over the work spindle, over the wheel spindle, on the base of the machine, or directly to the table.
Contact: Stocker & Yale, Inc.
133 Brimbal Avenue
Beverly, Massachusetts 01915
(617) 927-3940; Michael A. Lavey

The procurement and issue of any of the indicated sensory or other aids listed in several pertinent publications will allow an employer to fulfill the requirement of "reasonable accommodation" in the hiring of the handicapped.

MECHANISMS OF "REASONABLE ACCOMMODATION"

STATISTICS

As indicated previously, Section 503 of the Rehabilitation Act of 1973 requires employers to take affirmative action to hire and advance qualified handicapped persons and to provide reasonable accommodations within the limits of the company's resources and business necessity. Until the issue was studied, little was known regarding industry's interpretation of the requirement or what measures were taken in compliance. A study was conducted for the U.S. Department of Labor and was reported in June 1982 [137].

The findings revealed the following among firms employing a total of 512,000 workers, of whom 19,200 were disabled:

26 percent had to make no special accommodations at all for the disabled.
36 percent had to make accommodations for less than 10 percent of their handicapped workers.
38 percent had to make accommodations for 50 percent or more of their handicapped workers.

Kinds of Accommodations
19 percent were adaptations of the workplace, such as moving desks, changing from second to first floor, changing furniture to make for wider aisles, and so on.
15 percent involved special equipment or aids (readers for the blind, sign-language training for supervisors of deaf workers, braille equipment, and so on).
22 percent involved redesigning of jobs so that handicapped persons could fill them.
15 percent involved transfer to different jobs or special training in order to fill different jobs.
19 percent had to do with orientation of supervisors.

Accessibility
72 percent already had parking curb cuts.
64 percent had ramped entrances.
62 percent had general access throughout the plant.
67 percent had clear access to the personnel offices.
40 percent had audible/visible alarm systems.
31 percent had lowered drinking fountains.
29 percent had lowered telephones.
13 percent had braille marking in elevators, on doors, and so on.

Costs
51 percent of the accommodations cost absolutely nothing.
41 percent cost less than $500.
8 percent cost more than that amount because of the need for ramps, elevators, or special reading machines.
72 percent reported that the costs did not exceed their projections.

60 percent stated that the benefits far exceeded the costs.

The conclusion from the study was that accommodation most often was not something that was expensive or extensive or "a big deal." It was viewed as a practical and profitable management effort to make a worker more productive.

JOB ACCOMMODATION NETWORK (JAN)

Probably most helpful to employers undertaking steps in reasonable accommodation to meet the needs of impaired workers is JAN, the acronym for Job Accommodation Network, a service of the President's Committee on Employment of the Handicapped* (PCEH), supported by the National Institute of Handicapped Research and the Rehabilitation Services Administration. JAN is a data base that contains specific information concerning the performance of individual tasks by persons with limitations. The system allows employers to discuss with other employers those methods of accommodation that have proved successful in specific instances. The modes of accommodation are not theoretic or hypothetic but are real, having been field-tested and instituted in true work situations.

Operational since July 1984, JAN has gathered over 4,000 ideas for accommodation and has been of assistance to well over 300 organizations, including many of the so-called Fortune-500 companies. JAN is based at the University of West Virginia in Morgantown. Responding to telephone† inquiries are highly trained human-factors engineers, who ask the caller for details concerning the problem in need of solution. The job requirements are reviewed, and with a knowledge of the functional limitations of the new or returning employee, the data base is searched and the methods of accommodation successfully used in similar worker/work situations in other companies are found.

The data base prints out abstracts of these experiences, along with the names, addresses, and telephone numbers of the corporate officials who have reported them. The information is transmitted electronically to the company presenting the problem. Currently, because of federal support, there is no charge to users. The only requirement made is that employers share with the network their experiences with the aids or devices that have proved effective. This notification is accomplished through completion of JAN's Employer's Accommodation Input Questionnaire, a single-page form to be returned to JOB Accommodation Network, P.O. Box 468, Morgantown, WV 26505.

The success of the project is occasioned by the corporation-to-corporation interchange. Even though the state/federal programs in vocational rehabilitation date to the early 1920s, the relationship between the agencies and business has been "uneasy" [138]. Corporate personnel directors have felt that agency staff members did not understand the demands of commerce and industry, while the rehabilitative counselors sought some compassion from businesses rather than its "obsession with the bottom line." With the knowledge that another company has tried a device or method and met success, the manager is willing to try the ideas offered by the data base. The estrangement between agency and corporation is not there to block the utilization of the applicant or incumbent with a disability.

*Designated later as the President's Committee on Employment of People with Disabilities.
†JAN can be reached at (800) 526-7234, which is the equivalent number of (800) JAN-PCEH.

ARCHITECTURAL SPECIFICATIONS

In 1969, the Congress passed the Architectural Barriers Act (Public Law 90-480) that required certain federally owned, leased, or funded buildings and facilities to be accessible to physically handicapped persons. Five years later, an agency was created to enforce the law, and under Section 502 of the Rehabilitation Act of 1973, there was established the Architectural and Transportation Barriers Compliance Board. The act allows complaints to be filed regarding the lack of accessibility to federally owned or used buildings by physically limited personnel.

Certain architectural constraints have been developed to permit ingress by all persons, and some of these requirements follow:

Building entrances at ground level with unobstructed path of travel
32-inch (81.0 cm) door opening widths
Level thresholds to buildings and rooms
Sloping ramps instead of stairs (ratio 1:12 or 8.3 percent)
Safe, wide parking spaces close to buildings
Level walks with no curbs at crossways or from parking lots
Clear access to elevators and elevator buttons
Restrooms with wide stalls and with grab bars 33 inches high (82.5 cm)
Handrails on all stairways—extending 18 inches (45.0 cm) beyond top and bottom steps

Slip-resistant floors; carpeting with tight weave and low pile
Lower fountains and public telephones
Braille signs/signals and notices
Visual warning systems

Most jurisdictions have developed their own building codes to meet the requirements of the law, and specifications have been delineated regarding specific elements of the physical environment covering these entities.

The exact floor plans, suggested dimensions of facilities, and the like can be obtained from local municipalities* and by reference to established building codes or the *American National Standard Specifications for Making Buildings and Facilities Accessible to and Usable by Handicapped People,* ANSI A117.1-1980.†

SURVEYS OF THE HANDICAPPED

It might be necessary at times to determine the number of handicapped employees at a plant either to establish a baseline or to be able to detect growth in affirmative action efforts as they relate to the physically impaired. Probably one of the most recent surveys was conducted by the Du Pont organization [139].

Interestingly, Du Pont first examined the current business marketplace **myths** surrounding the hiring of disabled persons, which coursed as follows:

Insurance rates will skyrocket when one hires the disabled.
Considerable expense will be involved in making the necessary adjustments at the place of work.
Safety reports will be jeopardized.
Special privileges will have to be granted to the disabled.
Other employees will not accept the disabled.

None of the above holds true, and the experience of many companies has demonstrated the fallacy of these myths. Particularly untrue is the last one, for it has been shown that employees not only accept the disabled, but exceed all expected effort in helping orient newly hired impaired persons and usually develop close friendships with them. Of Du Pont's 135,000 employees, 2,745 were disabled, and the study showed that a high majority achieved average or better ratings in job performance, safety, and attendance.

While the findings are important, the focal point of this section is the provision of a classification for use in such a survey. The primary classifications follow [140]:

Vision impairment
Hearing impairment
Speech impairment
Impairment of special sense, other
Convulsive disorders
Mental retardation
Absence or loss of upper extremity
Absence or loss of lower extremity
Absence or loss of upper and lower extremities
Absence or loss of other structures or organs
Paralysis of extremities or trunk
Cerebral palsy
Orthopedic impairments, non-paralytic
Deformities of extremities and trunk
Vascular disorders
Metabolic disorders
Malignant disease
Respiratory disorders
Renal disease
Gastrointestinal disorders
Skin disease
Allergic (atopic) state
Blood disorder
Emotional disorder

Two other handicapping conditions remain for classification, but while they are not physical impairments they may limit the progress of the employee: undereducation and foreign national status without knowledge of English.

If a more detailed classification of malformations or anomalies is needed, see *SNOMED: Systematized Nomenclature of Medicine* [141] and International Terminology for the Classification of Congenital Limb Deficiencies, in *Atlas of Limb Prosthetics* [142], which actually is the report by Hector W. Kay.

LANGUAGE GOVERNING PERSONS WITH DISABILITIES

Many vocabularies have required straightening since certain minorities began to point out discrepant

*As excellent examples, see *An Illustrated Handbook of the Handicapped Section of the North Carolina State Building Code,* prepared for the Governor's Study Committee on Architectural Barriers and the North Carolina Department of Insurance Commissioner by R. L. Mace and B. Laslett. Raleigh: The North Carolina Building Code Council and the North Carolina Department of Insurance, 1974; and *Buildings Without Barriers: Planning with the Handicapped in Mind.* Edmonton, Alberta: Culture, Facility Development Branch, 1980.
†Prepared by the American National Standards Institute, 1430 Broadway, New York, NY 10018.

word usages that smacked of racism, sexism, or agism. As job categories have undergone change from fireman to firefighter and stewardess to flight attendant, as examples, other systems of terminology have been scrutinized and found wanting. Manus [143] in a brief but pointed writing entitled "Is Your Language *Disabling*?" directed attention to sensitive alterations in the "literature of exceptionality." While the demeaning designations of decades ago have fairly well disappeared from educated speech, certain indicated changes still remain unaltered. It is to be noted that the "Society for Crippled Children and Adults" is now the "Easter Seal Society," and "I.C.D." (International Center for the Disabled) has replaced the "Institute for Crippled and Disabled." To hasten the departure from "the hopelessness and insensitivity of the past," Manus [143] suggests these modifications:

Preferred	*Stigmatizing*
Serving clients	Servicing cases or clients
Serve clients	Service cases or clients
Client or patient or person	Case
Retarded person	Retardate
Person with paraplegic involvement	Paraplegic
Handicapped persons	The handicapped
Disabled persons or persons with disability	The disabled
Disabled persons (or child or adult)	Cripple(d)
Handicapped person (or child or adult)	Cripple(d)
Person with intellectual or emotional problems	Mental case
Blind person	The blind
Addicted persons	Addict

The terms to be ruled out, as Manus views them, depersonalize the individual, reify the disability, and equate the disabled person to disability or treat entire groups of people as objects or classes of objects.

Terms or expressions to be avoided because of their strong negative, derogatory connotations, as pointed out by the California Governor's Committee for Employment of the Handicapped [144], are the following: afflicted, cerebral-palsied, confined to a wheelchair, crazy, insane, crip, deaf and dumb, deaf mute, defective, deformed, limp, invalid, lame, maimed, paralytic, arthritic, epileptic, poor unfortunate, retard, spastic, spaz, stricken, victim, wheelchair-bound, and withered.

The elimination of deprecating labels will increase one's effectiveness as an agent in the adaptation and rehabilitation process of disabled persons. A 5-year (1975–1980) review of disabling language in four rehabilitation journals revealed that little progress had been made. There were 46 non-disabling-language titles versus 31 that contained "disabling" titles [145].

WHAT IS GOOD FOR CONGRESS IS GOOD FOR INDUSTRY

By way of increasing motivation toward greater employment of persons with physical impairments or functional limitations, it can be emphasized that in Congress, in 1982, there were the following members, all holding ranking positions or committee appointments, who had the conditions indicated [146]:

Senator Robert J. Dole: a paralyzed arm incurred during World War II combat service.

Senator John P. East: serves in a wheelchair.

Senator Daniel K. Inouye: lost an arm in World War II combat.

Senator Charles H. Percy: a hearing impairment incurred in World War II service as a gunnery officer.

Representative Charles E. Bennett: contracted polio while serving in the Philippine Islands during World War II.

Representative Tony Coelho: epilepsy.

Representative Claude D. Pepper: a hearing impairment.

Representative James H. Scheuer: had polio in his youth.

Representative Morris K. Udall: has a visual impairment and Parkinson's disease.

Representative Larry Winn, Jr.: has had a leg amputation.

UNIVERSAL POTENTIAL

That there is employment capability in nearly everyone with a limiting disorder is given emphasis by Harold Russell, who ended his first book *Victory in My Hands,* [147] with these words:

> People frequently marvel at the things I can do with my hooks. Well, perhaps it is marvelous. But the thing I never cease to marvel at is that I was able to meet the challenge of utter disaster and master it. For me that was and is the all-important fact—that the human soul, beaten down, overwhelmed, faced by complete failure and ruin, can still rise up against unbearable odds and triumph.

REFERENCES

1. Yankelovich, D. Counterculture vs. conservatism. *The Lamp* 54:8, Winter 1972.
2. Nicholi, A. M., II. Campus disorders: A problem of adult leadership. *Am J Psychiatry* 127:66, 1970.
3. Marti-Ibanez, F. The duty to rebel: Outlook on youth. *MD* 19:13, Feb 1975.

4. Douglas, J. D. *Youth in Turmoil: America's Changing Youth Cultures and Student Protest Movements.* Chevy Chase, MD: National Institute of Mental Health, Center for Studies of Crime and Delinquency, 1970.
5. Hendin, H. A psychoanalyst looks at student revolutionaries. *New York Times Mag,* Jan 17, 1971.
6. Somers, A. R. Violence, television and the health of American youth. *N Engl J Med* 294:811, 1976.
7. *Statistical Abstract of the United States 1985* (105th ed.). Washington, DC: U.S. Department of Commerce, Bureau of the Census, 1984. P. 600.
8. Hodgson, J. D. Address before the NAB National Youth Conference, Washington, DC, February 23, 1972. *News*—U.S. Department of Labor, Office of Information, Release 72-113, Feb 23, 1972. P. 5.
9. Rosow, J. M. Cited in *News*—U.S. Department of Labor, Office of Information, Release 71-167, March 24, 1971. P. 1.
10. *World Almanac and Book of Facts 1986.* New York: Newspaper Enterprise Association, 1985. P. 195.
11. Ely, T. S. Workplace hazards and young humans. *J Occup Med* 18:55, 1976.
12. *The Appointed Factor Doctor Service: Report by a Sub-Committee of the Industrial Health Advisory Committee.* London: Ministry of Labour, 1966. Pp. 1–2.
13. Herford, M. E. M. *Youth at Work: A Study of Adolescents in Industry by an Appointed Factory Doctor.* London: Max Parrish, 1957. P. 19.
14. Forssman, S., and Coppee, G. H. *Occupational Health Problems of Young Workers.* Geneva: International Labour Office, 1974.
15. *Older Americans Act of 1965, as Amended—History and Related Acts.* Washington, DC: U.S. Department of Health, Education, and Welfare, Office of Human Development Services, Administration on Aging, July 1979.
16. Age Discrimination in Employment Act of 1967, Public Law 90-202, 90th Congress, S. 830, (Dec 15) 1967, Sec.1(b).
17. *The Law against Age Discrimination in Employment.* Washington, DC: U.S. Department of Labor, Workplace Standards Administration, Wage and Hour Division, Sept 1970. P. 4.
18. Age-discrimination suit wins $425,215. *Los Angeles Times* II:7, March 24, 1985.
19. Population profile: Persons aged 25–64. *Stat Bull Metropol Life Insur Co* 66:20, Jan-March 1985.
20. Continued decline in mortality in the United States, Canada, and Western Europe. *Stat Bull Metropol Life Insur Co* 66:9, Jan-March 1985.
21. Gage, H. Ergonomics and the Aging Worker. In *Best's Safety Directory—1984.* Oldwick, NJ: Best, 1984. Vol. II, pp. 1033–1037.
22. Glorig, A. Personal communication, 1959.
23. Hanman, B. Publication unidentified.
24. *Older Workers: Myths and Reality.* Washington, DC: U.S. Department of Health and Human Services, Office of Human Development Services, Administration on Aging, 1984.
25. Louis Harris and Associates, Inc. *1979 Study of American Attitudes Toward Pensions and Retirement.* Additional commentary by Johnson & Higgins. New York: Johnson & Higgins, 1979. P. xv.
26. Gitelson, M. The emotional problems of elderly people. *Geriatrics* 3:135, 1948.
27. Manion, W. V. Why employees retire early. *Personnel J* 51:183, 1972.
28. Myers, R. I. Disability Retirement. Unpublished presentation, typescript, p. 4.
29. Brodsky, C. M. Compensation illness as a retirement channel. *J Am Geriatr Soc* 19:51, 1971.
30. Portnoi, V. Aging, natural death, and the compression of morbidity. *N Engl J Med* 303:1369, 1980.
31. Hodgson, E. S. Visual display units and spectacle provision. *Soc Occup Med Newsletter,* No. 38, March 1985. P. 19.
32. Morin, M. M., Pickle, L. W., and Mason, T. J. Geographic patterns of ethnic groups in the United States. *Am J Public Health* 74:133, 1984.
33. Drake, D. The Irish immigrants' fever. *Boston Med Surg J* 37:149, 1847.
34. Davey, W. N. Arden House: The unfinished edifice. *Am Lung Assoc Bull* 68:18, March 1982.
35. Lillington, G. A. Cited in Eradication of tuberculosis is possible by end of next century. *Int Med News* 15:16, May 15–31, 1982.
36. Tuberculosis—United States, 1984. *MMWR* 33:299, 1985.
37. Davidson, P. M. Tuberculosis: New views of an old disease. *N Engl J Med* 312:1514, 1985.
38. Nelson, H. TB rate among Southeast Asians, Latinos in U.S. higher than average. *Los Angeles Times* I:17, May 16, 1982.
39. Mandatory tuberculosis examination for first-time school enterers in Los Angeles County. *Los Angeles County Department of Health Services Public Health Letter* 7:1, Feb 1985.
40. Alexander, W. J., Harden, J. W., Weeks, J. D., et al. Boosted tuberculin reactions among Cambodian refugees. *JAMA* 248:1177, 1982.
41. Morse, D. L., Hansen, R. E., Swalbach, W. G., et al. High rate of tuberculin conversion in Indochinese refugees. *JAMA* 248:2983, 1982.
42. Powell, K. E., Brown, E. D., and Farer, L. S. Tuberculosis among Indochinese refugees in the United States. *JAMA* 249:1455, 1983.
43. Wyler, D. J. Southeast Asian refugees and malaria. *N Engl J Med* 293:203, 1975.
44. Jones, M. J., Thompson, J. H., Jr., and Brewer, N. S. Infectious diseases of Indochinese refugees. *Mayo Clin Proc* 55:482, 1980.
45. Wiesenthal, A. M., Nickels, M. K., Hashimoto, K. G., et al. Intestinal parasites in a community of Laotians. *JAMA* 244:2543, 1980.
46. Health status of Indochinese refugees—1981. *Physician's Bull* (Orange County [CA] Health Care Agency) 32:1, March 1982.
47. Barry, M., Craft, J., Coleman, D., et al. Clinical findings in Southeast Asian refugees: Child development and public health concerns. *JAMA* 249:3200, 1983.

48. Catanzaro, A., and Moser, R. J. Health status of refugees from Vietnam, Laos, and Cambodia. *JAMA* 247:1303, 1982.
49. Goodman, R. A., and Sikes, R. K. Hepatitis B markers in Southeast Asian refugees. *JAMA* 251:2086, 1984.
50. Epidemic conjunctivitis among Indochinese refugees. *MMWR* 29:353, 1980.
51. Frank, J. A., Jr., Hoffman, R. E., Mann, J. M., et al. Imported measles: A potential control problem. *JAMA* 245:264, 1981.
52. Gonococcal infections among Indochinese refugees—Thailand. *MMWR* 30:355, 1981.
53. Erickson, R. V., and Hoang, G. N. Health problems among Indochinese refugees. *Am J Public Health* 70:1003, 1980.
54. Davis, J. M., Goldenring, J., McChesney, M., et al. Pregnancy outcomes of Indochinese refugees, Santa Clara County, California. *Am J Public Health* 72:742, 1982.
55. Sudden unexplained death syndrome in Southeast Asian refugees: A review of CDC surveillance. *MMWR* 36:43SS, 1987.
56. Mortality in Southeast Asian refugees. *Physician's Bull* (Orange County [CA] Health Care Agency) 33:[6], 1983.
57. Baron, R. C., Thacker, S. B., Gorelkin, L., et al. Sudden death among Southeast Asian refugees. *JAMA* 250:2947, 1983.
58. Kirchhoff, L. V., and Neva, F. A. Chagas' disease in Latin American immigrants. *JAMA* 254:3058, 1985.
59. Richards, F. O., Jr., Schantz, P. M., Ruiz-Tiben, E., et al. Cysticercosis in Los Angeles County. *JAMA* 254:3444, 1985.
60. *A Rational Approach to Radiodiagnostic Investigations.* Geneva: World Health Organization, 1983. P. 16.
61. Nguyen, D. Culture shock: A review of Vietnamese culture and its concepts of health and disease. *West J Med* 142:409, 1985.
62. Ortiz, J. S. The prevalence of intestinal parasites in Puerto Rican farm workers in western Massachusetts. *Am J Public Health* 70:1103, 1980.
63. Anderson, J. N. Health and illness in Pilipino immigrants. *West J Med* 139:811, 1983.
64. Lock, M. Japanese responses to social change: Making the strange familiar. *West J Med* 139:829, 1983.
65. Lipson, J. G., and Meleis, A. I. Issues in health care of Middle Eastern patients. *West J Med* 139:854, 1983.
66. Wheat, M. E., Brownstein, H., and Kvitash, V. Aspects of medical care of Soviet Jewish emigrés. *West J Med* 139:900, 1983.
67. Leprosy on rise in U.S., primarily in immigrants. *Skin Allergy News* 11:8, July 1980.
68. Dreyfuss, J. Leprosy rise in county laid to immigration. *Los Angeles Times* V:25, Oct 14, 1983.
69. Goldsmith, M. F. "Imported" leprosy in U.S. *JAMA* 251:18, 1984.
70. Health status of the Cuban refugees. *MMWR* 29:217, 1980; Follow-up on the health status of the Cuban refugees. *MMWR* 29:255, 1980 and 29:343, 1980.
71. Demmi, L., and Doxsey, K. Encountering the recent influx of Cuban refugees in the emergency department. *J Emerg Nurs* 7:11, 1981.
72. Opportunistic infections and Kaposi's sarcoma among Haitians in the United States. *MMWR* 31:353, 1982.
73. Pitchenik, A. E., Russell, B. W., Clery, T., et al. The prevalence of tuberculosis and drug resistance among Haitians. *N Engl J Med* 309:162, 1982.
74. Pawson, I. G., and Janes, C. Massive obesity in a migrant Samoan population. *Am J Public Health* 71:508, 1981.
75. Fitzpatrick-Nietschmann, J. Pacific Islanders: Migration and health. *West J Med* 139:848, 1983.
76. Tuberculosis Among Hispanics in the United States—1980. *MMWR* 31:237, 1982.
77. Maduro, R. *Curanderismo* and Latino views of disease and curing. *West J Med* 139:868, 1983.
78. Horwitz, N. "Cockroach asthma" confirmed in Chinese immigrants. *Med Trib* 23:29, July 28, 1982.
79. Lin, T. Y. Psychiatry and Chinese culture. *West J Med* 139:862, 1983.
80. King, H., Li, J. Y., Locke, F. B., et al. Patterns of site-specific displacement in cancer mortality among migrants: The Chinese in the United States. *Am J Public Health* 75:237, 1985.
81. Tabor, M. Uses and limitations of male/female data. *Occup Health Saf* 50:38, Nov 1981; *World Almanac and Book of Facts 1986.* New York: Newspaper Enterprise, 1985. P. 108.
82. The mother of invention. *Shield* (Phillips Petroleum Co) 8:26, 1st Quarter, 1983.
83. *World Almanac and Book of Facts 1986.* New York: Newspaper Enterprise, 1985. Pp. 327, 329.
84. Number of working mothers now at record levels. *NEWS*—U.S. Department of Labor, Bureau of Labor Statistics, Release 84-321, July 26, 1984.
85. Abbott, E. *Women in Industry: A Study in American Economic History.* New York: Appleton, 1916. Pp. 49–50.
86. Braybon, G. *Women Workers in the First World War: The British Experience.* London: Croom Helm, 1981. P. 113.
87. Andrews, I. O. Work and maternity. *Proc Int Conf Women Physicians* 2:116, 1920.
88. Sappington, C. O. *Health Problems of Women in Industry.* Med Series Bull No. VII. Pittsburgh, PA: Industrial Hygiene Foundation, 1944. Pp. 1, 36–37.
89. *Putting Women in Their Place: The Federal Women's Program.* Washington, DC: U.S. Office of Personnel Management, 1979. Pp. 16–18.
90. *NASA Medical Newsletter.* No. 72-1. Washington, DC: National Aeronautics and Space Administration, June 1972. P. 2.
91. 52 job titles revised to eliminate sex-stereotyping. *News*—U.S. Department of Labor, Release 73-542, Nov 9, 1973.
92. Women blue-collar labor: The numbers grow. *Occup Health Saf* 52:23, Feb 1983.

93. Offshore . . . A woman's world, too. *Phillips Shield* #II:11, 1977.
94. Women shipbuilders: Just doing a job. *Manpower* 7:10, March 1975.
95. Woman's work? Just about everything. *Texaco Star* 61:12, Spring 1974.
96. McPherson, A. "Constructing" recognition for female laborers. *Occup Health Saf* 49:68A, March 1980.
97. *Women at Work: A Chartbook*. Bull. 2168. Washington, DC: U.S. Department of Labor, Bureau of Labor Statistics, 1983.
98. *The Myth and the Reality*. Washington, DC: U.S. Department of Labor, Employment Standards Administration, Women's Bureau, 1974.
99. Facts and fictions about working women explored: Several stereotypes prove false in national study. *ISR Newsletter* (Institute for Social Research, University of Michigan) 1:4, Autumn 1972.
100. Gries, M. R. Overcoming male myths and taboos. *Occup Health Saf* 50:58, Sept 1981.
101. Lawrence, J. F. Comparable worth: Worthy bid for fairness. *Los Angeles Times* V:1, May 19, 1985.
102. Pozdena, R. S. Women's wages. *FRB SF Weekly Letter* (Federal Reserve Bank of San Francisco), June 1984. Pp. 1–3.
103. Stellman, J. M. *Women's Work, Women's Health: Myths and Realities*. New York: Pantheon, 1977. Table 26, p. 191.
104. *A Woman's Guide to Apprenticeship*. Pamphlet 17. Washington, DC: U.S. Department of Labor, Office of the Secretary, Women's Bureau, 1980. P. 22.
105. Stillman, N. G. The law in conflict: Accommodating equal employment and occupational health obligations. *J Occup Med* 21:599, 1979.
106. Messite, J. Cited in Many of 5,700 chemicals on NIOSH list may affect reproduction. *Int Med News* 17:45, Feb 1–14, 1984.
107. *RTECS* (Registry of Toxic Effects of Chemical Substances)—1981–82 Edition. Cincinnati, OH: U.S. Department of Health, Education, and Welfare, Public Health Service, Centers for Disease Control, National Institute for Occupational Safety and Health, June 1983.
108. Curran, W. J. Dangers for pregnant women in the work place. *N Engl J Med* 312:164, 1985.
109. Le Clercq, G. R. Workplace reproductive risk: Corporate responsibilities. *Ann Am Conf Ind Hyg* 4:49, 1983.
110. Council on Scientific Affairs of the American Medical Association. Effects of physical forces on the reproductive cycle. *JAMA* 251:247, 1984.
111. Council on Scientific Affairs of the American Medical Association. Effects of pregnancy on work performance. *JAMA* 251:1995, 1984.
112. Council on Scientific Affairs of the American Medical Association. Effects of toxic chemicals on the reproductive system. *JAMA* 253:3431, 1985.
113. *Guidelines on Pregnancy and Work*. Chicago: American College of Obstetricians and Gynecologists, 1977.
114. Watson, A. P., and White, C. L. Workplace injury experience of female coal miners in the United States. *Arch Environ Health* 39:284, 1984.
115. Rosenberg, J., and Stellman, J. M. Women's protective clothing: Trends in sizing, designs and availability. *Ind Saf Hyg News* 18:14, May 1984.
116. PPE for women. *Occup Health* [Schering] 6:3, May/June 1982.
117. Tabor, M. Women in coal mines: PPE, where are you? *Occup Health Saf* 51:22, Jan 1982.
118. Kaplan, M. C. Task and tool design: It's a "man's world." *Occup Health Saf* 50:29, Feb 1981.
119. Ibrahim, M. A. The changing health status of women. *Am J Public Health* 70:120, 1980.
120. Haynes, S. G., and Feinleib, M. Women, work and coronary heart disease: Prospective findings from the Framingham Heart Study. *Am J Public Health* 70:133, 1980.
121. Haynes, S. G., Eaker, E., and Feinlieb, M. Cited in Type A men said to be at increased CHD risk if wife employed. *Int Med News* 15:33, May 1–14, 1982.
122. Waldron, I., Herold, J., Dunn, D., et al. Reciprocal effects of health and labor force participation among women: Evidence from two longitudinal studies. *J Occup Med* 24:126, 1982.
123. Slaby, A. R. Cited in Working women have somewhat better C-V status. *Int Med News* 15:36, May 1–14, 1982.
124. Kangilaski, J. Wives who work [increase] their HDL levels. *JAMA* 249:694, 1983; Correction. *JAMA* 249:1250, 1983.
125. Scully, D. *Men Who Control Women's Health: The Miseducation of Obstetrician-Gynecologists*. Boston: Houghton Mifflin, 1980.
126. Ruzek, S. B. How seriously are women's presenting symptoms taken? *Mobius* 1:66, 1981.
127. Crull, P., and Cohen, M. Expanding the definition of sexual harassment. *Occup Health Nurs* 32:141, 1984.
128. Mendelson, R. Sexual harassment. *Occup Health Nurs* 31:47, Nov 1983.
129. Sexual Harassment Guidelines. In *Time of Change: 1983 Handbook on Women Workers*. Washington, DC: U.S. Department of Labor, Office of the Secretary, Women's Bureau, 1983. P. 147.
129. *Information About . . . Women's Occupational Health Resource Center*. New York: The Center, [n.d.].
130. *United Nations Decade for Women, 1976–1985: Employment in the United States*. Report for the World Conference on the United Nations Decade for Women 1976–1985. Washington, DC: U.S. Department of Labor, Office of the Secretary, Women's Bureau, 1985. Pp. 65–69.
131. Blumenfeld, [N. I.], and Menkes, H. Cited in Differences between impairment, disability underscored. *Int Med News* 16:48, July 1–14, 1983.
132. Rehabilitation in the private sector. *J Rehabil*, July/Aug/Sept 1979.
133. Rehabilitation Xperts, 5271 Heil Avenue, Huntington Beach, CA 92649.

134. Ashton, P. C. Rehabilitation in a major corporate setting. *J Rehabil* 45:26, Jul/Aug/Sept 1979.
135. Haraguchi, K. L. Return-to-work programs: Emphasizing the positive. *Occup Health Saf* 51:20, Oct 1982.
136. Vocational rehabilitation activity showed steady and substantial growth during the past three years. *Calif Workers' Compens Instit Bull* 83-5, May 4, 1983.
137. Berkeley Planning Associates. *A Study of Accommodations Provided to Handicapped Employees by Federal Contractors: Executive Summary.* Prepared for U.S. Department of Labor, Employment Standards Administration. Berkeley, CA: Berkeley Planning Associates, 1982.
138. Bowe, F. Intercompany action to adapt jobs for the handicapped. *Harvard Bus Rev* 63:166, 1985.
139. *Equal to the Task: 1981 Du Pont Survey of Employment of the Handicapped.* Wilmington, DE: du Pont de Nemours, 1982.
140. Classification of impairment, by type and site. *Vital Health Stat* [10], No. 99, 1975. Pp. 51–56.
141. Cote, R. A. (Ed.). Developmental Malformation and Abnormal Product of Conception. In *SNOMED: Systematized Nomenclature of Medicine* (2nd ed.). Skokie, IL: College of American Pathologists, 1979. Sec. 2, pp. 121–133.
142. Kruger, L. M. International Terminology for the Classification of Congenital Limb Deficiencies. In American Academy of Orthopedic Surgeons, *Atlas of Limb Prosthetics*. St. Louis: Mosby, 1981. Pp. 501–517.
143. Manus, G. I. Is your language *disabling*? *J Rehabil* 41:35, Sept-Oct 1975.
144. *Language Guide on Disability.* Sacramento, CA: Governor's Committee on Employment of the Handicapped, 1984.
145. Boland, J. M. 1975–1980: Five long years or five short years? *J Rehabil* 46:40, Oct-Nov-Dec 1980.
146. "Able-disabled" congressmen cited. *Programs for the Handicapped* 5:14, Sept-Oct 1982.
147. Russell, H., and Rosen, V. *Victory in My Hands.* New York: Creative Age, 1949. P. 280.

18. DESIGN OF OCCUPATIONAL HEALTH FACILITIES

In Architecture as in all other Operative Arts, the end must direct the Operation. The end is to build well. Well building hath three Conditions. Commodity, Firmness, and Delight.

Sir Henry Wotton

In planning the physical plant of an occupational health service (OHS), it must be remembered that the facility is one in which the staff members spend their 8 workday hours and that it is an organizational unit to which employees come voluntarily for care or are directed to by surveillance mandates. The environment of a medical component can determine, to some degree, the progress that can be made by an employee/patient proceeding through a postillness or injury convalescence and the feeling that the worker has toward the employer. An attractive care setting can exude warmth and welcome without necessarily having to be ornate or demonstrative of the latest in chic interiors.

An OHS must be functional, but also it must be esthetically appealing and free from the prototypical or traditional look of the hospital.* Medical services in industry have changed since the early years of white walls and ceramic-tiled floors. Comfortable upholstered furniture has replaced the former wood benches of the clinic waiting room, and plantings and graphic art have helped to alter the frequent sterility of both consulting and treatment areas.

*Malkin [1] described the health care facility in these terms: "A critical look at our clinics, hospitals, and medical offices reveals that they are designed for ease of maintenance rather than human comfort. They seem resistant to human imprint—a definition of an institutional environment. The architecture, instead of embracing and welcoming inhabitants, seems to alienate and intimidate them. Hospitals, in particular, seem to be designed as a show of strength, fortresses against disease, which dwarf the individual and place him or her in a caste system in which the doctors and nurses are the ruling class and the patient or visitor is the serf. The language of the hospital is foreign to most people. They do not understand where to go or how to get there, and they need an interpreter to decode the medical jargon whispered all around them. It is not unlike a visit to a foreign country—nothing is familiar. The signage system in many hospitals is so inadequate and confusing that it only adds to the patient's or visitor's frustration and feeling of helplessness. It reduces the patient to a child who has to continually ask questions and beg for assistance."

As every contact with an OHS should be therapeutic, one avoids counterproductive elements in the design or decor of a unit devoted to highly personalized professional attention.

CONSTRAINTS

There are certain primary limitations present. The ideal space is not always available for the installation of an OHS, and managers are not universally convinced that the capital investment in a workable medical facility will be cost-effective. Often there is a "make-do" philosophy, and the area assigned for the development of the unit will be space not utilizable by the company in its operational scheme.

Planning the physical plant of the OHS cannot be undertaken with the complacent ease derived from previous design experience. One does not always know if there will be a vacant space available for a separate building or if management visualized conversion to a dispensary of an unused corner of an old shop. The kinds of areas adaptable to a new facility come in this variety of packaging: a separate building on unoccupied land, an addition to an existing building, a wing on a multiwing structure, conversion of a bay or two in a presently used manufacturing area, conversion of a set of vacated or to-be-vacated offices in the administration building, a partial or complete floor in an urban high-rise structure, and conversion of a World War II or older "temporary" building.* Because of this spectrum of starting points, one cannot always come in with an ideal

*One should be steeled against all possible suggestions or offers of space and buildings. The author had the provocative opportunity to test latent design skills when he was offered a building erected during the American Civil War for conversion to a dispensary that had to be "ultramodern," and that was an order.

plan—ideal as to orientation, size, location, adaptability, or accessibility. Great compromises have to be made. Nevertheless, some basic principles can be established and fought for to a degree proportionate to one's own strength.

Fulton [2] has listed the considerations needed in planning a department: (1) number of persons to be served, (2) number of shifts and number of employees working on each shift, (3) the scope and type of health care services to be rendered, (4) the character of the employees' occupations (and exposures), (5) the general layout of buildings and working areas, and (6) the policies of the management. Only with this information on hand can the initial design be conceived.

THE SITE

It is hoped that the medical unit will be as central as possible to the majority of employees. A numerical imbalance between white- and blue-collar workers, large buildings with automated processes and few workers, and the limitations of tall metropolitan buildings may negate this ideal placement. It is extremely convenient to be close to the employment function in the personnel department, yet this location may entail a long distance for the incumbent worker to come who has been injured at a far point. The most quiet area in the plant might be too removed from both the concentration of workers and the personnel office. As Pringle put it pithily some years back [3], "The ambulance room must, of course, be on the ground level, and be easily accessible to wheeled traffic. It is of no use having a beautifully appointed room, perched like an eyrie on a top floor, to which no stretcher can be taken, and from which nothing short of a helicopter will remove an unconscious patient, or stuck, like a jewel in a toad's head, right in the middle of a plant."

If centrality is sought, it must be determined that there will be no ingress to workers desiring to use the department as a passageway. A large medical department was designed and built in a new, attractive, huge nonmanufacturing structure, blocking, at either end of its area, two long corridors. It was anticipated that no one but patients would enter and leave through the two pairs of doors. Shortly after its opening, the dispensary portions of the corridors joined those of the remainder of the floor to become a continuum for heavy traffic on either side of the health service.

The orientation is of importance also because of the economy of heating and cooling. If a separate building is being planned, the climate will determine the siting of the structure. The least costly both to heat and to cool is a building with its long axis running east and west, with its major windows on the south. However, in the northern and colder regions, the building should be almost square, with the longer axis not over one and one-half times the shorter axis. In a temperate climate, to obtain optimum climatic effects, the building length should be one and one-half times its width and certainly not more than two and one-half times. Further, the long axis should not be more than 25 to 30 degrees off the east-west direction. If the structure is not air-conditioned, it should be placed to take advantage of the prevailing and local breezes for summer cooling. In the Southeast's hot and humid climate, the building should be oriented only with its major exposure a southern one, and the north-south/east-west ratio should be at least 1:1.5, with a desirable maximum of 1:3. This placement has the least cooling load in summer and a desirable winter heat gain. The heat and aridity of the Southwest require a nearly square building, and it should be located to block or slow the winds. The east-west axis should be long and preferably not more than one and one-half times the shorter one [4].

The only other factors germane to the site include access to adequate light and ventilation if the facility is being housed in a larger building and allowance for expansion if the plant population were to increase in size.

SIZE

Before considering the design, a brief note of space needs is in order. This factor is difficult to determine, for one usually is governed more by space available than that required. Fulton's writings and those of others should be consulted before planning [5–13]. Shepard [14] gives as a rough estimate 175 square feet for 200 employees and 300 square feet for 500 employees. Also he offers, as does McCahan [15], the estimate of 1 square foot of dispensary per employee up to 1000 employees (and this figure probably should include a minimum of 300 square feet). This level will be increased by the variabilities in programming, by the nature and variety of occupational health hazards present, the frequency of serious injuries, and the greater understanding of occupational health objectives by managers.

CONFIGURATION

Whether the OHS has its own building or is placed within a larger structure, any one of a variety of in-

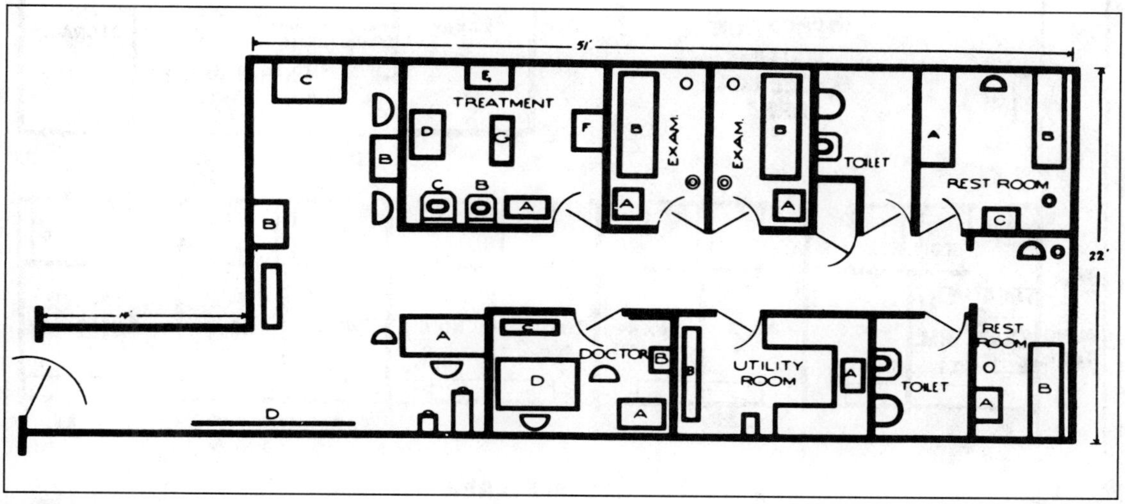

FIGURE 18-1. *Floor plan for medium-size occupational health service, exemplary of the single-corridor design. Waiting room: A. desk; B. table; C. couch; D. health literature rack. Doctor's office: A. files; B. cabinet; C. bookshelves; D. desk. Examination rooms: A. cabinet; B. examination table. Treatment room: A. cabinet; B. treatment sink; C. foot tub; D. utility table; E. cabinet; F. treatment chair; G. treatment table.*

terior layouts would be equally applicable. Simplest is the linear pattern, with individual rooms opening onto a long middle corridor. This plan would fit a single rectangular building or, for example, a long single-corridor wing along with other wings attached to the administration building. The advantage is simplicity in design, and there can be integrated into the arrangement of the rooms the concept of orderly work flow. A disadvantage is the total amount of walking that staff members have to do to see all patients or render all services. This activity has been given the approbrious title of "bunion derby." An example of this configuration is seen in Figure 18-1.

Variations of this single-line pattern are executed in the L-shaped and C-shaped structures. A good feature of either of these configurations is the opportunity of using the junction of the two corridors as the entrance and reception area, which by having a more central record area at a corner minimizes the distance to be traversed by the employee-patient and by the staff. Other designs are based on the T, H, closed H (joining the ends), X, or even the Greek cross configuration.

Most frequently, though, physicians are given an open area, and they then have to fit the needed facilities into the square footage available. This constraint necessitates inside corridors and inside work areas, which, with adequate ventilation and illumination, present no difficulties except to the rare claustrophobe.

Schowalter and Davis [17] have established as their goal in the design of medical units the provision of the following:

1. Patient-oriented facilities to allow bringing most services to the patient, rather than the patient to the services.
2. Privacy for the patient during examination and treatment.
3. Efficient use of medical equipment and floor space.

Meeting these objectives, the layout concept was carried out in the form of three primary functional areas, as seen in Figure 18-2:

1. Reception, waiting, and clerical area
2. Treatment and examination rooms
3. Medical staff areas and associated service rooms

Examples of various layouts are shown in Figures 18-3 to 18-5, from the smallest unit to one that can provide adequate medical services to a plant of many thousands of workers. While exact duplication may not be indicated, a scan of the floor plans may generate ideas for local replication of one or more modules. It must be mentioned that not all of the facilities illustrated are current. Some have undergone modification, others total change, because of altered needs, moves of headquarters, change of mission, or enlargement or deemphasis of the occupational health program. All of the physical layouts shown, however, were used at one time or another, and some are in current use.

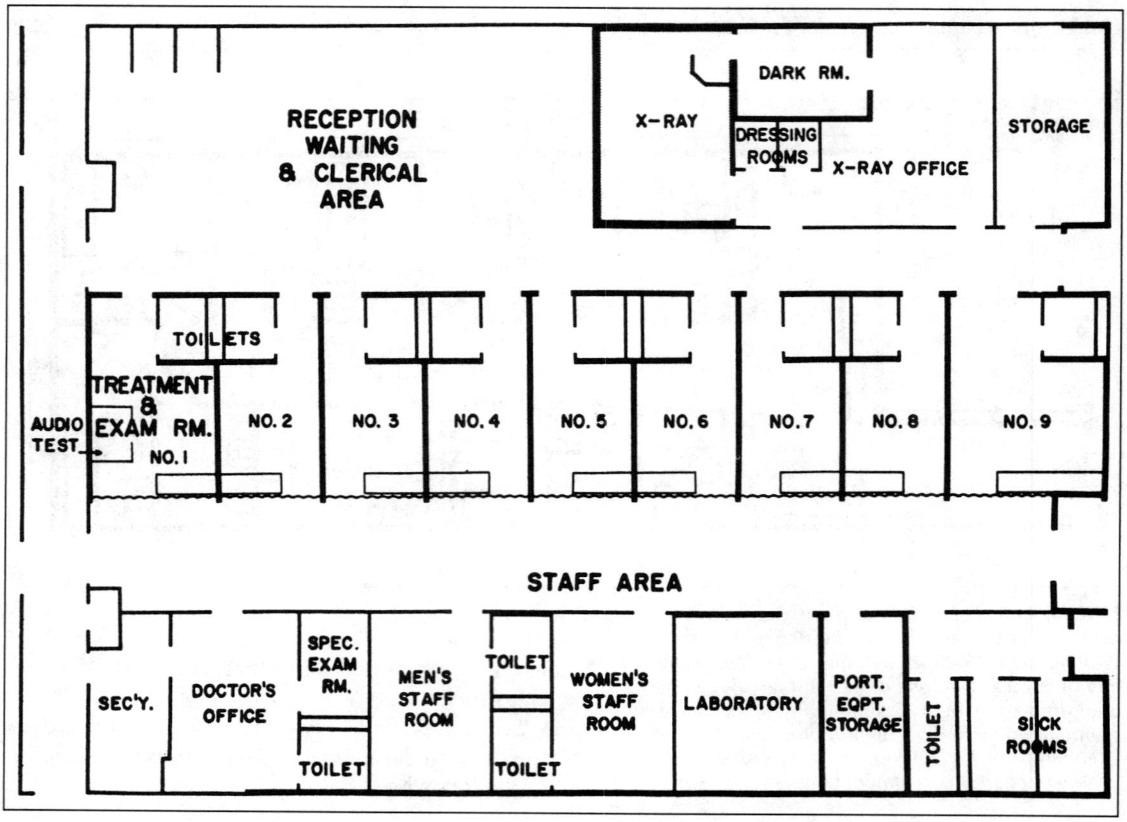

FIGURE 18-2. *Floor plan for occupational health service (72 × 96 ft) that served a workforce of approximately 7,000 at the Kansas City Works of the Western Electric Company. Three functional areas are delineated. (Reproduced with permission from Schowalter and Davis [17].)*

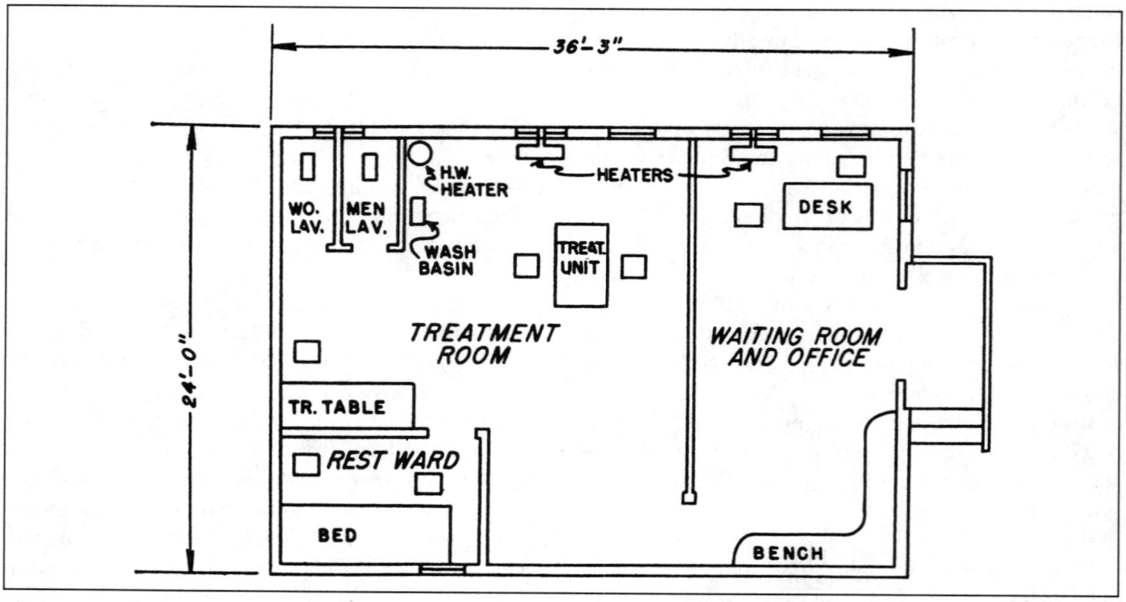

FIGURE 18-3. *Floor plan for small occupational health service of the type used by a single occupational health nurse.*

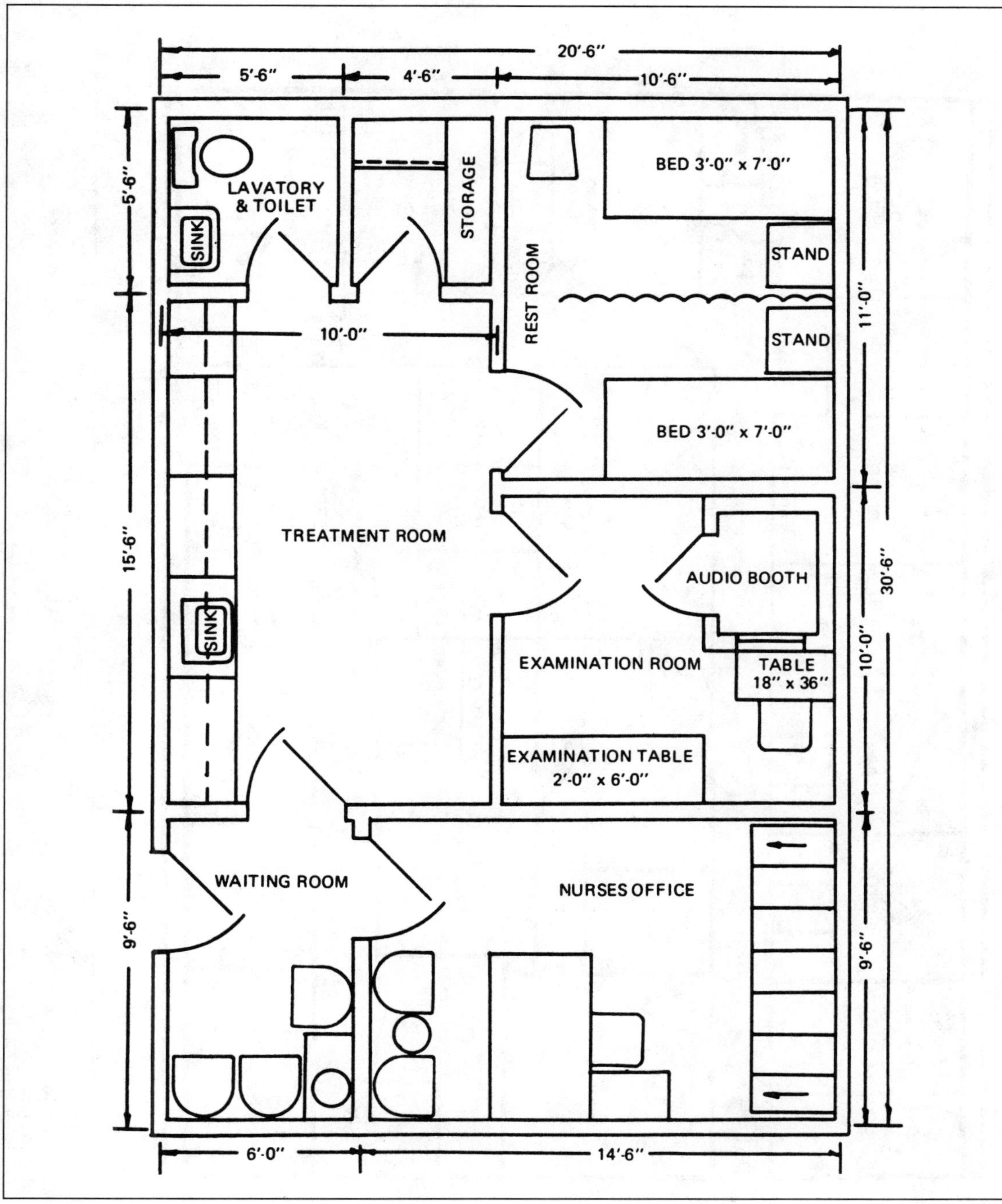

FIGURE 18-4. *Floor plan for occupational health service, 600 square feet, of a plant of 500 to 800 employees. (Reproduced with permission from Employers Insurance of Wausau.)*

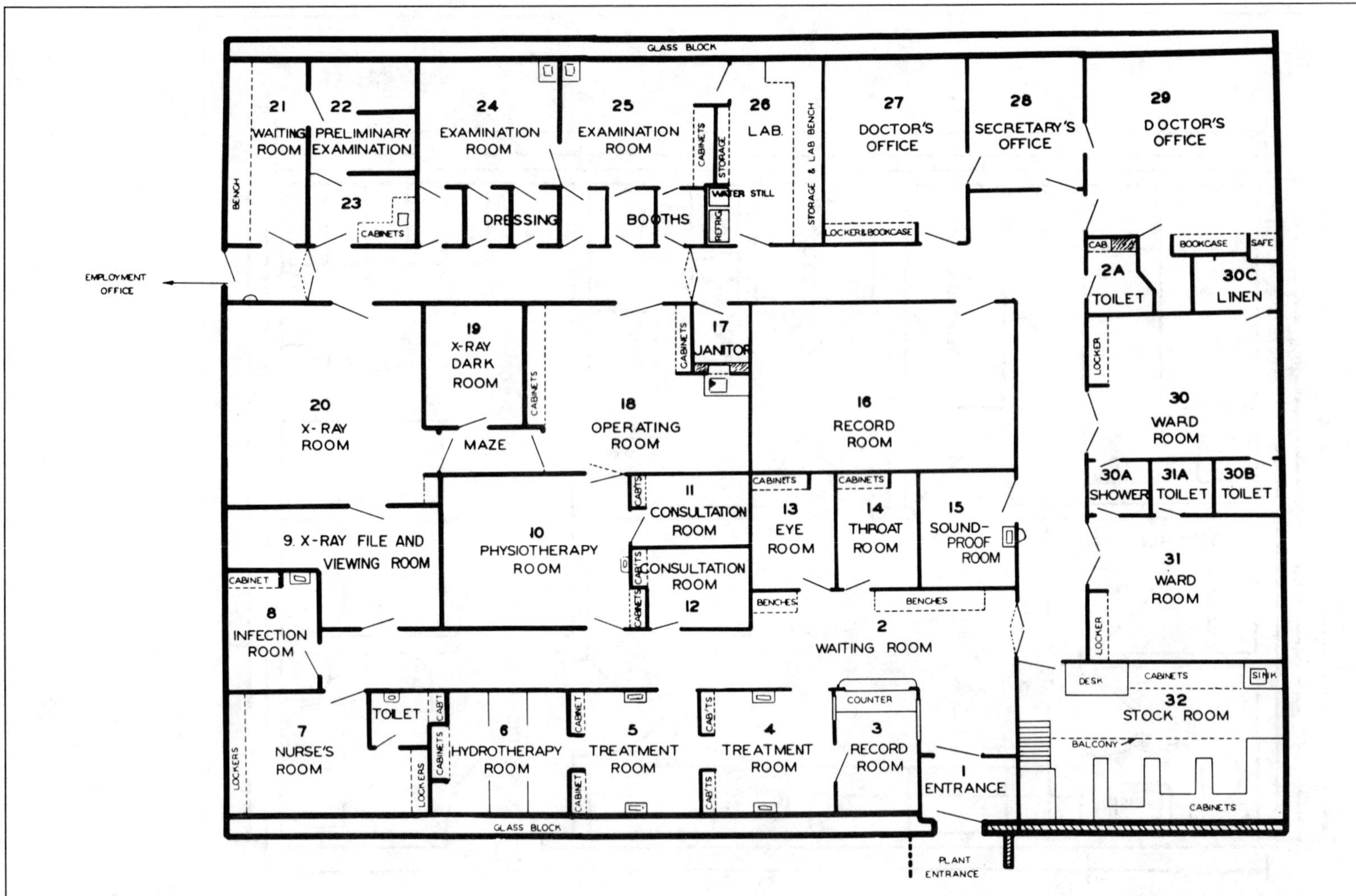

FIGURE 18-5. *Floor plan for occupational health service of a large company. The plan shows the separation of applicants for employment from employees requiring treatment. (Reproduced with permission from Irvin [9].)*

COMPONENT AREAS

The facilities of an OHS can be divided into a few broad classifications of functions. These elements are listed, with their constituent areas, to point up the kinds of activities and services rendered in many installations [18]. To be sure, not every unit will require space devoted to each of these functions, but all are listed to offer a check or reminder list to those professionals who, for the first time, are exploring the physical needs of a medical program.

RECEPTION OF EMPLOYEE-PATIENTS
Entrance foyer or vestibule
Waiting room
Reception deck

DOCUMENTATION OF SERVICES
Medical records room
Stenographic and clerical office
Document duplication room
Medical photographic unit
Computer facility

DIAGNOSTIC SERVICES
Consultation rooms
Examination rooms
Nurses' interview rooms
Audiometry booth(s) or room(s)
Vision testing room
Clinical laboratory
Electrocardiography room
Radiation monitoring room
Radiology office, viewing room, and file room
Radiographic examination room(s)
Radiology processing room
Special examination rooms (sigmoidoscopy or coloscopy, proctoscopy, gynecology)
Occupational hygiene laboratory

TREATMENT SERVICES
Major treatment room
Minor treatment rooms or cubicles
Clean emergency surgery room
Physical therapy room and cubicles
Counseling office(s) including EAP offices
Rest ward
Pharmacy or pharmacy storage
Occupational ophthalmic (optometric) service
Personnel decontamination unit with shower and entry and exit locks
Ambulance parking and transfer area

STAFF FUNCTIONS
Physicians' offices
Epidemiologist's offices
Secretarial and clerical offices
Medical library
Conference room
Equipment and supplies storage room
Custodial work and storage room
Staff lounge, change rooms, washing and toilet facilities
Sterilization and preparation room and linen stores
Occupational hygienist's office and staff offices
Chief nurse's office
Health educator's office
Health education preparation, stores, and display areas
Instrument room
Supply storage area

PATIENT'S FUNCTIONS
Washing and toilet facilities
Dressing booths (physical examination)
Dressing booths (radiology)
Specimen collection booths

SPECIAL PROGRAM FACILITIES
Dental hygiene unit
Podiatry unit
Toxicologist's office
Toxicologist's laboratory
Employee-patients' health library
Sanitarian's office

DESIGN CONSIDERATIONS

It must be remembered that in occupational medical programs there are variations in the services offered. Infrequently, complete care will be given through a prepaid plan, or rarely, because of geographic isolation, dependents of workers also will be served. Obviously, if the program includes dependent clientele, additional facilities will be needed, such as pediatric examination rooms, children's waiting room, a complete radiographic service, enlarged pharmacy stores, a greater gynecologic examination capability, and possibly an office for family planning. Special program activities will be carried out as determined by the presence of unusual health hazards, the existence of peculiarities in the work environment, specific ethnomedical factors in the workers, local cultural necessity, the age of the employees, or socioeconomic level of the workers.

Designers differ in their planning considerations,

and an observer cannot render judgment as to the correctness or incorrectness of a particular floor plan. Some medical directors separate examination facilities from areas devoted to treatment. The rationale is that it might be demoralizing for new employees who are awaiting examination to see the industrially injured being brought in for care. Other physicians feel that there must be a sharp division in the facilities established for male employees and those used by women. This kind of false schism is not followed in the offices of physicians in the community, and even in the suites of urologists and radiologists, both genders are given care, with appropriate attention to privacy where needed. Duplication of facilities is not indicated or practical.

It is advisable that there be a separate ambulance entrance, for patients just injured or suddenly felled by a cardiac event or cerebrovascular episode should not be wheeled by employees who are waiting to receive care. Not only is such a procedure upsetting to other patients, but also it can affect the attitudes of staff members attending to them.

Some OHSs have a single, common waiting room where all waiting patients are assembled. Such a setup can give the feeling of the casting activities, or "cattle calls," of Hollywood and can be extremely depersonalizing. If space and budget permit, smaller waiting rooms adjacent to the OHS sections to be visited are preferred.

SOME DESIGN APHORISMS

A department that is colorful and attractive without being ostentatious contributes to the value of the treatment.

Do not be afraid to "open up" the unit: Have open counters in place of windows in reception areas; remove a wall and put in a desk-high partition in front of a clerical area to make the dispensary seem larger and airier.

Use the necessary number of directional and identifying location signs, but do not use colored lines on the floor; they are redolent of the early days of the European immigration waves when few spoke or read English.

Give the custodians adequate room to store their supplies and clean work equipment.

A major treatment room can serve both men and women employees without breach of privacy; if privacy is needed, minor treatment rooms or dressing cubicles can be used.

A single rest ward with adequate cubicle curtaining around the beds precludes the cost of two such facilities (one for men and one for women).

Have a writing facility, small desk, or wall-affixed stand-up desk in every room where patients are examined or treated. This addition encourages prompt staff notations in the clinical records.

A common conference room (frequent euphemistic for coffee or lunch room) is better than one for nurses or physicians and one for other staff members; it permits continuous communication on an informal basis.

Keep the clean surgery clean, permitting no traffic, storage of unrelated items, or "dirty" surgical conditions.

If radioactive materials are used in quantity or at high levels by the company, maintain a decontamination unit.

If possible, have an emergency treatment room that can accept workers with occupational soiling and that provides immediate ingress from an ambulance; through appropriate ascending or descending ramping, the floor levels of the ambulance and the dispensary can be even.

Identify clearly the entrance to the OHS, and do not label it "First Aid" unless first-aid attendants only are on duty, as they are in many installations in Canada; further, do not confront entering employees with a puzzle of doors or windows, but let them read immediately where to report, for that moment is not the time for intelligence testing.

Always provide seating for employee-patients in treatment areas, so none need be treated while standing; fainting is frequent, even in the stalwart.

If counseling is carried on, be sure there is privacy. Single walls, without the thickness provided by studs, transmit rather than absorb sound; use acoustic tile and drapes, if necessary; some opaquing of window glass should be carried out, at least to eye level.

Whenever possible, use built-in cabinetry or other space-saving designs [19].

Provide locks on all storage areas of controlled drug items, maintain active inventories, and conduct frequent audits.

If there is emphasis on employment of the physically disabled, make sure that all wheelchair and crutch-using employees have a level floor or ramp ingress to the medical unit.

Do not place consultation or counseling rooms next to restrooms where the cacophony of sanitary-fixture flushing can break the spell of a developing rapport between counselor and employee.

Provide water coolers so that cold water can be used for the administration of oral medications in the OHS.

Establish several exits from the medical department,

and even though not always used, keep them accessible and clear.

Apply acoustic control to all noisy office machines.

Personalize the physician's or nurse's office.*

If consultation or interview rooms are small, they can be given depth through use of mirrored walls.

COLOR IN THE MEDICAL FACILITIES

As indicated previously, the OHS should be as pleasing a unit as possible for employees to visit. Decades ago, various colors made their entry, as they did in the coding of machinery, service lines, and hazardous areas. Colors can stimulate, depress, or do nothing at all. Light colors can, with appropriate assists by illumination, brighten interiors.

Certain colors should be avoided in an OHS. For example, primary colors can be too startling in an examination or treatment facility. Combinations of muted colors are restful, as is a succession of shades of a single color. The baseboard can carry the darkest shade, the wainscot or dado area a lighter shade, the remainder of the wall still lighter, and the ceiling the lightest shade of all or off-white. Rooms with an abundance of natural light can be painted with a shade of less reflectance value than a room with average natural light.

Lighter colors, apart from creating a more cheerful environment, invite cleaning more often. A semigloss surface on the wainscot will facilitate soil removal. Areas subject to considerable usage, such as doors, corridor walls, or chairs for patients whose work clothing carries considerable occupational soilage should be covered with a full-gloss surfacing to allow easier cleaning. Metal or ceramic tile on the walls will meet this need without requiring replacement or repainting.

Sinks and splashboards should be of stainless steel. While costly at the time of initial installation, the material is long-lasting in appearance and durability unless treated inadvertently with corrosives.

Flooring can present problems in choice. Whereas terrazzo has been used and is attractive, it can crack and fill with dirt. Asphalt tile gives some resilience, can be polished, and is available in a variety of colors. Such flooring can be polished with a revolving brush and fine steel wool so that wax, which produces a slippery surface, need not be used. Carpeting has proved impractical in treatment areas for it soon begins to show the polychromatic tattoo resulting from spillage of various liquid therapeutic preparations.

Drapes or curtains are more readily cleaned than venetian or even mini-blinds, and the use of glass-fiber fabric will allow extended use without necessitating cleaning. Frosted glass will provide the privacy needed in consulting or examining rooms, unless the OHS is in an isolated high-rise building where viewing of the activities is not possible. Even with visibility not possible in upper levels, certain patients still appreciate the concealment afforded by the treated glass, without having to occlude the light by closing the curtains or drapes.

CIRCULAR, WHEELSPOKE, AND CLUSTER DESIGNS

While not common to in-plant health service facilities, other designs are feasible and either have been suggested for or actually have been incorporated into contemporary buildings. It has been indicated that the rectangular dispensary building with the single control linear corridor demands considerable travel on the part of both the patient and the staff. To avert this time- and energy-demanding pattern, architects have devised the circular building, with a nurses' station at the hub and with rooms fitted between walls radiating from the central axis to the periphery of the structure. In the Scott and White Memorial Hospital opened in Temple, Texas, in 1964, three 8-sided towers in a clover-leaf arrangement characterized the building [20]. Nurse stations were placed in the center of the octagonal floors of each of the towers so that the staff members were within a few steps and equidistant from each patient's door (Fig. 18-6).

A somewhat similar idea was incorporated into an honorably mentioned architectural submission for a hospital [21]. The jury deemed the design "one of the most unusual and imaginative schemes submitted." The pattern differed from the Texas institution in that each of the four floors and basement had certain hospital functions (for example, records, radiology, utilities) in one circle surrounding a central well, while in a second outer circle there were placed patients' rooms, surgical and maternity suites, and staff locker rooms, among other facilities. A corridor circled the entire building between the inner and outer rings on two of the floors.

A variation of these building themes is seen in Figure 18-7, wherein the physician/staff corridors and

*Malkin [1] makes this observation: "The consultation room . . . should contain the doctor's personal memorabilia. Such items help the patient to see the doctor as a person with a family, hobbies, and interests outside of medicine. This reassures the patient that the doctor is a real person, not just a white coat with the stethoscope around the neck."

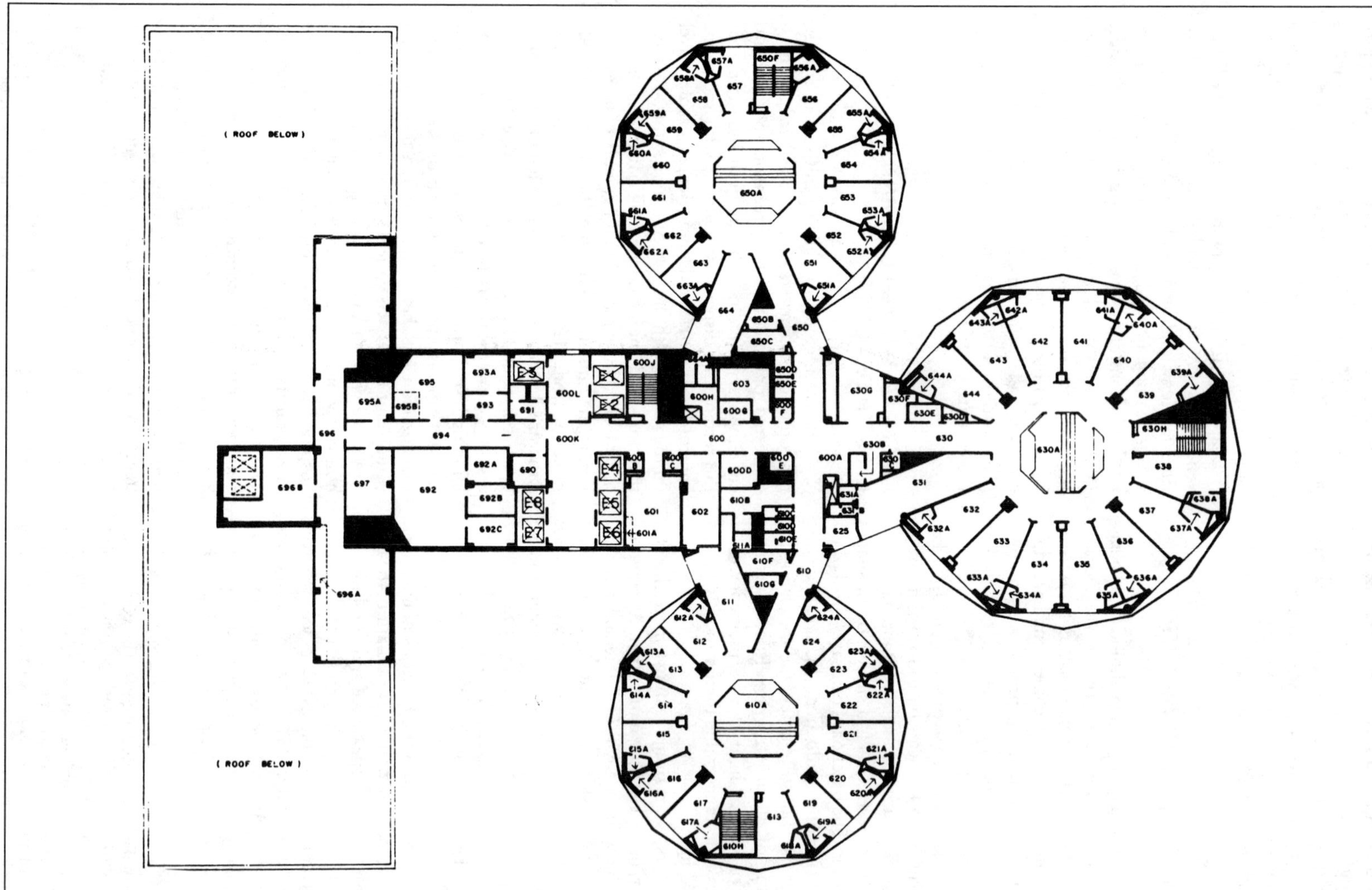

FIGURE 18-6. *Plan of the Hospital and Clinic Building, 6th floor, Scott and White Memorial Hospital, Temple, Texas; showing the 8-sided towers with centrally placed nursing stations. The concept can be adapted to the design of an OHS. (Reproduced with permission from the Scott and White Memorial Hospital. Courtesy of Donald W. Nelson.)*

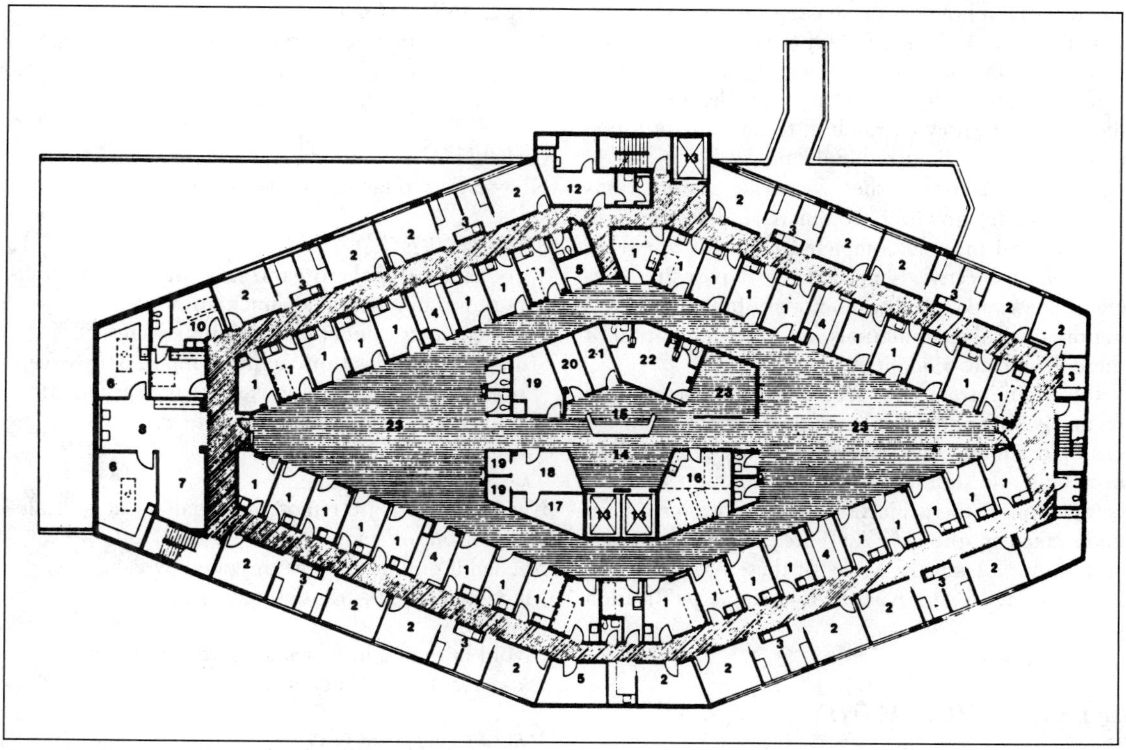

FIGURE 18-7. *Floor plan of the Miller Clinic of Nashville, Tennessee, showing the second floor and separate physician/staff and patient corridor. 1. Treatment room; 2. physician's office; 3. nurse's station; 4. clerk's station; 5. storage; 6. examination room; 7. recovery; 8. scrub/work area; 9. endoscopy room; 10. cystoscopy room; 11. closet; 12. physician's lounge; 13. elevator; 14. elevator lobby; 15. reception desk; 16. electrocardiography; 17. office; 18. patient education; 19. interview room; 20. audiometry; 21. vision testing; 22. specimen collection; 23. waiting area. (Reproduced with permission from* Hospitals *[31].)*

patient corridors are separate. A surgical area is at the end of one axis, and certain test facilities are located in a core unit, central to the entire facility. Expansion, when needed, will be carried vertically [22].

The reason for mentioning these concepts in design is that the principle can be extrapolated readily to an OHS. Records, clerical support, the clinical laboratory, and the like could be located centrally in a round building, and waiting areas, offices, examination rooms, library, health education, and like functions could be placed in the suites coursing circumferentially about the core. Rooms requiring considerable natural light would have it, and patients and staff would have a minimal distance to travel between functional units.

The author suggested in an earlier writing [23] the pentagonal design of an OHS, with a central record control unit at the core of the building and with five radiating wings coming off the 10-sided structure. Each wing accommodated a subset of related functions, and at three points on the periphery between outgoing spokes, there would be located wing secretaries. While nearly all patient-related activities were placed on the first level, a second floor provided locker/change room, conference room, child care, and medical director's and nutritionist's office space. Again, considerable natural lighting was provided, and the lengthy linear walk of the standardized dispensary building was avoided.

MOBILE UNITS

Some companies, in the past, have brought examination facilities to workers in the field at sites where it was infeasible for the employer to have a fixed health service station. This mode of care has been utilized in the petroleum industry in the United States [24,25], in the deserts of the Middle East [26], and as freestanding examination facilities brought to an employed population by a private medical enterprise [27]. A mobile unit has been designed for on-site pulmonary function testing [28], and commercial firms, particularly following the passage of the Occupational Safety and Health Act 1970, have offered either multitest screening or hearing or vision conservation services to industry nationwide. As most of these units are now extramural to an in-plant OHS, they will not be discussed in detail.

If an organization wishes to provide examinations in this mode, however, commercial designers and builders will provide completed units for whatever functional objective is needed, be it industrial hygiene, chest radiography, pulmonary functional evaluation, clinical examinations, or any combination of these diagnostic modalities.*

In certain instances where the work objective is of relatively short duration, construction of a dam for example, mobile units providing medical care have been built and stationed at the construction site until completion of the project. Such activities have been undertaken by the U.S. Air Force, by trade unions, and at music festivals. Many of these programs and facilities have been reviewed in a single publication [29].

THE COMPUTER FACILITY

Not shown in most of the designs depicted is the computer facility caring for occupational health and hygiene statistical and analytical data. In many of the contemporary medical departments, the function will be associated with the medical records section or the section on epidemiology. Certain design features must be observed if computers, word-processing equipment, or other new automated units are added to the OHS.

The checklist described by Eischen [30] includes the following categories for consideration in planning for a data processing activity.

OFFICE SPACE

Central computer configuration
- Computer's processor.
- Storage medium, usually a disk, possibly also a tape.
- Printer (usually stands alone).

Work stations, or CRTs.

ELECTRICITY

Determine voltage requirements.
Determine amperage requirements.
Regulator, if building subject to power surges.

*For example, Medical Coaches, Inc., Box 129, Oneonta, NY 13820-0129; Calumet Coach Company, 135 East 115th Street, Chicago, IL 60629.

AIR CONDITIONING

Temperature requirement: 60 to 80°F. (A basic rule—the computer can tolerate the same ambient temperature tolerated by the operator.)

CARPETING

Non-static-producing, to avoid paper jams.

FURNITURE

Work tables (for the organization of computer output and supporting documentation).
Filing cabinets (binder-held computer output).
Storage receptacles (for computer input, daily exceptions, and error conditions requiring special attention—may be in-bins or desktops).

TELEPHONE LINES

Needed if there are remote terminals—out of building or out of state.
Needed if on-line support provided by vendor.
Modems needed—translating devices—for each terminal.
(Avoid lines tied into switchboard, or one with even *one* extension—line must be separate.)

INSTALLATION DAY

The responsible person prepares the following:

Logs of material on disk files, material saved on backup media, files needed for various reports, and daily computer tools.
Schedule of daily/weekly activity.
Prepare a backup person.
Day before, check all items and supplies.
On day of arrival, check out diagnostic tests for individual components as well as integrated system.
Training of responsible person.

EXERCISE FACILITY

With the increase in wellness programs, some OHSs have added and equipped special exercise facilities. A few companies have added indoor or rooftop tracks in addition to exercise equipment. Such installations will require men's and women's locker, shower, and dressing room areas.

REFERENCES

1. Malkin, J. *The Design of Medical and Dental Facilities*. New York: Van Nostrand Reinhold, 1982.

2. Fulton, W. J. Medical department layout and design: The principles underlying industrial medical department planning, and their functional application. *Ind Med Surg* 27:1, 1958.
3. Pringle, P. The ambulance room in a small factory. *Practitioner* 169:173, 1952.
4. Physical factors in building a medical unit. *JAMA* 160:233, 1956.
5. Fulton, W. J. Medical department layout and design: Editing a proposed plan. *Ind Med Surg* 27:85, 1958.
6. Fulton, W. J. Reconstruction of the proposed plan. *Ind Med Surg* 27:179, 1958.
7. Fulton, W. J. Medium to smallest size medical departments. *Ind Med Surg* 27:333.
8. Bissonette, G. B. Planning for medium-sized medical department. *Am Assoc Ind Nurs J* 5:11, Feb 1957.
9. Irvin, E. A. Hospital layout saves time for patients and doctor. *Factory Management Maint* 105:123, 1947.
10. MacDiarmid, R. Planning a health center. *Med Bull* (Standard Oil of New Jersey) 15:96, 1955. Reprinted in *Ind Med Surg* 24:541, 1955.
11. Martin, C. E. A 500-employee medical department layout. *Ind Med Surg* 18:145, 1949.
12. Medical service in industry: Industrial medical department. *JAMA* 117:34, 1941.
13. O'Leary, D. J. Planning and equipping a large medical unit. *Am Assoc Ind Nurs J* 5:5, Feb 1957.
14. Shepard, W. P. *The Physician in Industry.* New York: McGraw-Hill, 1961.
15. McCahan, J. S. How to plan your medical department. *Mill Factory* 62:113, 1958.
16. *Operating Procedures for Industrial Dispensaries.* Army Service Forces Manual M210. Washington, DC: Headquarters, Army Service Forces, March, 1945, Fig. 9. Floor Plan, Dispensary F-H.
17. Schowalter, E. J., and Davis, L. E. A concept of industrial medical department layout. *J Occup Med* 4:667, 1962.
18. Capel, E. H. Design of industrial medical centers. *Med Bull* (Standard Oil of New Jersey) 20:406, 1960.
19. Felton, J. S. Space and labor saving devices in the industrial dispensary: I. Combination examination-treatment unit. *Occup Med* 3:560, 1947; II. Treatment unit. *Occup Med* 4:380, 1947; III. Multipurpose work unit for treatment room. *Occup Med* 4:387, 1947; IV. Clinical record distribution box for physician's office. *Arch Ind Hyg Occup Med* 4:426, 1951; V. Optical dispensing unit. *Arch Ind Hyg Occup Med* 4:432, 1951; VI. Multipurpose central clerical desk for treatment room. *Arch Ind Hyg Occup Med* 4:437, 1951; VII. Portable clinical laboratory equipment for field use. *Arch Ind Hyg Occup Med* 7:413, 1953.
20. An unusual shape's seen in center opened in Texas. *Med Trib* 5:21, 1964.
21. Circular hospital plan. *Mod Hosp* 79:51, 1952.
22. Design lines: Two medical clinics enhance efficiency and access to care. *Hospitals* 55:43, 1980.
23. Felton, J. S. Modernizing the medical facility in industry. *Ind Med* 16:291, 1947.
24. Crawford, W. S. The mobile examining unit. *Med Bull* (Standard Oil of New Jersey) 9:78, 1949.
25. Davis, K. Early diagnosis of disease at the place of work. *Ind Med Surg* 25:85, 1956.
26. Jones, S. A. The mobile medical unit in colonial work. *J Trop Med Hyg* 53:22, 1950.
27. Occupational health on wheels: Periodic physical examinations in mobile units. *Ind Med Surg* 24:383, 1955.
28. Glindmeyer, H., Weill, H., Jones, R., et al. Design and operation of a mobile pulmonary function laboratory. *J Occup Med* 16:584, 1974.
29. Craig, J. L. (Ed.). *First International Biomedical Engineering Workshop Series.* Workshop III, Technology for Mobile and Remote Medical Care Delivery, 15–21 October 1972, Dubrovnik, Yugoslavia. Washington, DC: American Institute of Biological Sciences, 1973.
30. Eischen, M. Computer coming? Here's how to get ready. *Mod Office Proced* 28:136, 1983.
31. Two medical clinics enhance efficiency and access to care. *Hospitals* 55:43, Nov. 16, 1980.

ABBREVIATIONS AND ACRONYMS

AAAS	American Association for the Advancement of Science
AACT	American Academy of Clinical Toxicology
AAIH	American Academy of Industrial Hygiene
AAOHN	American Association of Occupational Health Nurses
ABHP	American Board of Health Physics
ABMT	American Board of Medical Toxicology
ABOHN	American Board for Occupational Health Nurses
ACGIH	American Conference of Governmental Industrial Hygienists
ACIP	Advisory Committee on Immunization Practices
ACOG	American College of Obstetricians and Gynecologists
ADL	activities of daily living
AFD	appointed factory doctor
AHA	American Hospital Association
AIDS	acquired immunodeficiency syndrome
ALOSH	Appalachian Laboratory for Occupational Safety and Health
ANA	American Nurses Association
ANSI	American National Standards Institute
Anti-HAV	antibodies against the hepatitis A virus
Anti-HBeAg	antibodies against the hepatitis Be antigen
Anti-HBs	antibodies against the hepatitis B surface antigen
Anti-HBsAg	antibodies against the hepatitis B surface antigen
AOMA	American Occupational Medical Association
ARC	American Red Cross
ARS	antirabies serum, equine
ASFA	Aquatic Sciences and Fisheries Abstracts
ASP	associate safety professional
ASSE	American Society of Safety Engineers
BAT	Biological Abstracts on Tape
BCG	bacillus of Calmette-Guérin (vaccine)
BCSP	Board of Certified Safety Professionals
BEI	biologic exposure index
BLS	Bureau of Labor Statistics
BMI	body mass index
BSP	bromsulfophthalein
CABG	coronary artery bypass graft(s)
CAOHC	Council of Accreditation in Occupational Hearing Conservation
CAS	Chemical Abstract Series Registry
CBC	complete blood count
CDC	Centers for Disease Control
CEU	Continuing Education Unit
CHD	coronary heart disease
CHESS	Computerized Health and Environmental Surveillance System
CIH	certified industrial hygienist
CIHT	certified industrial hygiene technologist
cm	centimeter
CME	Continuing Medical Education
COHESS	Computerized Occupational Health and Environmental Surveillance System
COHN	certified occupational health nurse
COSTAR	Computer Stored Ambulatory Record
CPR	cardiopulmonary resuscitation
CPSA	Consumer Product Safety Act
CPSC	Consumer Product Safety Commission
CRPF	chloroquine-resistant *Plasmodium falciparum*
CRT	cathode ray tube
CRT	certified radiologic technologist

CSHO	compliance safety and health officer
CSP	certified safety professional
CVAs	cerebrovascular accidents
dB	decibels
dBA	decibel level as corrected by factors known as the "A" weighting network to indicate the sound level approximating the response of the ear
DBCP	dibromochloropropane
DCC	day-care center
DES	diethylstilbestrol
DEV	duck embryo vaccine
DOT	Department of Transportation
DRG	diagnosis-related group
DX	diagnosis
ECC	emergency cardiac care
ECG	electrocardiogram, electrocardiograph
ECHOES	Environmental, Chemical and Occupational Evaluation System
EHS	employee health service
EMBASE	Excerpta Medical Data Base
EMT	emergency medical technician
EOHS	environmental and occupational health and safety
EPA	Environmental Protection Agency
E-SRD	end-stage renal disease
FAA	Federal Aviation Administration
FDA	Food and Drug Administration
$FEF_{25\%-75\%}$	maximum-mid expiratory flow rate
FEV_1	forced expiratory volume—1 second
FEMA	Federal Emergency Management Agency
FIA	Federal Insurance Administration
FVC	forced vital capacity
FX	fracture
GGPD	glucose-6-phosphate dehydrogenase (deficiency)
GISO	General Industry Safety Order
HAV	hepatitis A virus
HBeAg	hepatitis Be antigen
HBIG	hepatitis B immune globulin
HBsAg	hepatitis B surface antigen
HBV	hepatitis B virus
HCM	health care management
HCP	hearing conservation program
HCW	health care worker
HDCV	human diploid cell rabies vaccine
HDL	high-density lipoprotein
Hg	mercury
HHA	Health Hazard Appraisal
HHS	Health and Human Services
HIS	Health Information System
HIV	human immunodeficiency virus
HSA	health status assessment
HSTS	high skin test strength (coccidioidin)
HTL	hearing threshold level
HTLV-III/LAV	human T-lymphotrophic virus type III/lymphadenopathy-associated virus
HWE	healthy worker effect
Hz	hertz (a unit of frequency equal to 1 cycle per second [CPS])
IARC	International Agency for Research on Cancer
ICD.9.CM	*International Classification of Diseases*, 9th revision, Clinical Modification
ICDA	International Classification of Diseases Adapted
ICS	Immigration and Customs Service
ID	intradermal
ID	identification
IG	immune globulin
IH	industrial hygiene
IHIT	industrial hygienist in training
IHSR	Industrial Hygiene Survey Report
ILO	International Labor Organization
IM	intramuscular
IMS	Information Management System
INH	isoniazid
INMARSAT	International Maritime Satellite System
IPAC	Immunization Practices Advisory Committee
IPV	inactivated polio vaccine
IV	intravenous
JCAH	Joint Commission on the Accreditation of Hospitals
JEP	job exposure profile
kHz	kilohertz
LAH	left anterior hemiblock
LBBB	left bundle branch block
LPH	left posterior hemiblock
LVN	licensed vocational nurse
MARS	Medical Analysis and Reporting System
MDCD	Manager, Division of Chemical Dependency

MEHI	Medical and Environmental Health Information System
MESA	Mining Enforcement and Safety Administration
mg	milligram
MI	myocardial infarction
MITAGS	Maritime Institute of Technology and Graduate Studies
ml	milliliter
MLIC	Metropolitan Life Insurance Company
mm	millimeter
MPP	manual of policies and procedures
MSDS	Material Safety Data Sheet
MTRC	Medical Telecommunications Response Center
NASA	National Aeronautic and Space Administration
NCHS	National Center for Health Statistics
NHCA	National Hearing Conservation Association
NIH	National Institutes of Health
NIOSH	National Institute for Occupational Safety and Health
NLM	National Library of Medicine
NMHSA	National Mine Health and Safety Academy
NOHIMS	Naval Occupational Health Information Monitoring System
NP	nurse practitioner
NSC	National Safety Council
NSPB	National Society to Prevent Blindness
OHC	occupational hearing conservationist
OHDPS	Occupational Health Data Processing System
OHIS	Occupational Health Information System
OHNP	occupational health nurse practitioner
OHP	occupational health program
OHSAC	Occupational Health and Safety Accreditation Commission
OHSS	Occupational Health Surveillance System
OPV	oral polio vaccine
OT	old tuberculin
OTA	Office of Technology Assessment
OTC	over-the-counter medications
PA	physician's assistant
PA-C	physician's assistant—certified
PAT	Proficiency Analytical Testing (program of NIOSH)
PC	protein C
PCEH	President's Committee on Employment of the Handicapped
PEL	permissible exposure level
PES	Professional Examination Service
PHA	passive hemagglutination (test)
PHPD	personal hearing protective device
PPD	purified protein derivative of tuberculin
PPD-B	PPD-Battey antigen (a research reagent)
PPD-S	International PPD Tuberculin Standard
PPM	parts per million
PRM-SDY	pyrimethamine-sulfadoxine
prn	whenever necessary
PSVT	paroxysmal supraventricular tachycardia
PSW	personal-service worker
RAC	risk assessment code
RAM	random access memory
RBBB	right bundle branch block
RFFIT	rapid fluorescent-focus inhibition test
RIA	radioimmune assay
RIG	rabies immune globulin, human
RN	registered nurse
RTECS	Registry of Toxic Effects of Chemical Substances
RTW	return to work
SAS	Statistical Analysis System
SC	subcutaneous
SCBA	self-contained breathing apparatus
SCUBA	self-contained underwater breathing apparatus
SGOT	serum glutamic oxaloacetic transaminase
SHD	state health department
SHIMS	Safety and Health Information Management System
SHIP	Seafarers' Health Improvement Program
SHP	safety and health person
SHS	student health service
SLM	sound level meter
SMR	standardized mortality ratio
SNOMED	Systematized Nomenclature of Medicine
SOAP	subjective findings, objective findings, assessment, plan
SPSS	Statistical Package for the Social Sciences

SSN	social security number
SSS	System Safety Society
STEL	short-term exposure level
TACT	Translation and Code Table
TCB	Testing and Certification Branch (Division of Safety, NIOSH)
Td	tetanus and diphtheria toxoids
TD	traveler's diarrhea
TDB	Toxicology Data Bank
TDF	Terminal Digit Filing
TIG	tetanus immune globulin
TLV-STEL	threshold limit value—short-term exposure limit
TLV-TWA	threshold limit value—time-weighted average
TSCA	Toxic Substances Control Act
TSP	total suspended particulates
TST	tuberculin skin test
TU	tuberculin unit
TVA	Tennessee Valley Authority
TWA	time-weighted average
USTS	usual skin test strength (coccidioidin)
UV	ultraviolet
VDRL	Venereal Disease Research Laboratories
VDT	video display terminal; visual display terminal
VEs	ventricular extrasystoles
WET	worker exposure tracking
WHO	World Health Organization
WPW	Wolff-Parkinson-White (syndrome)
YPLL	years of potential life lost

INDEX